Forensic Medicine for Lawyers

D1323604

This book is dedicated to the memory of

Elizabeth Hope Mason

who really enjoyed being associated with forensic medicine

Forensic Medicine for Lawyers

Fourth Edition

J K Mason, CBE, MD, LLD, FRCPath, DMJ, FRSE
Regius Professor (Emeritus) of Forensic Medicine,
Honorary Fellow, Faculty of Law, University of Edinburgh

With chapters by

M S Bruce, MB, ChB, MRCPsych, PhD
Consultant Psychiatrist in Addiction
Community Drug Problem Service
Royal Edinburgh Hospital

J S Oliver, BSc, PhD, CChem, FRSC
Senior Lecturer, Department of Forensic Medicine and Science,
University of Glasgow

Derek Chiswick, MB, ChB, MPhil, FRCPsych
Consultant Forensic Psychiatrist,
Royal Edinburgh Hospital, Edinburgh Healthcare NHS Trust

Butterworths
London, Edinburgh, Dublin
2001

United Kingdom	Butterworths, a Division of Reed Elsevier (UK) Ltd, Halsbury House, 35 Chancery Lane, LONDON WC2A 1EL and 4 Hill Street, EDINBURGH EH2 3JZ
Australia	Butterworths, a Division of Reed International Books Australia Pty Ltd, CHATSWOOD, New South Wales
Canada	Butterworths Canada Ltd, MARKHAM, Ontario
Hong Kong	Butterworths Hong Kong, a division of Reed Elsevier (Greater China) Ltd, HONG KONG
India	Butterworths India, NEW DELHI
Ireland	Butterworth (Ireland) Ltd, DUBLIN
Malaysia	Malayan Law Journal Sdn Bhd, KUALA LUMPUR
New Zealand	Butterworths of New Zealand Ltd, WELLINGTON
Singapore	Butterworths Asia, SINGAPORE
South Africa	Butterworths Publishers (Pty) Ltd, DURBAN
USA	Lexis Law Publishing, CHARLOTTESVILLE, Virginia

© Reed Elsevier (UK) Ltd 2001

All rights reserved. No part of this publication may be reproduced in any material form (including photocopying or storing it in any medium by electronic means and whether or not transiently or incidentally to some other use of this publication) without the written permission of the copyright owner except in accordance with the provisions of the Copyright, Designs and Patents Act 1988 or under the terms of a licence issued by the Copyright Licensing Agency Ltd, 90 Tottenham Court Road, London, England W1P 0LP. Applications for the copyright owner's written permission to reproduce any part of this publication should be addressed to the publisher.

Warning: The doing of an unauthorised act in relation to a copyright work may result in both a civil claim for damages and criminal prosecution.

Any Crown copyright material is reproduced with the permission of the Controller of Her Majesty's Stationery Office.

A CIP Catalogue record for this book is available from the British Library.

ISBN 0 406 91442 7

Typeset by Doyle & Co, Colchester
Printed and bound in Great Britain by Hobbs the Printers Ltd, Totton, Hampshire

Visit Butterworths LEXIS direct at: www.butterworths.com

Preface to the Fourth Edition

I am grateful to my publishers for commissioning a further edition of this book only five years since they took it under their wing. None the less, assuming that there is to be a similar interval between now and the need for a further edition, this preface must take on the semblance of the author's valediction.

Retrospection is inevitable at such times and it is interesting to look back at the book's progress and to compare the 'hand-book' format of the first edition with the 500 and more pages of the present. I sincerely hope that it has matured in more than size and that, as a result of my working more than 15 years in legal academia, it has become what it was always designed to be—a practical and wide-ranging review of the interplay between medicine and the law. At the same time, I would like it to be remembered that it was born of a very special teacher-student relationship and I am equally anxious that it has not moved too far from its natural home in the classroom in its efforts to remain just as well suited to the practitioner's office.

The pathology of trauma alters very little. What does change is the holistic environment within which the individual needs the protection of the law; the resulting evolution of the common law and the proliferation of statute law has been a major feature of the last five years. There is, as a consequence, far more black-letter law in this edition than in the last—this is, perhaps, especially so in relation to public health and to the physical environment. There have, however, also been changes of a more subtle nature in our social environment which I hope are reflected in the text. Our attitudes to marriage, reproduction and sex in general have developed rapidly. While we have regarded, say, identification of the dead as reaching its apogee in the major transportation disaster, we must now see genocide as taking pride of place. Changes have been taking place in our medico-legal systems—and who should doubt the need when we find a doctor to have been amongst the more ambitious of modern mass murderers? Indeed, it is on the reverse side of forensic medicine— the control of the medical profession—that there have been the most dramatic developments and I have found it necessary to expand this aspect considerably. We must also note the extension and altering direction of the drugs culture; in this respect, I welcome Dr Malcolm Bruce as the new author of the chapter on drug addiction.

v

The moral environment has also developed and its influence on forensic medicine has been far reaching—so much so that it is now impossible to dissociate medical ethics from medical law, especially at each end of life's spectrum. I have thought it right to devote a whole chapter to ethical problems, although it must not be supposed that this is in any way a substitute for the many textbooks which now relate specifically to the subject. At the same time, public opinion marches on and I have now consigned the once major topic of criminal abortion to a corner in history. The chapter on my much-loved subject of forensic serology is another casualty of the years; again, I would not suggest that the replacement sections on DNA do adequate justice to this major investigative advance, but this is not a book on forensic science. I have continued my resistance to the suggested inclusion of medical illustrations in what is, primarily, a text for lawyers; for those who really need them, I commend the third edition of *The Pathology of Trauma*, now edited by myself and Dr B N Purdue.

A number of colleagues have been kind enough to review specialised sections for me; these are acknowledged with gratitude in the text. Others have generously stepped into the breach at short notice to answer questions or to provide urgently needed materials. Among these are included my 'emergency assistant', Ms Maureen Sinclair; Dr Basil Purdue; Dr Diana Buchanan; Dr John Clark; Air Commodore SA Cullen; Dr P J Lincoln; Mrs Heather Cook of the BMA's Scottish Office; and Miss Amanda Finon of the GMC. Most particularly, I acknowledge the unstinting help from my research assistant, Ms Patricia Comiskey, as a result of whose efforts I can say with some confidence that the law is believed to be correct as at 31 August 2000. I am also deeply indebted to the Faculty of Law, University of Edinburgh, for a generous allocation from the Faculty Disbursement Fund. Finally, I express my appreciation of the courtesy and co-operation of the publishers—I hope they think it was worth it.

Edinburgh
October 2000   JKM

Preface to the First Edition

In my inaugural address to the University,[1] I defined forensic medicine as 'medicine applied to the protection and assistance of individuals in relation to the community'. This concept was based on the 'forum' as being a public place in which those responsible to the public in many spheres argued and defended their views rather than being limited to the criminal court.

It seemed to me that forensic medicine should be taught to medical students in this wide spirit whereas, paradoxically, it was the law students who, in having to decipher and understand the reports of their expert medical witnesses, needed the greater exposure to the details of pathology despite the fact that they had no medical background. I could find no textbook extant which would satisfy their particular needs; what follows is an attempt to fill the gap. One of the main difficulties has been to find the right pitch of knowledge and the book has, in the process of writing, settled into an outline of the LLB course in forensic medicine presently given at Edinburgh University. It is, however, hoped that it will still be found useful by practising advocates, solicitors, procurators fiscal and coroners.

I recently read a review which stated that 'the day of the single-author textbook has gone', and it is certain that multiple authorship ensures that each facet of the work is covered by an expert practising in that sphere: the single author attempting a wide range must lose a sense of immediacy.

In an effort to compensate for this, I have shown drafts of the majority of chapters to persons particularly well qualified to criticise and advise. Helpful criticism does not, however, necessarily mean approval and, lest naming one's reviewers might be taken as implying their shared responsibility for, and satisfaction with, the end result, I intend to express my thanks anonymously to the many members of the forensic fraternity, the academic staff of the Faculties of Medicine and of Law in Edinburgh University, the NHS officials, the government and local authority officers and others who have responded so kindly to my calls for help; my gratitude loses no sincerity in its generality.

Three special personal acknowledgments are, however, called for. Professor Keith Simpson and Mr Alistair R Brownlie have been good enough to read the whole manuscript from the point of view of the forensic pathologist and of the

1 *Ambitions for a Motley Coat* (1974), Inaugural Address No 56, University of Edinburgh.

vii

lawyer respectively. They have given invaluable advice although, again, it should be stressed that their participation does not necessarily imply agreement with the views expressed. Mr Charles N Stoddart has reviewed the text with particular reference to the legal technicalities. In doing so, he has not only improved the book's acceptability to lawyers but has also offered many helpful criticisms; he has my sincere thanks for undertaking a most time-consuming task.

I owe my secretarial assistant, Mrs Gladys Hamilton, a debt of gratitude for unstinting co-operation and much encouragement. A number of temporary assistants have had a hand in the typing but the great bulk of this has been undertaken by Miss Iris Falconer with great skill and good heart.

Finally, I have to thank my wife for letting it happen. At a time of our lives which was, for several reasons, difficult, she spent many lonely hours of televiewing without complaint; I hope this book is worthy of her memory.

Edinburgh
1978   JKM

Contents

Table of statutes

Table of cases

D

PAGE

PAGE

PAGE

S

T

Some terms used in medical evidence

The intention of this textbook is to give the lawyer a better understanding of the expert evidence provided by health care workers in both the civil and criminal courts and in consultation. A medical report that will be satisfactory to all interested parties cannot be written without using some academic jargon, and lawyers may well need an explanation of the phraseology that the medical witness uses. No apology is made, therefore, for an introduction that may seem unduly elementary to some readers but which may be useful, if only as a source of aides-mémoire, to others.

For anatomical descriptive purposes the human body should be regarded as standing erect with the palms of the hands facing forward (see Figure 0.1). Everything that can be seen in the mirror is then *anterior*, while that which cannot be seen is *posterior*. These views are related to the *coronal* plane—the plane that divides the body vertically through the shoulders. The vertical plane at right angles to this is the *sagittal* plane, and the sagittal plane that

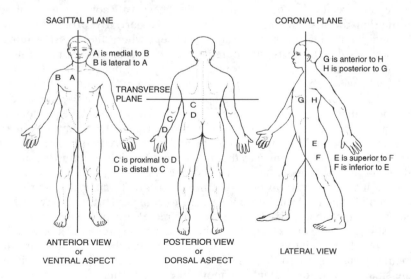

Figure 0.1 The planes of the body and some of the terms used for anatomical reference.

1

bisects the body into symmetrical left and right halves is the *midline*. If point A is on the same side of the body as point B and is nearer the midline, then A is *medial* to B and B is *lateral* to A. Thus, while the body as a whole has anterior, posterior and lateral aspects, the limbs have anterior, posterior, medial and lateral surfaces. The great toe is medial in man as in four-footed animals, but the human and primate thumb is on the lateral side of the hand.

Dividing the body horizontally results in the *transverse* section. From a section taken through the middle of the chest, one can move upwards towards the cephalic extremity and downwards to the caudal extremity. If one assumes that the limbs are extended to form an 'X', then point C is *proximal* to D if it is nearer to the midchest transverse plane than is point D and, at the same time, D is *distal* to C. These terms can, however, be used functionally rather than anatomically; thus, while anatomically the small intestine lies distal to the transverse colon, the former is functionally a proximal portion of gut.

Strictly speaking, the body has also a *superior* aspect which is seen from above and an *inferior* aspect which is the soles of the feet. The terms 'superior' and 'inferior' are, however, far more important as regards the surfaces of individual organs; all the above descriptions of the whole body are applicable to its component parts. Points on the body can also be described as superior or inferior to one another depending on whether they are nearer the head or the foot. The terms 'anterior' and 'posterior' can likewise be used relatively.

At its simplest, the body is divided into the head, the limbs and the torso. The interior of the head is the *cranial* cavity while the torso consists of the *thoracic* and *abdominal* cavities. The protection of these cavities differs markedly. The cranial cavity, which contains the brain, is surrounded by the rigid skull which, while giving a high degree of protection, is itself subject to shattering forces which can be propagated through its substance; once fully developed with its component bones fused, the skull also inhibits expansion of its contents. The thoracic cavity houses the heart and the lungs. The governing functional principle is that of elasticity. The contents have considerable freedom of movement and the chest wall consists of a mobile combination of ribs and muscle which is only partially protective. The abdominal cavity lacks a bony structure, except where the massive lumbar spine protects it posteriorly; its contents are, therefore, susceptible to injury both by penetrating and by blunt force. The major contents, which lie within an internal covering envelope, the *peritoneum*, include the stomach and greater part of the bowel, the liver and the spleen; these are loosely connected by ligaments and have considerable mobility. Those lying behind the peritoneum, including the pancreas and the kidneys, are more rigidly fixed but, in general, are better protected. The lower part of the abdominal cavity is bounded by the two pelvic bones and is known as the *pelvic* cavity which contains the urinary bladder and, in the female, the uterus and ovaries.

The ability of the various organs to move has great importance in relation to accidental injury. A mobile object can, to some extent, slide away from direct violence; the more fixed an organ is, the more susceptible it is to bruising and crushing. On the other hand, even the most mobile organ must be attached at some point to a relatively rigid structure. Organs that can move are thus particularly susceptible to shearing forces and to indirect injury; direct injury to the small bowel, for example, is more likely to be manifested in its fixed *mesentery* than in the mobile loops of gut. The size of the organ will influence the likelihood of its being directly affected—the liver is a good example—while the extent of air/fluid/solid interfaces will partly determine the damage likely to result from internal vibration and other stresses. The *elasticity* of the organ is another major determinant in this type of trauma, while the physical condition of an individual organ at the time of stress may affect its response—a diseased spleen, for example, is more likely to rupture than is a normal organ.

The solid portions of the body are composed of myriads of *cells* held together by *ground substance*. The cells are organised so as to form either *epithelium* or *connective tissues*. Malignant overgrowth of the former is known as *carcinoma* and, of the latter, as *sarcoma*. Epithelium either lines or cloaks the organs of the body. It is often specialised—for example, to secrete, as in the gut, or to waft particles (eg of dust); in the latter case, the epithelium is said to be *ciliated*. The skin is a most complex epithelium with many functions, perhaps the primary one of which is to retain the body fluids; thus, destruction of the skin by burning leads to a massive loss of fluid—the potentially lethal condition of *dehydration* leading to *surgical shock*. The *connective tissue* connects not only the various epithelia but also the major parts of the body—it includes fat, muscle, fibrous tissue including tendons and bones, the whole system being permeated by a network of blood vessels. The connective tissues are of great importance in the healing of wounds. When the continuity of part of the body, for example the skin, is interrupted, a variable quantity of bleeding takes place; this is partly stemmed by contraction of the cut ends of the vessels and by the pressure exerted by the extravasated blood and partly by the natural *haemostatic* mechanism present in the blood. Wandering tissue-repair cells then enter the bruise and the dead area is penetrated by new blood vessels which, in turn, provoke the appearance of young fibrous connective tissue cells. The vessels then age and the tissue becomes tough and bloodless, the result being a *scar*. The recognition of these stages is the basis of 'ageing' of wounds.

The blood itself is a specialised form of connective tissue which consists of cells and fluid; the latter is the *plasma*, which carries soluble foodstuffs and electrolytes, waste products and messenger substances, or *hormones*, which provide the body's system of communication between organs. The blood cells are described as being either red (*erythrocytes*) or white (*leucocytes*); the function of the former is the carriage of oxygen while the latter are, in general, concerned with the defence of the body against infection. Sarcomatous overgrowth of the white cells results in *leukaemia*, which will be described as being of various types according to the precise type of cell involved. *Platelets*, concerned with blood coagulation, also circulate in the plasma.

All cells other than the erythrocytes, which have no nucleus, consist of two main parts—the *nucleus* and the *cytoplasm*. The nucleus controls cell reproduction and contains 23 pairs of *chromosomes* which, in turn, for practical purposes, can be said to consist of *genes*; one of each pair of genes is derived from a parent. Normal cell division and tissue growth results from *mitosis* in which each chromosome reproduces itself; the two new cells therefore contain the same chromosomes as did their progenitor. The exception lies in the sex cells or *gametes*, spermatozoa in the male or ova in the female, which divide by a process of *meiosis* and contain only 23 single chromosomes; the fusion of two gametes thus results in a *zygote* with the normal nuclear configuration.

The genes contain the *deoxyribonucleic acid* (DNA) which determines the unique constitution of each individual—or of each pair of identical twins.

One pair of chromosomes dictates the sex of the subject. These sex chromosomes are designated X and Y. The presence of a Y chromosome in the pair indicates maleness.

In addition to describing the body on anatomical grounds, it is often useful to consider it systematically—that is, relating those parts which are functionally integrated irrespective of their position. These 'systems' are referred to frequently in medical reports and most are dealt with in greater detail in the opening chapter. In summary, the medical witness may refer to:

- The *nervous* system, comprising the brain and spinal cord (central nervous system) and the peripheral nerves.
- The *musculoskeletal* system, or the bones, tendons and muscles.
- The *cardiovascular* system, consisting of the heart and blood vessels.
- The *respiratory* system, running from the nose to the lungs and including the diaphragm and chest muscles.[1]
- The *gastrointestinal* system, which includes not only the gut from mouth to anus but also those organs whose function is to control the processing of food, ie the salivary glands, the liver and the pancreas.
- The *genitourinary* system. Although quite distinct functionally, the genital and urinary systems are commonly combined because of their close anatomical association. The genital system includes the ovaries, uterus, vagina and vulva in the female and the testes, ducts and penis in the male. The main components of the urinary system are the kidneys, the ureters, the bladder and the urethra, and the prostate gland in the male.
- The *lymphoreticular* system, which is responsible for many functions particularly related to defence against infection. The main solid organs are the spleen, the thymus gland and the numerous lymph nodes including specialised nodes such as the tonsils.
- The *endocrine system*, comprising those glands that control body function by secretion of hormones into the bloodstream. The most important from the forensic aspect are the pituitary, the adrenal and the thyroid glands.

All these systems are interlinked—all, for example, depend upon their component of the cardiovascular system and its contained blood, while the musculoskeletal system, in particular, cannot function in the absence of a nervous system. However, they form useful descriptive compartments in so far as the functional result of disease or injury within a system is immediately understandable.

Many medical terms are made up of the Latin names for the organ or tissue associated with a descriptive prefix or suffix. A selected list of these is given in Appendix A.

---

1   The intimate association of the heart and lungs leads to the frequent use of the term *cardio-respiratory system*.

1
Some aspects of applied anatomy and physiology

The cardiovascular system

Animal life depends upon the supply of oxygen to the tissues. This is the function of two biological systems—the respiratory system which collects or harvests the oxygen and the cardiovascular system which distributes it for consumption by the tissues. The two are closely interrelated, the common factor being the *erythrocytes* or red cells of the blood, of which there are about 5 million to the cubic millimetre of blood.

Red cells derive their colour from the pigment *haemoglobin*, a combination of iron and protein, the function of which is to accept oxygen in the lungs and to surrender it in the tissues. Maximum contact between the blood and the tissues is achieved at both these points by passing the blood through vessels that are approximately the diameter of individual red cells—these are known as *capillaries*. The extremely delicate nature of their walls allows controlled transference not only of gases but of water and salts or *electrolytes*; the system is very sensitive to oxygen deficiency and it is abnormal capillary permeability that is mainly responsible for the condition of *surgical shock*. This is an important concept—shock in medical terms is not a matter of mental distress; it is a profound biochemical disturbance which, triggered by capillary hypoxia (see page 488), leads to alterations in the distribution of body water and, particularly, of blood volume. Surgical shock is a condition of immense medico-legal importance as it occurs most commonly as a result of trauma; anything that reduces the peripheral blood pressure, such as haemorrhage or fluid loss due to burning, can precipitate the condition which is self-perpetuating—low peripheral pressure means oxygen starvation which leads to capillary damage, local fluid loss and increasing failure of the blood pressure.

The blood pressure that is commonly described in medical reports is measured in the arteries; its maintenance is a function not only of peripheral resistance but also of the pumping action of the heart. The pressure is described in two phases—the *systolic* pressure, which is the maximum achieved as a result of the heart beat, and the *diastolic*, which is the residual pressure maintained while the heart is refilling; in general, it is the diastolic pressure that reflects most accurately the level of strain upon the system.

5

The *heart* consists of specialised muscle tissue, the *myocardium*, and is enclosed in a fibrous sac, the *pericardium*. Essentially it consists of two separate pumps (see Figure 1.1), the left and right *ventricles*, which are fed with blood through non-return valves from the left and right *atria*. The size and weight of the heart are dictated largely by the condition of the ventricles which, in turn, depends mainly upon the peripheral resistance to the flow of blood. A ventricle that is coping with increased resistance will grow in bulk or *hypertrophy*; one that is failing to do so will *dilate*. These observations are, therefore, of great importance in assessing matters such as life expectancy in compensation cases. Blood passes from the ventricles to the tissues through *arteries*. The main artery of the body is the *aorta* which branches into vessels of descending calibre until the capillaries are reached. The capillaries then coalesce into tributaries or *veins* which ultimately form two main rivers—the *superior vena cava* coming from the upper part of the body and the *inferior vena cava* from the lower—which return the blood from the *systemic circulation* to the right atrium.

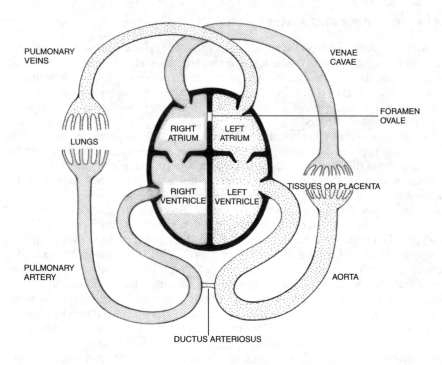

Figure 1.1 Diagrammatic illustration of the cardio-vascular system. The fetal connections used to bypass the lungs are shown in white.

All blood vessels have three coats—the *intima*, a normally thin lining which is subject to the degenerative change of atheroma; the *media*, a muscular coat; and the *adventitia* which is a loose covering responsible for the supply of nutriments to the vessel itself and for its stability in the body. Since the arteries are steadily decreasing in size, a considerable pressure must be maintained within them to ensure adequate blood flow; the arteries therefore have thick muscular walls. The situation in the veins, however, is that of a flowing river fed by tributaries; the walls are thin and the dark purple deoxygenated blood shows through them.

The blood returning in the venae cavae has given up much of its oxygen to the tissues and this must be replenished. It passes from the right atrium into the right ventricle and thence to the *pulmonary artery* which again divides until it forms capillaries within the lungs. These capillaries now surround the smallest air pockets, the *alveoli*. The partial pressure of oxygen in the alveolar air is higher than that in the blood; thus, oxygen passes to the blood which returns via the *pulmonary veins* to the *left atrium* thus completing the *pulmonary circulation*. The pulmonary capillaries are just as sensitive to changes in blood volume and oxygen content as are those of the systemic circulation; fluid loss from them results in *pulmonary oedema*, or water in the lungs, which, again, is self-perpetuating, in that displacement of the air in the alveoli by water decreases still further the supply of oxygen to the tissues.

The blood thus circulates in something of a figure-of-eight—that in the systemic arteries and pulmonary veins is oxygenated while that in the systemic veins and pulmonary arteries requires regenerating. Such a circulation will be useless to the fetus which has no access to atmospheric air. The lungs of the fetus *in utero* are, therefore, replaced by the *placenta*—a mass of capillaries derived from both the infant and the mother by means of which the former is supplied with oxygen as a 'tissue' of the latter; the pulmonary artery and veins are replaced functionally by the umbilical vessels. The fetal lungs must be bypassed and this is accomplished through two main mechanisms. First, the two atria are allowed to communicate through the *foramen ovale*. Some of the blood passes through this from the right atrium to the left atrium rather than to the right ventricle and pulmonary artery. Secondly, a connection, the *ductus arteriosus*, is established between the aorta and the pulmonary artery by means of which the great majority of blood pumped from the right ventricle can be diverted to the aorta and, thence, to the placental circulation. The ductus usually closes a few days after birth and the foramen ovale some weeks later. These points are of major medico-legal importance as so much forensic pathology revolves round the fetal and neonatal period and, in particular, around the post-mortem diagnosis of a 'separate existence'.

Damage to the heart or blood vessels results in haemorrhage, which is one of the most constant complications of trauma of all types. Its severity depends on three main factors. First, there is the size of the vessel. In this respect, the heart itself is the most important part of the system; otherwise, the larger the vessel damaged, the more dangerous to life is the injury. Second, the type of vessel is all-important—damage to an artery, subject to high internal pressure, will obviously be more dangerous than damage to a vein of comparable size. Third, there are the secondary effects, not only those resulting from oxygen deprivation in specific organs but also those due to occupation of space by extruded blood— thus, haemorrhage into the skull will have very different effects from the same amount of bleeding into the abdomen.

The *haemostatic* mechanism of the body—that is, its ability to control haemorrhage—rests first, on the properties of blood and, second, on the capacity of the vessels to contract, a matter of vascular health and size. The properties of the blood derive from two distinct sources—the *coagulation factors* and the *platelets*. The former, mainly designated by Roman numeral, are protein substances circulating in the plasma that take part in a complicated chain reaction when activated in the presence of calcium. The result of this reaction is to form *thrombin*, which then reacts with the circulating protein *fibrinogen* to form *fibrin* which is, in effect, the scaffolding of a clot. Deficiency of any factor can break the chain and cause one of what are collectively known as *bleeding diatheses*; for simplistic purposes, Factor II or prothrombin, Factor VIII, Factor IX and Factor I (fibrinogen) are the most important. The coagulation factors are synthesised in the liver; severe liver disease will therefore predispose to a bleeding condition. Deficiency of Factor VIII results in the hereditary disease *haemophilia* (lack of Factor IX is responsible for haemophilia B or Christmas disease). The function of the platelets is twofold. In the first place, they release substances that activate the coagulation mechanism and, secondly, they aggregate to form 'plugs' at the site of injury to a vessel and thus consolidate the fibrin clot. Excessive bleeding is, therefore, likely if platelets are absent—as happens in disease or poisoning of the bone marrow—or if they are abnormal.

The bleeding diatheses are medico-legally important in several ways. The response to injury will be abnormal—trivial wounds may result in severe haemorrhage or excessive bruising—and this will greatly influence their interpretation as to the time of infliction, the force used and the like. Secondly, the abnormal condition can be remitted by replacement of the deficient substance; it follows that failure to identify and neutralise the abnormal state before a surgical or dental operation might well be construed as negligent practice. Thirdly, replacement therapy is expensive, wasteful and not without its dangers; various and variant blood-borne viruses—of which the most notorious are the human immunodeficiency virus and the viruses of hepatitis B and C—appear without warning in blood and blood products and haemophiliacs were especially at risk in the period before diagnostic tests for their identification and measures to prevent their transmission became routinely available.

Blood coagulation and haemostasis occur normally only at the site of injury. The reverse of haemorrhage is the very dangerous condition of *intravascular coagulation* which occurs either locally in a diseased vessel or as a generalised condition resulting from severe surgical shock. A *thrombus* forms within the vessel; if this breaks off it becomes an *embolus*. Emboli can involve both the arterial and the venous blood systems. In the former case, they will lodge in the tissues; in the latter, they lodge in the lungs and cause the very important condition of *pulmonary thrombotic embolism*. The major significance of these abnormal states is discussed in Chapter 7. A system of blood factors, comparable to that involved in coagulation, exists in order to prevent the blood clotting in the normal circulation.

Cardiovascular damage may result from either indirect or direct trauma. The former is largely a matter of accidental injury and is described in Chapter 10. For present purposes, the most important causes of direct injury include stab wounds—when these are fatal, it is generally by virtue of penetrating the heart or a major vessel; incised wounds, when a major vessel is present under the surface—as at the wrist or in the neck; and gunshot wounds, in which damage is likely to be caused not only by the bullets but also by fragments of bone which act as secondary missiles.

Natural disease of the heart and blood vessels accounts for some 80% of the sudden deaths reported to the coroner or procurator fiscal. It provides a major preoccupation for the forensic pathologist and is discussed in detail in Chapter 7.

The blood

As has already been described (see page 3), the blood consists of two major fractions—the *cellular component* and the *plasma* in which the cells float. If the blood is clotted, the resulting altered fluid component is known as *serum*. Serum is technically easier to work with in certain laboratory examinations and it is common to speak loosely of 'serum concentrations'; but the substances measured will have been circulating naturally in the plasma.

The plasma is responsible for transport of carbon dioxide and of the products of ingestion and metabolism of fat, proteins and carbohydrates. It contains many of the mineral salts on which the biochemical balance of the body depends and also the hormones. The clotting factors, described above, are also present in the plasma which, normally, constitutes approximately 60% of the blood volume; a relative fall in this proportion leads to a viscous blood and local tissue hypoxia due to stagnation.

As described previously, the cells of the blood are divided into the red series (*erythrocytes*) and the white series (*leucocytes*) and there is also a platelet component (*see above*). The oxygen transport function of the first has been noted already. A relative lack of red cells constitutes *anaemia* which may result from haemorrhage or from an inability to form haemoglobin, usually because of a lack of its inorganic component, iron. There are other forms of functional anaemia which are important medico-legally. First, some poisonous substances convert the haemoglobin into forms that are less capable or incapable of accepting oxygen—the most important of these is carbon monoxide but there are other substances, particularly of an industrial nature, that achieve much the same end. Secondly, inherited abnormalities of the haemoglobin occur which are known as *haemoglobinopathies*; the best known of these is *sickle cell anaemia* but it is by no means the only member of the group.[1] The medico-legal significance of these diseases is not inconsiderable. First, sufferers from the conditions, which may be present in severe or mild form, are hypersensitive to low blood oxygen tensions arising from any cause—including, most significantly, anaesthesia; they are at some risk in air travel or in conditions of severe oxygen demand, a situation which might raise a valid defence when sudden death occurs during a struggle. Secondly, most of them show a strong ethnic distribution; they can, therefore, play a part in the interpretation of, say, of the Race Relations Act 1976.

The *leucocytes* are basically of two types—the *polymorphonuclears* and the *mononuclears*. The former constitute the body's tactical defence against acute infection; the latter are more akin to a strategic force which comes into action more slowly but whose influence persists for some time. The mononuclears are particularly responsible for the formation of *antibodies* and for the ability of the body to recognise a foreign intruder; an immediate reaction can thereby be set up should the intrusion be repeated. It is this system which is the target of the human immunodeficiency virus. Certain poisons—and some drugs in excessive amounts—suppress the formation of the white cells and the subject is then left prey to infections that would be repelled easily in normal circumstances.

The blood cells are formed in the *bone marrow* which is found in the centre of virtually all the bones of the body; any poison or ionising radiation that

---

1 Abnormalities may be structural—as in *sickle cell anaemia*—or qualitative—*thalassaemia*—resulting, for example, from the persistence of a fetal type of haemoglobin in the adult.

affects the bone marrow will affect the blood and its function. The bone marrow consists of cellular and fatty elements, the proportion of the latter increasing with age.

Effete blood cells must be removed and their important components preserved. This is mainly the function of the *spleen*, an organ which lies in the left upper abdomen covered by the lower ribs. It is one of those odd organs that are not essential to a normal life and its main medico-legal significance lies in the ease with which it is ruptured in vehicular accidents. Deliberate rupture of the spleen also once had a vogue as a method of murder in malarial areas, the organ being particularly fragile in that disease; nearer to home, it is also prone to traumatic rupture in the very common condition of glandular fever.

The spleen and bone marrow are parts of the *lymphoreticular system* which is completed by the *lymphatic* system of the ducts and glands responsible not only for the immune response of the body but also for the circulation of the extracellular fluid which bathes all the cells of the body. The lymphatic and cardiovascular systems are united where the main lymph duct empties itself into the larger veins of the upper thorax. Cancer cells are readily disseminated in the lymph and set up secondary deposits (*metastases*) when they are filtered in the lymphatic glands.

The respiratory system

Without oxygen, there is no enzymatic activity and the cells of the tissues will die. The requirement is urgent—the urgency depending on the sophistication of the cells concerned; the most sensitive cells of the brain will die if deprived of oxygen for some 10 minutes or even less. It is the function of the respiratory system to trap the oxygen which constitutes about one-fifth of the ambient atmosphere, to transfer it to the haemoglobin of the blood and to remove the main product of combustion—carbon dioxide—which circulates dissolved in the blood plasma.

Air is passed to the lungs from the nose or mouth, through the *larynx* to the windpipe or *trachea*. The larynx is protected by three bones or cartilages—the *hyoid*, *thyroid* (Adam's Apple) and *cricoid*—which are of very great importance in the post-mortem diagnosis of strangulation (see Chapter 13). The trachea splits into a left and a right main *bronchus* which, in turn, divide into *lobar bronchi*—one to each major lobe of the lungs. [2] The bronchi split into *bronchioles* which end in the air sacs or *alveoli* which, as we have seen, are surrounded by the pulmonary capillaries. The lungs are contained within two layers of a fibrous envelope—the *pleura*—which has two main functions; first, a negative pressure between the two layers serves to maintain the lungs in a position of expansion and, secondly, the surfaces combine to reduce the friction which would otherwise exist between the lungs and the chest wall; the formation of pleural *adhesions* is a frequent result of pulmonary disease.

Air is drawn into the lungs as the muscles of respiration—the chest muscles and the diaphragm—create a negative pressure. As compared with the heart, which is innervated by the autonomic system only, the lungs are directed by both the autonomic and voluntary nervous systems (see page 13)—we normally do not

---

2   The right lung has three lobes, the left only two. The right lung is therefore slightly larger than the left which must make way for the heart which lies in the left thorax.

consciously think about our respiration, but we are able to alter our breathing should we so wish. In the event of conflict, the autonomic innervation will succeed—it is very difficult to die from holding one's breath and, ultimately, an irrespirable medium, whether it be water or a poisonous gas, must be inhaled despite conscious resistance. Expiration requires no muscular effort and, in the event of respiratory failure, either positive pressure breathing must be applied— as when a patient is placed on a ventilator or in mouth-to-mouth resuscitation— or the whole chest must be subjected to artificial vacuum as in the near obsolete respirator.

In essence, the process of respiration is one of equilibrating the tensions of the various gases in the air and body fluids. If the oxygen tension is high in the alveoli and low in the pulmonary capillary blood, the gas will pass into the plasma and form oxyhaemoglobin in the red cells; if the oxygen tension is high in the capillary peripheral blood and low in the tissue fluids, oxyhaemoglobin will dissociate and the oxygen will be made available to the tissues. Similar principles apply to dissolved carbon dioxide. Tissue respiration is comparable to an engine boiler—the fuel is oxygen which is used to burn the foodstuffs to produce energy; the resultant 'ash' is represented by carbon dioxide. The analogy is elaborated in Figure 1.2 which also indicates the ways in which oxygen deficiency can occur.

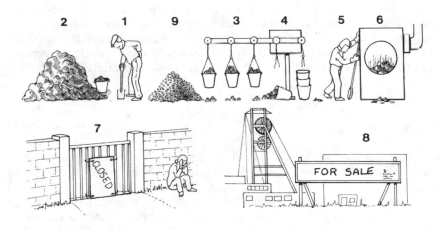

Figure 1.2 An illustrative concept of the respiratory system. A man (1) has to move coal (2) with a series of buckets (3) moved by an engine (4) to a stoker (5) who feeds the factory furnace (6) which represents the tissues of the body. Many things may interfere with the transport of the coal (2) which is supplied to the body in the form of *oxygen*:
1. The man may get tired = respiratory paralysis.
3. There may be insufficient buckets (red blood cells) = anaemia.
4. The bucket transporter may break down = heart failure.
5. The stoker may be ill = toxic hypoxia.
7. The factory gates may be closed to coal trucks = mechanical asphyxia.
8. There may be no coal = environmental anoxia.
9. So much dust may accumulate that the man cannot reach the buckets = lung disease.
In the end
6. The furnace goes out = death.

The lungs are continually attacked by dust particles present in the air and, normally, the specialised lining of the air passages can cope with this hazard efficiently. In certain circumstances, these defence mechanisms may be destroyed and the lungs will then become diseased as a result of exposure to the environment. The most common precipitating causes are smoking and atmospheric pollution. Alternatively, the lungs may be exposed to unreasonable quantities of dust which may, of itself, be dangerous—most of these *pneumoconioses* or dust diseases are industrial in nature and are discussed in Chapter 15.

Injuries to the lungs are generally of obvious type. They may be penetrated by instruments, by foreign bodies—for example, bullets—or by the ends of broken ribs. Two consequences arise. First the negative pressure in the pleural space may be broken and the lung collapses—not only does this lead to inefficient oxygenation of the blood but the immobile lung is a nidus for infection. Secondly, haemorrhage is inevitable and its severity depends on the size of the vessels involved. Blunt injury is commonly caused by crushing, as in vehicular accidents. Additionally, the large number of gas/fluid interfaces in the lungs renders them particularly sensitive to the passage of shock waves. Generalised pulmonary trauma is, thus, typical of falls from a height or of exposure to an explosive blast. The injuries consist of haemorrhage, laceration and destruction of the walls of the alveoli.

One of the most important medico-legal involvements of the lungs is that type of inflammation known as *hypostatic pneumonia* which is likely to follow enforced bed-rest after any injury. The lungs are inadequately expanded and oedema is common; the situation is ripe for the establishment of widespread infection. The less fit the subject, the more probable is the onset of pneumonia and the less likely is he or she to withstand the assault. The common fatal injuries in elderly persons are not those that are immediately lethal; they are those that entail lengthy periods in bed.

The nervous system

Anatomically, the nervous system is divided into the *central nervous system* (CNS) and the *peripheral nervous system* which involves all the nerves that pass out from the CNS to the remainder of the body. The CNS consists of the *brain* and *spinal cord*, the latter being divided into a number of segments related to the vertebrae of the spinal column; a major efferent or *motor* root and an afferent or *sensory* root pass through the lateral aspects of each vertebra. The motor and sensory nerve pathways pass respectively downwards and upwards in the spinal cord between the brain and the nerve roots appropriate to the area of the body they supply. It follows that damage to the spinal cord will result in functional abnormality of a *regional* distribution, the region affected being that which is supplied by nerve roots situated below the point of damage; thus, severance of the cord at the neck will result in paralysis of all four limbs (*quadriplegia*) whereas severance in the thoracic region leads to paralysis of the legs (*paraplegia*). Division of a nerve root, on the other hand, will show itself in a segmental distribution—either anaesthetic or paralytic—whereas damage to a peripheral nerve will cause similar changes either in a group of muscles (or wide area of skin) or in an individual muscle depending on the size of the nerve affected. One further major difference in response to injury must be noted. While some regrowth and recovery of function is possible in the peripheral nerves (the degree depending to some extent on the surgeon's skill) there is no true regeneration in the CNS;[3] this applies not only to the nerve fibres (akin to electric flex down which the impulses travel) but also to the nerve cells—or batteries—from which derive the ultimate nervous function; a child is born with the maximum number of brain cells it will possess and the decreasing mental capacity of senility is to some extent a measure of how these degenerate during life.

In the event of damage to the spinal cord, some functions can be retained through the medium of spinal reflexes which operate without the control of the brain; after division of the cord some useful reflex actions—such as the uncontrolled emptying of the bladder when it is full—may be established. Similar reflex reaction may be seen in the limbs when the brain itself is dead (see Chapter 12); it must, then, be distinguished from conscious movement which would, if present, be evidence of residual cerebral activity.

It is convenient to regard the central nervous system as a core running from the head to the 'tail' with nerve fibres carrying information and commands in both directions. The spinal cord forms the lowermost part and, above this, lies the hindbrain consisting of the *medulla* and *pons* where many centres organising the vital functions of the body—eg respiration—are situated; the pons is of very great medico-legal importance owing to the frequency with which it sustains fatal haemorrhage after head injury. There is then a narrow midbrain and, above this, the forebrain of which the central core is the *thalamus* and *hypothalamus* where, as a great simplification, the instinctive or animal processes are organised. Two major, bilaterally symmetrical, masses are connected to the centre core; these are the *cerebellum* which overlies and is part of the hindbrain and the *cerebrum* (covered by the *cerebral cortex*) which forms the major part of the forebrain. These masses are concerned with the more complicated functions of the body. The cerebellum essentially co-ordinates movements and posture. Anatomically, the cerebrum is divided into four lobes—the frontal concerned mainly with personality but also with the initiation of muscle movements, the parietal which is the area associated with sensation, the occipital concerned with vision and the temporal which is mainly associated with speech, hearing and equilibrium. Special areas within each lobe are related to special areas of the body, the important feature being that head injury can have reasonably predictable results.[4] The highly developed cerebral cortex acts in many ways as a controller of the instinctive thalamus. Thus, some drugs—and, in particular, alcohol—which appear to be stimulatory in nature are, in fact, depressants; the most highly developed part of the brain is most easily affected and this leads to diminished cognitive control of activity.

This concept of conscious control extends also into the peripheral innervation where, in addition to the nerve supply already described, all the organs are subject to nervous control through the *autonomic system*. This consists of two functional moieties—*sympathetic* and *parasympathetic* systems; the vagus nerve forms a major component of the latter. The autonomic system is responsible for all those activities that are subconscious—for example, the beating of the heart, the production of sweat, movement of the bowel, etc. By and large, its two

---

3   Clinical recovery of *functions* may appear when the, mainly, pressure effects of haemorrhage, oedema, etc, resolve.
4   Within the head, cranial nerves are given off to supply the head and the special senses and are analogous to the peripheral nerves of the spinal cord.

components are antagonistic; thus, it is the function of the sympathetic system to quicken the heart beat while impulses acting through the vagus nerve will slow it. This raises an important concept in forensic pathology—that of death due to cardiac inhibition resulting from reflex vagal activity.[5] Basically, a sudden and, particularly, an unnatural stimulation of the sympathetic nerves will lead to reflex compensatory action of the vagus nerve; this, being equally severe and unnatural, may so slow the heart as to paralyse it completely. The mucous membranes contribute a potent source of such dangerous reflexes but pressure on special centres of sympathetic activity—especially the *carotid sinus* in the neck or the *solar plexus* in the abdomen—may lead to a similar result.

Alternatively, stimulation of, say, the carotid sinus may result in unopposed hyperactivity of the sympathetic system itself, in which case, the heart muscle may be provoked into uncontrolled contractions or *ventricular fibrillation*. Both these mechanisms, which arrive at the same medico-legal end-point, can be subsumed under the title *neurogenic cardiac arrest* which is discussed further in Chapter 13.

The coverings of the brain and spinal cord are of great medico-legal importance. From without inwards, the brain is covered, first, by the skull and the cord by the component parts of the backbone. These rigid structures, designed to protect the delicate nervous structure from direct external violence, also have obvious disadvantages—there is no room for expansion or displacement of the contained organs and, if fractured, the broken bones themselves become potential lacerating instruments; skilled treatment of injury to the skull and spine is, therefore, a matter of urgency. Within its bony coverings, the CNS is surrounded by a tough membrane known as the *dura mater*. Large blood vessels flow between the bone and the dura; internally, numerous small veins drain into the *dural sinuses*. Head injury can therefore result in either *extradural* or *subdural* haemorrhage. The *arachnoid mater* is a thin membrane lying under the dura. A relatively wide space exists between this membrane and the *pia mater* which invests the brain closely. This subarachnoid space contains the *cerebrospinal fluid*, the main function of which is to give some leeway for expansion and to act as a water cushion for the brain, and also the main arteries as they pass from the neck to supply the brain substance; rupture of these vessels due to injury or natural disease results in *subarachnoid haemorrhage*. The thin pia mater invests the brain so closely that there is, effectively, no subpial space—any haemorrhage occurring in this area is of superficial *intracerebral* type. Deep intracerebral haemorrhage is often divisible into two types—petechial (or capillary), which is commonly associated with asphyxial states of all types, and massive, which may be traumatic in origin but is more likely to be due to natural disease. Intracranial haemorrhage is discussed in detail in Chapter 11.

A review of the nervous system is incomplete without consideration of the special senses but such a discussion is beyond the scope of this volume. It is obvious that the loss of a special sense is of particular civil medico-legal importance and that, of these senses, vision is not only the most important but is also, perhaps, the most vulnerable. In addition to penetrating wounds, partial or complete loss of vision due to trauma can result from damage to the outer covering (*corneal abrasion*), to infection due to the presence of foreign bodies, to intraocular haemorrhage and to *retinal* detachment; *sympathetic ophthalmia* is a particularly distressing situation in which the other eye may lose its function 'in sympathy' with

5   This will often be referred to in reports as 'vagal inhibition'—an unfortunate abbreviation for 'vagal inhibition of the heart action'. This is another reason why the less specific term 'neurogenic cardiac arrest' is to be preferred.

one that is damaged—this may, in fact, be an example of auto-immune disease (see below). Internally, the *optic nerve* may be damaged in association with fractures of the skull and, finally, blindness may result from damage to the occipital lobe of the cerebral cortex where the centres for vision are located—falls on the back of the head are, therefore, important in regard to vision. The importance of the eyes as a *cause* of death due to accidents—particularly vehicular—requires no emphasis.

The gastrointestinal system

The function of the gastrointestinal system is to accept food, digest it, store it, circulate it to the tissues in a form that provides a ready source of energy and to excrete unused residues. The whole process is controlled by a complex system of enzymes (see below).

The *alimentary canal* starts at the mouth and leads into the straight *oesophagus* which traverses the length of the thorax. The oesophagus opens into the *stomach* which, in turn, empties into the *duodenum* or first part of the small intestine. The *jejunum* and *ileum* form the second and third parts of the small intestine which is about 6 m (20 ft) in length and closely coiled within the abdomen. The large intestine consists of the *caecum* and its attached *vermiform appendix*; the ascending, transverse, descending and sigmoid *colon*; and the *rectum* which opens to the exterior at the *anus*.

The *peritoneum* lines the abdominal cavity and invests the small and large intestines. The envelope of peritoneum that is attached to the posterior abdominal wall and from which the small intestine is suspended is known as the *mesentery* and the major blood vessels lie within this. Tissues that lie posteriorly in the abdomen behind the mesentery are said to be *retroperitoneal* in position.

Constituents of food absorbed from the bowel are passed to the *liver* where they are both processed and stored. The liver is the largest organ in the body and occupies the upper right quadrant in the abdomen. It has numerous functions including the metabolism of carbohydrates, fats and proteins; the storage of a readily available source of energy (glycogen); the processing of waste material derived from breakdown of body tissue; the preparation of many of the substances essential for blood clotting; and the formation of bile which is stored in the *gall bladder* and passed into the intestine where it assists in digestion. Failure to secrete bile or to excrete it into the bowel shows itself as *jaundice*.

Ferments from the *pancreas* are also essential to digestion; this organ lies in the posterior part of the abdomen and empties its secretion into the duodenum.

The forensic importance of the gastrointestinal system is very great. The majority of poisons that are administered homicidally must be given by mouth; it follows that the primary symptoms of poisoning are commonly gastric or intestinal in nature and the early diagnosis of this form of crime depends greatly on the skill of the family doctor (see Chapter 21). The liver itself is also very sensitive to poisonous substances many of which are industrial in nature; jaundice is, therefore, an important sign of poisoning at work. Many drugs are detoxified in the liver; it may be the organ of choice at post-mortem examination for the identification and quantification of drug overdose. The function of the liver may also be greatly impaired by infection of the organ—when the condition of *hepatitis* is established. A proportion of these cases result from the 'hepatitis viruses B and C' which are transmitted from the blood of infected persons; the significance of these conditions in blood transfusion is discussed in Chapter 31. [6] Alcohol specifically affects the liver, the classic process running from fatty degeneration to fibrotic replacement and *cirrhosis* which results in liver failure and also in the more specific condition of *oesophageal varices* which may rupture and cause death from haemorrhage. It is, however, a feature of the damaged liver that it is capable of regeneration once the damaging agent has been removed.

The results of trauma to the bowel may be very serious. The contents of the bowel may be irritant—as in the stomach—or they may be heavily contaminated by bacteria—as in the large bowel. In either case, rupture of the viscus will result in severe damage to the abdominal cavity and death may follow due to shock (see page 5); stab wounds and gunshot wounds of the abdomen thus require urgent surgical treatment. The hollow organs are also sensitive to explosive blast, particularly if this is transmitted through water. The bowel itself is surprisingly resistant to blunt, non-penetrating trauma, but both the intestine and its mesentery can be ruptured when massive force is applied from outside over a limited area; the single lap-belt type of restraint used in commercial aircraft is a modern means of transmitting such forces during a crash.

The sheer bulk of the liver increases its susceptibility to penetrating injury but it is at its most vulnerable in crushing accidents or in conditions that set up severe vibrations in the body, such as falls from a height.

The pancreas, on the other hand, is well protected and is only occasionally injured. The organ is, however, prone to damage by disease in alcoholics and degenerative changes are found when cold injury occurs in the undernourished.

The urinary system

When considering the respiratory system, the body was compared to a furnace; following the same analogy, a mechanism for waste disposal or removal of the ashes is essential if the organism is not to be poisoned. Gaseous products of combustion are eliminated in the breath but soluble waste products circulating in the plasma of the blood are excreted in the urine, which is prepared and voided through the urinary system (see Figure 1.3).

This consists of a pair of *kidneys*, placed retroperitoneally in the abdomen with their upper portions covered by the lower ribs, from which pass a pair of tubes, the *ureters*. Each ureter drains into the *bladder*, a muscular reservoir whose outflow is protected by sphincters. Urine which is stored in the bladder is passed to the outside of the body through a single pipe—the *urethra*. The urethra in the female is short; in the male it is long and assumes a serpentine shape as it passes through the *prostate gland* and the *penis*. The opening of the female urethra lies close to the bacterially contaminated anus; ascending *cystitis*—or inflammation of the bladder—is, therefore, a common natural disease of women. Men, by contrast, are subject to the equally distressing condition of *prostatic hypertrophy*, which leads to stasis of the urine in the bladder and, again, infection.

6   These viruses—and the human immunodeficiency virus—can also be transmitted through the small quantities of blood remaining in hypodermic needles. 'Needle sharing' by drug abusers constitutes a major mode of spread.

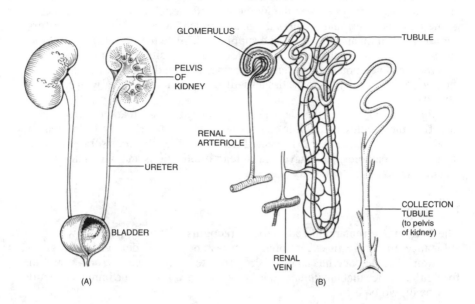

GLOMERULUS

TUBULE

PELVIS
OF
KIDNEY

RENAL
ARTERIOLE

URETER

COLLECTION
TUBULE
(to pelvis
of kidney)

BLADDER

RENAL
VEIN

(A)

(B)

Figure 1.3 The anatomy of the urinary system. (*a*) Macroscopic structure. (*b*) Microscopic appearance of a nephron. Note that the blood supplies the tubule after it has passed through the glomerulus.

The kidneys play a major part in the regulation of the body's biochemical status and have two further roles in the maintenance of health. First, as indicated above, there is the elimination of waste products. The primary mechanism of clearance is pressure filtration through a vast network of blood capillaries. It follows from this that any disease of the kidneys will have a profound general effect on the cardiovascular system; the most common adverse result is a raised blood pressure—the condition of *hypertension*. Disturbance of the blood pressure may, indeed, be the cause of death from a disease that started as a primary condition in the kidney tissues.

The excretory function with which this section is most concerned is based on the individual excretory units, the *nephrons* each of which consists of a *glomerulus* and a system of *tubules*. A glomerulus, of which there are approximately 2 million, is essentially a skein of blood capillaries enclosed in a capsule. The wall of the capillary acts as a semipermeable membrane—semipermeable because it will allow the passage of water and small dissolved particles but will retain particles of large molecular size, especially proteins. Filtration pressure, aided perhaps by diffusion, results in the appearance in the capsular space of what is effectively protein-free blood plasma. This contains not only waste products but also materials that are of value or even essential to the body, notably glucose and sodium; moreover, the body cannot lose all its water. Some sort of selective concentration is needed.

This is the role of the tubules which, from the functional aspect, can be divided into proximal and distal portions. The glucose, sodium and much of the essential water are reabsorbed in the former while complex reactions designed to regulate the degree of acidity of the blood take place in the latter. The distal tubules run into collecting tubules which act as tributaries to the ureters. The importance of clearly distinguishing between the glomeruli and the tubules is that the function of the latter is active and requires the use of much energy. They are, therefore, very dependent on an effective blood supply and, since the vessels to the tubules have already supplied the needs of the glomeruli, conditions at tubular level are ripe for the development of an 'energy crisis'; any condition that interferes with the free delivery of oxygen to the tissues will affect the renal tubules with particular severity.

Abnormal conditions that damage the glomeruli differ markedly from those affecting the tubules and, while the former have comparatively little medico-legal significance other than in respect of treatment, they illustrate some important principles of pathology that have widespread implications and which might well be considered at this point.

Immunity

The body has a remarkable capacity to recognise foreign materials within its substance and, save in exceptional circumstances, will defend itself against invasion. The defence mechanism is referred to as an *immune reaction* and the foreign substance that precipitates it is known as an *antigen*. The immune reaction may be of two types:

1. *Humoral*—this involves the formation of circulating antibodies which react specifically with antigens and can generally be demonstrated to do so in the laboratory.
2. *Cellular*—in which the body musters forces of migrant cells which will actively attack and either destroy or eliminate the intruder. It is this reaction which is primarily responsible for the rejection of transplanted tissues (see Chapter 12).

A major result of antigenic challenge is to stimulate the body's powers of recollection. Thus, the first intrusion causes comparatively gradual recognition followed by reaction. The pattern of the foreign substance is remembered, the templates of antibody production are retained and a second attack can be met by the immediate mobilisation of reserves. Repeated stimuli result in increasing immunity. Normally, this system is entirely to the body's advantage—it forms the basis, for example, of vaccination against various infectious diseases. Occasionally, however, the body may fail to distinguish between self and non-self, with disastrous consequences; this occurs in two basic ways. The first mechanism is incompletely understood but, possibly because of abnormal position rather than abnormal constitution, the body reacts against its own tissues without any stimulus from outside. This constitutes *auto-immune disease*—an example of which we have seen already but which has little forensic significance other than in relation to medical negligence by way of inadequate communication between doctor and patient (see page 474). As to the second form, it must be appreciated that antigens are molecular in nature and that any organised biological particle contains a number of antigens; individual antigens may, therefore, be common to substances of dissimilar nature. Once having recognised an antigen, the body will react to it similarly irrespective of mode of presentation. As an analogy, the body might remember being attacked by a villain armed with a willow bough; it will react violently and defensively to a subsequent friendly offer of a cricket bat.

Such a direct error of identification may occasionally result in severe disease of the glomeruli. Additionally, however, *immune complexes* are formed when a foreign antigen stimulates and combines with an antibody. These immune complexes—often associated with the *streptococcus* which causes sore throats—may become deposited on the glomerular capillary walls and establish a secondary reaction. The subsequent damage to the capillary walls and the efforts of the glomeruli to remove the deposited material result in *glomerulonephritis*, a diffuse condition in which all the glomeruli are equally at risk. Fortunately, in most cases the glomeruli return to normal and clinical recovery is the rule. Occasionally, however, the disease progresses and, after a variable time, the kidneys cease to function. Medico-legally, the importance is that treatment then depends on replacement by machine or transplant and this important subject is discussed later.

Frequently, in the less acute cases, the functional integrity of the glomerular filtration membrane is compromised and, as a result, the body protein is lost steadily into the urine—the condition known as the nephrotic syndrome. Few of the causes of the condition have forensic interest but it may be associated with certain medical treatments, particularly the use of drugs containing heavy metals.

Acute renal failure[7]

In contrast to conditions affecting the glomeruli, extraglomerular disease of the nephrons is a common complication of unnatural disease and is of special medico-legal interest.

The development of acute renal failure is intimately associated with shock—the medical definition of which was discussed on page 5. Essentially, shock is a matter of inadequate oxygenation of the tissues. The condition may arise from blood loss which, in turn, may be due either to bleeding or to destruction of the blood (haemolysis) within the body. Haemolysis may result from inherent enzyme deficiency diseases, autoimmune diseases, infection of the blood cells as in malaria or, occasionally, from the inadvertent precipitation of an immune reaction, the most obvious example of which is a mismatched blood transfusion. Oxygen lack may be induced during anaesthesia (see Chapter 31). Reduction of the plasma component of the blood may follow burning, severe surgical trauma or unusual conditions such as crushing of the muscles or sub-atmospheric decompression.

Acute renal failure may accompany any of these conditions. The medico-legal significance of this condition is twofold—first, nearly all the basic causes are unnatural and, secondly, the condition is recoverable in many cases provided that some mechanism can be substituted for the kidneys during a period of recuperation. This substitution treatment is known as haemodialysis, or 'the artificial kidney', in which the blood is diverted to a man-made membrane simulating the glomerulus. Passage of dissolved substances from the blood across this membrane can be controlled by altering their concentration in the

---

7   The condition was often referred to in the past as 'renal tubular necrosis'. This may, however, be a misnomer based on a faulty interpretation of autopsy findings.

'bath' fluid which takes the place of the filtrate in the glomerular capsule—in effect an 'osmotic gradient' can be established for any constituent of the plasma.

The kidneys sometimes fail to recuperate (treatment is notoriously difficult when the condition has been precipitated by burning) and haemodialysis carries hazards of its own including the increasing possibility of blood transfusion reactions and cross-infection between staff and patients—especially by the agents responsible for infective hepatitis. Generally, however, treatment is successful after a finite number of sessions.

By contrast, dialysis for the treatment of glomerular death must be continued throughout life. This process involves sustained and regular occupation of machines which are not limitless as to availability and are also expensive in bed space and nursing manpower; the tendency is to encourage home dialysis treatment—or alternative methods to haemodialysis such as peritoneal dialysis—despite the attendant difficulties associated with asepsis and other problems. Decisions as to treatment must involve socio-economic considerations and the treatment of chronic renal failure is a good example of the modern doctor's inability to treat many of his patients on purely medical criteria; much must nowadays involve a compromise with external factors. Organ transplantation is a more therapeutically effective—and cost effective—treatment for end stage renal failure but this is, itself, subject to even greater conflicts of supply and demand (see Chapter 12).

Both the glomeruli and the tubules may be involved in inflammation resulting from infection ascending from the bladder; this important subject is referred to later in this section.

Injury to the urinary system

The kidneys lie posteriorly in the body and are comparatively well protected by large muscle masses; they also lie in a good shock-absorbing bed of fatty tissue. Laceration by indirect trauma is, therefore, comparatively rare and the kidneys are not often torn in fatal accidents that inflict severe damage to other solid organs such as the liver and spleen. None the less, damage to the kidneys is surprisingly frequent in non-fatal automobile accidents—a situation probably associated with the great vascularity of the organs and consequent severe bleeding as a result of compression.

The kidneys are also prone to injury during violent attack. They are common targets in assaults by kicking—in which case very severe internal injury may be present in the absence of obvious external damage—and they may be involved in knifings. It is fortunate that the body can function perfectly well with only one normal kidney.

The ureters are well protected from external injury but, as they pass into the pelvis, they come close to the female generative organs; they are therefore at risk when the latter are subjected to surgical operation. The error of tying the ureters during gynaecological operations is well known and may occasionally be very difficult to avoid in the presence of widespread chronic inflammation.[8]

---

8   *Hendy v Milton Keynes Health Authority (No 2)* [1992] 3 Med LR 119 provides an example together with a useful distinction between medical misjudgment and medical negligence.

The bladder in both male and female is closely associated with the bones of the pelvis. Fracture of the pelvis—which results from a variety of accidents, such as those associated with transportation, falls from a height, crushing etc—is commonly accompanied by rupture of the bladder or of the urethra. Both these injuries are treatable by surgery but often the condition of the casualty dictates a delay in operation. The possibility is then raised of ascending infection of the urinary tract with consequent involvement of the kidneys as discussed below.

Bladder disorders of medico-legal importance

The bladder itself is controlled by the autonomic nervous system and the muscle is generally in a state of relaxation; distension results in reflex contraction and expulsion of urine. Autonomic urination is prevented by additional control of the external sphincter through the voluntary nervous system.

Since the nerve supply to the bladder sphincter originates in the lower part of the spinal cord, any injuries of the cord are likely to upset the capacity to control the act of micturition—the organ will revert to automatic action. Apart from the social inconvenience, the stage is then set for ascending infection of the urinary tract and it is not uncommon for the life of a paraplegic to terminate years after the spinal injury as a result of inflammatory destruction of the kidneys.

The different shape of the urethra in the male and female has a profound effect on the establishment of infection in the bladder. Thus, in the female, it is not difficult for organisms on the skin of the external genitalia to pass in retrograde fashion to the bladder, while the inherent laxity of the perineum predisposes to prolapse and inefficient emptying of the viscus. Inflammation of that organ (*cystitis*) is, therefore, common in women. The male urethra, by contrast, can protect the bladder from external invasion relatively well but the prostate gland is subject to enlargement of either a benign or cancerous nature. Obstruction to the flow of urine due to prostatism is a common accompaniment of later middle age; the resultant 'back pressure' may have serious effects on the kidneys themselves while the stagnation of urine induced is, as in the female, conducive to the establishment of infection; the process may be accelerated by the need to pass catheters into the distended organ.

Stagnation of urine leads to its prolonged contact with the inner wall of the bladder. Injurious substances that are excreted in the urine might be expected, therefore, to strike selectively at the bladder and this is indeed the case. Some hydrocarbons are active in the production of epithelial cancer (*carcinoma*) which may arise as a result of occupation (see Chapter 15).

Infection of the kidney

It is convenient to complete this section by returning to the kidneys themselves with a comment on inflammation due to infection. In the end, infection of the kidney probably results in as much glomerular destruction as does primary glomerular disease and, in contrast to the latter, inflammatory disease has considerable direct medico-legal significance. Thus, anything that facilitates the introduction of, or encourages the growth of, organisms within the bladder—including injury, surgery or simple instrumentation—may ultimately lead to severe disability or even to death.

The reproductive system

The male reproductive system consists of the twin *testes* which usually descend into the *scrotum* just before birth. The organs are formed of coiled tubules in which the *spermatozoa* (or male *gametes)* mature. A spermatozoon consists of a head (approximately 4 μm in length), a neck and a tail which is some 50 μm long. When stained, the head shows a typical dark nucleus at its base, an appearance that is quite characteristic even when the tail is lost. Some 400—500 million spermatozoa are shed with a normal ejaculation. The bulk of the seminal fluid is derived from the *epididymis*, one of which lies close to each testis; together they drain into the *vas deferens*. The vas deferens on each side opens into the *urethra* at the base of the bladder. Other small glands contribute to the total seminal ejaculate.

The female reproductive organs consist, first, of two *ovaries* which lie on each side of the pelvis. Each ovary has a finite store of eggs or *ova* (the female *gametes*) which greatly exceeds the requirements for the maturation each month—between the onset of menstruation and the menopause—of, normally, a single egg. The ovaries on each side are connected to the *uterus* by the *Fallopian tubes* down which the ova pass. There is a potential space between the ovary and the receptor end of the tube; occasionally, ova are fertilised and yet do not reach the uterus, in which case the dangerous condition of *ectopic pregnancy* is established. The outlet of the uterus is a tightly closed canal surrounded by the *cervix* which juts into the *vagina*. The vagina opens through the *vulva*. In the virgin state, the vaginal opening is protected by the *hymen*, a sheet of fibrous tissue with, usually, a small opening which will permit the passage of normal secretions. The size of the hymenal opening varies—it may be large originally or it may be dilated by tampons or masturbation. In general, however, the size is such that the first penetration by the penis results in laceration which is usually posterior in position; the distinction between the virginal hymen and one showing old or recent rupture is of obvious importance in accusations of rape. The vulva consists, internally, of a paired *labia minora* which join anteriorly and posteriorly as commissures. The posterior commisure is known as the *fourchette*; this again is likely to be damaged during forceful intercourse and during childbirth. The *labia majora* lie outermost; they are joined in front at the *mons veneris* but posteriorly dissolve into the tissues of the perineum.

In normal circumstances, spermatozoa injected into the vagina migrate to the Fallopian tube where a single male gamete fertilises the ovum, thus forming the *zygote*.[9] An unfertilised ovum will die in some two days but the fertilised ovum passes to the uterus where it is implanted some six days after fertilisation.[10] After about three months' development, a *placenta* forms which is attached to the growing fetus by the *umbilical cord*. The fetus is surrounded by a fibrous sac known as the *amnion* and floats in the *amniotic fluid*.

---

9 The female sometimes develops antibodies as a result of an immune reaction to her partner's spermatozoa. This is an important cause of childlessness which can sometimes be obviated by changing the spermatozoa (artificial insemination by donor) or by GIFT (see Chapter 17).

10 This process is copied artificially in the treatment of some forms of childlessness using *gamete intra-Fallopian transfer* (or GIFT). Alternatively, a zygote may be formed *in vitro* and inserted into the tube (ZIFT).

The birth process is started by contractions of the uterus and dilatation of the cervix, usually with rupture of the amnion. If the placenta becomes detached, the fetus will die and be expelled as a foreign body; it will be similarly rejected should the fetus itself die. Unnatural dilatation of the cervical canal will, of itself, cause the uterus to contract. Any of these situations can be simulated in order to procure abortion (see Chapter 18).

The endocrine system

The body contains a number of glands that discharge *hormones* into the bloodstream. These hormones have specific actions on various parts of the body; overproduction or failure of the *endocrine* glands can, therefore, result in disease or dysfunction of the target organs.

There are seven different glands secreting some 30 hormones which are commonly likened to an orchestra. The 'conductor' of the orchestra is the *pituitary* gland which lies in the base of the skull. The pituitary stimulates activity in many of the other glands but is itself sensitive to circulating hormones; once sufficient hormones are present in the blood, this servomechanism inhibits further stimulation. In addition to its supervisory function over the other glands, the pituitary itself controls growth, the secretion of urine and the contraction of the uterus during childbirth. Damage to the pituitary gland is, therefore, a very serious matter; it is a common result of fracture of the base of the skull and the gland may be damaged by the effects of haemorrhage after complicated childbirth.

The remainder of the endocrine glands, while vital to health, are of little medico-legal significance, but, as the names will certainly appear in autopsy reports, a brief description is given.

The *thyroid* gland lies in the neck and is responsible for mental and physical growth in childhood and for the general rate of metabolism in the adult—deficiency of thyroid hormone leads to cold and apathy, excess results in production of heat and hyperexcitability. The position of the thyroid renders it susceptible to bruising, which may be of considerable evidential value in cases of strangulation.

The *parathyroid* glands are small and closely associated anatomically with the thyroid. They control the distribution of calcium between the bones and the body as a whole.

The *adrenal* glands lie against the kidneys and are of immense importance to the body. Their central parts secrete *adrenalin* which affects the tone of the blood vessels and also the heart rate; its action is similar to that of the sympathetic nervous system. Adrenalin is secreted in response to sudden stress and, in effect, brings the body to a fighting trim in response to alarm. When given therapeutically, it has profound effects on the blood pressure and blood distribution; these must be considered in relation to death associated with surgical operations. The outer parts of the adrenal glands secrete the corticosteroids which control the salt and water balance of the body (and, hence, the distribution of the muscle/fat tissues), exert an effect on the metabolism of carbohydrates, influence the sex glands and are very much concerned with the response of the body to infection or other conditions resulting in inflammation. Corticosteroids can be used to suppress the immune response. Abnormalities of secretion are important in the expression of secondary sex characteristics—thus, an excess of virilising hormones in females leads to the *adreno-genital syndrome* which may lead to misdiagnosis of sex at birth or to an apparent change of sex at puberty (see Chapter 17).

The *pancreas* secretes the hormone *insulin*, absence of which causes the disease *diabetes* in which the storage of carbohydrate is inhibited and the blood contains large amounts of sugar—*hyperglycaemia*. The converse situation, *hypoglycaemia*, results from an excess of insulin. This is a rare natural condition but is an obvious hazard of the treatment of diabetes; considerable medico-legal importance attaches to 'automatic' behaviour whilst in a hypoglycaemic state—a problem which is discussed at page 405. Hypoglycaemia can be fatal and injection of insulin has been used as a refined method of homicide. Hypoglycaemia may, also, occur spontaneously in sensitive persons independently of insulin secretion; the syndrome closely simulates alcoholism and is still of some importance in the field of road traffic law.

The *testes* and the *ovaries* secrete hormones which, in the former, are concerned with the secondary sex characteristics and physique of maleness and, in the latter, with the control of menstruation and pregnancy and the control of female secondary sex characteristics; occasional cases of apparent sex change due to the excess secretion of feminising hormones are reported.[11] Similarly, the testes may fail to secrete androgens; an interesting variation, in which the secretion of androgens is normal but their action on the 'target organs' is inhibited, results in the medico-legally important condition of the testicular feminisation syndrome (discussed at page 235). A further important medico-legal connotation lies in the use of sex hormones in competitive sport (see Chapter 16).

The musculoskeletal system

This system consists of the bony skeleton (see Figure 1.4) to which the muscle masses are attached often through the medium of tendons. Those muscles which can be activated at will are known as *voluntary* muscles (or *striated* muscles, because of their appearance under the microscope). Many organs—for example, the bladder and bowel—are equipped with muscle that is not under conscious control and is therefore known as *involuntary* or, from its microscopic appearance, *smooth* muscle; such muscle is, however, an integral part of the system with which it is associated. Where bones articulate with one another in joints, the surfaces are covered with cartilage; cartilage is also formed at bony junctions when some mobility is needed—the prime examples being at the junctions between the breast bone and the ribs and between the two pelvic bones; such a union is known as a *symphysis*.

---

11 Scottish readers will be interested in the unique case of *X Petitioner* 1957 SLT (Sh Ct) 61 which was clearly misinterpreted at the time.

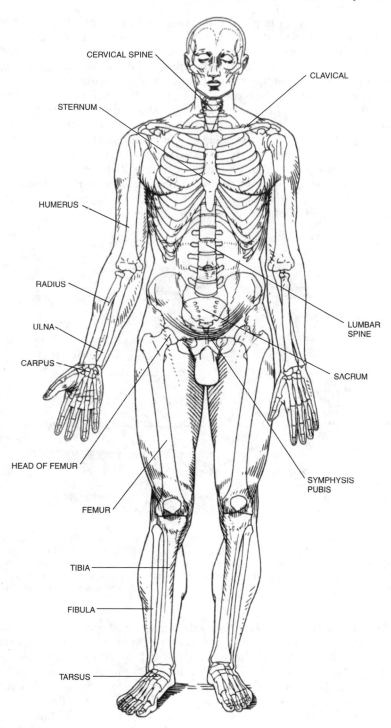

CERVICAL SPINE

CLAVICAL

STERNUM

HUMERUS

RADIUS

ULNA

CARPUS

HEAD OF FEMUR

FEMUR

TIBIA

FIBULA

TARSUS

LUMBAR
SPINE

SACRUM

SYMPHYSIS
PUBIS

Figure 1.4 The major relationships of the human skeleton. (From an original diagram by
Professor G J Romanes.)

The *skull* is divided simply into the vault, which covers the brain, and the base on which the brain rests. The base forms the anterior, middle and posterior *fossae* or cavities on each side in which the lobes of the brain are accommodated (see Figure 1.5). The skull rests on the spine which is formed of a number of individual vertebrae; the uppermost is known as the *atlas* bone—fracture of this bone is of great importance in the origin of the fatal, unnatural condition *traumatic sub-arachnoid haemorrhage*. The atlas and six small vertebrae form the *cervical* spine; below this are 12 *thoracic* vertebrae with which the ribs articulate posteriorly; five large vertebrae lying in the small of the back form the *lumbar* spine and below this are the fused vertebrae of the *sacrum* which makes up the rear wall of the pelvic cavity; the tail of the primates is represented by the small *coccyx*. The sacrum joins the two *pelvic* bones posteriorly; anteriorly the pelves are united at the *symphysis pubis* which allows for some expansion during childbirth but which is often split in severe accidents.

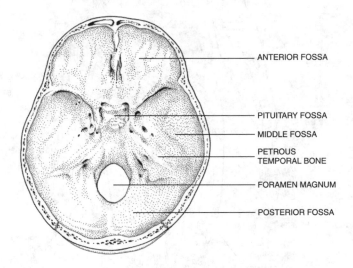

ANTERIOR FOSSA

PITUITARY FOSSA

MIDDLE FOSSA

PETROUS
TEMPORAL BONE

FORAMEN MAGNUM

POSTERIOR FOSSA

Figure 1.5 The inner surface of the base of the skull. The frontal lobes rest in the anterior fossae, the temporal lobes in the middle fossae and the cerebellum lies in the posterior fossae. The spinal cord passes though the foramen magnum. The weakest part of the base of the skull runs along the line of the petrous temporal bone through the multiple foramina and the pituitary fossa—recovery from fracture of the base can lead to permanent pituitary dysfunction.

The front of the chest is protected by the solid breast bone or *sternum* which is, again, a common casualty of accidental trauma. The shoulder girdle is formed by the *scapulae* or shoulder blades posteriorly and the *clavicles* or collar bones anteriorly. The *humerus* articulates with these to form the shoulder joint and, at the elbow, forms a joint with the two bones of the forearm—the *ulna* and the *radius* which is on the thumb side. The bones of the wrist are collectively known as the *carpus*, those of the hand as the *metacarpals* and those of the fingers the *phalanges*; the knuckles may, therefore, be either metacarpophalangeal or interphalangeal joints.

The thigh bone or *femur* has its large circular head embedded in the *acetabulum* of the pelvis. The hips must be wide in order to accommodate the massive leg muscles and the first part of the femur—known as the neck—must, therefore, adopt a relatively horizontal position before joining the main thigh bone at an obtuse angle which approximates, as will be seen later, more to a right angle in the female. The neck of the femur, which, effectively, carries the weight of the torso, is, thus, a mechanically weak point and is of great forensic importance owing to the ease with which it can be accidentally broken—especially in elderly women whose bones are becoming brittle; the condition then requires either prolonged bed-rest or the surgical insertion of a pin before the broken ends will reunite— conditions are ripe for death from hypostatic pneumonia or from pulmonary embolism (see pages 12 and 97). [12] The femur articulates at the knee joints with the large *tibia*, which lies medially in the lower leg, and with the slender *fibula* which lies laterally. Unlike the bones of the forearm, the bones of the lower leg cannot cross over—the foot cannot be pronated or supinated as can the hand. The bones of the ankle are known as the *tarsus* and include two particularly large individual bones—the *talus* and the *calcaneus* which have some importance in establishing the age of a stillbirth or neonate. The foot contains the *metatarsals* and the toes the *phalanges*.

The voluntary muscles are rarely described individually in post-mortem reports and need not be detailed at this point. Paralysis of individual muscles may be of great importance in relation to claims for compensation but, in those circumstances, far more information will be needed than could be provided in a book of this size.

The importance of fractures in virtually all aspects of forensic medicine is clear. Apart from their frequency in violence, they are demonstrable and readily presentable by means of X-rays (see Chapter 26), they can be 'dated' and many are of specific type; fractures are therefore discussed in regard to special situations throughout this book.

Otherwise, the major forensic significance of the skeletal system lies in its relationship to the identification of remains.

The bones of the body consist of calcium salts deposited in an organised fashion in a protein medium. Calcification and the laying down of bone in soft connective tissue begin in *centres of ossification* which are demonstrable visually and by X-ray at different times in individual bones. Although there is considerable biological variation, ossification centres are generally established in a regular order and with reasonable constancy so that their assessment can give a fair guide to the age of a fetus or young infant—it is only in these age groups that such early development is progressing.

Centres of ossification in the long bones are generally multiple and at least triple—one centre appearing in the shaft or *diaphysis* and one at each end or *epiphysis*. These must fuse in order to form adult bone and, again, this process is one of some regularity which extends throughout childhood and adolescence.

The individual bones of the skull unite in older age. This feature is, however, extremely variable.

---

12 Fracture of the neck of the femur is such an indicator of injury that procurators fiscal in Scotland and many English coroners will require all deaths associated with the lesion to be reported—even if the association is incidental.

The skeleton also gives considerable evidence as to sex. The bones of the female are, in general, less robust than are those of the male and the ridges formed where muscles and tendons are attached are less massive. Certain bones give particular indications of sex and, amongst these, the pelvis is pre-eminent, being designed to allow the passage of the fetus in the female. Other bones—notably the thigh bone and the skull—show particular sex differences, but the appearances are not always easy to interpret; the advice of a skilled anatomist will be found very valuable in all aspects of the identification of skeletal remains.

This is particularly true when estimating stature in life from the findings in one or two bones. The number of formulae which have been devised for this purpose testifies to the difficulties involved.

The application of the principles outlined above is described in greater detail in Chapter 3.

Biochemistry of the body

The cell is the basic building block of the body; the human body may consist of up to 5×10^{12} cells. To remain alive, each cell must manufacture energy from a series of chemical reactions that take place within the cytoplasm and are controlled by its nucleus. The sum total of these diverse chemical reactions taking place within a cell is known as cell metabolism and biochemistry defines and describes the nature of metabolism. The fuel for the metabolic process comes from ingested food, which consists of proteins, carbohydrates and fats; these are themselves composed of varying combinations of molecules of carbon, hydrogen and oxygen, with lesser amounts of nitrogen, phosphorus and sulphur. Energy is obtained and stored during the process of breaking down these compounds to carbon dioxide and water. This process requires a constant supply of oxygen (*aerobic metabolism*) although an alternative pathway (*anaerobic metabolism*) provides lesser amounts of energy for a limited time when oxygen is lacking. The energy thus provided has two main purposes—the maintenance of equilibrium and the manufacture of new material.

The metabolic processes are conducted in a fluid medium which is an aqueous solution containing chemicals that exist as electrically charged particles known as *electrolytes* or *ions*. The most important chemicals, in addition to hydrogen and oxygen, are sodium, potassium, chloride, calcium, phosphate, sulphate and bicarbonate. However, there is a difference in chemical composition between the fluid which is intracellular and that which is extracellular. To function properly, cells must sustain a difference across the membrane of the cell surface such that the fluid inside is more concentrated than that on the outside. This is effected principally by the constant pumping out of water and sodium, with a resultant perpetual requirement for energy. It is also necessary to ensure an environment within and around the cells that is neither acidic nor alkaline but is neutral as valued in units of pH. [13]

13 pH is a logarithmic notation of hydrogen ion concentration in a solution, with 7 representing neutrality. Acid solutions have a pH less than 7 and alkaline solutions have a pH greater than 7.

The second use for energy is in the acceleration of the chemical reactions of a constructive nature. The cell is in a constant state of turnover and not only must it keep manufacturing new components to replace those lost or broken down, but it may also have a specific function to store and release compounds. Many complex components are utilised in the formation of the ultrastructure of the cell, for there are numerous membrane-bound organelles—such as *mitochondria* and *lysosomes*—in its cytoplasm. These membranes are composed of proteins, sugars and fats. The most important, and also the simplest, components which are often attached to these membranes are *enzymes*. Enzymes are proteins having the property to accelerate chemical reactions; each cell must manufacture enzymes to accelerate the chemical pathways which are not only essential to maintain life but also for which the cell is particularly specialised (or differentiated). Regulation of the specific qualities and quantity of such enzymes is determined by information contained in the genes of the chromosomes. Errors in this information may occur, resulting in faults in or absence of particular enzymes, and these errors may be transmitted to succeeding generations via the chromosomes of the sex cells. Diseases due to such enzyme abnormalities are termed *inborn errors of metabolism*.

It is important to realise that interference with the enzyme functions within cells is directly responsible for the lethal effects of ingestion or inhalation of many poisons such as cyanide, arsenic and mercury. In the case of cyanide, the enzymes of the mitochondria are inactivated with subsequent blockage of oxygen transfer for metabolic processes. Other factors that influence the activity of enzymes are temperature, pH and, perhaps most importantly, the presence of specific substances in trace amounts. This last group are termed *'essential co-factors'* and may be simple chemicals such as magnesium or zinc, or may be more complex molecules known as *vitamins*. The vitamins, which are designated alphabetically, are either fat soluble (A, D, E and K) or water soluble (B, C) and are essential constituents of the diet.

While it is convenient to consider the biochemistry of the body at a cellular level, it is important to appreciate that an equilibrium must be maintained within and between the body fluid compartments, defined as intracellular, extracellular and vascular. For example, the concentration in the blood of glucose and calcium must be carefully monitored to remain within upper and lower limits. The endocrine system is principally responsible for controlling this balance, and achieves it by the elaboration of specific hormones. These hormones are secreted into the blood to be carried to distant tissues where they affect the functions of specific 'target' cells. Their release is, in turn, regulated by the level of the target-cell product in the vascular compartment. This 'feedback' control exists in order to maintain normal biochemical values. The function of individual hormones has been described above (page 23).

Another factor in the maintenance of biochemical equilibrium is the requirement to replace the water and electrolyte loss that occurs continuously (and often insensibly) in urine, faeces and perspiration. Situations in which this replacement assumes critical significance arise in the surgical patient who requires intravenous fluid therapy because of inability to receive or retain any food or fluid by mouth over a sustained period. Provision of this balance is further complicated by the change in general body metabolism that takes place in response to trauma, of which surgical intervention represents a more planned form. A distinct alteration in the nature of metabolic processes, to become destructive (*catabolic*) as opposed to constructive (*anabolic*), results in loss of important nutriments, electrolytes and water. These changes are hormonally induced and constitute a reaction to stress—the so-called preparation for fight or flight. The observed decrease in body temperature in the period after trauma provides a further index of the profound alteration in body metabolism. [14]

Deoxyribonucleic acid (DNA)

Probably the most important development in forensic science in the last fifteen years has been the introduction of the concept of DNA profiling. The theory behind this is that each person has a genetic make-up which, excluding identical twins, is unique to that individual. If, therefore, we could demonstrate that pattern in cells, it would be proof that those cells were derived from that individual. Moreover, this highly specific pattern would be identical in all his or her nucleated cell types—the pattern derived from, say, the cells of the hair follicles would be the same as that found in the white blood cells. There is no intention in this book to extend discussion to forensic science and DNA profiling is very firmly a matter for the scientist; nevertheless, the subject is so bound up with forensic medicine— particularly the medicine of sexual offences—that some mention of the fundamentals is needed. The practical applications are discussed in greater detail at page 296.

The vast majority of the cells of the body consist of cytoplasm which surrounds the nucleus—the main exceptions are the red blood cells which have no nucleus. The nucleus contains the chromosomes which dictate our inherited characteristics. Essentially, the chromosome is a very long, coiled helix of DNA. Each is connected to a complementary chromosome and the pair form a double helix; the two strands of the helix are held together by the specific pairing of nucleotide bases. [15] These bases are combined as triplets (ie three bases) which are known as codons—a codon being responsible for the production of a specific body protein in the cytoplasm of the cell. An aggregation of codons becomes a gene which, in turn, is responsible for a specific inherited characteristic. The forensic significance of the genes is discussed further at page 271.

Only 3–5% of DNA is responsible for the coding of proteins; the intervening stretches are not transcribed. Most of this non-coding DNA lying between the genes consists of base sequences which are apparently non-functional; this so-called 'satellite' or 'repetitive' DNA is repeated in the same sequences throughout the chromosomes in a pattern that is specific for the individual. It is also transmitted from parent to child in a recognisable fashion (see Chapter 18).

The demonstration of this individual pattern is a matter of very sophisticated technology. From the lawyer's point of view, it is sufficient to say that, by means of a radioactive 'DNA probe', the DNA pattern of the subject under study can be

---

14 The outcome of injury largely depends upon the body's biochemical capacity to adjust to the new situation, which is thus of major forensic importance. For a full review, see D N Baron 'The Chemical Pathology of Trauma' in J K Mason and B N Purdue (eds) *The Pathology of Trauma* (3rd edn, 2000).

15 There are two groups of base: the purines—adenine (A) and guanine (G)—and the pyrimidines—cytosine (C) and thymine (T). A always pairs with T and G always pairs with C. In point of fact, thymine is replaced by uracil (U) in ribonucleic acid (RNA) which is responsible for 'copying' DNA.

revealed by autoradiography in a form which has been aptly likened to the 'bar code' that is now attached to most pre-packed goods for sale. The original correspondence of two biological specimens is confirmed by the correspondence of their two 'bar codes'.[16] The technology and uses of DNA profiling are being continually improved and extended; some references to these are made at appropriate places in the book.

16 The technique was described originally by A J Jeffreys, V Wilson and S L Thein 'Individual-specific "Fingerprints" of Human DNA' (1985) 316 Nature, London 76.

2

Comparative medico-legal systems

All countries have developed methods of primary inquiry into sudden or unnatural death. The major systems from which these derive can be simply described as the English, or Coroner, System and the (European) Continental System. The further distribution of these throughout the world largely follows the pattern of early colonial expansion. The Scottish procurator fiscal has absorbed features of both these systems; it is, therefore, convenient to leave discussion of that office until the others have been described.

The coroner

The office of coroner in England and Wales developed from the twelfth century, at which time the coroner was largely responsible for supervising the material interests of the Crown in criminal cases. As these could well be affected by the status of the dead person and by the precise conditions surrounding the death, the coroner's office became intimately concerned with the investigation of suspicious deaths; the identity of the deceased was always fundamental, the coroner had to view the body[1]—at the locus if possible—and inquests were held with juries. The financial connotations of sudden death gradually relaxed, or were diverted to other offices, and the position of the coroner declined until it was revived in the Middle Ages. At that time, the coroner's attention was specifically directed to the establishment or exclusion of criminality, a principle that persisted until the nineteenth century and which still motivates the procurator fiscal's office in Scotland.

It was not until 1860 that coroners could fairly claim that they were free to act independently of outside influences, and the election of coroners was abolished in 1888. The modern coroner is appointed by the Local Authority under the Coroners Act 1988, s 1. He must be medically or legally qualified and be of at least 5 years standing in his profession; he is independent of the government and is solely responsible for his actions—only the High Court can give him instructions. Many of the more controversial aspects of his office have been gradually whittled away although the requirement to hold his inquiries in public remains.[2]

1 A duty abolished only by the Coroners Act 1980. See, now, Coroners Act 1988, s 11(1).
2 Evidence given from behind a screen is still regarded as being heard in public: *R v HM Coroner for Newcastle upon Tyne, ex p A* (1998) 162 JP 387.

The present system was established in the Coroners Act 1887, which stated (s 3(1)):

> 'Where a coroner is informed that the dead body of a person is lying within his jurisdiction, and there is reasonable cause to suspect that such person has died either a violent or an unnatural death, or has died a sudden death of which the cause is unknown, or has died in prison, or in such place or under such circumstances as to require an inquest in pursuance of any Act, the coroner, whether the cause of death arose in his jurisdiction or not, shall, as soon as practicable, issue his warrant for summoning not less than 12 nor more than 23 good and lawful men to appear before him at a specified time and place, there to inquire as jurors touching the death of such person as aforesaid.'

The 1887 Act was significantly amended by the Coroners (Amendment) Act 1926 which, in particular, empowered a coroner to order a post-mortem examination if he had reason to suppose that a death occurring within his jurisdiction was a sudden death of which the cause was unknown and that the examination might prove an inquest to be unnecessary. The 1926 Act also restricted the coroner's mandate when dealing with deaths due to homicide and his power to charge a named person with murder, manslaughter or infanticide was removed by the Criminal Law Act 1977, s 56.

These, and several other statutes, have now been consolidated in the Coroners Act 1988 while the secondary legislation is to be found in the Coroners Rules 1984.[3] As a result, the coroner must now hold an inquest when there is reasonable cause to suspect that the deceased:

(a) has died a violent or unnatural death;
(b) has died a sudden death of which the cause is unknown; or
(c) has died in prison or in such a place or in such circumstances as to require an inquest under any other Act.[4]

It is to be noted, particularly, that the authority to order a post-mortem examination prior to deciding whether or not to hold an inquest extends to the situation in which it is uncertain whether the death was violent or natural and that the examination may be directed to solving the problem;[5] condition (b) above must be read with this in mind. As a result, more than 70% of deaths reported to the coroner are now disposed of without inquest.

A duty at common law rests on 'any person about the deceased' to inform the coroner of circumstances that indicate the need for an inquiry. Otherwise, there is no legal obligation on a doctor to report a death directly to the coroner although, in practice, he commonly does so when he judges it necessary;[6] the more cumbersome, although technically correct, process is to annotate a completed certificate of cause of death to the effect that the coroner has been informed of the death—but this can confuse the relatives. The statutory duty to do so is vested in the Registrar of Deaths.[7] The circumstances in which he must refuse to register a

---

3 SI 1984/552.
4 Coroners Act 1988, s 8(1).
5 Coroners Act 1988, s 19. *R v Greater Manchester North District Coroner, ex p Worch* [1988] QB 513, [1987] 3 All ER 661, CA.
6 Many coroners distribute a list of cases suitable for direct reporting. One example is reproduced in Appendix C.
7 Registration of Births and Deaths Regulations 1987, SI 1987/2088, reg 41.

death without reference to the coroner are set out in Appendix B. The only other statutory duty to report directly to the coroner is imposed on Governors of Prisons, Borstals, Detention Centres and other similar institutions.

On being informed of a case that he considers to be within his jurisdiction, the coroner has certain options open to him. He can decide that no further action is called for; in this case, he notifies the registrar to accept the certificate of death granted by the medical practitioner. He can order a post-mortem dissection and, if he decides as a result of this that no further investigation is required, he himself may certify the cause of death as indicated by the autopsy; this coroner's certificate invalidates any previous medical certificate as to the cause of death. In any other circumstances, he may hold an inquest and he must do so in the circumstances detailed above; it has now been confirmed that the coroner conducting the inquest may make use of an assessor who should not, however, combine his role with that of an expert witness.[8] An inquest must be held with a jury only when it is suspected that death:

1. occurred in a prison or in such circumstances as to require an inquest under any other Act;
2. occurred while the deceased was in police custody, or resulted from an injury caused by a police officer in the purported execution of his duty;
3. was caused by an accident, poisoning or disease notice of which is required to be given under any Act to a government department, to any inspector or other officer of a government department or to an inspector appointed under s 19 of the Health and Safety at Work etc Act 1974;[9] or
4. occurred in circumstances the continuance or possible recurrence of which is prejudicial to the health or safety of the public or any section of the public.[10]

Condition 4 is obviously open to interpretation, but the governing principle is that the case should be put before a jury if a recurrence could be prevented or safeguarded against as a result of action taken by some authority.[11] The Act does not preclude the coroner from summoning a jury in the case of, for example, a road-traffic accident if he thinks it necessary, but he is very greatly restricted in a case of murder, manslaughter, infanticide, causing death by dangerous driving or suicide in which there may have been abetment. In the event of a person being charged with such offences connected with the death of the deceased, the coroner must accede to a request from the Director of Public Prosecutions to adjourn his inquest; the coroner need not resume the inquest after the relevant criminal proceedings but, if he does so, the finding of his inquest must not be inconsistent with the outcome of those proceedings.[12]

The function of the coroner and/or his jury is now tightly constrained. Neither can express an opinion on any matters other than who the deceased was and how,

  8 *R v HM Coroner for Surrey, ex p Wright* [1997] QB 786. The procedure may, therefore, be similar in both England and Scotland (see p 39 below).
  9 Note that the Reporting of Injuries, Diseases and Dangerous Occurrences Regulations 1995, SI 1995/3163 may be altered without reference to the Coroners Act.
 10 Coroners Act 1988, s 8(3). This applies even though the death occurred abroad: *Re Neal* (1997) 37 BMLR 164.
 11 *R v HM Coroner at Hammersmith, ex p Peach* [1980] 2 All ER 7.
 12 Coroners Act 1988, ss 16 and 17.

when and where the deceased came by his or her death.[13] A list of recommended conclusions open to the coroner's inquest is given in Appendix D. Even so, no coroner's verdict may be framed in such a way as to suggest civil liability or criminal liability on the part of a named person.[14] As to the former, it is clear that difficulty may arise when 'lack of care' is included in the conclusion. Despite the coroner's overarching duty to investigate the facts 'fully, fairly and fearlessly',[15] 'how' a deceased came by his death, means 'by what means' and not 'in what broad circumstances'; the verdict including 'lack of care' is to be distinguished from a supposed claim in negligence at common law. It has been suggested that, for the avoidance of doubt, the term 'lack of care' should be replaced by 'neglect' and, then, used only when there is a direct association between the lack of care and the death.[16]

As to the latter, restriction of the embargo to a named person allows for the verdict of 'unlawful killing' and, in the event of evidence of unlawful killing coming to light during the inquest, the case must be adjourned and the Director of Public Prosecutions must be given the necessary details. Thus, a coroner's verdict of unlawful killing is generally unsatisfactory and has no practical value—it would more logically be replaced by an open verdict. Effectively, the coroner and his jury may *explore* facts bearing on civil and criminal liability while the prohibition in r 42 applies only to the *verdict*.

After giving his verdict, the coroner provides the registrar with a certificate after inquest which includes the circumstantial as well as the medical causes of death. Statements signed by both the witness and the coroner are known as depositions and can be used in subsequent legal proceedings, provided that they were taken in the presence of the person who is accused at any later criminal trial.

The Committee on Death Certification and Coroners headed by Judge Brodrick made it abundantly clear that, in their judgment, it is the accurate certification of the cause of death that has become the most important function of the coroner: 'Today [1971] the role of the Coroner as an investigator of crimes against the person has become a relatively insignificant one'.[17] This view has been underpinned by subsequent legislation. In practice, while very nearly a quarter of all deaths occurring in England and Wales are dealt with by the Coroners' Service, natural disease accounts for at least 75% of the cases currently examined by coroners' pathologists.

Northern Ireland[18]

Northern Ireland has a coroner's system but it differs from that in England in a few important respects. The coroners operate under the Coroners Act (Northern Ireland) 1959 and the rules made thereunder. Coroners are appointed by the Lord Chancellor in England and they have to be practising solicitors; the coroner for

---

13 Coroners Rules 1984, r 36. In *R v HM Coroner for North Humberside and Scunthorpe, ex p Jamieson* [1995] QB 1 it was said that 'how' was restricted to 'by what means' and not 'in what broad circumstances'.
14 Coroners Rules 1984, r 42.
15 *R v Surrey Coroner, ex p Campbell* [1982] QB 661.
16 *R v HM Coroner for North Humberside and Scunthorpe, ex p Jamieson* [1995] QB 1, CA.
17 *Report of the Committee on Death Certification and Coroners* (1971) Cmnd 4810, p 130.
18 This note has been kindly edited by Professor J Crane.

Greater Belfast is full-time but the other six coroners are part-time. The cases coming within their jurisdiction are clearly stated in s 7 of the Act:

> 'Every medical practitioner, registrar of deaths or funeral undertaker and every occupier of a house or mobile dwelling and every person in charge of any institution or premises in which a deceased person was residing, who has reason to believe that the deceased person died, either directly or indirectly, as a result of violence or misadventure or by unfair means, or as a result of negligence or misconduct or malpractice on the part of others, or from any cause other than natural illness or disease for which he had been seen and treated by a registered medical practitioner within twenty-eight days prior to his death, or in such circumstances as may require investigation (including death as the result of the administration of an anaesthetic), shall immediately notify the coroner within whose district the body of such deceased person is of the facts and circumstances relating to the death.'

This section also places a duty on a number of people, including doctors, to report these deaths to the coroner, and the doctor's duty in this regard is reinforced by the legislation governing death certification which requires a doctor to complete a death certificate *only* when he has seen and treated the deceased for the fatal illness within 28 days of death, knows the cause of death and knows it to be entirely natural. In all other circumstances the coroner must be informed and no death certificate may be issued.

The coroner's functions are similar to those of his English counterpart save that, whereas the latter must hold an inquest on all unnatural deaths, the 1959 Act, s 13, only requires that he *may* do so; in practice, he generally does do so. Section 8 of the Act provides for the involvement of the local police in the investigation of the circumstances of the death. A police officer carrying out this duty is thus acting as a coroner's officer. However, the coroner has jurisdiction only when the death takes place or the body is 'found' within his district; thus, he has no jurisdiction when a person dies overseas and the body is repatriated to Northern Ireland.

One significant difference is that, instead of returning a simple verdict such as accident, misadventure etc, the Northern Irish coroner or his jury must make 'findings' in the form of a concise statement as to the cause of death. The same rules disbarring the coroner from expressing any opinion on questions of civil or criminal liability apply. As in England and Wales, there is a rule against self-incrimination but, additionally, there is a statutory rule which provides that a person suspected of causing a death cannot be compelled to give evidence.

The government provides a full-time forensic pathology service with four forensically trained pathologists to assist the coroners in these investigations. About 1,400 coroner's autopsies are carried out annually. This service—and its counterpart dealing with forensic science—are provided to coroners without charge.

The system in Europe

It is impossible to generalise about the comparable systems in Continental Europe—the procedures for investigating sudden and unexpected death vary not only from country to country but also within national boundaries.

A legal code based on Roman law operates in many states and, as a result, the medico-legal system is almost expressly designed to obviate the need for post-mortem dissection. In general, deaths that are due to violence or that cannot be certified are reported to the police, who are often represented by a lawyer—the *procureur*, *magistratura*, etc. A selected doctor—comparable to the British police surgeon—is called upon to make an external examination, the purpose of which is to exclude the possibility of criminality; further action is improbable once this has been achieved.

If the case is a serious one, the responsible Judge—eg *juge d'instruction*, examining magistrate—appoints a qualified specialist in forensic medicine to make a further external examination and, as a result of this, an internal autopsy may be authorised. The widespread establishment on the Continent of medico-legal institutes very often results in the provision of opinions that are backed by several individuals of high repute. The magistrate or his equivalent is normally responsible for certification of the cause of death in those cases falling within his disposal; this function is assumed by the higher court in criminal cases.

Interesting systems have developed in Scandinavia. There is no uniformity but the principles are based on direct co-operation between the police and specialised forensic pathologists (with the interposition of a public health officer in Denmark), the performance of autopsies by two doctors, reporting to the court rather than to the prosecution or defence and the authority of a higher forensic medical body. One side effect is that forensic pathologists very rarely go to court to give evidence and, if they do, they are there as advisers to the court rather than as witnesses for one or other side. The system has been perfected in Denmark, where medico-legal reports can be referred to the Medico-Legal Council at the request of the court or of either side. The medical intricacies are then thrashed out by experts in private and the opinion of the council is binding.

The medical examiner

The medico-legal system of many of the United States rests on the office of medical examiner. This has much in common with the European system, with the major difference that the investigation of sudden and suspicious deaths is the responsibility of a medical rather than a legal organisation. Thus, a single medical man inspects the locus of death, decides the need for internal autopsy and, in many instances, performs the post-mortem dissection himself. Only when his inquiries are complete and these indicate the possibility of criminality does he notify the district attorney of his findings although, in the meantime, a close liaison has been maintained with the police.

His powers of investigation are wide but his jurisdiction is very limited; two courses are open to him—he can either issue a death certificate and dispose of the case or refer the case to the prosecutor.

Scotland—the procurator fiscal

The office of the procurator fiscal in Scotland was unknown, other than in the ecclesiastical courts, until about the time of the Reformation. The public prosecutor, a concept clearly imported from France, first appeared in the Burghs in the middle of the sixteenth century and the practice of appointing such officials spread rapidly. The office was formally recognised as one of service to the Crown in 1746 and became financially independent of fines collected about a century later. Modern procurators fiscal are appointed by the Lord Advocate. Their function is to receive reports from the police of all crimes committed in their districts—and to direct the police in their task;[19] additionally, the fiscal prepares the Crown case in criminal trials committed to the High Court and conducts the prosecution in the Sheriff's Court. It follows that the procurator fiscal must be a lawyer and is very unlikely to be also medically qualified. The main responsibility of the fiscal for the purposes of this chapter is to investigate any sudden, violent, suspicious or accidental death or any other death that is reported to him. A list of reportable deaths is given in Appendix E. Although some of the items on this list are clearly associated with public health or with the possibility of civil negligence, it remains true that the basic medico-legal function of the fiscal is to exclude criminality; establishing the precise cause of death is not his duty.

As in England and Wales, the statutory responsibility to report appropriate deaths to the fiscal rests with the registrar[20] but, by common usage, most of his preliminary information stems from the police, medical practitioners or the next-of-kin, the last two often working through the medium of the first. The fiscal will then call for a report from the 'sudden deaths' officer (a member of the police force) and from the police surgeon who will have examined the body externally; these reports will include information as to the medical history of the dead person. The fiscal will invite the police surgeon to grant a death certificate if he decides that no further inquiry is needed; the system clearly operates very much more smoothly when there is a close working relationship between the fiscal and his medical adviser.

Should the fiscal decide, or should he accept the advice of the police surgeon, that it is necessary, he will authorise a post-mortem dissection giving one of the following reasons for so doing:

1. that his inquiries cannot be completed unless the cause of death is fully established;
2. that there are circumstances of suspicion;
3. that there are allegations of criminal conduct;
4. that death was associated with anaesthesia in connection with a surgical operation and the fact that all precautions were taken must be established.

The dissection is carried out by two doctors whenever the circumstances give grounds for suspicion or suggest the possibility that criminal proceedings may follow; it is only necessary for one pathologist to give evidence in court.[1] The fiscal's pathologist may issue a death certificate after the autopsy.

The fiscal's inquiries are conducted in private. In the event that further proceedings are likely, he has the power to precognosce material witnesses. Precognition implies the private interrogation of witnesses which will amplify their preliminary statements and which will form the basis of the fiscal's final report to Crown Counsel in whom is vested the ultimate decision as to what

19 *Smith v HM Advocate* 1952 JC 66 at 71-72.
20 Registration of Births, Deaths and Marriages (Scotland) Act 1965, s 28.
 1 Criminal Procedure (Scotland) Act 1995, s 281(2).

proceedings, if any, are to follow upon a death. However, not every death reported to a fiscal needs to be reported to Crown Counsel. The great majority of sudden deaths will be free from suspicion and may be cleared by the fiscal upon his own responsibility; a list of those conditions that must be reported by him to Crown Counsel is given in Appendix F. Precognitions are informal and the evidence is not usually taken on oath, although it may be. The defence have a right to precognosce witnesses but they may have to visit a witness to take the statement which he is, then, under a duty to give to them. An unwilling witness can be cited to attend court at a trial even though he or she failed to attend for precognition.

Outwith criminal proceedings—in which, it will be noted, privacy is maintained until the hearing in the definitive court[2]—the fiscal's inquiries can be made public by way of the Fatal Accidents and Sudden Deaths Inquiry (Scotland) Act 1976.

Under s 1(1), the procurator fiscal for the district with which a death is most closely associated must apply to the Sheriff for the holding of a Public Inquiry under the act when:

'(a) *(i)* it appears that the death has resulted from an accident occurring in Scotland while the person who has died, being an employee, was in the course of his employment or, being an employer or self-employed, was engaged in his occupation as such; or

(ii) the person who has died was, at the time of his death, in legal custody; or

(b) it appears to the Lord Advocate to be expedient in the public interest that an Inquiry under this Act should be held into the circumstances of the death on the ground that it was sudden, suspicious or unexplained, or has occurred in circumstances such as to give rise to serious public concern.'

Public inquiries are mandatory in respect of deaths detailed in s 1(1)(a) but whether or not one is held under para (b) is entirely within the discretion of the Lord Advocate; serious public concern might, for example, attend cases of alleged negligence in hospital, accidents involving public transport, etc.[3] Any person with an interest may make representations to the Lord Advocate that an inquiry should be held. Such representations will be considered but the Lord Advocate's decision is final—although, as with all public administrative decisions, being subject to judicial review.[4] The sheriff sits without a jury but an expert assessor may be appointed at the request of any properly interested party. No witness can be compelled to answer any question indicating that he is guilty of any crime or offence. The sheriff determines as to when and where the accident and the death(s) took place, their cause or causes, the reasonable precautions that might have prevented the accident, any defects in the system of working that contributed to the accident and any other relevant facts. The determination of the Sheriff is not admissible in evidence in any judicial proceedings, of whatever nature, arising out of the accidental death. To avoid duplication, a fatal accident inquiry will not be held in certain circumstances—eg when a public inquiry by an inspector of the Health and Safety Executive is being undertaken.[5] The Act applies to fatal accidents resulting from North Sea operations.

2   The situation in England and Wales has approximated to that applying in Scotland since the passing of the Criminal Justice Act 1967.
3   Between 1% and 2% of deaths reported to the fiscal come to Fatal Accident Inquiry; some 15% of these will be associated with medical mishap.
4   *Lothian Regional Council v Lord Advocate* 1993 SLT 1132n.
5   Health and Safety Inquiries (Procedure) Regulations 1975, SI 1975/335.

Systems in some parts of the Commonwealth

Australia[6]

In common with the majority of Commonwealth countries, Australia, a federation of six states and two territories, has retained much of the common law of England and the office of Coroner. Understandably, in the some 200 years since the first British settlement in what is New South Wales, Australian law and practice has diverged from that in England. The states and territories developed from six former colonies. These federated in 1901 creating the Commonwealth of Australia; thus, there is a similarity but no uniformity in the legislation governing coroners.[7]

New South Wales, Victoria, South Australia and Western Australia have a state coroner system in which there is a recognised hierarchy. Queensland, as yet, has no state coroner. In the Northern Territory, there is a Territory Coroner with a deputy in Darwin, both of whom also sit as magistrates.[8] In Tasmania and in the Australian Capital Territory, the Chief Magistrate also sits as Chief Coroner. In an interesting example of Commonwealth/State co-operation, the Western Australian State Coroner is responsible for Cocos (Keeling) and Christmas Islands, both of which are Commonwealth Territories.

One important difference between Australian coronial law and practice and that of England is that, in the former, any person who has knowledge of a 'reportable' death must inform a coroner or a member of the appropriate police force of the fact. The Australian coroners' powers of entry and of seizure have been defined and extended. The power to commit has generally been withdrawn. If it becomes clear during an inquest that a crime has been committed in relation to the death, Australian coroners are required to refer the matter to the Director of Public Prosecutions or to the Commissioner of Police of the Northern Territory.

Coroners utilise members of the relevant police forces as investigators in all states and territories. There are specialist officers in New South Wales and Western Australia who are dedicated to the Coroner's Court as investigators, while remaining under the disciplinary and administrative control of the respective Commissioners of Police. In the latter state, the Attorney General has the statutory power to appoint persons other than police officers as coronial investigators.

Recent amendments to the relevant Acts in New South Wales, Victoria and Western Australia have provided a legislative power of objection for the senior available next-of-kin where that person may wish to prevent a medico-legal autopsy being performed on the dead body of a relative.[9] The coroner may accept the objection and find as to the cause of death in the absence of an autopsy; alternatively, he or she can refuse to accept the objection. In that case, the next-of-kin may appeal to the State Supreme Court for a ruling. While coroners may have a regard for the religious beliefs of the nest-of-kin, an objection based purely on religious grounds

6   A note kindly revised by Professor J Hilton.
7   The relevant statutes include: Coroners Act 1980 No 27 (NSW) (amended in 1993); Coroners Act 1985 (Vict); Coroners Act 1957 (as amended) (Tasmania); Coroners Act 1975 (SA); Coroners Act 1920 (as amended) (WA); Coroners Act 1993 (NT); Coroners Act 1958 (as amended) (Qd); Coroners Ordinance 1956 (ACT).
8   Any magistrate may sit as coroner in most jurisdictions.
9   The hierarchy in seniority of the next-of-kin is defined in the relevant Coroners Acts.

will fail—at least in New South Wales.[10]   Occasional difficulties arise from an objection that is sustained—the Supreme Court of Western Australia found that a child had died from the Sudden Infant Death Syndrome despite that diagnosis being one that can, by definition, only be made after a comprehensive autopsy.[11]

The appointment of grief counsellors, either to Institutes of Forensic Medicine or to Coroners' Courts, has been a relatively recent development.   The skilled services offered by these counsellors has proven valuable both to the relatives of the deceased and to the coroners.

Medico-legal annual autopsy rates remain in all states at approximately 10 per 10,000 population.   Coroners in New South Wales occasionally sit with a jury when they consider it desirable or when a jury is requested by an interested party—such a request is binding on the coroner.   Coroners' juries have been abolished in all other jurisdictions.

Although the office of coroner is entrenched and is generally working well in Australia, the prospect of its being replaced by a medical examiner system is raised from time to time.   Such a movement is unlikely to gain much momentum so long as the coroners are seen to be discharging their role of protecting the public from untimely violent or unnatural death through the use of the autopsy and the inquest.   However, as in other fields of human endeavour, personal idiosyncrasy may intrude from time to time.   As yet, however, this has not yet proved any real threat to the integrity of the coronial system overall and it continues to enjoy a fair measure of public confidence.

New Zealand[12]

Primary medico-legal responsibility rests with the coroner, whose function is similar to that of his English counterpart—that is, to decide who died, when and where and from what cause.   He has no authority to commit for trial.   The current overall autopsy rate is of the order of 6,000 per year from a population of 3.1 million—or just under 20 per 10,000 population.   The distribution of autopsies, however, varies considerably with the locality; thus, out of 80 coroners, only four have a caseload in excess of 500 per year.   The Justice Department has recommended that all autopsies for the coroner should be carried out by specialist pathologists; while usually acceding to this, the coroner may choose his own pathologist—an option that is generally subject to agreement with the police authority in cases of suspected homicide.   Public inquests can be dispensed with but the opportunity to do so is generally taken only when death has been shown by autopsy to be from natural causes.

New legislation was introduced by the Coroners Act 1988 (with amendments in 1989, 1992 and 1994), the main object of which was to eliminate unnecessary autopsies—particularly those arising from the reluctance of doctors to certify the cause of death.   A further objective was to facilitate the early release of the bodies of Maoris in deference to their cultural needs.   Interpretation of the Act has not, however, been uniform and the net result of the legislation has been to reduce the number of autopsies by some 10%.

10 *Abernethy v Dietz* (1996) 39 NSWLR 701; *Morris v Hand* (1997) unreported, No 300/97, per Dowd J.
11 *Unchango; Re death of Unchango (Jnr); ex p Unchango (Snr)* (1997) 95 A Crim R 65.
12 Based on information kindly supplied by Dr Ken Thomson.

Canada[13]

The Federal Government of Canada has no overriding authority over the medico-legal system, which is established on a provincial basis.

The coroners' system operates in Ontario (the Coroners Act 1990) where there is a full-time Chief Provincial Coroner and two Deputy Provincial Coroners, one of whom is responsible for inquests and the other for investigations. Under them are eight regional Coroners and each city or district has one or more investigating coroners; there are 320 investigating coroners in Ontario, all of whom are appointed by the Provincial Government and must be fully registered medical practitioners. The coroner visits the scene of death and carries out a full investigation of all cases notified; as a result, an autopsy is requested in some 35% of these. Inquests are, in some cases, mandatory—eg when death occurred in custody or was due to a construction site, mining or railway accident; otherwise, an inquest may be ordered by the coroner investigating the case or by the Chief Coroner. Inquests are heard with a jury and the bases for their being called are generally similar to those described under the Fatal Accidents and Sudden Deaths Inquiry (Scotland) Act 1976; the coroner is generally motivated by a concern for public safety. The jury cannot make any finding of legal responsibility.

In the Province of Quebec, the Chief Coroner and his deputy are legally qualified and are appointed by the Provincial Government. There are two types of coroner throughout the Province. Approximately 100 investigating coroners are medically qualified and investigate each reported death; there are also legally qualified coroners whose responsibility is to preside over all inquests.

Alberta, by contrast, has created a medical examiners system. The Chief Medical Examiner is based in Calgary and the Deputy Chief Examiner in Edmonton. Each pathologist/medical examiner has a staff of part-time medically qualified assistants who function somewhat similarly to coroners. Post-mortem dissections are carried out either by or on behalf of the Chief Medical Examiners in major hospitals. Inquiries are held into selected cases before a provincial judge. Somewhat similar systems operate in Manitoba, Nova Scotia and Newfoundland.

British Columbia, Saskatchewan, New Brunswick and Prince Edward Island use lay coroners as do the three Northern Territories. In British Columbia they are appointed by the Provincial Government and have the same quasi-judicial responsibilities as have the coroners in Ontario. They are carefully selected and are frequently retired police officers or registered nurses who act as their own investigators; they are, however, supported by forensic pathologists and by a large number of other experts who are retained on contract with the coroners' service. The coroner's office also has a legal counsel on staff who advises on all judicial issues. In-hospital and other clinical death investigations are carried out by trained nurse investigators working in conjunction with the pathologists. A report of inquiry, which will include appropriate recommendations, is issued by the coroner in each case. Inquests are held only when there is 'public concern' and they are mandatory when death occurred in custody. The inquests are formal; witnesses are initially examined by the coroner's counsel and most interested parties are represented by counsel.

13 This note kindly revised by Professor J A J Ferris.

The Far East

Malaysia and Singapore retain the coroners' system but this has adapted pragmatically to prevailing circumstances.

The coroners' system in Singapore[14] can be taken as an example of practice in conditions of exceptionally high-density population. All magistrates and district judges are gazetted as coroners and take turns of one month's duty as field coroners, who view cases in the mortuary or attend on-site investigations. The field coroners assist the State Coroner, whose tenure of office is one year. Thus, coroners are legally qualified and, as in England, all unnatural, unexpected, violent and accidental deaths are reportable to him along with deaths from unknown causes and deaths following therapeutic and diagnostic procedures. The coroner's statutory mandate is to determine who died, when, where and from what cause and if there is someone responsible for the death. The coroner can refer the case to the Public Prosecutor in the event of a verdict of causing death by a negligent act.

About 3,200 cases are reported to the coroner annually; between 70% and 80% of these are subjected to autopsy (about six medico-legal autopsies per 10,000 population per year). The coroner is assisted by a forensic pathologist when deciding as to the scope of post-mortem examination and the need for autopsy. Although there are various religious objections to autopsy, the coroner's decision is final and binding. Death is due to unnatural causes in 50% to 60% of the autopsied cases.

The coroner can dispense with an autopsy if the death results from natural causes and is substantiated by adequate medical records; thus, in the remainder of the referred cases, a death certificate is issued without autopsy and a public inquiry is not held. An open public inquiry must be held in all other cases unless the case goes directly to a criminal court.

Malaysia, by contrast, is a predominantly rural country. The primary medico-legal system operates less precisely and it is understood that, in general, the decision as to post-mortem examination rests with the investigating police officers; dissections are not carried out on cadavers of persons of the Muslim faith.

India[15] and Sri Lanka[16]

The medico-legal systems of both India and Sri Lanka reflect the original Indian penal code compiled by Lord Macaulay in 1844.

The Indian Coroners' Act 1871 was repealed in 1999 and thus the coroner's inquest, which was being followed in the metropolitan city of Mumbai (formerly Bombay), came to an end. The three existing coroner's courts in the city were disbanded and replaced by eight centres designed to streamline the system and to facilitate post-mortem dissections. Thus, the medico-legal system is now uniform all over India and is governed by s 174 of the Indian Code of Criminal Procedure. Two types of inquests are followed: police inquest and magistrate's inquest.

Any officer-in-charge of a police station who receives information that a person has committed suicide, or has been killed by another or by an animal or by machinery, or by an accident, or has died in such circumstances as raise a reasonable suspicion that some other person has committed an offence, must immediately inform the

14 This note kindly revised by Dr Cuthbert Teo.
15 Information kindly updated by Dr R S Bangal.
16 Based on information kindly supplied by Professor M L Salgado.

nearest executive magistrate empowered to hold an inquest and must proceed to the place where the body of the deceased person is lying. There, he must make an investigation in the presence of two or more respectable inhabitants of the neighbourhood and must draw up a report of the apparent cause of death, describing such wounds, fractures, bruises and other marks of injury as were found on the body, and stating by what weapon or instrument, if any, such marks appear to have been inflicted. The report is signed by the police officer and sent immediately to the district or the sub-divisional magistrate.

A magistrate's inquest is held only in cases of major public interest or when important problems of law and order are involved; these generally relate to deaths in custody. When any person dies while in police or judicial custody, the nearest magistrate empowered to hold an inquest may hold an inquiry into the cause of death, either instead of or in addition to the investigation held by the police officer. The magistrate can also have the body of any person who has already been interred disinterred and examined if he considers it expedient in order to discover the cause of death. Wherever practicable, the magistrate must inform the relatives of the deceased and allow them to be present at the inquiry. The magistrate does not sit with a jury but he can appeal to the public for help in the investigation process.

In general, a forensic pathologist becomes involved only when a dead body is sent to him for autopsy by the police or the magistrate. This is obligatory in the case of all sudden, unnatural, unexpected and unexplained deaths. The number of autopsies performed varies from centre to centre; about 5,000 are undertaken annually in a city the size of Pune. But it will be appreciated that it is very difficult to generalise about a country that is so vast and so diverse as is India.

The Sri Lankan penal code dates from 1883. Deaths due to suicide and accident, those associated with animals or machinery and sudden deaths of which the cause is unknown are investigated by way of inquest. These are conducted in Sri Lanka by inquirers into sudden death who are appointed by the Minister of Justice. Inquirers in the principal cities are qualified in law but, elsewhere, they may be practitioners of Ayurvedic medicine or educated laymen; thus far, no MB qualified practitioner has applied to become an inquirer. Although inquirers may be properly referred to as coroners, they do not have the authority of English coroners. It is to be noted that inquirers do not hold inquests in cases of homicide; inquests into deaths occurring in prison or police custody and in mental or leprosy hospitals must be conducted by a magistrate.

Both inquirers and magistrates may call upon any qualified medical practitioner to assist them by performing an autopsy; judicial medical officers— who are specialists in forensic medicine and who combine the duties of forensic pathologist and police surgeon—will assist when required. The police always assist at an inquest, a report of which must be sent by the inquirer to the magistrate of the area. The law requires that anyone who knows of a sudden, unnatural or suspicious death must report it to a police officer.

An analysis of the various systems

Although the reader will have formed his or her own opinions, it is not out of place to present a brief review of the advantages and disadvantages of the systems described. Before doing so, a cause of some confusion must be removed. Much suspicion of the coroners' system has been based on the nature of this office in the

United States. In practice, the office of coroner in the United States has little more than nominal similarity with that in the English system, the coroner in the United States being generally elected or a political appointee. He may be unqualified either medically or legally although this is now very rare. Thus, there is some basis for distrust of the system but this is insufficient reason for extrapolating that the English coroner would be better replaced by a medical examiner.

The system which operates in England and Wales has been criticised on the grounds that it often publicises many cases which are of no public concern. The dispensation provided by the Coroners Act 1988, s 19 has done a great deal to dispel this objection but, nevertheless, there are instances—of which suicides are the most prominent[17]—in which much unnecessary distress must be given to relatives; it is also doubtful if many of the run-of-the-mill domestic accidents merit public investigation. It cannot be denied that a system which virtually imposes post-mortem dissection on nearly a quarter of persons dying is likely to be unpopular and, in the current socio-medical climate, the necessary retention of organs which might have a bearing on the cause of death is likely to be viewed with suspicion.[18] For these and other reasons, the Home Office has published a Charter covering the coroners' service.[19]

The coroner's place in the investigation of those deaths which *merit* greater publicity must also be questioned. A number of deaths are statutorily subject to investigation by specialist authorities—in particular by the Health and Safety Executive.[20] The coroner's inquest in such cases does little more than duplicate the work involved and, thereby, open up the road to ambiguity; there seems little reason why its findings in such cases should not be confined to the identification of the dead. Moreover, irrespective of specific statute, Ministers can, and do, call for public inquiries into cases of major concern;[1] the possibility of confusion here has been recognised and, as in the case of criminal proceedings, the coroner must now adjourn his inquest pending the result of any public inquiry and, should it be reopened, the findings must not conflict with those of the inquiry.[2]

An equal, if not greater, objection to the system can be based on the anomaly that, while the coroner is required to investigate deaths which occur in increasingly complex conditions within an increasingly litigious society, his remedial powers are now negligible. The general public find it hard to understand this and recourse to judicial review of coroners' decisions is now commonplace. Judicial review is available either by way of the Rules of the Supreme Court Act 1981, s 31 or the High Court may intervene through the powers of the Attorney General to order another inquest under the Coroners Act 1988, s 13. Satisfaction for the applicant is, however, by no means guaranteed. In the first place, the remit of the Divisional Court is limited to consideration of procedural error, legal irregularity or unreasonableness of the decision; secondly, the court is inherently reluctant to take further action unless it was likely that it would serve a useful purpose and

---

17 D R Chambers 'The coroner, the inquest and the verdict of suicide' (1989) 29 Med Sci & L 181.
18 At the time of writing, the retention of children's hearts, albeit for research rather than medico-legal purposes, has caused something of an uproar and has resulted in a public inquiry.
19 Home Office circular 285/99.
20 Health and Safety at Work etc Act 1974, s 14 (see p 220). See also, for example, Regulation of Railways Act 1871; Civil Aviation Act 1982, s 75.
 1 Tribunals of Inquiry (Evidence) Act 1921 - although this is rarely invoked and less 'official' grounds for setting up an inquiry are used far more frequently.
 2 Coroners Act 1988, s 17A, inserted by the Access to Justice Act 1999, s 71.

that this could be achieved without undue difficulty;[3] and, thirdly, in quashing a verdict, the High Court has no power to substitute its own findings but can only order a new inquest to be held either by the same or by another coroner in the same administrative area.[4] If the public have been disenchanted by one inquest, they are hardly likely to be satisfied by being offered another.

At the more prosaic end of the coroner's tasks, the undoubted trend towards his role of adjusting the records of the registrar leads to a very high autopsy rate with a potential limitation of standards while, at the same time, excluding an important segment of natural disease from clinicopathological research. From whichever angle one looks at it, there is a strong case for reconsideration of the structure and function of the coroners' system—perhaps restyling it on a two-tier basis with the investigation of the more important cases being undertaken by way of a superior judicial inquiry.[5] A system which was effectively established in 1887 is unlikely to function ideally in the modern world.

As to the system operating in Scotland, the rigid interpretation of the fiscal's function to exclude criminality would lead to undue constriction of the pathological service and, in practice, a much wider spectrum of sudden death is examined by dissection; even after selection by external examination, natural disease accounts for some 55% of deaths in which a fiscal's autopsy is performed—from about 5% of the total deaths in Scotland—and the proportion is increasing as a result of the funding of academic departments of forensic medicine by the Crown Office.

At present, however, it seems that neither of the major systems in the United Kingdom addresses ideally its function of eradicating conditions that operate against the public interest. As has been discussed, the power of the coroner's court in this respect is almost nominal. There is greater scope in Scotland under the 1976 Act but this avenue of life-saving propaganda is used surprisingly seldom. For example, some 800 road deaths occur annually in Scotland, yet such deaths are rarely the subject of a fatal accident inquiry. Thus, while the fiscals' service strikes a fair balance between the deployment of available resources and providing value to the public, support to community health might be still further improved by greater use of the public inquiry.[6]

It is difficult to complete this section without drawing attention to the great attractions of Scandinavian forensic medical practice, particularly as regards the presentation of expert medical evidence in the higher courts. The acceptance of a wholly objective assessment by a superior medical authority eliminates the sometimes unhappy suggestion of partisanship on the part of witnesses; of perhaps greater importance, it ensures that expert evidence is treated as a whole and unwitting omissions, which may compromise justice, are avoided.[7]

3   See eg *R v HM Coroner for Inner London North District, ex p Linnane* [1989] 2 All ER 254.
4   Coroners Act 1988, s 13(2). For recent examples, see *R v HM Coroner for Inner West London, ex p Dallaglio* [1994] 4 All ER 139 (possibility of unconscious bias on the part of the coroner); *R v HM Coroner for Coventry, ex p O'Reilly* (1996) 35 BMLR 48 (reliance on oral rather than written evidence).
5   For elaboration of this, see D R Buchanan and J K Mason 'The Coroner's Office Revisited' (1995) 3 Med L Rev 142. The government may, in fact, be thinking along these lines in respect of major disasters: D Millward 'Coroners Face Loss of Power' *Daily Telegraph*, 10 July 1997, p 12. For general criticism, see S M Cordner and B Loft '800 Years of Coroners: Have They a Future?' (1994) Lancet 799.
6   Expansion of the service is limited in practice by the number of available Sheriffs.
7   See, for the classic example, L Blom-Cooper 'A miscarriage of justice – English style' (1981) 49 Med-Leg J 98. See also the opinion delivered by Lord Emslie LJ-G in *Preece v HM Advocate* [1981] Crim LR 783.

3

Identification of the dead and of remains

In normal circumstances, there is little or no doubt as to the identity of a dead body brought to the mortuary. Formal identification is made by a close relative or associate by way of a visual examination. There is a tendency—particularly in the medico-legal ambience—to substitute direct vision by the television camera; while this represents a praiseworthy attempt to spare the relatives' feelings, the present author doubts if it achieves this objective and suggests that it may, in fact, introduce a note of uncertainty to the procedure. Be that as it may, there is generally little difficulty and this is especially so if the identification is corroborated.

Major problems of identification of the dead arise in two ways and these require rather different methods of solution. First, there is the identification of the single currently unknown body. The most difficult scenario involves one that is discovered in some place unrelated to habitation—the classic example being the body discovered in a wood or a shallow grave. Such subjects may well have died by criminal means and are often decomposed. It may be that no immediate clues to identity are available and the problem will, therefore, be one of deductive identification—fitting a name to a body. If, on the other hand, a body is discovered in a house, there is, at least, a possibility that it is a cadaver of a person associated with that house and, in the initial stages, the identification team can work from that premise. The problem is then the much simpler one of fitting a body to a name; only when the probable names have been excluded does one have to revert to the random situation.

The second, and quite distinct, problem relates to the major disaster. Even here, the topic is not quite homogeneous—the identification of a large number of victims of a flood is likely to be more difficult than in the case of a train accident which, in turn, may well be more complex than is the air disaster, in which an accurate list of those presumed killed is usually available. It is very unlikely that any effort will have been made to inhibit identification in such cases and—other than in aircraft accidents, when extensive mutilation and burning is likely—the bodies will probably be found in a reasonably preserved condition; at least some clues as to likely identity will be to hand and, in particular, circumstantial evidence in the form of clothing, documents, jewellery and the like will be available. Identification in the mass is a matter of fitting a number of bodies to a number of names that are known with varying certainty.

The methods used in various conditions will certainly overlap but, for descriptive purposes, it is convenient to discuss primary characteristics, comparative methods and circumstantial means of identification and to relate these to the random body, to the single body of likely identity and to the mass disaster.

The purposes of identification

Excluding such philosophical concepts as the right of every free-born person to an identity after death, which has been implied from the United Nations Declaration of Human Rights, the identification of an otherwise unknown dead body is needed, first, in the field of criminal investigation; the chances of apprehending a criminal are greatly increased once the identity of the victim has been established. Secondly, many important procedures in the civil field—eg grant of probate, resolving of partnerships and the general administration of estates—depend upon accurate identification; failure in this respect may result in a delay of seven years or more before death can be presumed.[1] In disasters of an explosive nature, the process of identification might well have to be limited to establishing the total number of deaths and this may be one way by which the standard period required for presumptions of death may be acceptably shortened.[2] Thirdly, there are purely social reasons for assigning a correct name to a dead body—many people have an understandable affection for the remains of their next-of-kin and certain religions have strict rules as to the disposal of the dead which sometimes conflict with those of the state in which the death occurs.[3] Finally, accurate identification of the fatal casualties and correlation of their injuries with their environment in transportation accidents—particularly those involving airlines—may greatly assist the accident investigation authorities, either in relation to the cause of the accident or as to the prevention of fatal injury in the future.

Identification of the single unknown body

Proof that the remains are human

Surprising as it may seem, mistakes as to the human or animal origin of skeletonised remains are not uncommon at first assessment. At least one murder investigation has been mounted because a bear's paw was mistaken for a human hand, and bones are often referred to forensic departments suspected as being the remains of human infants but which are, in fact, derived from middens. Such errors are, however, generally corrected rapidly: in case of doubt, the opinion of a specialist anatomist should always be sought and be backed, if necessary, by DNA analysis (see page 54 below).

1   Cestui Que Vie Act 1666, s 1; Matrimonial Causes Act 1973, s 19(3); Presumption of Death (Scotland) Act, 1977, s 1.
2   In both jurisdictions the time limit can be waived if there are good indications that a person died at a particular time—eg when an aircraft is lost over the sea: E E Sutherland *Child and Family Law* (1999) p 50.
3   See, for example, A R Gatrad 'Muslim Customs Surrounding Death, Bereavement, Postmortem Examinations, and Organ Transplants' (1994) 309 BMJ 521.

A more difficult situation arises when only soft tissues or unidentifiable bones are available; it may then be necessary to invoke immunological evidence. Proteinaceous tissues of all animal species, including humans, contain antigens (see page 18) which are more or less specific to that species.[4] Artificial antibodies may be prepared to these antigens which can, thereby, be identified in the laboratory. The commonest method is to precipitate the antigen/antibody complex and, for this reason, the test is often referred to as a 'precipitin test', the details of which are not needed here. It is clear, however, that such a test depends upon protein still being present. It is, therefore, less likely to be useful when it is most needed—that is, in the identification of skeletonised remains.[5] Such tests are simple and inexpensive. The technology has, however, largely been taken over by the more specific procedures involving DNA.

Determination of sex

It may be difficult to establish the sex of a body by cursory superficial examination even in the absence of severe burning or putrefaction. Unisex fashions in hairstyle and clothing contribute to the difficulty. Problems may arise from congenital deformities of the genitalia while a surprising number of persons have undergone gender reassignment surgery which may be of partial type (see transsexualism, page 235 below). Such difficulties can, however, be overcome relatively easily provided that the body is not severely damaged and that the possibilities are born in mind.

Early putrefaction and burning short of combustion may actually accentuate secondary sexual characteristics—particularly the size of the breasts. On the other hand, severe burning, putrefaction and the ravages of animals may destroy the genital region. The sex can then generally be determined by the finding of either a uterus in the female or a prostate gland in the male; these organs are among those in the body that are most resistant to putrefaction and also to destructive forces such as a bomb explosion. In the event of complete skeletonisation, the sex of the dead person can be derived, with varying degrees of certainty, from a study of the total skeleton or from individual bones. Many bones show *comparative* differences between male and female but the pelvis very often provides definitive indications of sex (see Figure 3.1).

Many sophisticated measurements can be made to this end but only a general summary is needed for present purposes. Essentially, the female pelvis is adapted to supporting the fetus and facilitating its passage during childbirth. Thus, the female pelvis is wider and squatter, with a far straighter sacrum, than is found in the male; the dorsal surface of the pubic bone also becomes pitted during childbirth. An accuracy of 95% or more is claimed for the determination of sex from the pelvis. The wide hips of the female dictate a more acute angle between the neck and shaft of the femur than is needed in the male in order to bring the knees together; the thigh bone is perhaps the most valuable of the long bones that may be available for sexing—provided the ethnic origin is known, an accuracy of some 80% can be obtained from examination of the femur alone. Sex differences are also notable in the skull, which is one of the bony specimens most frequently

4   There may be some cross-reaction between closely related species but this is of little
    practical importance in human forensic medicine.
5   Bone does, however, retain protein for a considerable time. In general, it can be said that
    a bone which is completely free of a 'greasy' feel is likely to be more than ten years old.

presented to forensic departments. The features that are sought include the round orbits and more vertical forehead of the female; the greater surface area of the mastoid process in the male; and the prominent supraorbital or eyebrow ridges that are a feature of masculinity. The examination of the skeleton is invaluable in the identification of the converted transsexual in that the original structure of the bones cannot be altered by surgery.

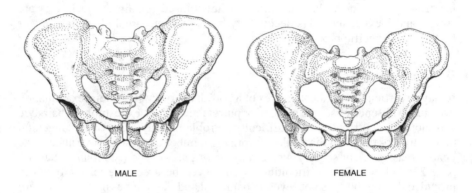

MALE   FEMALE

Figure 3.1 The pelvic bones of the male (left) and the female (right).

Determination of age

A superficial examination in the presence of putrefaction or burning can result in gross error as to the age of a cadaver; objective parameters are needed. The condition of any remaining organs may provide these but again, the skeleton can give very useful clues. The significant findings in the bones depend to a large extent on the age group; it is convenient to consider the fetus and neonate, the adolescent, and the adult as separate categories.

The fetus and neonate

Objective evidence of age at this stage is to be obtained from the development of the bones and, in particular, from the presence of certain centres of ossification; these have been described on page 27 and a representative list is given in Appendix G. The most important centres are those that distinguish the fetus that is legally capable of being born alive (24-week pregnancy)[6] and the full-term fetus (see Chapter 19 for details). Although it is simple to demonstrate these centres at autopsy, the most objective, and permanent, record is obtained by the routine radiological examination of unidentified fetuses. Anomalous appearances occur in individual centres but, at this stage of development, the *overall* picture can produce an accuracy of ± month.

6   Still-birth (Definition) Act 1992.

In childhood and adolescence

The most useful information, up to the age of 20, is given by the joining of the epiphyses to their shafts (Appendix H). Although such unions generally follow in a definite chronological order, the variations in individuals are wide and, certainly when using a single observation, an accuracy greater than ± 2 years can rarely be claimed. The accuracy increases pari passu with the number of observations made and numerous attempts have been made to sum these mathematically, allowances being made for 'weighting' the relative accuracy of the individual observations. Such considerations are for the anthropologists.

Adult life

The ageing of an unknown body becomes progressively more difficult once adulthood is attained. The union of the basi-sphenoid junction in the base of the skull is said to occur with some constancy around the old legal age of maturity— 21 years. Otherwise, while the sutures of the vault of the skull close in a relatively regular order, union does not commence until approximately the age of 35[7] and, even then, the findings are subject to wide variation. Moreover, the skull consists of inner and outer tables of bone; the sutures in the former close significantly earlier than those of the outer table. It is improbable that the skeletal remains of an adult can be 'aged' any closer than within one decade—and this is an optimistic assessment.

Other gradual changes associated with use, such as the angle of the jaw bone, occur as part of the natural process of ageing; the presence of disease states either in remaining soft tissues or in the bones may give general indications of age but only within very wide limits.

Ageing from the teeth

In the experience of nearly all observers, the most valuable indication of age from infancy to adulthood can be obtained from the teeth. The subject is discussed in detail in the section on forensic odontology (Chapter 28).

Determination of stature

The determination of the stature in life from post-mortem remains is fraught with difficulty. Even if the whole cadaver is available, a direct measurement has its own inaccuracy as the body in life measures some 2.5 cm (1 in) less than the body when dead. There is also the complication of age. Men in a developed society continue to grow up to the age of 21 or slightly more. After the age of 30, however, the natural processes of senile degeneration result in an average decrease in stature of something of the order of 0.6 mm (1/40 in) per year.[8]

On the other side of the coin, it has to be remembered that the exact height of an individual during life is available only rarely—it is far more likely that no more than a subjective assessment or, at best, a fairly rough measurement will be forthcoming. It follows that tables or mathematical formulae designed to assess

---

7 An exception is the interfrontal suture which closes in childhood.
8 M Trotter and G C Gleser 'The Effect of Ageing on Stature' (1951) 9 Amer J Phys Anthropol 311.

the in-vivo stature of a person from incomplete remains are likely to be of limited value in the identification of the single unknown body no matter how much work has gone into their preparation.

Subject to that proviso, the bones of the lower limb provide the best evidence, and the more bones that are examined, the narrower will be the range within which is put the final estimate of living height. Taking everything into consideration it is doubtful whether an accuracy of greater than within 2.5 cm can ever be achieved by studying individual bones and this, again, may represent considerable overconfidence; the interested reader is referred to the classic specialised monographs.[9]

In practice, it is probably best to use simple calculations which give a rough estimate but which do not pretend to scientific accuracy. A useful rule of thumb is that the humerus (arm bone) is 20%, the femur (thigh bone) 27% and the tibia (lower leg bone) 22% of the subject's height in life. The spine, if available, is some 35% of this and the distance between the outstretched fingertips approximates to the total height.

The use of comparative methods

The problem of allotting a body to a probable name is very much simpler because information concerning many characteristics individual to the presumed person is likely to be available. The matter is then one of comparing these with the findings in the cadaver. It is not necessary to discuss here such obvious characteristics as colour of hair or eyes, save to point out that these may alter considerably after death. The forensic medical practitioner will, however, be much concerned with the provision of medical information in relation to identity.

Medical information

Recognisable disease states, evidence of past surgical procedures, deformities and tattoos can be included under this general heading.

The value of the past medical history depends very much on the nature of the information. Thus, a history of cardiac pain in a missing person is relatively useless as restriction of the coronary circulation or, indeed, damage to the heart muscle, is discovered at post-mortem examination in a very high proportion of persons beyond middle age. A history of gall bladder disease might, on the other hand, be much more significant. A combination of evidence—eg severe arthritis of the spine together with disease of the thyroid gland—will provide far greater probability of identification than would be suggested by the sum of those diseases present in the population as single entities.

Similar considerations apply to surgical procedures. A history of removal of the appendix is unhelpful save, perhaps, in distinguishing between two nameable bodies (see below); partial removal of the female genitalia is less common but would certainly be insufficient evidence by itself on which to base an identification. Each case requires individual assessment as to significance and, again, a combination of surgical procedures may provide virtually incontrovertible

9   Eg W M Krogman *The Human Skeleton in Forensic Medicine* (1962).

evidence of identification. The presence of surgical prostheses—particularly if X-ray or other in-life records are available for comparison—may provide evidence that would satisfy even the most sceptical. Old fractures, which can also be compared by X-ray, can be very useful.

Deformities may also be common or rare. They may be congenital—that is, present from birth—or acquired. Very often, they provide little more than confirmatory evidence of identification made on other grounds.

Tattoos present some interesting problems in identification. First, it has been pointed out that many tattoos are of standardised pattern and the presence, say, of a heart pierced by an arrow cannot be regarded as proof of identification. Secondly, the investigator must be wary of descriptions of tattoos; what may be a clear illustration to one party may be quite differently interpreted by another. It is, however, fair to say that so long as an adequate description of tattoos in life is available—particularly in the form of photographs—they may provide excellent evidence of identification. It is of practical importance that, although tattoos may be superficially obscured by the carbonisation of burning, scrubbing the area may reveal an easily identifiable pattern in the deeper dermal tissues.

Personal identification

Three methods of positive, personal identification are outstanding— fingerprinting, dental comparison and DNA (*deoxyribonucleic acid*) profiling.

The science of dactylography or fingerprinting is one for the expert and is outside the province of this book. Indeed, for present purposes, fingerprints have a limited use in identification since permanent records are available in the United Kingdom only for those who have been involved in criminal proceedings.[10] The main value of fingerprints in the identification of a body from the general population depends on the opportunity to compare the prints from the cadaver with those on the personal possessions of the supposed person—a method that is particularly useful in the context of the major disaster. The practice of removing the hands from cadavers for the sole purpose of comparative fingerprinting has been severely criticised;[11] while the coroner has full authority to conduct his investigation to the extent he considers necessary, this does seem to be a method of doubtful necessity which must be distressing to relatives of the deceased. The preservation of heel or sole prints in those who are at risk of sudden death with mutilation—eg airline crews—is less emotive than is fingerprinting and is not restricted by statute; it is also probably of more practical value, as the feet are commonly preserved from burning by boots or shoes.

The importance of dental identification has been recognised for many years. Dental reconstruction of one sort or another is widespread in the populations of developed countries[12] and records are readily available where the dental service

---

10 It used to be that fingerprints taken in the course of a criminal investigation had to be destroyed if there was no conviction. Exceptions to the rule are, however, now in place (Police and Criminal Evidence Act 1984, s 64(3A); Criminal Procedure (Scotland) Act 1995, s 18(4)).

11 Eg in the inquest into the deaths arising from the 'Marchioness' disaster: R Williams 'Families Furious at Coroner's Decision' The Scotsman, 18 March 1995, p 3. See *R v Inner West London Coroner, ex p Dallaglio* [1994] 4 All ER 139 at 145 per Simon Brown LJ.

12 The same could not be said of the so-called underdeveloped countries, where dental disease is comparatively rare; effectively, there is nothing in the mouth to 'compare'.

is of high quality. The methods involved in and the limitation of dental identification are discussed in Chapter 28. It is enough to say here that the method is wholly dependent on the quality of record-keeping by practitioners and that the certainty of identification increases in almost geometrical progression with the number of positive correlations present. Ultimately, a comparison of ante- and post-mortem charts may be as personalised a method of identification as is a fingerprint, although the dedicated police officer will always be unhappy that there are no internationally recognised criteria on which to certify a dental identification. A comparison of X-rays taken before and after death may, however, provide evidence of identification which will satisfy even the most sceptical. Table 3.1 indicates some of the relative merits and demerits of dactylography and odontology as methods of identification.

TEETH	FINGERPRINTS
Fire resistant	Destroyed by fire
Durable	Subject to putrefaction
Records readily available	Limited recording
'Compatible inconsistencies' due to incomplete charting	Unchanging
No acknowledged criteria of proof	Well-established criteria
Useless without records	Possible value of personal possessions in absence of records

Comparative dental X-rays are as personalised as
are comparative fingerprints

Table 3.1 Some advantages and disadvantages of dactylography and odontology as methods of identification (see also Chapter 28)

Although the identification of tissues and of tissue-containing fluids has been greatly affected by the introduction of DNA profiling (for which, see page 296), the process has serious limitations in respect of the identification of remains. In the first place, it depends, again, on comparison and it is, at least, unlikely that base-line material will be available—other, perhaps, than in hair roots recovered from a potential subject's hair brush. Against this, there could be circumstances in which it would be possible to identify a man by, say, testing his children and, thus, proving paternity and identity (see page 242). In addition, however, the process requires the DNA to be in relatively unadulterated form; it is, effectively, only following extensive mutilation in the fresh state that a body would be so affected by post-mortem changes as to be unidentifiable by ordinary means and yet contain useable DNA.[13] None the less, suitable specimens should be removed when available and stored in optimal conditions against the possibility of future need; increasingly sophisticated methodology is steadily extending the scope for analysis of partially degraded material.

13 Though a great deal depends on the sophistication of the scientific method: W Goodwin, A Linacre and P Venesis 'The Use of Mitochondrial DNA and Short Tandem Repeat Typing in the Identification of Air Crash Victims' (1999) 20 Electrophoresis 1707. There is no attempt in this book to analyse the scientific methodology of DNA typing.

Identification in a major disaster

The identification of a large number of casualties poses many organisational problems which vary, to a large extent, with the nature of the disaster. It may be that the subjects are well preserved but that there is little knowledge of their origin, as may occur in a rail accident; they may be relatively unclothed and severely carbonised, as in a hotel fire. The aircraft accident is, perhaps, the least uncommon form of mass disaster and, by virtue of its unforeseeable and varied location, it is certainly likely to present the most urgent logistical problems to both the investigators and the medico-legal authorities.[14] Although the passenger complement is likely to be well known, its international composition will raise particular difficulties for those responsible for identification and repatriation of the deceased. The aircraft accident can be taken as a model for mass disaster investigation so long as it is appreciated that it involves certain unique features. Differences are likely even within the general category of 'aircraft accident'— thus, one accident may present as a problem involving structural disintegration while another may approximate to a mass cremation.

The secret of accurate, rapid identification of mass casualties lies in the organisation. The essential is to establish a 'commission of identification' which, on the one hand, is receiving information about missing persons and, on the other, is being advised of observations on the dead bodies from various sources. The scheme is illustrated in Figure 3.2. The standardised documentation form introduced by the International Criminal Police Organisation in order to achieve this objective has been criticised on many counts but it is used widely; alternative forms, which have been recommended by the International Civil Aviation Organisation, are used by the Air Accident Investigation Branch of the United

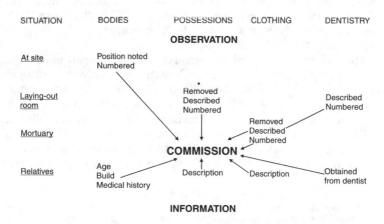

Figure 3.2 Diagrammatic representation of the identification commission established for a major disaster. Sources of observation and information are shown. The importance of numbering the bodies—and of maintaining a single set of numbers—is emphasised.

14 For an example of the effect on a medium-sized hospital, see C T Doyle and M A Bolster 'Medico-legal Organisation of a Mass Disaster—the Air India Crash' (1992) 32 Med Sci Law 5.

Kingdom.[15] Whatever type of documentation is used, the process of identification is essentially one of sorting through numerous 'information' files and attempting to 'marry' these to 'observation' files. The use of computerised information has been recommended and, indeed, put to good use;[16] the present writer has always believed that the flexibility of manual systems is to be preferred when conditions are likely to vary. It is recognised, however, that information technology and computer literacy among the population as a whole are improving so fast that this may no longer be valid; modern disaster plans should, at least, consider the inclusion of computer facilities.

The main difference between identification in the mass and identification of the single unknown body lies in the enforced use in the former of much circumstantial evidence. Thus, a large amount of preliminary or 'primary' identification is done on the basis of documents carried and on the presence of recognisable jewellery and clothing; jewellery, being fire resistant, is especially valuable in this context.

The use of such circumstantial evidence requires much care—it is, for example, essential to ensure that possessions attributed to a given body in the furore of cadaver retrieval were, in fact, incontrovertibly associated with that body. Vagaries such as exchange of tickets and the widespread use of chain-store clothing must be accepted as potential hazards. It is, therefore, very important that any circumstantial evidence should, whenever possible, be confirmed by an alternative method, preferably one involving 'personal' identification. Of these, dental evidence is of outstanding importance; medical evidence, particularly if it is of an unusual nature, has a significant part to play. The value of DNA typing in the major disaster depends very much on the conditions of the disaster and is subject to the limitations discussed above at page 54. It will be needed most when there is severe mutilation of the bodies—but this is the circumstance in which degradation of the material is most likely.[17] The most practical limitation of the method lies in its cost. Each test currently costs some £350 and several tests may be needed for each subject; few medico-legal authorities are likely to enthuse about such expenditure unless it is essential.

Visual identification, the standard 'personal' method of many police forces, is highly suspect in the context of a mass disaster. Not only may recognisable peculiarities be erased or mimicked but the observers are often under such emotional stress that they are particularly prone to unwitting error. It is generally far better to present next-of-kin with a maximum of three bodies, ideally already identified by other means, when subjecting them to the ordeal of recognition. The enforcement of visual identification could be regarded as inhumane in the majority of aircraft disasters;[18] it is, however, in many ways surprising how often

---

15 The use of these forms was originally described by P J Stevens in A K Mant (eds) *Modern Trends in Forensic Medicine—3* (1973).

16 Eg T Solheim, S Rønning, H Bjørn and P K Sundnes 'A New System for Computer Aided Dental Identification in Mass Disasters' (1982) 20 Forens Sci Internat 127.

17 See R Fernando and P Vanezis 'Medicolegal Aspects of the Thai Airbus Crash near Kathmandu, Nepal: Findings of the Investigating Pathologists' (1998) 19 Amer J Forens Med Path 169. B Ludes, A Tracqui, H Pfitzinger et al ' Medico-Legal Investigations of the Airbus A320 Crash upon Mount Ste-Odile, France' (1994) 39 J Forens Sci 1147 comment on the usefulness of DNA testing *when all conventional identification methods have failed* (my emphasis).

18 The display of polaroid photographs of the victims has been found to be a useful expedient in disasters not involving severe burning or facial mutilation.

relatives will insist on that harrowing experience—it would, then, be quite improper to deprive them of what is undoubtedly their right to assure themselves of the identity of their near kin.

In recent years, the accurate identification of the victims of a major disaster has come to assume paramount importance and, certainly, the medico-legal authorities are under great pressure to complete this task and to return the bodies to the next-of-kin. While, so far as is known, it has not yet happened, it is not difficult to foresee a successful action in negligence following inaccurate identification—or even on the grounds of undue delay in release of the bodies. The latter would, of course be measured by acceptable practice and, in this respect, the significance of the autopsy findings to the overall accident investigation should never be overlooked. Premature release of identified bodies before the maximum investigative information has been obtained must be deprecated; the accidental death of a close relative is always a personal tragedy—but the tragedy can, to an extent, be mitigated if a full investigation serves to prevent a similar occurrence in the future. Satisfying the public on this issue may be one of the most distressing tasks that befall the medico-legal authorities.[19]

---

19 It was, for example, publicly suggested that the accident site on Mount Erebus following the 1979 disaster should be declared 'holy ground' and the bodies left in situ: P B Herdson and J K Mason 'The Role of Pathology in Mass Disasters' in J K Mason and B N Purdue (eds) *The Pathology of Trauma* (3rd edn, 2000) ch 3.

4

Post-mortem changes and the timing of death

For present purposes, death is defined as the irreversible failure of the cardiovascular system. A functioning heart and competent blood vessels are essential for the transport of oxygen, without which the body tissues must die; on the other hand, the heart, which functions under autonomous control, may continue to beat and nourish the tissues when natural respiration—which depends upon an intact brain stem—has ceased or been suspended and has been replaced by machine. It will also distribute the blood for several minutes if the brain stem sustains unnatural injury—the judicial hangings of the past were apposite examples. Thus, in normal circumstances, the state of the cardiovascular system provides the most useful distinction between true life and death. It is accepted that total death of the persona must await the irrecoverable death of the brain, which will be delayed for some 15 minutes following cessation of the circulation; nevertheless, the *practical* application of the concept of 'brain-stem death' arises only in relation to artificial survival and is considered in Chapter 12.

The main function of the doctor called to the locus of an unexplained death is to decide that death has taken place and to pronounce life extinct; other considerations must take second place. This decision may be difficult in the event of grossly diminished cardiac output—as may occur in hypothermia or in drug-induced central depression of the vital functions, and even more so when the not uncommon combination of the two arises.[1] Some form of cardiac activity, even if demonstrable only by special techniques, is always present when death is apparent rather than real but the conditions under which the police surgeon is working will almost certainly be less than ideal. However, once life has been pronounced extinct, the next step is to decide on the time of death—the importance of which in the investigation of suspected homicide scarcely needs emphasis.

Given the definition of death that has been adopted above, the changes that occur after death can be deduced from a review of the functions of the cardiovascular system. The cessation of oxygen transfer results in cellular death. Those components of the cell that are most sensitive to hypoxia—the enzyme systems—

---

1 In the particular conditions of an emergency call to a sudden death—as may occur on a train or in an aircraft—the doctor must also decide whether or not to attempt resuscitation. This is by no means a foregone clinical obligation, given the fact that *some* degree of hypoxic brain damage will have occurred (see Chapter 13).

will be first affected. After a variable period of residual activity, energy production ceases and the body cools. Blood which has been circulating is now stagnant and settles under the influence of gravity. There is a final attempt at metabolism in an environment increasingly deprived of oxygen (*anaerobic metabolism*) and waste products accumulate where they are formed; the ground substance of the body degenerates and the individual cells lose cohesiveness. In the absence of an effective bloodstream, the body is defenceless, and bacteria, whether derived from within or without the corpse, are left to multiply at the expense of the tissues—the process of putrefaction is set in train and may be augmented by the flesh-eating larvae of various flies. The process of skeletonisation may be hastened by carnivorous animals and, ultimately, the skeleton itself may crumble to chalky dust. These changes can be used in an attempt to estimate the length of time the body has been dead but, ultimately, the attempt can scarcely be regarded as successful.[2]

The timing of death

The first 24 hours

It is only within the first 12–18 hours that any reasonable accuracy can be expected as to the time of death. Even then, it is important that the basic inaccuracies inherent in any biological phenomenon are appreciated. The solution of a murder by way of pathological demonstration that death occurred at 0010 rather than 2350 may look well in fiction but has no place in reality.

The estimate of the time elapsed during the first 12 hours after death is based mainly upon the body temperature. Theoretically, this temperature falls according to a sigmoid curve; numerous attempts have been made to liken the body to an experimental cylinder to which the laws of physics can be applied without reservation. However, no matter how many variables are introduced into a mathematical calculation, accuracy cannot be guaranteed in a practical situation.

Some of the factors that must influence the rate of cooling are illustrated in Figure 4.1 and include:

1. The body *temperature* at the time of death. Conditions that tend to raise the temperature at the time of death—for example, infection or cerebral haemorrhage—will result in an artificially short estimate of the post-mortem interval based on temperature recordings; hypothermic and algid states will produce the opposite effect.
2. *Clothing.* The rate of fall in body temperature of a reasonably clothed body is approximately two-thirds that of a naked one.
3. *Body insulation.* A fat body is better insulated against heat loss compared with a lean one, while those with a large surface area in relation to the body weight will cool faster than will those of more massive physique; thus children and the aged will always cool faster than will well-nourished adults.
4. *Convection currents.* A body will cool faster in moving air than does one in a closed environment. The effect may be considerable.
5. The *environmental temperature* is a variable that will always affect the rate of cooling, but the time taken for the body to reach either a high or a low ambient temperature is the same because the rate of fall will be correspondingly slow or fast.

2   Innumerable papers have been written on the subject. The most comprehensive source is to be found in B Knight (ed) *The Estimation of the Time since Death in the Early Postmortem Period* (1995).

6. The *isothermic* or *plateau* stage. It will be appreciated that these factors will not only influence the rate of cooling but will also dictate the length of time taken for the body to *start* to cool (point B in Figure 4.1). It will also be noted that the shorter is the actual time since death, the greater is the mathematical significance of this unknown variable.

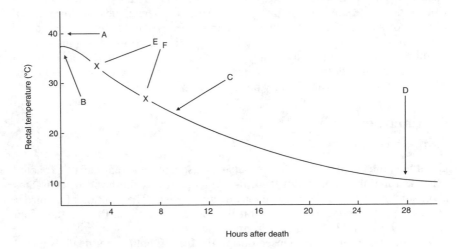

Figure 4.1 The uncertainties in the post-mortem body temperature.
A = The deceased's temperature in life.
B = The isothermic stage, greatly dependent upon the body's insulation.
C = The rate of fall which is influenced by the environmental conditions.
D = The room temperature.
In the event, two readings taken at E and F and extrapolated to 37°C will give as accurate a result as is likely to be obtained.

While it might be possible to compute a formula that would accommodate the measurable variables, no such formula could take into account unknown variations such as the effects of moving the body before measuring the temperature, changes in environmental temperature and the action of draughts. Figure 4.2 illustrates a serious attempt to overcome these difficulties while, at the same time, confining the technology to that which would be reasonably available to workers in the field; it will be seen that, despite the research involved, the best accuracy that can be invoked is of the order or ± 2.5 hours.[3] Attention has also been drawn to the work of Henssge;[4] Figure 4.3 reproduces his nomogram which takes account of the body weight and also introduces various empirical 'corrective factors' related to ambient variables such as clothing and air movement. The present writer has no experience of using this method but it is noteworthy that the author claims no greater accuracy than ± 2.8 hours.

3   L M al-Alousi 'Multiple-probe thermography for estimating the postmortem interval: II. Practical versions of the triple-exponential formulae (TEF) for estimating the time of death in the field' (2000) J Forens Sci, in press.
4   C Henssge 'Death Time Estimation in Casework. 1. The Rectal Temperature Time of Death Nomogram' (1988) 38 Forens Sci Internat 209.

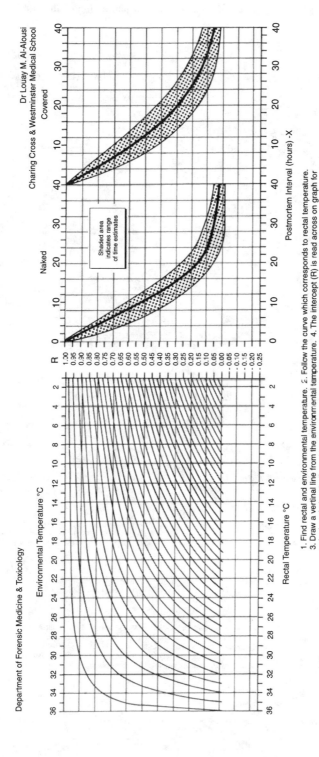

Figure 4.2 al-Alousi's nomogram for estimating the post-mortem interval (by kind permission of the author).

Figure 4.3 Henssge's time of death nomogram (by kind permission of the author).

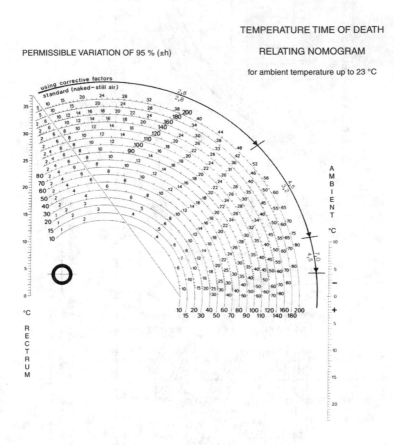

TEMPERATURE TIME OF DEATH

RELATING NOMOGRAM

for ambient temperature up to 23 °C

PERMISSIBLE VARIATION OF 95 % (±h)

The nomogram expresses the death-time (t) by:

$$\frac{^{T}\text{rectum} - ^{T}\text{ambient}}{37.2 - ^{T}\text{ambient}} = 1.25 \exp(B \times t) - .25 \exp(5 \times B \times t); \quad B = -1,2815 \,(\text{kg}^{-.625}) + .0284$$

The nomogram is related to the chosen standard i.e. naked body extended lying in still air. Cooling conditions differing from the chosen standard may be proportionally adjusted by corrective factors of the real body weight, giving the corrected body weight by which the death-time is to be read off. Factors above 1.0 may correct thermal isolation conditions and factors below 1.0 may correct conditions accelerating the heat loss of a body.

HOW TO READ OFF THE TIME OF DEATH
1. Connect the points of the scales by a straight line according to the rectal and the ambient temperature. It crosses the diagonal of the nomogram at a special point. 2. Draw a second straight line going through the center of the circle, below left of nomogram, and the intersection of the first line and the diagonal. The second line crosses the semi-circles which represent the real or the corrected body weights. At the intersection of the semi-circle of the body weight the time of death can be read off. The second line touches a segment of the outermost semi-circle. Here the permissible variation of 95% can be seen.
Example: Rectal temperature 26.4°C; ambient temperature 12°C; body weight 90 kg. Result: Time of death 16 ± 2.8h.
Statement: The death occurred within 13.2 and 18.8 (13 and 19) hours before the time of measurement (with a reliability of 95%).
Note: Use the evaluated mean ambient temperature of the period in question (e.g. contact the weather station).
Recommendation: If the values of the mean ambient temperature and/or the body weight (see 'corrective factors') are called in question, repeat the procedure with other values which might be possible. The possibly wider range of death-time can be seen in this way.

REQUIREMENTS FOR USING THE METHOD
−   no strong radiation (e.g. sun, heater, cooling system)
−   no strong fever or general hypothermia
−   no uncertain severe changes of the cooling conditions during the period between the time of death and examination (e.g. the place of death must be the same as where the body was found).

EMPIRIC CORRECTIVE FACTORS OF THE BODY WEIGHT FOR BODIES OF AVERAGE WEIGHT (REFERENCE: 70 KG)

dry clothing/covering	in air	Corrective Factor	wet through clothing/covering wet body surface	in air	in water
		0.35	naked		flowing
		0.5	naked		still
		0.7	naked	moving	
		0.7	1-2 thin layers	moving	
naked	moving	0.75			
1-2 thin layers	moving	0.9	2 or more thicker	moving	
naked	still	1.0			
1-2 thin layers	still	1.1	2 thicker layers	still	
2-3 thin layers		1.2	more than 2 thicker	still	
1-2 thicker layers	moving or	1.2	layers		
3-4 thin layers	still	1.3			
more thin/thicker	without	1.4			
layers	influence	...			
thick bedspread		1.8			
		...			
+ clothing combined		2.4			
		2.8			

Note: For the selection of corrective factor (c.f.) of any case, only the clothing or covering of the lower trunk is relevant! Insulating bases (e.g. thick foam upholstered base) slow down the cooling even of naked bodies up to c.f. of 1.3; bases which accelerate the cooling (e.g. concrete base of a cellar) require c.f. round .75 for naked bodies or reduce c.f. for clothing by 0.1 to 0.2 units.

Provided the corrective factor chosen is 1.4 or above the following table should be consulted if the real body weight differs greatly from the reference of 70 kg since there is a

DEPENDENCE OF THE CORRECTIVE FACTORS OF THE BODY WEIGHT UNDER STRONGER INSULATION CONDITIONS
real body weight [kg]

4	6	8	10	20	30	40	50	60	70	80	90	100	110	120	130	140	150
									1.3								
1.6	1.6	1.6	1.6	1.5					1.4					1.3	1.2	1.2	1.2
2.1	2.1	2.0	2.0	1.9	1.8				1.6				1.4	1.4	1.4	1.3	1.3
2.7	2.7	2.6	2.5	2.3	2.2	2.1	2.0		1.0			1.6	1.6	1.6	1.5	1.4	1.4
3.5	3.4	3.3	3.2	2.8	2.6	2.4	2.3		2.0		1.8	1.8	1.7	1.6	1.6	1.5	1.5
4.5	4.3	4.1	3.9	3.4	3.0	2.8	2.6	2.4	2.2	2.1	2.0	1.8	1.8	1.7	1.7	1.0	1.0
5.7	5.3	5.0	4.0	4.0	3.5	3.2	2.9	2.7	2.4	2.3	2.2	2.1	1.0	1.0	1.8	1.7	1.6
7.1	6.6	6.2	5.8	4.7	4.0	3.6	3.2	2.9	2.6	2.5	2.3	2.2	2.1	2.0	1.9	1.8	1.7
8.8	8.1	7.5	7.0	5.5	4.6	3.9	3.5	3.2	2.8	2.7	2.5	2.3	2.2	2.0	1.9	1.8	1.7

Example. Real body weight 20 kg. Chosen corrective factor (reference 70 kg) 1.6. Use a corrective factor of 1.9 resulting in a corrected body weight of 38 (40) kg.

REFERENCES: MARSHALL T K, HOARE F E (1962): Estimating the time of the death. J Forensic Sci 7: 56-81; 189-210; 211-221. HENSSGE C (1988): Death time estimation in case work, I. The rectal temperature time of death nomogram. Forensic Sci Int 38: 209-236. HENSSGE C (1992): Rectal temperature time of death nomogram: Dependence of corrective factors on the body weight under stronger thermic insulation conditions. Forensic Sci Intern 54: 51-66. ALBRECHT A et al (1990): On the application of the rectal temperature time of death nomogram at the scene of death. (German, summary in English). Z Rechtsmed 103: 257-278.

The question then arises as to whether it is better to adopt a relatively simple approach and, at the same time, freely admit its limitations. The old standard, or 'rule of thumb', routine has been to accept an average fall in temperature of 1° C per hour (or 1.5° F per hour). The resultant 'time' is then modified either by the use of a correction factor based on the ambient temperature or, often more usefully, by personal assessment of the conditions at the locus of death. In practice, it is surprising how the variables may cancel each other out—a person in a cold room will wear more clothes which may themselves mitigate the effects of draughts, etc. A more attractive alternative, as indicated in Figure 4.1, is to assess the actual fall in temperature over a period and extrapolate from this; even so, this fails to allow for the 'plateau' period[5] and does not take into account the variance in the shape of the curve with time. Clearly, such methods are likely to give the wrong rather than the right answer. None the less, it is abundantly clear that even the most

5   Although one could add an arbitrary figure, say 1½—2 hours, to account for this.

sophisticated formulae—including techniques which involve multiple points of measurement—will result in wide variations; it is at least arguable that it is better to take the simple road to inaccuracy rather than to complicate the journey.[6]

It is everywhere agreed that temperature measurement loses all meaning once the temperature of the body has decreased by 85% of its original difference from that of the environment. Moreover, the above considerations apply only to bodies found on land. As would be expected, cooling of the body is more rapid in cold water although, here again, much will depend on the quantity and the flow of the medium.

The stomach contents

The emptying of the stomach as a means of estimating the time of death has led to many famous forensic duels in the witness box—and, probably, also to miscarriages of justice in reported cases from Australia and Canada.[7] Little need be said beyond the now accepted fact that stomach emptying depends on so many variables as to be useless as a measurement per se. That is not to say that inspection of the contents of the stomach need not be undertaken in the absence of a suspicion of poisoning; the mere fact that a meal of given consistency is present may, at least, be sufficient to indicate a time at which the deceased certainly *was* alive.

One to three days

As the enzymatic processes of the body fail, so too does the elimination of waste products. The tissues of the body become altered in consistency and the most prominent evidence of this is found in the phenomenon of *rigor mortis*. Biochemically, this is associated with a massive increase in the lactic acid content of muscle; clinically, the resultant stiffening and shortening of the muscle fibres presents as a fixation of the joints which can be broken down only by force.

Rigor results from reduction of the chemical constituent of the muscles known as adenosine triphosphate. The stiffening of the muscles commences when the level of this substance is reduced to 85% of the normal but the process is not demonstrable clinically until some time has passed. All muscle fibres are affected but stiffening will be demonstrable earliest in those bundles of smallest mass; joints supplied by very large muscle groups will be affected the slowest.

In theory, therefore, one would expect the muscles of the face to be the first to demonstrate rigor. The larger muscles would then become involved, the arms appearing stiff before the knees and hips. In practice however, this order is not always maintained. The condition is apparent some 5–7 hours after death and is usually established throughout the body in 8–12 hours. The muscles remain in rigor until the processes of degeneration and putrefaction cause secondary laxity. Rigor has been observed to disappear clinically in much the same anatomical order as it became established but, again, the process is variable. The body is

6   Indeed, current research indicates that modern sophisticated methods offer no obvious advantages over the 'rules of thumb': L Nokes 'Analysis of algorithms in actual cases' in B Knight (ed) *The Estimation of the Time since Death in the Early Postmortem Period* (1995).
7   For reviews, see M Horowitz and D J Pounder 'Gastric Emptying—Forensic Implications of Current Concepts' (1985) 25 Med Sci Law 201; F A Jaffé 'Stomach Contents and the Time of Death. Reexamination of a Persistent Question' (1989) 10 Amer J Forens Med Path 37.

generally free of rigor some 36 hours after death, but it is by no means uncommon for the condition to persist for four days. Relating the degree of rigidity to the body temperature will help to indicate the phase of the rigor 'cycle'.

Theoretically, the degree of distribution of rigor should give a useful indication of the time elapsed since death but, in practice, a phenomenon that depends upon biological processes is inevitably capricious in its presentation. Its onset is accelerated in conditions leading to an ante-mortem excess of lactic acid in the tissues including, in particular, exercise or a pyrexial illness. It will come on slowly, if at all, in persons whose muscle is degenerate, as in those who have suffered wasting illnesses; children demonstrate the phenomenon far less readily than do adults and rigor may never appear in a dead infant. The rate of onset of rigor depends to some extent upon the ambient temperature; it will be accelerated in the summer months and retarded in the winter. The best that can be realistically expected from a consideration of rigor mortis is a 'time of death' at the centre of a bracket of probability extending over some 6–12 hours—and this only over a very limited total period.

Certain conditions simulate rigor mortis but are easily distinguished. The most common of these is cold stiffening; a body that has been placed in the refrigerator is virtually beyond assessment as to rigor. At the other end of the scale, intense heat will result in shrinkage and stiffening of the muscles; the effects of the heat should be readily seen on the skin but, even so, errors have been made in the distant past with serious consequences.[8]

Cadaveric spasm deserves a mention although it is far less common than might be supposed from a review of the literature. This is a contraction of the muscles which is probably mediated by the central nervous system when death occurs in conditions of high emotional tension; it is instantaneous and permanent until putrefaction occurs. The most common manifestation is seen in the hands, which may be found grasping some object, particularly one that gives some hope of support.[9] Cadaveric spasm may occasionally involve the hand which has held a firearm used suicidally. The medico-legal diagnostic importance of this is more theoretical than practical as the phenomenon must be very rare.

Attempts have been made to improve the timing of death during this difficult period by investigating other biochemical changes that occur in the body after death. For obvious reasons, the parameters must be simple to measure and resistant to putrefaction; effort has therefore been primarily concentrated on the changes in the distribution of inorganic salts found in those fluids that classically remain sterile after death—in particular the cerebrospinal fluid and the vitreous humour of the eye. The level of, say, potassium alters with time after death and does so very nearly in mathematical progression in a single individual. The variations between individuals are, however, so wide as to eliminate any real hope of improvement in the accuracy of the timing of death by the routine use of such laboratory investigations.[10]

---

8 Eg L Blom-Cooper 'A Miscarriage of Justice—English Style' (1981) 49 Med Leg J 98.
9 The writer's most vivid recollection is of a severed hand still clutching an aircraft seat-belt.
10 See, among may other papers, J G Farmer, F Benomran, A A Watson and W A Harland 'Magnesium, Potassium, Sodium and Calcium in Postmortem Vitreous Humour from Humans' (1985) 27 Forens Sci Internat 1. A most authoritative review of the subject is to be found in J I Coe 'Post-mortem biochemistry of blood and vitreous humour in paediatric practice' in J K Mason (ed) *Paediatric Forensic Medicine and Pathology* (1989) ch 13.

Beyond the third day—putrefaction

The process of putrefaction begins with death but only becomes manifest after a few days. Again, many variables have to be considered, particularly the condition of the body before death, the temperature and humidity of the environment and the relative sterility of the area. Thus, the bodies of persons who have died while suffering an acute infection or of those subjected to open injury will decompose faster than the norm; particularly rapid changes occur in dead bodies that are allowed to lie in bed under activated electric blankets.

Generally, there is discoloration of the abdominal skin in two to three days and swelling of the tissues, with the formation of blisters, towards the end of the first week. At this point, the veins—especially those close to the abdomen, such as in the upper thighs—become swollen and stained; the process is known as 'marbling'. Gross disfiguration is present in some three weeks. Partial liquefaction is commonly evident in the body at the end of a month. It will be seen that, other than in the first few days, when the changes are surprisingly constant, an estimate of the time of death in a putrefied body can generally be given only in terms of weeks.

Putrefaction of the body is normally delayed in water unless this is heavily contaminated by sewage. In ordinary circumstances, an immersed body will tend to float after a week to ten days but this will be greatly modified by clothing and water temperature; in deep cold water a body may not surface for some three weeks or, indeed, may never do so. There is a similar retardation of putrefaction in coffins in which bursting of the body, an almost invariable accompaniment of putrefaction in the open, is an uncommon finding.

Some features of putrefaction are of forensic importance. Muscular, and particularly fibrous tissues are resistant and certain organs—for example, the uterus and the prostate gland—may be recognisable for a considerable time; this is of obvious importance in identification. Vascular walls tend to resist decomposition and evidence of coronary insufficiency can often be discovered when the general appearances would suggest that a search would be unlikely to be rewarding; this will be particularly so if calcification has occurred.

The combination of destruction of the blood and formation of gas may lead to the issue of bloody fluid from the orifices. The appearances may closely simulate those of ante-mortem haemorrhage and must be interpreted with caution. Genuine blood clots, however—such as those which may have arisen in the cranial cavity—may persist and be readily recognisable as such for some time.

Finally, there is the problem of the body that appears to have resisted decomposition to an unusual degree. This may happen as a natural phenomenon in the closed environment of the coffin. Nevertheless, it has long been held that the finding of such a cadaver should raise the suspicion of poisoning by metallic compounds; in the writer's opinion, an association between preservation and poisoning can be relegated to folklore—and as being of minimal importance in modern times.

Two well-known modifications of the normal process of putrefaction require mention. The first of these is mummification where, in the presence of drying conditions and the absence of bacterial contamination, the tissues may become desiccated rather than putrefied. Ultimately, the mummified tissues may be reduced to powder but, in the meantime, the general format of the body may be remarkably preserved. The bodies of infants, which are relatively sterile internally, tend to mummify very readily.

Secondly, there is the formation of adipocere which results from the transformation of the normal fluid fats of the body to solid compounds. This variant of putrefaction may occur in any tissue containing fat, predominantly if associated with moist conditions; it is therefore prevalent in bodies recovered from the water and in bodies exhumed from coffins. Adipocere adheres to the bone, the result being that, even after the skin has disintegrated, the body may retain recognisable characteristics of importance in identification; injuries to soft tissues may also be preserved. The presence of adipocere almost invariably means that the body has been dead for some weeks if not months.

Skeletonisation

Ultimately, all the soft tissues of the body will decompose, the tendons and other highly fibrous tissues being most resistant.

The time for complete skeletonisation is extremely variable and depends not only on the natural processes of decomposition but also upon predators from the insect and animal worlds—and from fungi and other moulds. The author has seen two bodies reduced to skeletons within their clothing in a light aircraft which remained undiscovered for two months in an English summer; it is doubtful if such rapid skeletonisation would occur in winter. Probably the main determinant is the degree of exposure to carnivorous animals and dipterous larvae. The former are also important in that their activities may well simulate ante-mortem injury; the clue to diagnosis lies not only in the pattern of injury but also in the absence of any vital reaction.

Although the time can be much shorter, it is probably fair to estimate a skeleton with which are associated remnants of fibrous tissue as having been dead for approximately one year, but from this point estimates of the intervals since death can be assessed in brackets only of years or even decades. The environment is all-important—bones many hundreds of years old have been discovered well preserved, particularly in dry caves. Numerous scientific techniques, including some of considerable sophistication—such as the analysis of radioactive carbon—have been introduced for the dating of skeletons but are beyond the scope of this book.

Hypostasis

Pooling of stagnant blood is known as hypostasis. The gravitational distribution of the blood becomes evident on the skin and contrasts vividly with the pale exsanguinated portions; the condition of post-mortem lividity is established. Similar changes occur in the internal organs where it is important that they are not confused with ante-mortem haemorrhage, for example in the lungs.

Post-mortem lividity, can be seen within one to two hours after death—and sometimes even earlier—and is generally fully established in 6–12 hours. At this point, although the fluid blood itself may be displaced later, there is sufficient staining of the tissue to maintain some evidence of hypostasis irrespective of the subsequent position of the body. Sustained pressure prevents pooling of the blood and it is common to find that generalised lividity of the back is notably absent from the buttocks and shoulder blades which take the main weight of the recumbent body. A general absence of lividity should raise the expectation of exsanguination due to severe internal bleeding.

Hypostasis begins as soon as the circulation ceases. Its demonstration is of relatively little value as a method of timing the interval since death although— taken in conjunction with other signs—it has some use in this respect during the first six hours.[11] Moreover, post-mortem lividity is the first *visible* sign of death and some jurisdictions insist that it be present before a certificate of death is issued. Its main forensic significance, however, lies in establishing the position of the body after death and, particularly, in demonstrating that it has been moved. In the event that the position has been altered after staining of the tissues has been established, the examining doctor may discover either a dual distribution of lividity or a distribution that is incompatible with the locus as presented to him. Either finding must raise the possibility of outside interference—a typical example being when a body has been confined in the boot of a car and dumped some hours later.

There are two conditions that require differentiation from lividity. The first of these, bruising, is a relatively simple decision. Apart from the fact that bruises are commonly localised, they are, by definition, the result of bleeding into the tissues as opposed to stagnation of blood in the vessels. A rather more difficult situation arises in the distinction between hypostasis and the congestion of an asphyxial death; this has considerable practical significance. Thus, a baby dying in the prone position will show a facial distribution of lividity with pallor over the pressure points—the centre of the forehead, the tip of the nose, the chin and cheek bones. The contrast between this appearance and that of congestion of the face resulting from an asphyxial death due to suffocation may be difficult to appreciate.

The colour of the lividity also provides evidence as to the mode of death. No great reliance can be placed on its 'blueness'—or de-oxygenisation—as all deaths are, ultimately, anoxic in type. A lividity of bright red colour, however, indicates the presence of fully oxygenated blood which is typical of death in the cold or of exposure to cold after death. Cyanide poisoning gives a rather similar result. Perhaps the most well-known example of this type of observation is the diagnosis of poisoning by carbon monoxide. The cherry-pink colour is usually obvious when sought in a good light. Chemicals and drugs which convert the haemoglobin of the blood into methaemoglobin will produce lividity of a dark-brown hue; the same result follows poisoning by some aromatic hydrocarbons.

Post-mortem artefacts

Artefacts—or simulated ante-mortem injuries—resulting from efforts at resuscitation are not uncommon. Heat, be it in the form of direct application or resulting from electrical stimulation, is the most common form encountered. It is perfectly possible to produce burns in a dead body, but these can be differentiated by the absence of so-called vital reactions—that is, the defensive reactions of the living body to injury. The most immediate vital reaction to a burn is dilatation of the surrounding capillaries which shows as an area of redness diffusing into the

11 Recent colorimetric work has, however, suggested that the rate of change in the degree of hypostasis may correlate with the time of death up to 48 hours after death: P Vanezis and O Trujillo 'Evaluation of Hypostasis using a Colorimeter Measuring System and its Application to Assessment of the Post-mortem Interval (Time of Death)' (1996) 78 Forens Sci Internat 19.

normal skin colour. Blisters formed before death contain more protein than do those arising post-mortem. Infiltration of the area by white blood cells is evident microscopically in a few hours and, later, there is repair by connective tissue cells (*fibroblasts*). None of these signs will be present in a burn inflicted after death.

A very common series of artefacts result from attempted resuscitation by external cardiac massage. The breastbone is almost invariably bruised if not dislocated and fractures of the ribs are often caused. The difficulty in distinguishing such injuries from those inflicted during life on purely pathological grounds lies in the self-evident fact that *efficient* cardiac massage simulates a functioning circulation. Any bruise or fracture caused by this means will, therefore, closely resemble ante-mortem injury. The same will be true of the microscopic changes which accompany bony fracture; these are discussed at page 149.

As discussed above, severe post-mortem injuries may be inflicted by carnivorous animals or crabs on land and by fish or shellfish in water—the last may bare exposed parts to the bone in a matter of days. Infestation and accelerated destruction of decomposing tissue by larvae of dipterous flies and of beetles is so common as to deserve special mention. It has forensic significance in that entomology has been used on numerous occasions in an attempt to assess the time interval since death. Thus, the insects present can be correlated with their known preferred breeding habits while the age of the larvae and the number of generations can give further information as to the time of death.[12] Their assessment is more complicated than would appear theoretically and is certainly a matter for the expert who should, ideally, collect his own specimens in the post-mortem room and at the locus.

Finally, traumatic injuries inflicted on the dead body must be mentioned. A body lying on a roadway may be damaged by vehicles whose drivers are genuinely ignorant of having done so. Post-mortem injuries are outstandingly associated with bodies in the sea where buffeting on rocks by the waves, contact with ships' propellers, grappling in fish nets and the like may result in a confused picture. The important practical point is that the possibility of such sources of injury must be considered in relation to the locus of discovery of the body.

12 Among large numbers of publications, see M L Goff, A I Omori and K Gunatilake 'Estimation of postmortem interval by arthropod succession' (1988) 9 Amer J Forens Med Pathol 220.

5

Legal disposal of the dead

With one minor exception,[1] it has been illegal since 1836 in England and Wales to dispose of a body unless the death has been registered. There is a wider relaxation of the general rule in Scotland which was designed to take into account the difficulties of communication that used to exist in parts of the country but, in the event of burial before registration, the person in charge of the cemetery must notify the registrar of the occurrence. The current legislation relating to disposal of the dead in Great Britain is contained in the Births and Deaths Registration Act 1953, as amended, and in the Registration of Births, Deaths and Marriages (Scotland) Act 1965. In either case, legal disposal begins with medical certification.

Medical certification of the cause of death

Although the general layout of the certificate conforms in each case to the international system of certification of the cause of death, there are some important differences of practice in England and Wales and in Scotland.

In England and Wales, there is a statutory duty laid upon the doctor who attended the deceased during the terminal illness to issue a medical certificate of the cause of death.[2] This obligation does not cease simply because the case is one reportable to the coroner. The correct procedure is for the doctor to issue the certificate, personally report the case to the coroner and initial the box printed on the reverse of the certificate to indicate that he has done so; the Scottish certificate also has a facility for noting that the procurator fiscal has been informed. The practice of reporting the death to the coroner or procurator fiscal and taking no further action is commonly adopted but has no foundation in law; conversely, there is no absolute obligation on the English doctor to inform the coroner—to pre-empt the registrar in this duty is only a way of saving valuable time.[3] The reverse of the current English certificate of cause of death

1   A registrar in England and Wales may issue a certificate for disposal before registering the death if he has received written notice of the death from a qualified informant and has received a medical certificate of the cause of death—provided the death was not one that should have been reported to the coroner.
2   Registration of Births and Deaths Regulations 1987, SI 1987/2088.
3   By contrast, there is a common law duty on the Scottish doctor—in common with any member of the public—to inform the procurator fiscal if he has reason to believe that there are grounds for doing so.

indicates five broad categories of death which the coroner needs to consider and which should, therefore, be reported; in summary, these are deaths due to violence, deaths the cause of which is unknown, those contributed to by drugs, poisons or abortion, operative or anaesthetic deaths and those associated with employment.

The English medical certificate requires the certifying doctor to state the date on which he last saw the deceased alive and, in common with the Scottish certificate, to indicate whether or not the body was seen after death and, if so, by whom. The certifying doctor does not have to view the body after death,[4] but in the absence of such precaution, the registrar must refer the case to the coroner if the remainder of the certificate indicates that the doctor had not seen his patient during the last 14 days of the patient's life.[5] The doctor in England and Wales further certifies that he was in medical attendance during the deceased's last illness; if no one can so certify—a situation that often obtains in holiday periods—there can be no medical certificate and, ipso facto, the case is referred to the coroner.[6]

A 'Notice to Informant' is attached to the English certificate and the doctor is required to furnish this forthwith. The medical certificate may be sent without delay to the registrar but, since the death cannot be registered in its absence, it is often handed to the informant together with the notice.

A certificate of neonatal death—which goes under the rather lengthy title of 'Medical Certificate of Cause of Death of a Live-born Child Dying within the First Twenty-eight Days of Life'—is in use in England and Wales.[7] Effectively, this bridges the gap between the standard death certificate and the certificate of stillbirth (see below) and contains information relevant to both the deceased and to the health of his or her mother. The disposal of the form is the same as for the certificate of adult death. No similar certificate is used in Scotland.

The most important respect in which the Scottish process of medical certification varies from that in England is that, in Scotland, there is no requirement upon the certifying doctor to have been in attendance during the last illness. Under the Births, Deaths and Marriages (Scotland) Act 1965 Act, s 24(1) it is proper for any doctor who is able to complete the certificate 'to the best of his knowledge and belief' to do so. While this has the great merit of removing a large number of manifestly natural deaths from the intricacies of the medico-legal system, it carries some disadvantages; many doctors are unwilling to certify a cause of death of which they are not quite certain while, on the other hand, the procurator fiscal has no wish to accept the English coroner's responsibilities as to the accuracy of the mortality statistics. It is possible for a certificate to be couched in such terms as 'death from natural causes, probably . . .', which is regarded as a generally satisfactory compromise. There is nothing in the certificate relating to the last time the deceased was seen alive; it follows that there is no obligation on the registrar to refer a case to the fiscal for reasons similar to the English '14-day

---

4   But he would be well advised to do so. There are many recorded instances of bodies being discovered alive in the mortuary (eg Law and Science 'Apparent Death—Complete Recovery' (1981) 21 Med Sci Law 228).

5   Many coroners extend this rule to include *all* deaths where the deceased was not seen during the last 14 days of life (see Appendices B and C).

6   It is customary for a relatively junior member of staff to complete the certificate when a patient dies in hospital. Both the English and Scottish certificates now request that the name of the consultant responsible for the case be supplied.

7   Registration of Births, Deaths and Marriages (Amendment) (No 2) Regulations 1985, SI 1985/1133.

rule'. A practical advantage of the system is that the certificate can be signed competently by a pathologist who has established the cause of death at autopsy; this has to be done if the case has been referred to the fiscal—and the fiscal's pathologist may complete the certificate on the basis of an external examination alone if he feels able to do so.

There is no 'Notice to Informant' on the Scottish certificate. The certificate as to the cause of death must be transmitted either to a qualified informant or to the registrar within seven days of the death.[8] Illustrations of the various certificates are shown in Appendix I.

The informant

Persons qualified and liable to act as informants in England and Wales include a relation of the deceased present at the death, in attendance during the last illness or residing in the subdistrict where death occurred; a person present at the death; the 'occupier' of the house or any inmate of the house if either knew of the happening of the death; or a person causing the disposal of the body. If death occurred outside a house, informants may include any relative of the deceased having knowledge of the necessary particulars; any person present at the death; any person who found the body, who is in charge of the body or who is causing the disposal of the body. The 'occupier' includes the chief resident officer of a public institution.

In Scotland, the duty to give information of particulars of death devolves, in succession, upon any relative of the deceased; any person present at the death; the deceased's executor; the occupier of the premises where the death took place; or any other person having knowledge of the details to be registered. If the deceased's home is unknown, any person finding the body, including the police involved in the investigation, has a duty to inform the registrar but all such deaths are then reportable to the fiscal.

Registration

The importance of registration of a death is often inadequately emphasised. The registrar must be informed even in the unusual situation of a body being buried without registration; cremation without registration is not permitted (see below). When the coroner holds an inquest, he must send the necessary particulars to the registrar within five days of its completion. In the event that the coroner adjourns his inquest at the request of the Director of Public Prosecutions, he must send a certificate to the registrar giving such particulars as are required for registration 'so far as they have been ascertained'.[9] The distressing delay in registration imposed by criminal proceedings is thus very much reduced and brings English practice into line with that existing in Scotland.

Otherwise, registration can be completed only when the full details required by the Acts of 1953 and 1965 are supplied; the process thus provides an essential back-up service in the detection of secret homicide.

---

8   The death certificate can also reflect current national interests. The English certificate, for example, asks for information as to the relationship of the death to employment; the Scottish version is specifically concerned with any association with pregnancy.

9   Coroners Act 1988, s 16(4).

Informants, other than the coroner, must attend personally at the registry and provide the necessary information within five days of the death in England and within eight days in Scotland; the registrar will then issue a certificate for disposal after registration.

Burial

Almost incredibly, there is no general statute that requires any individual to dispose of a body and there is nothing that says that a body must be buried or cremated. There is, however, an obligation at common law 'in the nature of a public duty' that rests on persons in possession of a dead body to dispose of it in a manner suitable to the estate.[10] There is a common law right to be buried in one's parish churchyard but, again surprisingly, there is nothing that dictates that a person be buried in a recognised graveyard.[11] A person cannot will how his or her body is to be disposed of; no directions are binding on the executors on whom the responsibility rests.[12] The local authority must take the responsibility when no other arrangements have been made[13] but, otherwise, only the general health laws govern the method of disposal; thus, the burial or cremation of a body may be ordered by a magistrate should its retention above ground be considered a danger to health.[14] The provision of burial grounds is now the responsibility of Burial Authorities,[15] but, surprisingly, national laws restricting the position of cemeteries have been repealed; such matters are now subject only to by-law regulation. Burial outside England requires the authority of the coroner;[16] the procurator fiscal must authorise the removal of a body 'firth of Scotland' if the death has been subject to his inquiries—otherwise, the body is simply accompanied by a Certificate of Registry of Death in Scotland. Some difficulty is introduced when a body is removed from Scotland to England and the death was one which would have been subject to inquest had it occurred in England. Strictly speaking, the coroner is then bound to hold an inquest and the matter is discussed briefly at page 79 below. Common sense, however, boggles at the need for two legal officers of the same Crown to investigate the same death and the problem appears to be solved on the basis of pragmatic co-operation.[17]

After burial or cremation, a notification that the body has been disposed of must be delivered to the registrar within 96 hours of the event. Failing such

10 *Rees v Hughes* [1946] KB 517. Preventing the burial of a body is also an offence at common law: M Hirst 'Preventing the Lawful Burial of a Body' [1996] Crim LR 96.
11 The reader who would enjoy a smile is referred to B Hilliard 'Last Rights' (1997) 147 NLJ 1566 which also contains some little known facts as to burial at sea.
12 *Williams v Williams* (1882) 20 Ch D 659; *Conway v Dalziel* (1901) 3 F 918. The exceptions to this rule lie in the Human Tissue Act 1961 and the Anatomy Act 1984.
13 National Assistance Act 1948, s 50(1) and Public Health (Control of Disease) Act 1984, s 46. The obligation exists once it is apparent that no other arrangements are being made: *Secretary of State for Scotland v Fife County Council* 1953 SLT 214.
14 Public Health Act 1936, s 162; Public Health (Scotland) Act 1897, s 69
15 Local Government Act 1972, s 214.
16 Removal of Bodies Regulations 1954, SI 1954/448, modified by Removal of Bodies Regulations 1971, SI 1971/1354.
17 For full discussion, see I H B Carmichael *Sudden Deaths and Fatal Accident Inquiries* (2nd edn, 1993), pp 227-230. There is no reciprocal difficulty because, whereas the coroner must investigate the death of a body lying within his jurisdiction, the fiscal is responsible only when the circumstances of death were associated with his district.

advice within 14 days of registration, the registrar must, after inquiry, report the matter to the appropriate Community Physician (or Specialist in Community Medicine).[18]

Exhumation for medico-legal purposes

Exhumation is an unpleasant procedure, particularly if the body has been buried only recently, and one that engenders considerable emotion. Although the practice is, as a result, very strictly controlled, there are occasions when the re-examination of a body already buried may be of overriding importance either to the state, as in the case of suspected criminality, to insurance companies or to individuals when civil actions for damages are contemplated or when identification is disputed. A coroner in England and Wales may authorise exhumation of a person buried within his jurisdiction either for the purpose of holding an inquest, or of discharging any other of his relevant functions. He may also do so in connection with criminal proceedings relating to the death of the body exhumed, or to the death of another person that is related to the circumstances surrounding the death of the person to be exhumed.[19] In all other cases, permission must be sought from the Home Secretary.[20] Something of the order of two medico-legal exhumations are carried out annually in England and Wales; even before the widening of the powers enjoyed by the coroner, only a minority of these were carried out under licence from the Home Secretary.

In Scotland, the person requiring the exhumation, whether it be the procurator fiscal or a member of the public, petitions the sheriff to that effect. In the former instance, the sheriff must notify the next-of-kin of the deceased, who are given the opportunity to make objections at a hearing. If the petition is granted, the sheriff will issue a warrant for exhumation. In the latter, the remains are regarded as sacred and the grave is protected against disturbance at least until the process of disintegration is complete. The sheriff may, however, authorise disinterment and reinterment prior to this in the light of necessity—eg if a road needs widening; otherwise, the rule is adhered to very strictly.[1]

In the case of exhumation in anticipation of criminal proceedings, presumptive identification is made by the superintendent of the graveyard consulting his records and by the undertaker's recognition of the coffin and of the internal wrappings. Whenever possible, relatives should be asked to confirm the name on the identifying plaque.

Many exhumations authorised for the purpose of establishing the precise cause of death are concerned with suspected poisoning. It is then incumbent upon the pathologist in charge of the operation to obtain a full series of control specimens which can be analysed for the poison along with the tissues from the body. These

18 Registration of Births and Deaths Regulations 1987, SI 1987/2088, r 51.
19 Coroners Act 1988, s 23.
20 Burial Act 1857, s 25. An ecclesiastical faculty is needed whenever a body is removed from consecrated ground; the requirements are treated fairly liberally: *In re Durrington Cemetery* [2000] 3 WLR 1322. A licence is not required when the sole purpose is to remove the body from one piece of consecrated ground to another: *Re St Luke's (Holbeach Hurn); Watson v Howard* [1990] 2 All ER 749. Local authorities have special powers of removal and reinterment (eg Town and Country Planning Act 1990, ss 238,239).
1 *Nicholls v Angus Council* 1997 SCLR 941.

include earth from above, around and below the coffin, the wood and any fluid from inside the coffin, and portions of the burial robes. It is also advisable to collect further control specimens of soil from a distant area of the cemetery. Parallel analyses will provide valuable evidence as to the possibility of any poison having entered the body from outside after burial rather than having been ingested before death.

There is considerable onus on the pathologist to make a particularly thorough examination of exhumed bodies; so far as is known, no request for a second exhumation has ever been granted.

Cremation

As a reflection of its finality, cremation as a method of disposal of the dead is carefully regulated.[2] Cremation is the ultimate method of concealing a crime; on the other hand, it has certain advantages over burial as a legal method of disposal of the dead. Moreover the modern operation of the coroners' (and fiscals') system has greatly reduced the opportunity for the concealment of homicide. Any regulations must therefore be so designed as to permit without undue hindrance a process that is in the public interest and yet, at the same time, safeguard that interest in respect of criminality. The Cremation Acts 1902 and 1952 constitute the law in both England and Wales and in Scotland. It is re-emphasised that the discretionary powers under which a body can be buried without certification as to the cause of death and prior to registration of the death do not apply to cremation— the process of cremation cannot be set in motion until the registration of the death is complete. Subject to that proviso, the regulation of cremation can be described conveniently by way of the forms that must be completed before it can be allowed:[3]

Form A. This constitutes an application for cremation which sets out, inter alia, the relationship of the applicant to the deceased, the wishes of the next-of-kin, the details of the death, an affirmation to the effect that there is no reason to suspect foul play or the need for further examination of the body and a statement by those who have been in medical charge of the deceased. The application must be countersigned by a householder who knows the applicant.

Form B. This is the certificate of the medical attendant who has 18 questions to answer relating to the mode and cause of death, the scope of his attendance on the deceased, operative treatment and nursing care in the recent past. The doctor must certify that he has no reason to suppose that further inquiry is needed and he must also affirm that he is not related to nor has he a pecuniary interest in the death of the deceased. Despite its comprehensiveness, Form B does not replace the medical certificate as to cause of death; the latter is essential for the registration of the death whereas Form B is related only to the process of cremation.

---

2   In contrast to the surprisingly lax attitude to burial, the Cremation Regulations 1930 prohibit the burning of human remains in any place other than a crematorium which must be certified for the purpose (Cremation Act 1952, s 1). In England and Wales, similar regulations now apply to the burning of body parts removed during the course of post-mortem examination: Cremation (Amendment) Regulations 2000, SI 2000/58.

3   Regulations as to Cremation 1930, SR & O 1930/1016, r 8. The identical regulations for Scotland are to be found in Cremation (Scotland) Regulations 1935, SR & O 1935/247. Several amendments have been made to both and are incorporated in the main regulations.

Form C. This is a confirmatory medical certificate which must be completed by a practitioner of at least five years' standing who has no family or professional relationship with the practitioner signing Form B. He must state whether he has seen the body and whether he has made a careful external examination. There is no statutory requirement for him to have done so but the regulations clearly indicate the need; a negative answer would certainly result in the rejection of the certificate. There is provision for stating whether or not he has performed a post-mortem dissection. There are five questions relating to his having questioned various categories of person as to the circumstances of the death; there must be a positive reply to at least one of these. Finally, the certifying doctor must affirm that he is satisfied as to the cause of death.

Form C can be dispensed with if the patient died in hospital where he was an in-patient and a post-mortem examination was made by a pathologist who would have been qualified to complete Form C; the practitioner completing Form B must, in these circumstances, know the result of the post-mortem examination before giving his certificate. [4]

Form F. This form is completed by the medical referee (a medical officer nominated by the crematorium and appointed by the Home Secretary or the Scottish Ministers). The signature confirms that the referee is satisfied that the regulations have been complied with, that the cause of death has been established and that no further examination is required; cremation of the remains is authorised.

The Cremation Act gives very wide powers to the referee. He can complete Form C himself; he can withhold Form F without giving reasons and can make any inquiries he thinks fit; he can report the case to the coroner or procurator fiscal; he can also invite a pathologist to perform a post-mortem examination or make such an examination himself. In the last circumstance, the person performing the autopsy completes *Form D*, which will then replace Form C and will also override Form B. In the event that the case has been reported to the coroner or procurator fiscal, the certificate of those officials, *Form E*, replaces Forms B and C and clears the case for the medical referee. Form E may be issued before the conclusion of the medico-legal inquiries but, in England and Wales, it does not state the cause of death; it does not replace either the coroner's death certificate or Certificate after Inquest. The version of Form E provided by the procurator fiscal does indicate the cause of death but, notwithstanding, a normal certificate of cause of death must also be provided by his medical adviser. Surprisingly, a body that has been buried for not less than a year may be disinterred and cremated without further documentation or authorisation; the situation is subject only to the requirements for exhumation. [5]

It is clear that the regulations are designed to prevent the concealment of criminality as it is generally understood and, in this, they are probably successful. It is equally clear that success depends upon the good faith of the doctors involved in their application. Without this, the system will fail and it will fail most dramatically when the doctors themselves are the targets of the regulations. This has been shown recently in the notorious case of Dr Shipman, who was convicted

4   Cremation (Amendment) Regulations 1985, SI 1985/153; Cremation (Scotland) (Amendment) Regulations 1985, SI 1985/820—incorporated in the main regulations as reg 8A.
5   Regulations as to Cremation 1930, reg 13.

of the murder of 15 or more patients, the majority of whom were cremated.[6] If the case does nothing else, it emphasises the importance of the roles of the second certifying doctor and of the medical referee in the regulation of this method of disposal of the dead.

The Anatomy Act 1984

This Act governs the retention of a body for the purposes of use in an anatomy school. The Human Tissue Act 1961 extended the scope of, but did not replace, the Anatomy Acts 1832 and 1871, which are now repealed by that of 1984. Although many of the terms of the two Acts are very similar, the 1961 Act raises issues of far more general application and is discussed in detail in Chapter 12. The 1961 Act takes precedence over the 1984 Act should there be any apparent clash over their application.[7]

In general, the disposal of a body through the dissecting room is subject to the dissection being conducted only by a licensed person in a licensed establishment. Given that the deceased has expressed a wish during life that his or her body be so used,[8] the person lawfully in possession of the body can authorise an examination in accordance with the request. The power of veto of a spouse or relative which existed under the previous Anatomy Acts even when the deceased had bequeathed his body has, thus, been withdrawn. In the absence of a directive, the person lawfully in possession of the body may authorise an examination unless the deceased is known to have objected or the spouse or a relative objects; in this instance, the 'person lawfully in possession' means the hospital authority or the management of a similar institution in which the death occurs.[9] The body cannot be possessed without a valid certificate of the cause of death and it must not be dissected unless the death has been registered. Records of receipt and disposal of the body must be kept and retained for five years after disposal[10]—and further records must be kept of any parts retained under s 6 of the Act after the anatomical examination is concluded. The body can be held only for such a period as adequate preservation of the body can be maintained. Final disposal after examination must be, so far as is practicable, according to the wishes of the deceased or any surviving relatives. The body must be disposed of either by burial or cremation; in the event of cremation, a special *Form H* must be completed.

A major medico-legal distinction between the Anatomy Act and the Human Tissue Act is that, whereas the former is specially designed for the provision of teaching material to medical schools, dissections under the latter must be carried out by registered medical practitioners. It is also noticeable that, in contrast to the 1961 Act, the 1984 Act specifies offences under the Act.[11]

---

6 C Dyer 'Tighter controls on GP's to follow doctor's murder conviction' (2000) 320 BMJ 331. See also the case of *R v Cox* (1992) 12 BMLR 38, in which a doctor was convicted of the attempted murder of a patient who had already been cremated.

7 Anatomy Act 1984, s 1(5).

8 This may be in writing at any time or orally in the presence of two witnesses during the terminal illness (s 4(2)).

9 *R v Feist* [1858] Dears & B 590. The situation is clarified in s 4(9) of the 1984 Act (see Chapter 12 for further discussion).

10 Anatomy Regulations 1988, SI 1988/44, reg 2, as amended by Anatomy (Amendment) Regulations 1988, SI 1988/198.

11 Anatomy Act 1984, s 11; Anatomy Regulations 1988, reg 5.

The disposal of stillbirths

A stillbirth is defined as a child that issued from the mother after the 24th week of pregnancy and that did not at any time after being expelled from its mother breathe or show any sign of life.[12]

The pathological distinction between stillbirth and perinatal death is discussed in Chapter 18. We are concerned here only with the regulations surrounding the actual disposal of the body; these are governed in England and Wales by the Births and Deaths Registration Act 1953, s 11 and in Scotland by the Registration of Births, Deaths and Marriages (Scotland) Act 1965, s 21. The process is essentially similar under both statutes.

The body of a stillbirth cannot be disposed of without a valid medical certificate of stillbirth which, throughout Great Britain, can be completed by virtue of the certifier either having been present at the birth or having examined the body following information as to its birth. The certificate may be signed by a registered medical practitioner or by a certified midwife. In the event of the registrar being in any doubt as to whether the child was born alive, the case must be reported to the coroner or to the procurator fiscal; in practice, many cases are reported direct when the certifier thinks it necessary. There is provision under both jurisdictions for a declaration by the informant that the child was stillborn when, for some reason, there is no professional person available to provide a certificate. (See Appendix I.)

A stillbirth is, technically, a birth rather than a death. The informant therefore has 42 days in England and 21 days in Scotland to register the event. Stillbirths do not come within the compass of the Human Tissue Act and, in the present state of the law, must be buried or cremated. Disposal is contingent upon the issue of a Certificate for Disposal or of the appropriate' coroner's or fiscal's certificate. The medical referee can authorise the cremation of a stillbirth provided he is satisfied it has been registered,[13] specially adapted Forms A and F are then used. There is no requirement for the superintendent of the place of disposal to notify the registrar of disposal of a stillbirth—as there is in the ordinary case of death—unless the body has been buried without a certificate of registration. It scarcely needs mention that, if a child has survived birth for even a fleeting time, certificates both of birth and death are required—the 'neonatal' certificate as to cause of death is then used.

The disposal of fetuses

There is no law as to the disposal of a fetus that is expelled dead from the mother before the 24th week of pregnancy. There is no requirement for registration and the method of disposal must simply comply with current standards of proper public behaviour and with the various Public Health Acts. Fetuses of this type are not subject to the restrictions of the Human Tissue Act and may be retained for scientific purposes, but there are serious ethical problems. The subject has been addressed by the Polkinghorne Committee,[14] which clearly suggested that the dead fetus was entitled to respect and that any research involving it should be subject to consideration by a research ethics committee. It was also recommended

12 Still-Birth (Definition) Act 1992.
13 Regulations as to Cremation 1930, reg 15.
14 *Review of the Guidance on the Research Use of Fetuses and Fetal Material* (Cmd 762, 1989)

that the consent of the mother, but not that of the father, should be obtained before any research or therapeutic use of fetal tissues was undertaken; no distinction in this respect was to be made between dead fetuses derived from therapeutic abortion and those resulting from natural miscarriage.

A major area of legal doubt still surrounds the rights of parents to have a fetus properly buried.[15] The superintendent of the burial ground is hardly likely to object if asked for such a service but he must be concerned lest he is illegally burying an uncertified stillbirth. There is no reason why a doctor should not provide a certificate to the effect that the body is *not* that of a stillbirth; there is anecdotal evidence that this is being done increasingly often but, of course, neither the procedure nor the certificate have any legal backing as things stand.

Otherwise, although there is no legal obligation to do so, it is suggested that the hospital should ascertain the wishes of the mother as to the disposal of fetal remains in order to avoid the possibility of giving offence. Even then, compliance may be impossible; there is no doubt that this is an area where guidance is certainly required—possibly in the form of further amendment or clarification of the Cremation Regulations.

Disposal of bodies returned from outside the United Kingdom

Although the procedure is not quite uniform—any differences depending upon the actual country in which death has occurred—the disposal of bodies returned from outside the United Kingdom follows generally similar principles.

The death is certified according to the regulations of the country in which it occurred and, usually, the death certificate is accompanied by further certificates as to freedom from infection and to embalming. The papers are notarised by the Consul, who may also add his own certificate.

In the event of burial in the United Kingdom, all the documents are referred to the registrar of the area where the body is to be interred. Since the death has already been registered abroad, the registrar will then issue a Certificate of Non-liability to Register which, in effect, takes the place of the usual Disposal Certificate. Notification of disposal is still required within 96 hours of the event. No Certificate of Non-liability is required in Scotland where burial is controlled by the appropriate cemetery authority. If the next-of-kin wish for a cremation, an application must be made on Form A which is sent, with all the relevant documents, to the Home Office or the Secretary of State whence a licence to cremate is provided.

It is now clear that, despite the fact that both the death and the cause of death occurred abroad, the coroner for the district in which the body lies must hold an inquest if the circumstances were such that one would have been held had the death occurred in England or Wales.[16] While it is certainly true that post-mortem

---

15 Respect for the fetus is gaining momentum elsewhere. See, for example, L Kallenberg, L Forslin and O Westerborn 'The Disposal of the Aborted fetus—New Guidelines: Ethical Considerations in the Debate in Sweden' (1993) 19 J Med Ethics 32. On the other hand, it has been held in the United States that to impose a choice of methods of disposal of a fetus on a woman is to influence her unduly in her choice of abortion: *City of Akron v Akron Center for Reproductive Health Inc* 462 US 416 (1983).

16 *R v West Yorkshire Coroner, ex p Smith* [1983] QB 335, interpreting what is now the Coroners Act 1988, s 8(1). The coroner in Northern Ireland is under no such obligation.

examinations conducted abroad are often incomplete by British standards, [17] this does not necessarily mean that the overall investigation of the death was inadequate; conducting two investigations seldom does any good and may well lead to confusion. Moreover, it means that the coroner must, for example, inquire into the deaths of, say, those servicemen killed in action abroad who are repatriated while having no jurisdiction over those buried on site. [18] Quite what would happen in the event of a major war in which fatal casualties were repatriated is uncertain, but it seems that this interpretation of the Act is ripe for review at parliamentary level. [19]

17 M A Green 'Sudden Death of British Nationals Abroad' (1979) 19 J Forens Sci Soc 1.
18 P Victor 'Friendly Fire Victims Unlawfully Killed' The Times, 19 May 1992, p 1. The Oxford coroner was, effectively, called upon to pronounce on the tactics of a modern battle.
19 For discussion, see D Buchanan and J K Mason 'The Coroner's Office Revisited' (1995) 3 Med L Rev 142.

6

The spread of communicable disease: some aspects of public health

Epidemiology is the study of the determinants and mode of distribution of disease. All natural disease is to some extent subject to outside influences but communicable disease is that type that can most obviously be controlled by legislation.[1] Community health is therefore a part of the general spectrum of forensic medicine, and virtually all the early university chairs in forensic medicine combined medical jurisprudence with public health—and it has long been the author's belief that criminality should be regarded as no more than a facet of forensic medicine rather than as its *raison d'être*. Actions in tort or delict may well be based on transference of disease, while the doctor who fails to diagnose exotic disease may be sued in negligence—an aspect of forensic medicine that has come to greater prominence with the availability of cheap, world-wide travel facilities. Some understanding of the spread of communicable disease should be available to the lawyer concerned with medical aspects of the law; it is the purpose of this chapter to present this in outline.

Environmental disease

There is no doubt that a proportion of human disease is attributable to the environment in which we live and much of this is beyond human control—the undoubted association between tumours of the skin and over-exposure to sunlight is a good example; there is nothing our legislators can do to offset such hazards. A major part of environmental disease, however, can be attributed to the discharge of man-made pollutants into the atmosphere, water or soil. While this can be extensively controlled by legislation, it is, essentially, a matter of environmental poisoning and is discussed under that heading in Chapter 21; disease of this type cannot be regarded as communicable in the ordinary sense of the word. Increasing interest is, however, being shown in environmental disease which is distributed by the individual. Such conditions are readily amenable to legislation and are very likely to be the source of litigation—but they are difficult to classify. It is here suggested that the man who distributes noxious gases through his defective car engine is 'communicating' disease in much the same way as the man who distributes pathogenic organisms through his

1   And has been for 150 years beginning with An Act for Promoting Public Health 1848.

sputum. Thus, it is not inappropriate to introduce the concept here but, although there are other apposite examples, it is proposed to limit discussion to the most topical and contentious issue of passive smoking.

Passive smoking has become a major medico-legal concern. The issue turns on the assumption that if, as there is no doubt, smoking is a direct cause of disease, then it is probable that the secondary smoking of other people's tobacco will also cause disease—and that those who contaminate the environment will be liable for so doing. There are many who still doubt such an association and who, as a corollary, regard the prohibition of smoking as an interference with personal liberty.[2] The scientific situation was summed up in the words of the Australian Hill J:

> 'I am prepared to accept that many of the underlying studies . . . would not be accepted by all, and perhaps by even a majority of scientists, as rigorous proof in accordance with scientific method.'[3]

None the less, there is considerable evidence in favour[4] and, of greater pragmatic importance, the courts of many jurisdictions will accept the proposition. This is particularly evident in Australia where, while declining to evaluate the statistical evidence themselves, the judges of the Federal Court have accepted, on appeal, that there *is* some association between passive smoking and respiratory disease including lung cancer[5]—although the minority opinion was, in general, able to accept only an exacerbative rather than a causative relationship. Large class actions have succeeded in the United States and there has been at least one success in the United Kingdom.[6] One must agree with Brahams, who suggested that the only issue in the future is likely to concern the time at which employers should have banned smoking in the workplace.[7]

Passive smoking may also have an effect on the fetus. There is increasing evidence that maternal smoking is a significant factor in the aetiology of 'cot deaths' (see page 276).[8]

Organisms responsible for infectious disease

The common concept of communicable disease is, however, that of disease which is passed by way of organisms from person to person. Organisms capable of causing human disease vary greatly in habit and in size. Ascending from the smallest, the groups that are of greatest concern include the following.

2   See eg *Boddington v British Transport Police* [1999] 2 AC 143, HL.
3   In *Tobacco Institute of Australia Ltd v Australian Federation of Consumer Organisations Inc* (1992) 111 ALR 61 at 114.
4   There is a mass of literature in support. Morling J gave a wide-ranging review of the early studies in *Australian Federation of Consumer Organisations v Tobacco Institute of Australia Ltd* (1991) 98 ALR 670, FC but this is not included in the report; it is available on the Internet, which is well worth a visit.
5   *Tobacco Institute of Australia Ltd v Australian Federation of Consumer Organisations Inc* (1992) 111 ALR 61. Discussed by S Chapman and S Woodward 'Australian Court Decision on Passive Smoking Upheld on Appeal' (1993) 306 BMJ 120.
6   *Bland v Stockport Metropolitan Borough Council* (1993) reported by C Dyer 'UK Woman Wins First Settlement for Passive Smoking' (1993) 306 BMJ 351.
7   D Brahams 'Passive Smoking' (1993) 341 Lancet 552. As indicated in *Waltons & Morse v Dorrington* [1997] IRLR 488.
8   See J Golding 'The Epidemiology and Sociology of the Sudden Infant Death Syndrome' in J K Mason (ed) *Paediatric Forensic Medicine and Pathology* (1989) ch 9.

The viruses

The characteristic of these minute organisms is that they are incapable of a free existence and must live as true parasites within living tissue. As a corollary, viruses can be grown in the laboratory only in cultures of live tissues. The importance of viral disease is increasing both absolutely and relatively as the potency and range of antibacterial agents increases. Examples of virus disease include rabies, measles and AIDS (see below);[9] several of the more serious modern sexually transmitted diseases are viral in origin. Many of the 'new' virus diseases that are being discovered probably result from animal organisms adapting to a human environment; it is the fear of inducing this that inhibits adoption of many of the potential 'break-throughs' in medical treatment—especially xenotransplantation or the use of animal organs as human replacements (see page 163 for a short consideration).

The bacteria

These unicellular organisms of great simplicity are omnipresent. Those that cause disease are described as *pathogenic* and those that produce a purulent reaction are *pyogenic*. Bacteria exist in various shapes—the round *cocci* which, inter alia, cause sore throats, boils and pneumonia; the rod-shaped *bacilli*, which include the organisms responsible for typhoid fever and tuberculosis; the curved *vibrios*, which are responsible for cholera; and the coiled *spirochaetes*, which cause several diseases additional to syphilis. The *anaerobic bacteria* form a group that is of special importance in forensic medicine; they will grow only in the relative absence of oxygen and proliferate particularly well in wounds, causing tetanus and gas gangrene. Bacteria that are not pathogenic in their normal habitat may produce disease when displaced in the body so called *opportunistic infection* of which serious infection of the kidney by the normally innocuous *E. coli* is a good example.

The classification of bacteria is, however, not as simple as it may seem, as the majority of species exist in multiple *strains* of varying pathogenicity; moreover, each strain may become pathogenic for no apparent reason other than an unidentified variation in the micro-environment. It is for this reason that we have epidemics of disease due to generally harmless bacteria such as *E. coli*.

The protozoa

These are more sophisticated unicellular organisms which cause many diseases of world-wide economic importance, including malaria, sleeping sickness and the bowel disease amoebic dysentery.

The fungi

These are branching organisms of simple type which are increasing in importance as they may flourish in severely ill patients, particularly those on antibacterial treatment.

The helminths or worms

These take many forms and vary from those that are scarcely visible to the naked eye to others that are several metres long. They are often of considerable medico-legal

9   Slightly different viruses, known as *Rickettsiae*, cause the typhus group of fevers.

importance due to their close association with food and its preparation and, in some instances, with occupation. Many have no more than a nuisance value but others—for example, one tapeworm of dogs which causes hydatid disease in man—are potentially dangerous to life; the pork tapeworm may cause an intractable form of epilepsy. Whether or not a helminth is dangerous to life depends, to a large extent, on whether it spends its larval stage within the human tissues—in which case, serious disease may result; adult worms which infest the liver may, however, also cause serious disease.

The prions

Neurological disease due to prions has recently achieved notoriety in the form of bovine spongiform encephalopathy (BSE) in animals and Creutzfeldt-Jakob disease (CJD) in humans. The nature of prions is currently uncertain although they appear to be abnormal proteins which are either inherited or result from sporadic mutations. They are transmissible both from human to human—eg in infected human growth hormone[10]—and animal to human—eg by eating infected meat – and, as such, are of very great importance in public health. The field is, however, mercifully limited at the moment.

The spread of communicable disease (see Figure 6.1)

If a disease is to spread, the responsible organism must be passed from person to person. The simplest way in which this can be done is by *direct contact*, when the organism must be either on the skin or in secretions that are passed directly from person to person. The most obvious examples of such contact diseases are those that are sexually transmitted and the infectious skin diseases. *Blood-borne* disease can be regarded as a variation on contact disease; the organism is spread from person to person by the exchange of infected blood via either transfusion or contaminated hypodermic needles.

Otherwise, human-to-human transfer of disease depends upon excretion of organisms and this can take several routes—particularly via the sputum, the urine and the faeces. Sputum does not necessarily mean the mass of phlegm seen in sufferers from bronchitis but includes the more important invisible spray known as *droplets* that is spread each time a person coughs; in so far as this can be directly inhaled by others, droplet infection is a matter of *proximity contact* and is fostered by conditions of overcrowding with inadequate ventilation. Urine is a vehicle for surprisingly few communicable diseases—typhoid fever is of the most immediate concern in the Western hemisphere but, on a world-wide basis, the condition of schistosomiasis, due to a worm, is a far more important source of morbidity. Contrastingly, the faeces may contain large numbers of pathogenic organisms—not only those associated with the many infectious bowel diseases but also those that become pathogenic when displaced—for example, when contaminating wounds, including the *anaerobic bacilli*.

An excretion that is passed may remain on the hands and any organisms can then be transferred to the utensils or food of others—the role of the food handler in the transmission of disease is of great importance. Alternatively, the excretion may be passed into the water supply—either localised, as into a well, or generalised, as into a stream or river; sporadic disease in the locality, or explosive

---

10 A whole issue of Butterworths Medico-Legal Reports is devoted to the resultant litigation: *Creutzfeld-Jakob Disease Litigation* (2000) 54 BMLR 1.

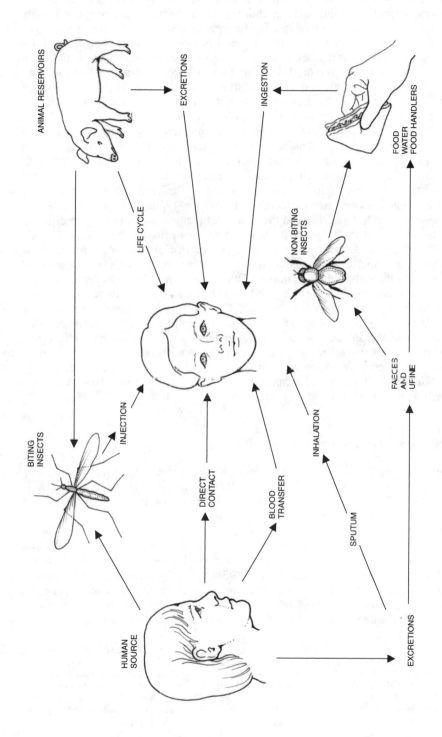

Figure 6.1 Schematic representation of the spread of disease due to microbiological organisms.

epidemic disease involving a whole distant community may then arise. The major contribution of the public authorities to the health of the people probably depends upon the provision of an efficient system of sewage disposal. Otherwise, the excretions may dry and become incorporated in dust; control of those pathogenic organisms that are resistant to desiccation is a major problem within institutions—it is the standard route of cross-infection of patients in hospital. Finally, infected excretions may be transferred to foodstuffs by insects, of which the house-fly was once the most important; its virtual eradication from developed societies is a major factor in improved public health.

The organisms responsible for many communicable diseases are not excreted but remain in the blood. Transfer from case to case must then depend upon either direct exchange of blood as in transfusion or needle-sharing or on the action of blood-sucking insects; the importance of *insect-borne disease*[11] is vast in the world as a whole but slight in temperate climates. Pandemics of arthropod-borne disease, among which are included yellow fever, typhus, plague, malaria and sleeping sickness, have changed the course of history, and it is only an efficient public health system that prevents their recurrence or limits their effects. Certain arthropod-borne diseases are essentially human in distribution—louse-borne typhus fever, which is associated with overcrowding in conditions of poor personal hygiene, is the outstanding example. Others, however, depend upon an animal reservoir—the most historic example being the rat as a source of bubonic plague by way of its associated fleas. Human diseases that are animal dependent are known as *zoonoses*. Zoonoses may also persist by means of a direct association between man and animals. Some are industrial in nature—for example, the infective jaundice of sewer workers or hydatid worm disease of sheep farmers—but the most urgent contact zoonosis is undoubtedly rabies—a disease particularly apposite to the theme of this chapter because its control in Great Britain, at least up till now, rests almost entirely on legislation.[12]

The control of communicable disease

The general methods for control of infectious disease are clear from the foregoing paragraphs. First, one can attempt to eliminate—or, in human instances, isolate—the source of infection; secondly, knowing the mode of spread, an effort can be made to break the chain at some vital point; thirdly, one can use artificial means to promote immunity in the population.

Statutory powers to achieve these ends are contained in the several Acts and regulations pertaining to public health; the main United Kingdom legislation is contained in the Public Health Acts 1936 and 1961 and the Public Health (Scotland) Acts 1897–1945. Many of the powers are wide and far beyond the ambit of the individual—they include adequate supervision of housing, the control of sewage, drainage and water supplies, the whole range of inspection and control

---

11 Using the word in a colloquial sense. Ticks and mites which also transmit disease are not, zoologically speaking, insects; a better general term is 'arthropod-borne disease'.

12 Animal Health Act 1981, s 17; Rabies (Importation of Dogs, Cats and other Mammals) Order 1974, SI 1974/2211, as amended. At the time of writing, serious consideration is being given to the modification of controls whereby animals that have been immunised may be imported or reimported. See Pet Travel Scheme (Pilot Arrangements)(England) Order 1999, SI 1999/3443.

of foodstuffs, the control of important biological goods likely to be infected, such as animal bones or skins, and the quarantining of animals.[13] The United Kingdom law as it affects individuals is now consolidated in the Public Health (Control of Disease) Act 1984 and the Public Health (Scotland) Act 1897.

Much current attention is focused on what are described as exotic diseases—that is, diseases that are imported from abroad. They may be of little or no public concern—if a visitor becomes ill with malaria it will not be communicable in Britain because the insect carrier, the anopheles mosquito, has been so reduced in number as to be ineffective; this, in turn, is the result of efficient public health measures.[14] Some exotic diseases, by contrast, may have relatively severe consequences—a person with typhoid fever, for instance, could infect a number of contacts before discovery; they could also be catastrophic—a classic example would be the importation of yellow fever into an area where the mosquito vector was present in sufficient numbers to start an epidemic. Even in parts of Britain it could be a matter of very great concern if a human or animal case of plague were introduced into an area where rats and fleas abounded.[15] The control of exotic disease is largely a matter of port health control;[16] while the control of shipping has been practised successfully for very many years, the problems are accentuated by the widespread use of air travel—aircraft can transport infected insects and persons incubating disease will reach their destination before becoming overtly ill. Special regulations[17] are applied to aircraft and, in those parts of the world at special risk, control is exercised on an international basis.[18] Other contact zoonoses are controlled either by prohibition of imported animals or compulsory quarantining—measures that are available only to an island state.

These major concerns are of little interest in the present context. Of greater immediate importance is the fact that certain control measures impinge upon the rights of the individual and also on the doctor/patient relationship—the various regulations strike what may be seen as an uneasy balance between coercion of the individual and the needs of the State.[19] This is particularly so in the case of the acquired immune deficiency syndrome which has such legal ramifications as to merit a short section to itself.

13 See also Environmental Protection Act 1990, as amended.
14 Most exotic diseases are specifically treatable and diagnosable in the laboratory. It would now be considered negligent to fail to take the necessary steps to make a diagnosis, despite the infrequency of the disease; extensive damages have, in fact, been awarded for such mistakes: *Langley v Campbell* (1975) Times, 6 November, is an example.
15 All ships must be in possession of either a Deratting Certificate or a Deratting Exemption Certificate; certificates are valid for six months (International Health Regulations (1969) art 54). A Community Health Physician who finds that an excessive number of rats are dying must report the matter: Public Health (Infectious Diseases) Regulations 1988, SI 1988/1546), reg 11.
16 Public Health (Ships) Regulations 1979, SI 1979/1435.
17 Public Health (Aircraft) Regulations 1979, SI 1979/1434; Public Health (Aircraft) (Scotland) Amendment Regulations 1974, SI 1974/1017.
18 International Health Regulations 1969 (amended 1973 and 1981 by the World Health Organization) cover cholera, plague, smallpox and yellow fever. These, together with leprosy, malaria and rabies contracted in Great Britain and viral haemorrhagic fever are subject to special, immediate reporting to the Chief Medical Officer (Public Health (Infectious Diseases) Regulations 1988, SI 1988/1546, r 6).
19 For an analysis, see P Old and J Montgomery 'Law, Coercion, and the Public Health' (1992) 304 BMJ 891 or, more recently, M Brazier and J Harris 'Public health and private lives' (1996) 4 Med L Rev 171. The problem was vividly illustrated in *Birmingham Post and Mail Ltd v Birmingham City Council* (1993) 17 BMLR 116.

Blood-borne viruses

The last two decades have seen the increasing importance of, and the emergence of, viruses which have the dual properties of being transmitted mainly by blood transfer and by sexual intercourse. These include the hepatitis viruses B and C (HBV and HCV) and the human immunodeficiency virus (HIV), which is ultimately responsible for the acquired immune deficiency syndrome (AIDS).[20] HBV is transmitted relatively easily and can cause liver disease which may well prove fatal. Transmission of HIV is comparatively difficult but, so far as can be determined, once established, it nearly always results in AIDS which is, currently, a fatal disease despite the improvements in drug therapy which seem, at least, to delay the development of the clinical disease.

HBV, HCV and HIV are transmitted in blood which is introduced parenterally—that is, by injection through the skin. Although many people have been infected using contaminated blood, or blood products, for transfusion, the amount of blood needed to initiate the diseases is minute; drug abusers who share needles are, therefore, particularly at risk and, in some areas, the drug abusing population constitutes the major reservoir for HIV infection and subsequent AIDS.

The Human Immunodeficiency Virus

The HIV is, however, an unusual organism in that its spread is markedly, though increasingly less obviously, associated with male homosexuality. HIV infection is, therefore, intimately tied to problems arising from anti-discrimination legislation based on gender which, in the United Kingdom, is to be found in the Sex Discrimination Acts 1975 and 1986. More men are infected with HIV than are women. Thus, it could be indirect discrimination, and, therefore, unlawful to reject a man for employment because he tested positive for HIV infection unless the employer could show good cause for so doing. In point of fact, it would probably be unlawful on general grounds, to do so as it has been specifically condemned by the Council of Europe speaking through its Ministers of Health.[1] Discrimination against the symptomatic patient is covered under the Disability Discrimination Act 1995 where AIDS is classified as a 'progressive condition'. A person so affected is regarded as disabled when he or she is impaired—but not to the extent of a *substantial* adverse effect—if the condition is one that is likely to progress to the latter state.[2]

Other immediate medico-legal aspects of HIV infection stem from the inevitably fatal outcome of AIDS. Thus, for example, a person who tests positive for HIV will never obtain a life insurance policy and may well be denied a mortgage for house purchase. Moreover, the mere fact that a man has been tested for HIV infection may stigmatise him as leading a life-style which some regard as involving increased health risks and others would view with disapproval. The result has been that AIDS has been treated quite unlike any other communicable disease and the normal public health measures to combat an epidemic have not been applied.[3]

20 There are theories as to AIDS which cast doubt on this proposition—they are, for example, given some credence in South Africa; the vast majority of microbiologists would regard these alternatives as unacceptable.
1 *Conclusions Concerning AIDS and the Place of Work* Document OJ 1989 C28. See *A (supported by Union Syndicale, intervening v Commission of the European Communities* (1994) Times, 30 June.
2 Disability Discrimination Act 1995, Sch 1, para 8(1).
3 For a critical approach, see R Danzinger 'An epidemic like any other? Rights and responsibilities in HIV prevention' (1996) 312 BMJ 1083.

This is seen, first, in testing for the condition. Thus, although AIDS may well come within a differential diagnosis, the probable majority opinion is that conditions surrounding the disease are so unique that, notwithstanding consent to venepuncture having been obtained, it would be an assault to include a test for HIV in a diagnostic series without obtaining *specific* consent to do so.[4] This raises the problem of children who cannot consent to or refuse testing. Compulsory testing of infants has been instituted in some jurisdictions;[5] the paramount interests of the child would probably result in court ordered tests in any disputed case in the United Kingdom.[6] Secondly, confidentiality is taken to extreme lengths so that it is even doubtful if those placed at risk—for example, the infected person's partner—are entitled to be informed of that risk;[7] it is also widely held that not even the patient's general practitioner may be informed of his condition against his will. As a corollary, HIV infection and AIDS are not notifiable diseases (see below) although local authorities must provide reports on the situation to the responsible minister.[8] Thus, the greater part of knowledge as to the spread of HIV now comes from anonymous testing of defined groups, such as pregnant women, which is scarcely a substitute for the rigorous application of epidemiological methods. It is, however, to be noted that the majority of developed countries have adopted similar policies; so far as is known, only Cuba takes an opposing view. The problem of confidentiality for the infected health care professional is addressed in Chapter 30.

The advent of AIDS has, however, reopened the question of liability for knowingly transmitting sexually transmitted disease—the answer to which is still uncertain in the United Kingdom. Civil liability would depend on, first, whether a duty of care exists between two persons having sexual intercourse; although this is well established in the United States, it can only be regarded as probably so in the United Kingdom.[9] Second, there is the problem of consent. A general consent to intercourse would probably elide any action in battery.[10] The

4 This is the view supported by the British Medical Association; it is not, however, accepted universally. For an excellent review of opinions, see J Keown 'The Ashes of AIDS and the Phoenix of Informed Consent' (1989) 52 MLR 790. The pragmatic answer is that the GMC *has* found a doctor guilty of serious professional misconduct for doing so: C Dyer 'GP reprimanded for testing patients for HIV without consent' (2000) 320 BMJ 135.

5 Eg Ryan White CARE Act Amendments (1996), s 7(b)(3), USA.

6 Applications to test a child under the Children Act 1989 have to be made to a High Court Judge of the Family Division: *Re X (a minor)(HIV tests)* [1994] 2 FLR 116. See now *Re C (a child) (HIV test)* [2000] Fam 48, Fam D; [1999] 2 FLR 1004, CA, where tests were ordered in the face of parental objection.

7 The General Medical Council states that the only exception to the general principle, that the patient's request for privacy should be respected, arises where the doctor judges that the failure to disclose would put the health of any of the health care team at serious risk: General Medical Council *HIV and AIDS: the ethical considerations* (1995).

8 AIDS (Control) Act 1987. The minister can also order the hospitalisation and, if necessary, the detention of sufferers from AIDS (though not from uncomplicated HIV infection): Public Health (Infectious Diseases) Regulations 1988, SI 1988/1546), reg 5. For discussion, see M Brazier and M Lobjoit 'AIDS, Ethics, and the Respiratory Physician' (1990) 45 Thorax 283.

9 Based on extra-judicial statements by Lord Brandon quoted in K Litton and R James 'Civil Liability for Communication of AIDS—A Moot Point' (1987) 137 NLJ 755. Also discussed in J Taitz 'Legal Liability for Transmitting AIDS' (1989) 57 Med Leg J 216.

10 This ignores the question of whether it is legally possible to consent to sustaining a serious injury by way of disease: *A-G's Reference (No 6 of 1980)* [1981] QB 715. From the reverse angle, it would be rape to force a woman to have unprotected sex if she was consenting only to intercourse with the use of condoms: *R v Shaw (Grenville Charles)* [1997] 2 Cr App Rep (S) 206.

plaintiff could, however, maintain that she did not consent to intercourse with an infected person; a civil action in negligence might be available on the grounds that consent was, thereby, flawed—an argument that is based on the doctrine of 'informed consent' (see page 473).[11] The difficulties of proving causation would be very great in the case of AIDS, which takes many years to develop, though the same objection might not hold if the disease was, say, gonorrhoea with its short incubation period. Attributing criminal liability to transmitting disease has always been a suspect policy[12] and it would be difficult to do so in England given the restrictions of the Offences Against the Person Act 1861[13]—the best, but still dubious, line might be to charge 'administering a destructive or noxious thing' (s 24). The difficulties are such that several jurisdictions have introduced new and specific legislation[14] and this would seem to be the route favoured in the United Kingdom by those who see the need for criminal sanctions.[15] It is very doubtful if current government policy would support any such movement as regards sexual intercourse; recklessly risking the spread of disease by other means might, however, be a different matter—a surgeon who operated for three years knowing he was infected with HBV has been imprisoned for one year.[16]

Notification of infectious disease

As indicated above, the isolation of infective cases is an effective way of controlling human infectious disease; moreover, the original source of a disease can often be traced through a knowledge of those thereby infected. Both these public health control measures depend primarily upon notification of cases.

A number of diseases are statutorily notifiable to the local authority by the practitioner in charge of the case. Strangely, the Public Health (Control of Diseases) Act 1984, s 10 contains only an archaic list to which food poisoning is added by s 11. A far longer list of diseases which are affected by the 1984 Act has been achieved by regulation;[17] the combined list is reproduced in Appendix J, from which it will be seen that the scope of regulation is not uniform. The comparable list in Scotland derives from the Infectious Disease (Notification) Act 1889, as

11 For major discussion, see R O'Dair 'Liability in Tort for the Transmission of A.I.D.S.: Some Lessons from Afar and the Prospects for the Future' (1990) 43 Current Leg Prob 219.
12 See R Porter 'History Says No to the Policeman's Response to AIDS' (1986) 293 BMJ 1589.
13 The very old case of *R v Clarence* (1888) 22 QBD 23, in which a man who infected his wife with gonorrhoea was found not guilty both of inflicting grievous bodily harm and of assault occasioning actual bodily harm, would not necessarily be followed today. The government now seems prepared to consider criminalising the intentional transmission of disease but not reckless transmission: Home Office *Violence: Reforming the Offences Against the Person Act 1861* (1998).
14 Eg Public Health Act 1991, s 13 (NSW) which invokes the concept of informed consent in criminalising the transmission of sexually transmissible disease; Public and Environmental Health Act 1987, SA.
15 S Bronitt 'Spreading Disease and the Criminal Law' [1994] Crim LR 21. Convictions for criminal negligence have been successful in serious cases in Canada. See eg *R v Mercer* (1993) 84 CCC (3d) 41.
16 *R v Gaud*, Southwark Crown Court, 1994 reported by C Dyer 'Surgeon Jailed for Infecting Patients' (1994) 309 BMJ 896. The charge, presumably *faute de mieux*, was that of committing a public nuisance; the severity of the sentence may reflect the serious deceptions also involved. Another doctor has been disciplined by the GMC: C Dyer 'Doctor who refused HIV test is struck off register' (1997) 314 BMJ 847
17 Public Health (Infectious Diseases) Regulations 1988, SI 1988/1546, reg 3, Sch 1.

amended by the Public Health (Scotland) Act 1945 and the resultant regulations;[18] there are some minor differences and it is, therefore, shown separately as Appendix K. Neither list is exhaustive, as the local authority or the health board has the power to add to the printed list when local conditions indicate the need or desirability.[19] The end result is that there can be no question of a binding confidentiality between doctor and patient in this respect (see Chapter 30); this statutory type of breach of confidence illustrates two important points of principle in medical ethics—first, the 'need to know' quality of the person to whom confidential information is disclosed[20] and, secondly, the precept that is thus established that the public need is likely to take precedence when it is in conflict with that of the individual.

But statutory powers go deeper than this. It is an offence for a person knowing he has an infectious disease to expose others to that infection (1984 Act, s 17) or to carry on with his occupation when likely to do so as a result (s 19). A local authority can request a person to stop work if he is suffering from enteric fever, dysentery, diphtheria, scarlet fever, acute inflammation of the throat, gastroenteritis or undulant fever.[1] In the absence of consent, a justice or a sheriff may order a healthy person from a building in which he is considered at risk, he can make a hospital order and he can require a person to be detained in hospital if housing conditions are unlikely to be satisfactory upon discharge; clearly, however, such an order may be difficult to enforce. Perhaps the quickest preventive measure lies in the authority to order a medical examination of a person thought to be suffering from or to be the carrier of a 'notifiable' disease,[2] if it is considered to be in the interest of the person himself, his family or the public in general. Control of the carrier state is most important (1984 Act, s 36; 1968 Act, s 72). In this condition, a person feels perfectly well, yet is excreting pathogenic organisms—the state may be a hangover from an overt attack of the disease but, equally commonly, the carrier will never have been aware of being infected.[3] He may therefore resent compulsory medical treatment, but the devastation that could be caused by a typhoid carrier who persistently polluted a water supply or who was engaged in food handling of any sort needs no emphasis. Carrier states are notoriously difficult to treat and, in the event of failure, the local authority is empowered to compensate a person who has suffered any loss by agreeing to abandon work (1984 Act, s 20; 1968, s 71).

A number of other statutory safeguards of public health are available. For example, food handlers who are suspected of carrying disease must be reported to the local authority.[4] A non-patrial entering the country for a period of six months

18 Public Health (Notification of Infectious Diseases) (Scotland) Regulations 1988 (SI 1988/1550), added to by SI 1989/2250.
19 Public Health (Control of Disease) Act 1984, s 16; National Health Service (Scotland) Act 1972, s 53.
20 This is actually laid down in the 1988 regulations, reg 12.
 1 Public Health (Control of Disease) Act 1984, s 20(1A) inserted by Food Safety Act 1990, s 59, Sch 3, para 28. The Scottish equivalent lies in the Health Services and Public Health Act 1968, s 71(2).
 2 Public Health (Control of Disease) Act 1984, ss 35, 36. The extent of the effect of the 1984 Act on the various diseases is, however, variable—see Appendix J. The English legislation of 1984 is very similar to the Scottish Acts of 1897 and 1968 as they have evolved; it has not been thought necessary to footnote the latter unless there is a significant difference.
 3 The specific exclusion of the carrier state of AIDS—that is, HIV positivity—from the regulations exemplifies the importance placed by the authorities on privacy as to the condition.
 4 1988 Regulations, Sch 4, paras 2 and 5. The relevant diseases are typhoid, paratyphoid and other salmonella infections, amoebic and bacillary dysentery and staphylococcal infection likely to cause food poisoning.

or more is normally referred to a medical inspector for examination. The immigration officer should refuse entry if the medical inspector advises that it would be undesirable for him to be admitted. He may also refuse entry if the passenger declines to submit to a medical examination.[5] Two sections of the 1984 Act are of particular relevance to pathology. Section 44 states that every person having charge of the body of a person who has died from infectious disease, who could well be the pathologist or his mortuary keeper, must take such steps as are reasonably practicable to prevent persons coming unnecessarily into contact with or proximity to the body. Section 48 empowers a Justice of the Peace to order removal of a body from any building to a mortuary if retention of the body constitutes a hazard to others; the body must then be disposed of within a specified timetable.

Immunisation

There can be no doubt as to the efficacy of mass immunisation as a method of controlling infectious disease. At the same time, no immunity procedure is entirely without risk; controversy centres on the right balance being struck between, on the one hand, the effectiveness and the risk of vaccination against a particular disease and, on the other, the chance of contracting that disease and its short- and long-term effects both on the individual and on the public. A good illustration is provided by smallpox. This very severe disease could have wreaked havoc if re-introduced into Britain and, consequently, preventive vaccination was at one time compulsory; the procedure had, however, a recognisable mortality and morbidity of its own. By the middle of this century, other control measures had become so effective that the risks of vaccination were considered to outweigh the dangers of contracting the disease and compulsion was abandoned in 1971; the eradication of smallpox remains probably the greatest achievement of the World Health Organization.

Nevertheless, a voluntary immunisation programme is still an essential part of the control of many infectious diseases; within the United Kingdom, immunisation is recommended as a routine against diphtheria, tetanus, whooping cough, poliomyelitis, measles, tuberculosis and rubella.[6]

Immunisation is of two types—active and passive. In the former, the body is presented with either an attenuated (made-safe) live strain of the wild pathogenic organism or with a killed form. This vaccine acts as an antigen which stimulates the formation of antibodies, which are then ready to repel the antigen when it presents again in its natural disease-provoking form; antibody production can be boosted by repeated doses of the vaccine and is, therefore, long lasting. In passive immunity, the body is supplied with preformed antibodies; the action is short and is designed only to combat the actual or supposed entry of a dangerous organism before it can take hold in the body.

Active immunisation—that type of inoculation or vaccination given in childhood or before travelling to an infected area—has a number of hazards, many of which are now only theoretical. The recipient may have a completely unforeseeable idiosyncracy to the injection and may sustain a severe allergic

---

5   Statement of Changes in Immigration Rules 1994, paras 320-321. See also Immigration Act 1971, s 4, Sch 2, para 7.
6   Standing Medical Advisory Committee for the Central Health Services Council *Immunization against Infectious Diseases* (1972).

shock. More commonly, the organisms in the vaccine may reactivate an abnormal condition present in the recipient—classic examples are skin eczema after vaccination against smallpox and convulsions after whooping-cough immunisation. The vaccine may cause a modified form of the disease it is intended to prevent—some children, for instance, suffer what is apparently a mild attack of measles following inoculation. In the case of live virus vaccines, the growth may not be pure—yellow fever vaccines that are grown on eggs may contain viruses that have been infecting the eggs themselves. A more serious, though similar, possibility arises when the virus has been attenuated in animals, in which case, natural animal viruses may become contaminants; this is of special significance when primates closely related to man have been used. Such complications have been virtually eliminated in modern manufacture. Of greater practical importance is the possibility that antibodies may be provoked not only to the desired antigen, but also to the medium in which it is prepared. Thus, the original form of anti-rabies vaccine was grown in nervous tissue; there was a possibility that anti-nervous tissue antibody could be formed in the recipient with disastrous results within his own brain.[7]

A further danger lies in the potential effects on pregnancy. This is a hazard almost specific to those vaccines composed of living viruses; these may cause abortion or, more seriously, may damage the growing fetus if given within the first three months of intrauterine life. This last possibility is particularly evident in immunisation against German measles, a fairly predictable chance in that the only purpose in immunising is to prevent a true attack of the disease during childbearing. The likelihood of damage to the fetus is such that a guarantee of contraception for at least 60 days is required of a woman before she can be immunised against rubella.[8]

Formidable though the contraindications may seem, the risks of immunisation must be contrasted with the dangers of inadequate control of the relevant diseases; looked at in this way, the hazards as a whole are very slight.[9] Nevertheless, complications do occur and raise difficulties when public policy is involved; the Vaccine Damage Payments Act 1979 represents a pragmatic solution to the problems. Under this very limited statute, a lump sum[10] is payable to a minor who can be shown to have been severely disabled as a result of vaccination carried out as part of the public health campaign.[11] The same sum is payable when the damage was inflicted before birth or to a person who is affected through contact with another who has been immunised.[12] This legislation does not exclude the

---

7 The vaccine is now produced in duck embryos or in human diploid cells.
8 The congenital rubella syndrome has been a frequent cause for so-called 'wrongful birth' actions—in which the mother claims that she would have had a termination had she been properly advised—and 'wrongful life' actions—whereby the neonate who has been accidentally infected is effectively claiming that he or she was deprived of the right to be aborted. Actions of the latter type will not succeed in the United Kingdom: *McKay v Essex Area Health Authority* [1982] QB 1166.
9 Although, clearly, the balance need not necessarily be the same. Diphtheria immunisation is, for example, virtually without risk while the disease is extremely dangerous; vaccination against cholera is again without risk but its protective value is very slight.
10 Now £40,000: Statutory Sum Order 1998, SI 1998/1587.
11 For discussion of the causal link, see R Goldberg 'Vaccine Damage and Causation —Social and Legal Implications' (1996) J Law Soc Scot 100.
12 Vaccine Damage Payments Regulations 1979, SI 1979/432, reg 5A. The vaccination procedures covered involve immunisation against diphtheria, tetanus, whooping cough, poliomyelitis, measles, rubella, tuberculosis, smallpox and any other disease specified by regulation including mumps and *Haemophilus* influenza type B, SIs 1990/623, 1995/1164.

application of the wider social security provisions for disabled persons,[13] nor does it inhibit an action for damages in the event of medical negligence (see Chapter 30). Such negligence would be shown only if the doctor had failed to follow accepted practice—for example, it might be suggested as being negligent to immunise against whooping cough a child who was known to suffer from convulsions, or to continue with a course of vaccination when the first dose had precipitated a convulsion.[14] Even so, the balancing of the risks of contracting the disease against the risks of its prevention is a matter of clinical judgment; negligence would be difficult to prove in the majority of cases.[15]

Persons travelling abroad present a special problem. There are two types of active immunisation involved—those procedures undertaken for the obvious benefit of the individual, of which immunisation against poliomyelitis and typhoid fever are good examples, and those that are required by the health authorities of the countries to be visited before entry is permitted. The former category poses little difficulty. If a woman is pregnant or has an infant child and wishes to travel to an area in which an immune state would be desirable but, at the same time, involves an injection that might present an above-average risk to her fetus or child, she should be warned of the dangers both of immunisation and of travel while non-immune and should be given appropriate advice including that of postponing her travel. The choice is then up to the patient within the terms of 'informed consent' as discussed in Chapter 31. Travel to countries that insist on certain vaccinations poses difficulty if it is necessary during high-risk periods. In certain circumstances, such as travel from an area known to be free of a particular disease, a certificate giving a valid reason for non-vaccination may be acceptable; in other cases, for example, in travel from an area where yellow fever exists to one where it could be introduced, a period of quarantine on arrival may have to be accepted. The problem is, however, of less practical importance than might be supposed; a real risk for the fetus from the international requirements probably exists only in the case of smallpox vaccination and this is no longer required for travellers.

The dangers of passive immunisation are of a different type but are very real. Antibodies are produced in the blood of animals. Therefore, when an antibody is injected, foreign antigens derived from the animal are also introduced and an immune reaction of varying severity may be established. This is of wide forensic importance due to the frequency with which anti-tetanus antibodies need to be given after wounds of all sorts. In many cases it might be at least arguable that the dangers of passive immunisation were greater than the likelihood of contracting tetanus; but in the event of misjudgment, it would be difficult to defend an accusation of negligence in the light of previous decisions.[16] Such dilemmas should, in practice, become very much rarer if the official policy of active immunisation against tetanus in childhood is widely followed—the correct procedure in a wounded person who has been previously immunised is to boost the active immunity with a fresh dose of antigen; this carries no risk of an untoward species reaction.

13 Social Security and Child Support (Decision and Appeals), Vaccine Damage Payments and Job Seekers' Allowance (Amendment) Regulations 1999, SI1999/2677.
14 For advice as to vaccination in difficult circumstances, see *Thomson v James* (1996) 31 BMLR 1, QBD, revsd (1997) 41 BMLR 144, CA.
15 The major hurdle being that of causation: *Bonthrone v Secretary of State for Scotland* 1987 SLT 34; *Loveday v Renton* [1990] 1 Med LR 117. But a case has succeeded in the Supreme Court of Ireland: *Best (an infant) v Wellcome Foundation Ltd* (1992) 17 BMLR 11— based, inter alia, on the application of common sense.
16 For example, *Coles v Reading and District Hospital Management Committee* (1963) 107 Sol Jo 115.

7

Sudden natural death

The mechanism of sudden natural death

Between 75% and 80% of the cases coming to autopsy at the hands of the English coroner's pathologist are found to have died from natural causes. Even in Scotland, where a high proportion of such deaths are certified without dissection, many medico-legal post-mortem examinations fail to disclose anything unnatural. The proportions differ very much from city to city and, particularly, as between city and rural areas; even so, a diagnosis of death due to natural disease is likely to be made in more than half of the fiscal's cases that are examined internally. These cases, therefore, form an essential part of forensic medicine, both in their own right and also because it is impossible to appreciate properly the medico-legal interactions between trauma—particularly that due to accidents—and incapacitating disease without a knowledge of the mechanisms underlying the latter.

For present purposes, 'sudden death' is defined as unexpected death following so rapidly from the onset of symptoms that the cause of death could not be certified with confidence by a medical practitioner who was asked to review the case. While the present author feels that the risk is exaggerated, it has to be admitted that it is this type of death that is most likely to conceal a 'secret homicide'—and, as we have already noted (at page 76), this is particularly so if the person responsible is a health care professional. Sudden death of this sort is almost entirely a matter of disease of the cardiovascular system[1] and will be discussed as such, first in relation to the immediacy of death and, secondly, as to the age of those affected.

In order of increasing suddenness, death may be due to haemorrhage from vessels, to peripheral blockage of vessels or to inhibition of the heart's action (see Figure 7.1).

The mode of death due to *haemorrhage* depends on two main factors—on the size of the vessel that bleeds and, when internal, on the ability of the cavity

---

1   In one study of sudden natural death carried out in London, 66.5% of the deaths were due to heart disease and a further 27.6% were due to non-cardiac cardiovascular disease: A C Thomas, P A Knapman, D M Krikler and M J Davies 'Community Study of the Causes of "Natural" Sudden Death' (1988) 297 BMJ 1453. Although this study is relatively old, there is no reason to suppose that the figures are very different today.

involved to accommodate the blood shed and of the contained organs to continue to function normally. The effects of bleeding from a small vessel should be less than from a larger one but, given the same size of small vessels in the cranial cavity and in the abdomen, the effect in the latter may be slight while it may be lethal in the former because of the resulting compressive effects on the brain.

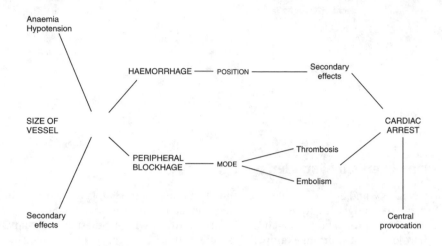

Figure 7.1 Factors involved in sudden death related to the cardiovascular system.

The effect of *blockage of a peripheral vessel* is determined by the nature of the part deprived of blood, by the size of the vessel blocked and by the method of occlusion. The primary effect of arterial occlusion on an organ or area is to deprive it of oxygen; the secondary effect on the body as a whole depends on the function of that organ. Thus, a man can well survive a portion of his spleen being deprived of blood, but closure of a vessel supplying the respiratory centre in the brain will cause immediate death. The effect of the size of vessel is obvious—one might be able to withstand the sudden elimination of a lobule of lung, but sudden obstruction of a main pulmonary artery would almost inevitably be fatal. Three main processes lead to blockage of an artery. The slowest in effect is restriction of the lumen due to thickening of the wall. This process is one for which the body is often able to compensate by the development of new vessels—known as a collateral circulation. An urgent need for extra oxygen in the organ supplied by the vessel or a very rapid exacerbation of the restrictive thickening may result in sudden incompetence; the subject is discussed later in the context of coronary disease. A faster method of preventing blood flow is provided by local *thrombosis*, that is, abnormal clotting of the blood within a vessel.[2] Generalised (or disseminated)

---

2   Normal thrombosis is, of course, an important constituent of the control of bleeding. Abnormal, intravascular thrombosis—and, particularly, venous thrombosis—can be precipitated by relative stasis of the local circulation, local injury to the vessel wall and abnormality of the clotting mechanism (known collectively as Virchow's triad). The conditions are likely to coincide in the post-operative state.

intravascular coagulation occurs in surgical shock and in other conditions but the common presentation considered here is that of a single clot forming round a localised area of damage to the vessel lining. Clots of this type may arise in arteries or in veins. In addition to the dangers inherent in obstructing what may be a vitally important vessel, such as a cerebral or coronary artery, conditions are set up for the third and most rapid form of blockage which is known as *embolism*. In this condition, fragments of preformed clot break off. If this occurs in an artery, the particles are forced into vessels of decreasing size until they lodge and cause a sudden deprivation of blood to the parts beyond, the process being known as *infarction*—death of a particularly sudden type will occur if a major cerebral vessel is embolised.[3] If the clot that disintegrates is located in a vein, it passes to the right side of the heart where, if large enough, it will occlude the main pulmonary artery but, if smaller, will pass into the lung until it can go no further; this is the condition of *pulmonary embolism* which is a common cause of death in persons immobilised in bed, and whose blood tends to clot in the leg veins as a result.[4]

The heart action may be inhibited by any of these processes. The heart itself may perforate, in which case the blood held within the pericardial sac stifles the normal heart action mechanically—this condition is known as *cardiac tamponade*. There can be blockage of the coronary vessels, which supply the heart muscle, either by thickening of the walls, by thrombosis or by embolism. The feature distinguishing these occlusions from those occurring in peripheral vessels of comparable size is that sudden deprivation of oxygen in even a small area of heart tissue which is vital to its rhythmic function inhibits the action of the heart as a whole; the contractions become ineffective, the condition of *ventricular fibrillation* is set up and the tissues throughout the body are immediately deprived of oxygen. Additionally, any disease of the heart muscle—whether it be inflammatory, toxic or simply due to excessive imposed loads—may, at a particular moment, become sufficiently severe to stop the heart beat and to cause sudden death. Finally, inhibition of the heart through abnormal stimulation of its regulatory nerves must be mentioned; the concept of vagal inhibition of the heart action, which was introduced on page 14, is referred to at many points in this text.

These various processes are likely to present at different times in life; the underlying causes of sudden death must be related to age if their forensic significance is to be appreciated.

In infancy and early childhood

Death in this age group is discussed in detail in Chapter 19. Many sudden infant deaths are associated with congenital cardiovascular malformations; the presence of these will have been known previously and death will not be unexpected— they are, therefore, beyond the definition of sudden death that is adopted here. This age group, into which the important group of so-called 'cot deaths' occurs, provides the exception to the rule that sudden unexpected death is almost entirely

3   This may occur when thrombus has formed in the left side of the heart due to valvular disease of the heart.
4   Strictly speaking, this type of embolism should be referred to as thrombotic embolism. Embolism by itself is a generic term for the process whereby vessels are blocked by particles of any sort. Thus we have conditions such as fat embolism, air embolism or embolism by particles of tumour etc, but the origins in each instance are quite distinct.

associated with the cardiovascular system. Although it has been suggested that some 'cot deaths' may be due to primary disease of the heart, this is plainly not the common cause. A proportion of these baffling cases may be due to fulminating viral infection and, certainly, many sudden deaths in early childhood do result unequivocally from infection—either of the brain (meningitis), the lungs (pneumonia) or the bowel (enteritis). Such disease states can progress very quickly; allegations of negligence on the part of the doctor may well be made on the grounds of his or her failure to attend the child with sufficient haste—and this will be particularly so should the child die or be severely handicapped as a result.[5] The pathologist's role will then be critical. He may well be able to ascertain the cause of death but he will be asked to go further as to the *reason* for the death. The extent and severity of the disease process may provide some indications as to the treatability of the condition but, as applies in so many aspects of forensic pathology, the pathologist does well to remember that, save in unusual circumstances, he is not a clinician.

In the young adult

Bleeding in the form of subarachnoid haemorrhage is, perhaps, the most important process under this heading and, since subarachnoid haemorrhage is also a frequent result of injury, the cases are of particular medico-legal significance.

The common form of naturally occurring subarachnoid haemorrhage is of congenital origin. As a result of malformation of the muscle wall, balloon-like swellings, known as *berry aneurysms*, form in the cerebral arteries at the base of the brain, most commonly at one of the comparatively abrupt, geometric junctions in the area. The wall of the aneurysm is thin and is liable to rupture. The resulting pressure effect of the extruded blood is particularly concentrated on the vital centres of the brain and can cause sudden unexpected death. Often, it is the death rather than the symptoms that is sudden—the steady build-up of pressure due to a relatively slow leak of blood may cause a severe headache for several hours but such premonitory signs are often overlooked.

The distinction between natural disease and injury as a cause of subarachnoid haemorrhage is not always a simple matter. Trauma may rupture even normal cerebral vessels; although there is some difference of opinion among various researchers as to the true cause-and-effect relationship, it is logical to suppose that abnormally weak arteries could be damaged by abnormally slight force. Similarly, while most berry aneurysms rupture in the absence of a permanently raised blood pressure, it would be hard to deny the probability that a transient rise in pressure could predispose to 'blow-out'. The contribution of an altercation to such a death may therefore be doubly difficult to interpret.[6] Aneurysms may be so small as to be invisible and, occasionally, it may be impossible to demonstrate a specific bleeding point; it has to be said, however, that one can be found more

5   In *Stockdale v Nicholls* [1993] 4 Med LR 190 a practitioner was sued for failing to attend and sending his practice nurse to see to a sick child; the court found him not to be negligent. Irrespective of an action in negligence, the physician who fails to attend a sick patient may be accountable to the health authority and, subsequently, to the General Medical Council.

6   There is a tendency not to prosecute such cases in the English courts. A very useful, although rather old, review of this difficult subject is by B Knight 'Trauma and ruptured cerebral aneurysm' (1979) i BMJ 1430.

often than not and failure to do so must raise a suspicion of an unnatural cause for the discovered haemorrhage—injury to the neck is particularly important in this respect (see Chapter 11).

The inclusion of the condition in a section devoted to the young adult does not imply that it does not also occur in older age groups; it most certainly does, and studies have drawn attention to the increasing average age at which spontaneous subarachnoid bleeding occurs.[7] The incidence in older persons is increased by rupture occurring in cerebral vessels damaged by the degenerative disease of atheroma. Death is surprisingly often associated with straining on the lavatory pan.

Intracerebral haemorrhage is rare in young persons. When it occurs, it is likely to be due to bleeding into a tumour of the brain which may be primary but which is more likely to be secondary to a tumour of the genital system. Haemorrhage into cerebral tumours is a more common cause of death in elderly persons, secondary deposits from the stomach and lung being the most common findings.

Acute haemorrhagic deaths in young women may result from bleeding due to growth of the fetus in an abnormal position—the so-called *ectopic gestation* which results from the ovum 'losing its way' or being 'held up' in its passage to the cavity of the uterus. Such catastrophes have been largely eliminated by modern antenatal care but, despite the virtual disappearance of criminal abortion, it is still probably true that, from the medico-legal point of view, sudden death in a young woman should be suspected of being associated with pregnancy until proved otherwise.

Apart from such relatively obvious causes, the diagnosis of natural sudden death in young persons may present considerable difficulty. In some instances, the deaths appear to be due to one of a group of primary diseases of the heart muscle collectively known as cardiomyopathies. Occasionally, a toxic origin may be shown for such diseases—alcoholic cardiomyopathy is a good example; more often there is an abnormality of growth, one side of the heart being greatly enlarged. This condition is known as *asymmetric hypertrophic cardiomyopathy*. Either side of the heart may enlarge. One possible mechanism of death is that an enlarged left ventricle occludes the outlets into the great vessels but, alternatively, the increasing bulk of muscle may outstrip the capacity of the coronary arteries to supply the muscle mass with oxygen, a concept that is discussed further below. Dysplasia, or degeneration of the right side of the heart is, also, not infrequently associated with sudden death in apparently healthy athletes.[8] On other occasions, 'inflammation' of the heart muscle, so-called *myocarditis*, has been invoked as a cause of obscure deaths. The condition may be due to true infection, usually of viral type, to an allergic reaction or to disorders of the endocrine system— eg overactivity of the thyroid gland. These abnormalities can be diagnosed only by a microscopic examination and are characterised by collections of white blood cells in the muscle of the heart. While such a finding may satisfy some observers, others are sceptical of their true significance; the distinction between findings that are causative of death and those that are purely incidental is discussed in Chapter 10.

7 D A L Bowen 'Ruptured Berry Aneurysms: A Clinical, Pathological and Forensic Review' (1984) 26 Forens Sci Int 227.
8 A Coumbe, A L Perez-Martinez, A W Fegan and I R Hill 'Arrhythmogenic right ventricular dysplasia (ARVD): an overlooked and underdiagnosed condition?' (1997) 37 Med Sci Law 262.

Often, nothing significant is found and sudden deaths in young adults may be as obscure as are cot deaths in infants.[9] Such a situation arises, again, in fit young people who have recently taken part in athletic pursuits. In the author's experience, a relatively common feature appears to be an enlargement of the spleen suggesting convalescence from a recent infection—possibly infectious mononucleosis or glandular fever. Microbiological studies are, however, consistently negative, and the cases remain as a distressingly inexplicable group. Rather than certify death on extremely tenuous grounds in order to satisfy the registrar, it would be better to classify such cases under, say, 'sudden unexplained death in young adults'; such a policy would at least serve to stimulate research into an unexplored field.[10]

In later years

Sudden death in late middle age is dominated by degenerative changes in the vessels of the cardiovascular system.

The main degenerative change is atheroma, in which the wall of the vessel is replaced by fatty material which, breaking down, leaves a greatly weakened structure. In the absence of surrounding support, the tendency is for such a diseased vessel to dilate—an aneurysm is formed. The commonest site is in the abdominal aorta—rupture is progressive and the symptoms of abdominal pain may well result in the patient's admission to hospital; death is, however, eventually very rapid as the blood intended for the lower limbs is poured into the abdominal cavity. Almost instantaneous death may result from a rather similar process known as 'dissecting aneurysm'—so-called because the blood passes *within* the wall of the vessel before being released. This occurs predominantly at the origin of the aorta; the blood may sometimes be forced back into the pericardial sac and sudden death is due to cardiac tamponade.[11] Deep vessels in the brain may be weakened by atheroma and, in the event of rupture, will cause intracerebral haemorrhage, while massive haemorrhage into the intestine may follow erosion of a vessel at the base of an ulcer in the stomach or duodenum; such deaths are only occasionally entirely unheralded.

Rupture of arteries is more likely in the presence of a raised blood pressure—hypertensive heart disease is a potent cause of sudden death in this age group. Apart from the peripheral catastrophes that may occur, the heart itself—which enlarges in order to perform more work—may 'outgrow its strength' and suddenly fail, a mechanism that is discussed below. High blood pressure is not, however, the only cause of steady enlargement of the heart; disease of the heart valves—in particular, narrowing (*stenosis*) or incompetence of the aortic valve—may provoke

9 'SUDS' is particularly well—although not exclusively—recognised in Asian and Middle Eastern communities but, here, as in cot deaths or 'SIDS'—the sudden infant death syndrome—the unexpected death occurs in sleep: M A Elfawal 'Sudden unexplained death syndrome' (2000) 40 Med Sci Law 45.

10 See M J Davies 'Unexplained Death in Fit Young People' (1992) 305 BMJ 538. See also *Inquest into the Death of Alan Massie*, Warrington, reported by, inter alia, D Skentelbery 'Junior Doctor Died of Natural Causes, Says Coroner' (1994) 309 BMJ 1530. It is to be noted that the coroner found this case to be so important that he used his option of reporting the matter to the Department of Health (see Chapter 2).

11 A comparison of the two main forms of aneurysm is made in: D Fothergill, D A L Bowen and J K Mason 'Dissecting and Atherosclerotic Aneurysms: A Survey of Post-mortem Examinations, 1968-1977' (1979) 19 Med Sci Law 253.

the same effects. Valvular disease of this type is, however, now relatively uncommon as compared with 50 or 60 years ago. Physiological abnormality of the heart valves still occurs and is a recognised cause of death; the lawyer may be confronted with the diagnosis of *floppy mitral valve* which is the paradigm of such conditions—but, again, the mere presence of such a valve is no proof that it caused death.

Coronary heart disease

The subject of coronary heart disease has been left until last because its ability to kill is almost all-embracing in its age span—deaths from this cause have been reported in men aged 19 and, indeed, the younger the subject, the more likely is the first 'coronary attack' to be fatal.[12] Death from coronary heart disease is, however, most common in the period of life from age 45 onwards and, from that point, it becomes the commonest single cause of death in most industrialised countries. It is by far the most important cause of sudden death and there are very few other causes of instantaneous death. Inevitably, a high proportion of such cases are reported to the coroner or the fiscal. Some understanding of the disease process is essential to the lawyer because of its frequent appearance in pathology reports; the disease also has important associations with accidents, particularly of industrial or vehicular type, and many insurance companies attach much significance to coronary artery disease in relation to life expectation and compensation.

The heart, like any other muscle, depends on an efficient blood supply to provide it with energy. But, whereas most muscles have a comparatively simple action, the heart must contract constantly and rhythmically. This sophisticated action is controlled by aggregations of nerve tissue known as 'nodes', from which extend 'bundles' of conducting tissue; if any of these specialised areas are deprived of oxygen, the muscle as a whole will beat in an arrhythmic fashion—ventricular fibrillation is established and the efficient pumping action ceases. It follows that localised ischaemia of the heart muscle may cause instantaneous death. Deprivation of oxygen in other than an essential area will cause localised ischaemic death of muscle but, very often, this dead area can be repaired by the process of fibrosis or scar formation. A 'coronary attack' has been survived, but the heart wall may be thinned and dangerously short of blood—a pathological process that has struck once is likely to do so again; a person in this situation is, therefore, a bad risk in respect of certain occupations. Oxygen deprivation of a large area of muscle is likely to be fatal because insufficient useful tissue remains; death in such circumstances may be a longer process than it is when a vital area is involved.

The blood supply to the heart is carried by the left and right coronary arteries which normally are of adequate bore. But, for reasons that are not entirely understood, most persons' coronary arteries silt up as a natural process of ageing—the condition is that of progressive coronary atheroma. The process is something like the furring of hot-water pipes but, in the case of the arteries, the atheromatous

12 Death from coronary disease in young persons is sometimes genetically determined by way of the disease 'familial hypercholesterolaemia'. It is probable that most coronary disease is genetically affected but, in this case, the genetic influence is of the multifactorial type that is equally determined by the environment (see page 272).

material, which consists of fat and connective tissue, is laid down *within* the inner lining of the vessel.[13] The body's main defence against the process lies in the establishment of a collateral circulation, which is effective so long as the occlusive process is slow. But this may not always be so. The thick atheromatous plaques require a blood supply of their own and, not infrequently, the walls of the minute vessels will give way—the condition of *intramural haemorrhage* is established and the bore or lumen of the vessel is *suddenly* occluded. Very often, the plaques degenerate without haemorrhage and a necrotic 'abscess' forms which may itself rupture, leading to sudden *atheromatous restriction* of the lumen; in each case, bursting results in *disruption of the intima* which may form a valve-like obstruction to the flow of blood. Finally, the blood in contact with a diseased area tends to clot in situ and the process of *coronary thrombosis* is superimposed on coronary atheroma.[14] The significance of thrombosis in sudden cardiac death is to some extent controversial. Although it is common lay practice to speak of coronary occlusion as thrombosis, the two conditions do not necessarily go hand in hand. It has been stated that thrombi are found less commonly in cases reported to the coroner or fiscal than in those dying in hospital, but the degree of disparity depends on such variables as preselection of cases for dissection and the intensity of search. Thrombosis is, however, not *essential* to the post-mortem diagnosis of a coronary death—many of these are physiological in nature and may be due to localised spasm of the arteries. Similarly, the anatomical result of ischaemia of the muscle—infarction—is not always seen at autopsy; death due to ventricular fibrillation may have been too rapid for the formation of visible changes. The possibility that many apparent thrombi are, in fact, post-mortem in origin must also be considered although it is an academic rather than a practical problem—post-mortem clots are unlikely to form in the absence of a significant ante-mortem abnormality.

The above description refers to acute coronary insufficiency arising at a specific point in the arterial tree. An equally common situation is that in which a sudden increase in cardiac effort is demanded—due either to a physical or to an emotional stimulus—and in which the diseased circulation is unable to expand so as to satisfy the immediate need for increased oxygen; this is the typical situation in the witness who collapses in the witness box. Inadequacy of this type is particularly prevalent in those in whom the atheromatous process has advanced to calcification, with consequent rigidity of the arterial walls, and in those whose arteries have been severely affected by heavy smoking. These cases pose a difficulty in pathological interpretation—death is due to a failure of response, and the circulation will have the same appearance after death as it would have done had it been possible to examine it in life; much of the diagnosis must rest, therefore, on the circumstantial evidence or, if none is available, on the absence of any other cause of death. At the end of the day, however, it has to be, and has long been,[15] said that the pathologist, faced with a physiological death, will attribute death to

13 There is now relatively convincing evidence that alcohol protects the individual from 'coronary death': eg R Jackson, R Scragg and R Beaglehole 'Alcohol Consumption and Risk of Coronary Heart Disease' (1991) 303 BMJ 211. More recently, M Bobak, Z Skodova and M Marmot 'Effect of beer drinking on risk of myocardial infarction: population based case-control study' (2000) 320 BMJ 1378.
14 There is very strong correlation between death from coronary disease and smoking. Smoking has a profound effect on coagulation of the blood.
15 See the archetypal work on the subject: T Crawford *Pathology of Ischaemic Heart Disease* (1977) pp 23 and 77.

the one anatomic abnormality he can find—coronary atheroma—and will give the cause of death as 'coronary insufficiency' in order to satisfy the needs of the coroner or fiscal; the pathologist supposes that this is true but there is often no positive evidence that it is an accurate assessment.

This physiological type of coronary death relates in the main to inadequate arteries supplying a heart of normal size. Much the same situation will obtain if normal-sized arteries are required to maintain a heart of abnormally increased bulk. Potential examples of this have already been noted—the heart in hypertension, suffering from the effects of valvular disease or enlarged due to cardiomyopathy. Persons so affected are living dangerously, because a sudden requirement for oxygen may be beyond the immediate capacity of the relatively small vessels. Sudden death can result but, again, the findings at autopsy will need careful interpretation. The processes are illustrated in Figure 7.2.

Many of the natural sudden deaths described thus far are precipitated by the need for increased cardiac output. Major forensic significance therefore attaches to the conditions leading to that demand because these must be regarded as the basic cause of dying. Thus, the association of disease and death at work is of far-reaching importance in relation to benefits under the Social Security Act; this is discussed in Chapter 15. Disease may also cause vehicular accidents which are discussed in Chapter 10, but falls in the house, drowning and many other types of apparently violent death may be precipitated by natural disease. Natural disease is clearly of importance in the evaluation of homicide. Severe disease discovered in a man dying during a fracas may provide grounds for a plea to reduce a charge of murder to one of manslaughter or culpable homicide. It may, contrariwise, aggravate an offence. In a case seen by the author, a man seated in a locked parked car was threatened by a passer-by—he died suddenly and autopsy revealed extensive coronary disease with fibrosis of the heart muscle; although there had been no physical contact, the assailant was convicted of culpable homicide.

If the foregoing represents the normal sequence of events, it might be asked, 'Why do so many coronary deaths occur during sleep?' The answer is unclear. It has been suggested that lowering of the blood pressure, which occurs during the early stages of sleep, may predispose to the formation of thrombi (or clots) within diseased and narrowed vessels. But it has also been shown that the blood pressure rises erratically during sleep, possibly associated with dreams, and the effect is a subconscious demand for increased oxygen supply. Such cases do not necessarily invalidate the general hypothesis discussed above.

Causes of sudden death other than cardiovascular in adults

In practice, only two conditions merit space under this heading.

Asthma can undoubtedly cause sudden death. The incidence of death is rising although it is still relatively uncommon. Severely affected persons may enter a condition of grave respiratory difficulty known as *status asthmaticus*. This may occur, but it is not essential to the valid attribution of death to asthma as sufferers seem to be unduly susceptible to sudden collapse.[16] It has long been suggested

16 For a good overall review, see E R McFadden and E L Warren 'Observations on Asthma Mortality' (1997) 127 Ann Int Med 142. An asthmatic death raised an interesting aspect of coroners' law. In *R v Poplar Coroner, ex p Thomas* [1993] QB 610, a delay in the arrival of an ambulance did not alter the fact that death from a severe asthmatic attack was of natural type.

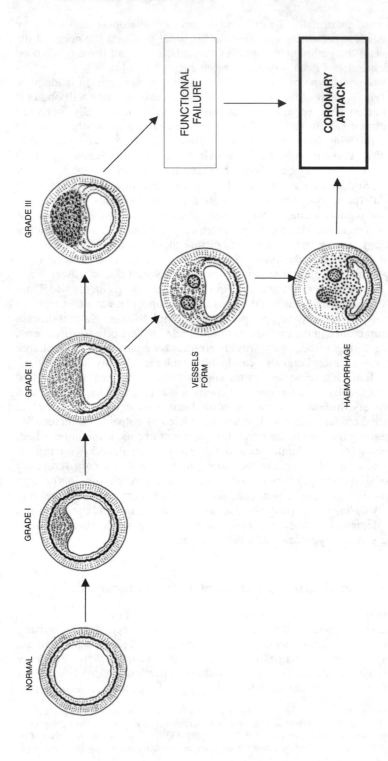

Figure 7.2 Development of a coronary attack. Atheroma forms, Grade II disease representing more than 50% restriction of the lumen. The plaque becomes vascularised and haemorrhage results in sudden occlusion. Alternatively, calcified arteries may not be able to dilate to satisfy an urgent need for increased blood supply. It should be noted that simple Grade II disease may lead to insufficiency if the muscle mass of the heart increases without an increase in vessels.

that these deaths may, in fact, be due to the general use of potent drug therapy rather than to the underlying condition, and certainly this is an aspect that should be investigated whenever such a case presents; the problem attracted a deal of media attention following an 'epidemic' of asthma mortality in New Zealand.[17]

Epilepsy is in a rather similar category. *Status epilepticus*, a long-sustained epileptic attack, is a well-known cause of death. But epileptics are subject to sudden death in the absence of such obvious symptoms and, again, the pathological diagnosis is then, essentially, a matter of exclusion and history-taking.[18] This form of sudden natural death is additional to the extrinsic dangers of an epileptic attack, such as falling from a height or drowning.

17 There is considerable debate as to whether the deaths were, in fact, mainly attributable to the drug fenoterol: N Pearce, R Beasley, J Crane et al 'End of the New Zealand Asthma Mortality Epidemic' (1995) 345 Lancet 41.
18 In one series, 34% of sudden deaths in young adults were attributed to epilepsy: F K Bennani and C E Connolly 'Sudden unexpected death in young adults including four cases of SADS: a 10-year review from the West of Ireland (1985-1994)' (1997) 37 Med Sci Law 242.

8

Wounding

The law

From the purely medical aspect, anything that entails damage to the body tissues can be described as a wound, but it is more colloquial to speak of an accidental wound—or any wound caused other than by an instrument—as an injury; a wound is an injury inflicted by another party or is self-inflicted. Medically speaking, wounds and injuries are a single pathological entity. A division of injuries on legal grounds is to some extent artificial and, since the basic problem in the pathology of violence is to distinguish between accident, suicide and homicide, it is almost impossible to discuss one category to the exclusion of the other two. For the purpose of this chapter, wounds are defined as injuries arising from an assault. So far as is possible, self-inflicted and accidental injuries will be discussed only in relation to differential diagnosis; some overlap is, however, inevitable.

The law on wounding in England and Wales is governed by the Offences Against the Person Act 1861 which itemises various offences.

Wounding or causing grievous bodily harm with the intent to do so or with intent to resist lawful arrest are considered in s 18, while s 20 describes the offence of maliciously wounding or inflicting grievous bodily harm either with or without the use of any weapon or instrument. Injury may be 'inflicted' with or without the corollary of an assault,[1] injury 'caused' without the use of force can be indicted under s 18 provided it is intended and grievous. Assault occasioning actual bodily harm is the subject of s 47. Sections 42 and 43 have now been repealed and the separate common law offences of assault and battery are now confirmed as such by the Criminal Justice Act 1988, s 39.[2] An assault may involve no more than causing a person, either intentionally or recklessly, to anticipate immediate violence;[3] a battery, however, involves the infliction of personal violence—albeit

---

1   *R v Wilson* [1983] 3 All ER 448.
2   But it seems that battery can be subsumed under assault if it makes for rationality: *R v Lynsey* [1995] 3 All ER 654.
3   *R v Ireland; R v Burstow* [1997] 4 All ER 225, HL—silent telephone calls constituted an assault.

no more than an unwanted touching.[4] Assaults and batteries which involve no element of aggravation may, of course, be actionable at civil law.[5] The nature of a wound is not defined, but there is case law[6] to indicate that a wound must involve a break in the whole skin, which would include a similar injury to a contiguous mucous membrane.[7] The point is relatively unimportant, as the alternative charges of causing actual or grievous bodily harm will cover bruising or more serious injuries such as may result in fracture without skin damage.[8]

In Scotland, an assault is an attack on the person of another for which punishment is not specified in any rule. An assault is, however, aggravated, for example, by the use of firearms, stabbing or by throwing corrosive substances. An assault that causes injury is likely to be more severely punished than is one that does not. Assault 'to severe injury' may be libelled, ie specified in the indictment, and it is a very severe aggravation to assault 'to the danger of life'—which can be specified whether or not there were injuries.[9] The attack can be direct, indirect or simply one involving threatening gestures—provided that it is sufficient to cause alarm. In general, there must be intent to do harm although it remains an offence to cause injury recklessly.[10]

Murder—the ultimate in wounding—is defined in England as the unlawful killing of a reasonable creature in being with malice aforethought, either express or implied.[11] In Scotland, voluntary murder is simply murder committed intentionally. The English concept of 'constructive malice'—that is, unintentional killing while committing some other offence—has been abolished[12] and the offence is now that of manslaughter. In Scotland, the difference between involuntary murder—that is murder committed without the intention to kill—and culpable homicide is blurred; in general, the former must be accompanied by 'wicked recklessness'—unintentional killing short of this is culpable homicide. The Scottish concept of 'reckless murder' has no place in English jurisprudence where intention is essential to the crime—although it is sufficient that the intention was to cause grievous bodily harm only.[13] This chapter is concerned, however, not so much with the law on homicidal wounding as with the general, non-specific, body responses and pathological evidence that may follow wounding or injury; specialised injuries, such as those due to heat or gunshot, are discussed in separate chapters (14 and 9 respectively).

4 *Collins v Wilcock* [1984] 3 All ER 374, in which an exception was made for 'all physical contact which is generally acceptable in the ordinary conduct of daily life' (per Goff LJ at 378). While consent may form a defence to mere assault, it is restricted when the assault involves bodily harm: *R v Brown* [1994] 1 AC 212. But see *R v Wilson (Alan Thomas)* [1997] QB 47 where there was 'no aggressive intent' between husband and wife.
5 No such distinction is made in Scots law where a criminal assault is generally taken to involve an element of 'attack'.
6 *R v M'Loughlin* (1838) 8 C & P 635.
7 By contrast, intraocular haemorrhage resulting from a blow without damage to the cornea was *not* considered to be a wound in the legal sense: *C (a minor) v Eisenhower* [1984] QB 331.
8 *R v Wood* (1830) 1 Mood CC 278.
9 *Kerr v HM Advocate* 1986 SCCR 91. See T H Jones and M G A Christie *Criminal Law* (1992) p 177.
10 *HM Advocate v Harris* 1993 SCCR 559.
11 The rule under which death must occur within 'a year and a day' has been repealed: Law Reform (Year and a Day Rule) Act 1996.
12 Homicide Act 1957, s 1.
13 An aspect of the law which is subject to much criticism. See *A-G's Reference (No 3) of 1994* [1998] 1 Cr App Rep 91 at 102 per Lord Mustill.

Bruises

Even though the skin is not broken, the subcutaneous tissues—those beneath the skin—may be damaged by blunt violence; the resulting extravasation of blood from broken vessels constitutes a bruise (Figure 8.1).

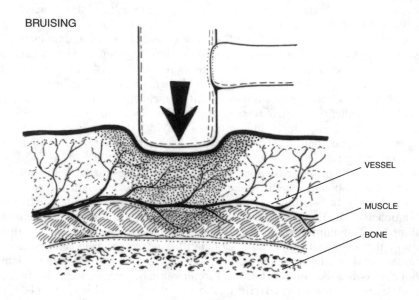

BRUISING

VESSEL

MUSCLE

BONE

Figure 8.1 Bruising. Subcutaneous capillaries may rupture when the skin is struck by a blunt object with insufficient force to break the skin; blood is then extruded into the surrounding tissues. A bruise is, therefore, a form of subcutaneous laceration.

Bruising results from bleeding *into* the tissues. A wound caused by a clean cut with a knife seldom results in bruising as the blood escapes through vessels that are damaged only on the edges of the cut. Bruising can, however, surround a laceration of the skin if that breach has been caused by a blunt object; in that case, there may be damage to the vessels internal to the cut surface and blood will escape in both directions. The extent of bruising is, in general, inversely proportional to the sharpness of the object inflicting a wound.

The appearances of bruising without laceration of the skin are not uniform and depend on several factors. First, the part involved is important—the more lax the tissue, the easier it is for the blood to spread; the tissues around the eye, for example, will bruise far more readily than will the firm tissues of the back—hence the characteristic widespread 'black eye'. Secondly, there is the age of the person— blow for blow, children and old people bruise more easily than do young adults or the middle aged; an assessment of the force involved must take these factors into consideration. Thirdly, extravasated blood will move along the tissue lines of least resistance; the *shape* of a bruise may thus have, and probably will have, little relation to the agent causing it and its shape may change with time. Along with this, the *position* of a bruise may vary with gravity; indeed, a deep bruise of, say, the thigh muscles may be invisible on the surface until the blood racks down the fascial planes and presents beneath the skin of the knee.

Thus, the external evidence of bruising may alter with time; it is often most valuable to re-examine the victim of an alleged assault some 24 hours after an inspection made shortly after the event—bruises that were indistinct or even invisible may, by then, have become quite defined. Some bruises may never appear on the surface. This is particularly true over flat bones such as the skull when, should the head strike or be struck by a relatively soft structure, maximum damage to the vessels may be effected against the hard underlying bone; bleeding will then be internal rather than visible at the surface and the extent of a head injury must not be assumed on the basis of an examination of the scalp alone.

The *degree* of bruising is further influenced by the physical state of the injured person, irrespective of age. The physiological limit to a bruise is set by the body's capacity to plug the injured vessels and to clot the escaping blood. Persons with inborn coagulation factor deficiencies, of which haemophilia, itself rare, is the best-known form, or with a diminished number of platelets, with abnormalities of the small blood vessels or with liver disease will bleed more readily than normal and may give a false impression of the severity of injury.

Capillary blood is dark red; recent bruises will be maroon to purple in colour. The tint darkens and browns as oxygen is removed and, soon, the enzymes of the body begin to change the contained haemoglobin into bile pigments; as a consequence the bruise of a few days' age takes on a greenish hue which, as it disperses, changes to yellow. It is often stated that the cycle takes about one week, but this is so dependent upon the size of the extravasation and upon the factors discussed above that accurate 'dating' of a single bruise is by no means a simple matter. The medical witness will be able to provide far more valuable evidence as to timing when this is of a comparative nature—it is often perfectly possible to state that one given bruise or set of bruises is older than another. This is of obvious importance in cases of alleged assault in which it is important to eliminate those injuries that are of no immediate concern: such comparative evidence achieves greatest importance in the analysis of injured children (see Chapter 19) or of the abused elderly. A feature of the natural elimination of bruises is that some free iron is commonly left in the area, and this is readily demonstrable under the microscope. Thus, a more objective method of ageing bruising—and wounds of all types involving haemorrhage—is theoretically available after post-mortem dissection. Unfortunately, the appearances are again variable, and it is scarcely possible to do more than generalise. It is probably safe to say that it is not usual to find iron-containing pigment in a bruise that is less than three days old.[14] The method is of considerable value in distinguishing cerebral haemorrhage that is the *result* of an accident from natural haemorrhage—which could have been accruing for some time and which may have *caused* the accident.

Bruises arising in the subcutaneous tissue seldom cause significant damage unless they become infected. Bruising may, however, affect deeper tissues. Thus, a bruise within the eyeball may cause permanent blindness and the possible fibrous reactions to bruises of vital organs—say, for example, bruising involving the coronary circulation of the heart—may cause physical effects some time after

14 B Knight *Forensic Pathology* (2nd edn, 1996) p 165.

the original injury. Deep bruises which, by virtue of the size of the vessels involved, amount to frank haemorrhage may have severe immediate and long-term effects which are also influenced by the function of the structure involved—bleeding into the brain, for example, may cause irrecoverable damage to the nerve cells. The back is a particular area where severe bruising may be missed at autopsy unless the tissues are incised.

All authorities are agreed that bruises can be produced after death. Such bruises will probably be of small size and will certainly require a disproportionate degree of force to cause them; in the event of doubt, microscopic studies designed to demonstrate the persistence or absence of enzymatic processes may on occasion distinguish ante- from post-mortem lesions. It is often only possible to say that such bruising occurred 'at or about the time of death'.

Abrasions

An abrasion occurs when the outer skin is damaged but the deeper layers remain intact. Although little harm is caused to the body as a whole, rupture of vessels of minute size within the relatively rigid epidermis may result in long-term and relatively faithful reproduction of the object causing the abrasion; it follows that such injuries are of major diagnostic importance.[15]

Abrasions may result from a frictional movement between the skin and an object or to simple pressure on the skin; in either case, the damage may be *ante mortem* or *post mortem*.

Moving abrasions will not replicate the pattern of the offending object but will give evidence, first, of the direction of the abrasive force. Thus, by visualising the 'pile-up' of epidermis at the far end of an abrasion, the pathologist can give evidence as to the direction of a blow or of contact with the ground in, say, a pedestrian street accident. Parallel, linear abrasions 1-3 mm in width are suggestive of having been caused by finger-nails; they may confirm the fact of an assault, they may give evidence as to the relative positions of attacker and attacked and they may serve to identify or exclude a suspect by demonstrating finger span or abnormalities of the fingers or finger-nails. These abrasions must be distinguished from 'knife-point' abrasions, which may also be made, for example, by gem stones. Such markings are thin (< 1 mm), generally straight and often form a criss-cross pattern. They may be self-inflicted, generally with a view to a claim to having been assaulted, in which case they are of remarkably uniform depth; it is, however, surprising how often injuries actually sustained in an assault can appear to have been self-inflicted.

Impact abrasions, without relative movement, often reproduce closely the object causing the injury. Examples include the imprints of weapons, boots or parts of an automobile; even if clothing intervenes and makes its own imprint, the shape of the abrasion may indicate its cause. An outline of a contact object will appear when skin having loose underlying connective tissue is struck; the abrasion is then caused by friction between the *edges* of the instrument and the *wall* of the skin which is compressed (Figure 8.2).

15 Even in the absence of skin damage, ante-mortem 'blushing' of the vessels beneath a pressure point may leave a distinct pattern, eg following a slap.

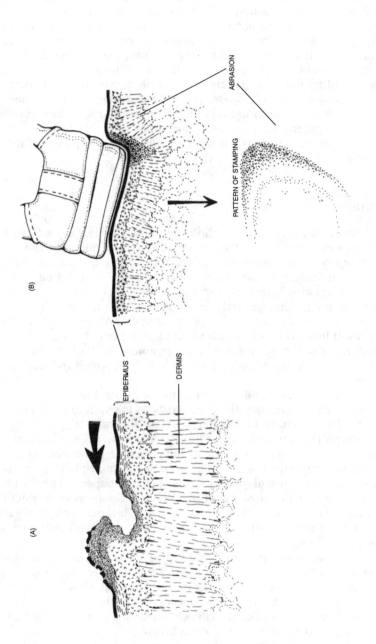

Figure 8.2 Abrasions of the skin. (*a*) Horizontal. The object struck moves along the surface and the broken epidermis 'piles up' as the force is applied. The direction of force is, thus, evident for some time after the event. (*b*) Vertical. As the skin is depressed, it is abraded by the sides of the striking object. A fairly faithful contour impression of the object remains. Contour bruising may also be seen.

Abrasions inflicted coincidentally with or after death merit special mention. They are devoid of vital reaction and take on the appearance and texture of parchment; wide areas of 'parchmenting' may result from contact with a flat object. Such post-mortem 'pressure' abrasions are very common in vehicular accidents, and are found in bodies recovered from the sea that have been pounded on the rocks. They must be distinguished from the rather similar picture produced by the post-mortem application of heat or other forms of localised desiccation. In either case, the 'parchmenting' is the product of extruded tissue fluids which form a thin scab. Very similar appearances follow slippage of the epidermis as a result of manhandling the cadaver in the mortuary; this can be a serious cause of confusion to the pathologist who performs a 'second' autopsy.

Lacerations

Strictly speaking, any breach in the whole skin thickness is a laceration. It is customary, however, to confine the term to a breach of the skin caused by direct blunt injury or by tearing or shearing forces; a laceration caused by a sharp object is an incised wound or a stab wound (see Figure 8.4 below).

Lacerations resulting from blunt force must involve crushing of the skin as a prelude to splitting. They generally occur over a bone that lies close to the skin with little intervening soft tissue, eg in the scalp. A blow over the cheek bone may result in a laceration; an identical blow 2.5 cm (1 in) below on the cheek itself might well cause no more than an abrasion. Perhaps the classic laceration due to blunt injury is the boxer's 'cut eye', which is found in the eyebrow area.

The essential features that define a laceration due to blunt injury are the presence of associated bruising, the irregularity of the split and the manifest crushing or tearing damage to structures *within* the split (Figure 8.3)—an incised wound will merely divide them neatly. A laceration cannot, therefore, give as much evidence as to the shape of the causative instrument as can an abrasion, but the two often coexist. The presence of multiple lacerations of generally similar type, particularly if they are closely grouped but not identical in direction, must raise the suspicion of foul play. Lacerations as here defined can seldom be suicidal unless they result from a fall; remarkable motivation would be needed to produce self-inflicted lacerations with blunt instruments—but this has been seen.

Lacerations due to kicking are generally multiple and are concentrated around the ear and side of the neck. Other selective sites for kicking, such as the abdomen, may well not show breaks in the skin as there is no underlying bone against which it can be crushed. Even so, the elasticity of the skin of the abdominal wall or loin predisposes to the characteristic feature of the kicking injury—that is, the unusual extent of deep bruising.

Lacerations due to tearing or shearing are very common in vehicular accidents. They are often accompanied by severe damage to the underlying muscle or even bone. The extreme example is the very frequent spiral laceration of the leg involving all the tissues, which is caused by savage twisting of the limb which is held firm while the torso is free to move.

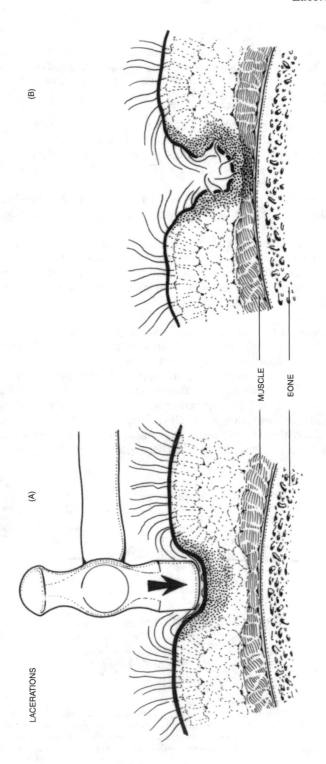

Figure 8.3 (*a*) The skin will split if it is compressed between an object and bone with sufficient force. (*b*) The split will, however, be irregular, there will be associated bruising and surface elements will be forced into the deeper parts of the lesion.

Incised wounds

Incised wounds result from the use of a knife-edge of any type including, for example, broken glass. The danger of such a wound depends upon the position and its depth; a deep incision of the buttock may cause little more than discomfort, whereas a comparatively superficial cut in the wrist may prove fatal due to division of a major artery.

Incised wounds may be accidental—often sustained in the kitchen—but, as such, are seldom serious. A most common problem, however, is to distinguish cutting injuries that are self-inflicted with suicidal intent from similar dangerous injuries sustained as a result of an aggravated assault. The major points of distinction include:

- The position of the incision. The neck is the most common site for both homicidal and suicidal incisions. Those in the wrist are, however, almost diagnostic of suicide.
- Suicidal injuries to the neck are nearly always multiple and show evidence of altering determination, some incisions being superficial while one, or perhaps two, are deep and lethal. True, a suicide may be resolute at first attempt but the murderer is unlikely to be tentative; homicidal incised wounds are, therefore, commonly both severe and of similar depths.

Incised wounds are not infrequently inflicted for the purpose of maiming or disfiguring rather than killing. Intended as punishment, they are nearly always made on the face; deep self-inflicted wounds in this location are very rare save in the presence of severe mental derangement or as a form of ritual disfigurement. A specific incised wound of different type may be found on the fingers, the palm of the hand or the extensor surface of the forearm; such injuries, often irregular in distribution and depth, commonly represent attempts at self-defence, and strongly indicate that other wounds on the body are homicidal in nature. Bruises, or even lacerations, may also be found on the forearm when the 'defence' has been against assault with a blunt weapon.

INCISION

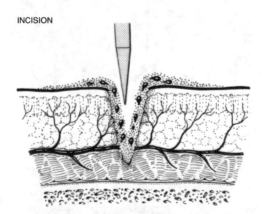

Figure 8.4 Incision. In some cases, there is a graduation from laceration to incision—a blow from a blunt axe will, for example, show features of both. In the typical incision from a sharp instrument, however, the wound is clean cut, there is no bruising and the vessels are divided to give rise to severe bleeding to the *exterior*. No superficial material is forced into the wound.

Pathological findings designed to demonstrate the direction of the cut are often difficult to interpret. The 'exit' end is almost bound to be shelving; the 'entry' wound may well be precipitously deep in homicide or shelving towards the centre when self-inflicted, but the appearances must be very variable and will also be modified by the shape of the part that is cut. Serious injuries are almost bound to be multiple and a major difficulty is, then, to distinguish a homicidal wound from superimposed superficial and deep suicidal lesions.

Chopping injuries

We have seen that blunt weapons cause lacerations and sharp-edged instruments cause incisions. Injuries due to blunt edged weapons form an intermediate group which can be referred to as chopping injuries.[16] The most likely weapons of this type include spades and poorly maintained axes. Injuries will almost certainly be homicidal—and, therefore, multiple—and the head is the most probable target.

The precise appearances will depend almost entirely on the bluntness of the weapon—they can, however, usually be considered as incisions with lacerated edges. It has been pointed out that many of the traditional chopping instruments—such as the panga or the kukri—are finding their way into street violence. When specifically sharpened for the purpose, such weapons can cause devastating injuries including transection of bones.

Penetrating wounds

A wound can be described as penetrating if its depth exceeds its width. When the superficial characteristics of such an injury are those of an incised wound, it is a stab wound; it is customary to restrict the term to injuries inflicted by pointed instruments, eg a needle, a knife or a bayonet. Like most wounds, stab wounds can be homicidal, suicidal or accidental.

Accidental stab wounds are invariably single unless the offending instrument has multiple penetrating points; an accidental fall on to the points of a garden fork or a spiked railing could provide multiple stab wounds of symmetrical pattern, identical direction and equal depth. It may be difficult to distinguish accident from suicide or homicide when there is evidence of only a single thrust. Much will depend upon the findings at the locus of death and on the position and direction of the wound. The site of a suicidal stab wound must have been accessible to the dead person and, in practice, the great majority of single suicidal stab wounds are in an elective site, occasionally deep in the neck, but more commonly following the path of the classic Japanese method of self-immolation running upwards from below the ribs to penetrate the heart.

Homicidal or otherwise aggressive stab wounds have always been a common feature of forensic practice. Knives are omnipresent, they can be carried relatively easily—especially, say, in a sock beneath trousers—and it is not difficult to maintain that their carriage was for legitimate purposes. The control of knife-carrying is, therefore, difficult but many attempts to do so by statute have been

---

16 A useful term introduced by B N Purdue 'Cutting and Piercing Wounds' in J K Mason and B N Purdue *The Pathology of Trauma* (3rd edn, 2000), ch 9.

made. Thus, any knife can be classed as an offensive weapon for the purposes of the Prevention of Crime Act 1953, s 1[17]—which prohibits the carrying of an offensive weapon in a public place without lawful authority— although, in general, whether there was an intention to use it to cause injury is a question of fact to be decided in the individual case. Some types of knife are, however, clearly designed for attack or defence and are, therefore, in a different category. Thus, the manufacture, sale and possession of flick-knives or gravity knives is proscribed in the Restriction of Offensive Weapons Acts 1959[18] and a flick-knife is now deemed in law to be an offensive weapon per se.[19] The widest restriction is found in the Criminal Justice Act 1988, s 139, which makes it an offence to be in possession in a public place of any article that has a blade or is sharply pointed other than a folding pen-knife;[20] s 141A criminalises the sale of such knives, including axes and razors, to persons under the age of 16.[1] Restrictions in Scotland extend to the carriage of a folding bladed or pointed instrument of a length greater than three inches (7.5cm).[2] Despite such regulation, it is the experience of the majority of forensic pathologists in Great Britain that stabbing is by far the most frequent form of murder in an urban environment.

Single homicidal stab wounds are comparatively rare, as most wounds leave the victim capable of resistance for a measurable time during which the blow is repeated; single homicidal wounds are, therefore, often associated with a drugged, drunk or sleeping victim and are almost always aimed at the heart. Occasionally, single homicidal wounds may cause difficulty by reason of their unusualness. In a case seen by the author, a man's body was picked up from his front garden and treated as a supposed sudden natural death; it was not until the body was being undressed in the mortuary that a single stab wound was noted in the right loin— very rapid death had resulted from transfixion of the aorta. It may be reasonable in such atypical cases to question the intention to kill and to accept them as instances of involuntary murder, manslaughter or culpable homicide.

Multiple stab wounds are very strongly suggestive of voluntary murder. When a suicide inflicts several wounds upon himself, the earlier wounds are likely to be shallow—a close grouping of the injuries is likely unless the suicide results from religious frenzy or other mental imbalance. Multiple murderous stab wounds show, by contrast, a more uniform degree of force, several being potentially lethal— they are often widely spaced and of different directions unless the repeated stab wounds have been inflicted on an unconscious body. Caution must, however, be exercised in ensuring that all multiple stab wounds are attributable to the same

17 Defined as any article made or adapted for use for causing injury to the person, or intended by the person having it with him for such use by him or by some other person (Public Order Act 1986, s 40(2)). For Scotland, see Criminal Law (Consolidation) (Scotland) Act 1995, s 47, as amended by Offensive Weapons Act 1996, s 5.

18 As amended by Restriction of Offensive Weapons Act 1961 and the Criminal Justice Act 1988, s 46.

19 *R v Simpson (Calvin)* [1983] 3 All ER 789; *Tudhope v O'Neill* 1982 SCCR 45. See also *DPP v Hynde* [1998] 1 All ER 649 for butterfly knives.

20 Forgetfulness is not a defence: *Crowe v Waugh* 1999 SCCR 610. Section 139A of the 1988 Act and s 49A of the 1995 Acts as introduced by the Offensive Weapons Act 1996, s 4, make special provisions for school premises.

 1 Introduced by the Offensive Weapons Act 1996, s 6. Marketing a knife in a way that suggests it is suitable for combat, or that stimulates its use as a weapon, is controlled under the Knives Act 1997.

 2 Knives Act 1997, s 10.

weapon. It is not uncommon for members of gangs to inflict individual injuries, possibly with a view to confusing the subsequent investigation. Many such injuries may be either non-fatal or inflicted after death; the pathologist may, therefore, be faced with a decision as to which was the wound that caused death.

In any event, evidence will be drawn from the pathologist as to the nature and shape of the weapon, either to assist in the search for, or for purposes of comparison with, a suspect article. As with all wounds, the sharper the instrument, the less tissue damage and bruising will be found. A stab by a knife will produce a clean incised wound which, by virtue of the elasticity of the skin, will stretch into an ellipse. A double-edged weapon will normally produce a symmetrical surface pattern, whereas one with a single edge may show relative blunting of one end, or a boat shape, of the entry slit. The knife may, of course, have been withdrawn at an angle—in which case, the skin at one angle of the incision may show relatively superficial injury. A knife may also have been plunged more than once through the same opening which can, as a result, take on a cruciate appearance; an unusual appearance in the skin should, however, indicate the need to consider an unusual instrument. All authorities are agreed that differential contraction of the skin and subcutaneous tissue may, on occasion, give a misleading impression of the cross-section of the weapon used.

The breadth of the wounds must be measured with the edges opposed. In general, the weapon—and, in particular, a knife—cannot be wider than this so long as the natural taper of the point is taken into consideration and the width is related to the depth of the wound; rocking or twisting the knife, however, may produce a wound that is larger than its maximum width. Similarly, the depth of the wound is unlikely to be longer than the full length of the weapon; a false indication of length may be obtained if the body surface has been compressed by the blade guard, as may particularly be the case in wounds of the abdomen. A stab wound seen where the skin is relatively stable and incompressible—as in the chest—will sometimes demonstrate bruising or abrasion due to the blade guard. As opposed to this, a knife with a pronounced choil, or shoulder between the blade and the ricasso which fits into the handle, may tear the skin outwards if plunged in to its full extend. Despite the obvious need for caution, the accurate measurement of a number of stab wounds in a single body may enable the pathologist to give a reasonably accurate description of the likely size and shape of the blade of the weapon used, especially if it was a knife (see Figure 8.5).

The direction of the stab may also be important in establishing how the knife was held. The direction of the blow—and the attitude of the victim—can be gauged by passing a metal rod through the various incisions made in the fascial membranes and organs in the course of penetration; measurement of wounds in the pericardium and pleara, for example, may also give the most accurate indication of the width of the knife. Clearly, however, this may distort the shape of the wounds and it should not be done until they have been properly measured and recorded; it must also be remembered that the direction of penetration is being assessed with the body in a supine position, whereas the wounds are likely to have been inflicted while the victim was erect. Estimating the strength with which the blows were struck is extremely difficult. An opinion must take into account the clothing of the victim although, unless one is dealing with, say, thick leather, this makes surprisingly little difference. To find that the wounds extended 'up to the hilt' is to assess the results of force rather than its degree. Deep penetration of the tissue by a sharp, pointed instrument is relatively easy; the main resistance

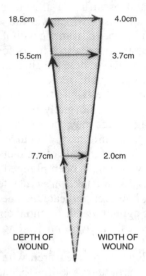

18.5cm   4.0cm

15.5cm   3.7cm

7.7cm   2.0cm

DEPTH OF   WIDTH OF
WOUND   WOUND

Figure 8.5 The shape of a knife assessed from the appearance of three stab wounds of different depth. The actual knife was of remarkably similar shape, although the point was curved.

to penetration is provided by the skin and, clearly, the less pointed is the weapon, the greater will be that resistance. Once the skin has been passed, a knife will slip through the tissues with relative ease; it would be within the power of practically any adult to inflict a lethal wound using a pointed knife of one of many types which are unrestricted as to sale.

The mode and cause of death after wounding

Rapid death resulting from incised or stab wounds is usually due either to haemorrhage or to damage to a structure that is vital to life; death may occasionally be caused by air entering a broken vein.

Haemorrhage is by far the most common of these potential causes of death and will be much more severe if an artery is penetrated than if only veins are affected; the speed of death will depend upon the size of the vessel involved and on the secondary effects of the accumulation of blood. It is difficult to inflict a stabbing injury of 15 cm depth without lacerating an artery of at least moderate calibre, and the direction of most homicidal stab wounds results in their frequent termination in the heart, aorta or major pulmonary vessels. Death is often very rapid, but it pays to be cautious in interpretation as some remarkable periods of survival have been recorded . This is especially so in respect of penetration of the heart, where conditions are unusually complex. Many so injured will die rapidly from haemorrhage but, quite often—in, perhaps, a large minority of cases—the wound in the pericardium will at least partially close itself by the formation of blood clot; this possibility is denied to the elderly person who has no pericardial sac due to the presence of healed pericarditis. On the other hand, complete closure of the pericardium will lead to accumulation of blood within the sac and to the potentially fatal condition of cardiac tamponade; survival for sufficient time to reach the operating theatre thus depends on an uneasy, and scarcely assessable, balance between haemorrhage and haemostasis. Haemorrhage from non-penetrating incised wounds need not be severe unless a major artery lies superficially at the site if injury—the most obvious example of such an area is on the flexor surface of the wrist which, accordingly, is a favourite site for suicidal incision.

Rapid death due to interference with the function of structures other than blood vessels is rare and is confined to special situations. Thus, stab wounds at the nape of the neck may result in near instantaneous death, with minimal haemorrhage, due to the destruction of the vital centres in the medulla of the brain stem. Incised wounds of the trachea or larynx may lead to collapse of the neck structures with valve-like obstruction of the main airway; more probably, the airway will be blocked by blood or impacted tissues. Incised wounds of the neck may, in fact, result in many modes of death—vagal inhibition of the heart, airway obstruction, air embolism, venous bleeding from the jugular veins or arterial bleeding from the carotid arteries; consequently, the length of the agonal period may be particularly difficult to assess.

Death attributable to wounds or injuries occurring some time after the event presents no special features. Among other complications, those of prolonged immobilisation—pneumonia or pulmonary embolism—or of reduction in blood volume—in particular acute renal failure—may arise and must be regarded as logical sequences of the original assault in the absence of proof of intervening medical negligence. Even this may not affect the question of causation as the original wounding needs only to have played a significant part in the death for the charge of murder to be relevant;[3] the negligent medical act would constitute a novus actus interveniens only if it was wholly dissociated from the wounding.[4]

---

3   The well-known case *R v Jordan* (1956) 40 Cr App Rep 152, in which a prosecution for manslaughter failed because of incorrect medical treatment, appears to have been an exception which was decided on its own special facts and is a bad precedent.
4   As was the case in *R v Smith* [1959] 2 QB 35; *R v Cheshire* [1991] 3 All ER 670, CA.

9

Injury and death due to firearms and explosives

The law

The law relating to firearms is statutory throughout Great Britain and is contained, in the main, in the Firearms Act 1968 which has been heavily amended. A firearm is defined in s 57(1) of the Act as any lethal barrelled weapon of any description from which any shot, bullet or other missile can be discharged.[1] Personal firearms are of three categories—the smooth-bore weapon, or shotgun, rifled weapons—which include revolvers, 'automatic' pistols and rifles—and, in certain circumstances, air weapons.[2] Shotguns were devised primarily for the sport of killing small animals; rifles, while being used in some forms of sport hunting, eg deer stalking, were mainly perfected for the killing of man. The regulations governing the possession and use of rifled weapons are, accordingly, far more strict than apply in the case of shotguns. Section 1 defines, by exclusion, those weapons that it is unlawful to possess without simultaneously holding a firearm certificate.[3]

No one under the age of 14 may acquire or use any firearm or ammunition unless as a member of a recognised club, or when in a shooting gallery using miniature rifles or air weapons; but an airgun can be used under supervision by an adult over 21 in a private place. Persons over 14 may be given or lent an airgun, or a 'Section 1' firearm subject to the possession of a firearms certificate, but sale to a person below the age of 17 is prohibited; the possession of an assembled shotgun under the age of 15 is subject to supervision by an adult over the age of 21. The carriage of an airgun in a public place by a person under the age of 17 is prohibited unless the gun is securely covered.

Certificates to possess and use an airgun are not required but, in addition to it being illegal to sell such a gun to anyone under the age of 17, it is also unlawful

1 It thus includes a number of unusual weapons—eg a spear gun operated by elastic: *Boyd v McGlennan* 1994 SLT 1148.
2 *Castle (John) v DPP* (1998) Times, 3 April. It is not necessary for the prosecutor to prove the weapon is lethal.
3 The offence is one of strict liability: *R v Steele* [1993] Crim LR 298; *Smith v HM Advocate* 1996 SCCR 49. By reason of the Firearms Act 1982, the rules relating to firearms are extended to imitation firearms—that is, those having the appearance of a Section 1 firearm or that are readily convertible into such a weapon.

to present a young person under the age of 14 with an airgun for his possession. The relaxation of certification does not apply to 'specially dangerous air weapons'—defined as pump-action air rifles having a kinetic energy greater than 16 J (12 ft lb), or 8 J (6 ft lb) in the case of pistols—which are classified as 'Section 1' firearms.[4] Smooth-bore guns (not being an airgun) having a barrel not less than 60 cm long, and with a bore not exceeding 5 cm, are not Section 1 firearms, and their possession is regulated by the issue of shotgun certificates which are obtained from the local police; there are no further restrictions on the acquisition of shotguns by persons over the age of 17 and, in certain circumstances, shotguns can be used without a certificate being held—the most important of these being when the gun is borrowed from a person with a certificate and is used on his private property. It is an offence to shorten the barrel of a shotgun to less than 60 cm;[5] the resultant 'sawn-off shotgun' would be a Section 1 weapon and its possession restricted to the granting of a firearm certificate.

Whereas it is generally only necessary to be 'of good character' to qualify for the issue of a shotgun licence, a person seeking a firearm certificate must not be of intemperate habits, of unsound mind or for any reason unfitted to be entrusted with firearms. The chief constable must be satisfied that the applicant has a good reason for acquiring a firearm and that its acquisition would not be prejudicial to public safety or to peace. Very few categories of person are exempt from firearm certificate requirements—the commonest are members of approved rifle clubs and cadet corps and race starters at athletic meetings; persons in the service of the Crown or in the police are exempt although subject to rigid regulation by their parent authorities. The possession of certain specially dangerous weapons— eg automatic repeating rifles or weapons discharging a harmful liquid gas—is prohibited without the specific authority of the Secretary of State.[6]

Shotguns are, therefore, widely distributed and, despite the regulations, legally held firearms are responsible for a substantial number of deaths; aside from those held by the criminal fraternity, the illegal possession of firearms is fairly widespread—the illegality often not being appreciated. A number of specific offences relating to the use of firearms are created by the Firearms Act 1968. These include:

- The possession of a firearm or ammunition with intent to endanger life and also, in Scotland, to cause serious injury to property[7] or to enable another person to do so (s 16).
- Having possession of a firearm or imitation firearm with intent to cause, or to enable any other person to cause, any person to believe that unlawful violence will be used against him (s 16A).[8]
- Using a real or imitation firearm to resist arrest or possessing a firearm or imitation firearm at the time of committing (or being arrested for) a 'specified offence' (s 17).

4 Firearms (Dangerous Air Weapons) Regulations 1969, SI 1969/47. Guns activated by compressed carbon dioxide are included (Firearms (Amendment) Act 1997, s 48).
5 Firearms (Amendment) Act 1988, s 6.
6 Firearms Act 1968, s 5, added to by Firearms (Amendment) Act 1988, s 1, Firearms (Amendment) Act 1997, s 1; Firearms (Amendment) (No 2) Act 1997, s 1. This includes self-loading air pistols (1968 Act, s 5(1)(ab)) and small calibre pistols (s 5(1)(aba)) under 'rifled guns'.
7 Removed in England by the Criminal Damage Act 1971, s 11(8).
8 Inserted by the Firearms (Amendment) Act 1994, s 1.

- Trespassing with a firearm[9] (s 20).
- Carrying in a public place without lawful authority or reasonable excuse a loaded shotgun or any other firearm whether loaded or not together with appropriate ammunition (s 19).[10]

To wound or cause grievous bodily harm with intent to do so by any means—which includes shooting—is a statutory offence in England and Wales.[11] In Scotland, wounding by shooting is a serious aggravation of an assault.

Gunshot injuries are of major pathological interest in that they can be interpreted with considerable objectivity; the pathologist can often give opinions that are soundly based and that are particularly valuable both to the police and to the lawyer.

Airgun injuries

Unless the pellet penetrates some vital spot, such as the eye or the brain, severe injuries from the normal airgun or air pistol, with a muzzle velocity of 80–105 ms^{-1}, are unlikely. None the less, pellets travelling at a speed of more than 110 ms^{-1} when discharged from more powerful guns will generally penetrate skin and even bone;[12] the effect of those fired from air weapons described as especially dangerous may be comparable to those from small bullets from a rifled firearm. Due to their relatively low velocity, airgun pellets rarely fragment. Beyond this, injuries due to air weapons do not merit a separate description.

Shotgun injuries

Shotguns are normally smooth barrelled and may be single or double barrelled.[13] The barrel of the former or one barrel of the latter may be tapered towards the muzzle—a manufacturing process known as *choking* which serves to lengthen the period during which the shot is restrained in a compact mass. The calibre of shotguns is expressed in unusual terms. When the diameter of the barrel is less than ½ in (1.25 cm), the calibre is given by that diameter—eg 'four-ten' means a barrel diameter of 0.410 in; guns larger than this are measured by 'bore'—or the number of spherical lead balls exactly fitting the barrel that go to make 1 lb. An 8-bore is therefore a larger and more powerful gun than is the common 12-bore.[14]

The shotgun cartridge consists of a cardboard or plastic cylinder attached to a brass plate which contains the primer. The main powder charge used to be separated

---

9 *Grace v DPP* [1989] Crim LR 365 gives an interesting discussion as to what constitutes a firearm.
10 This, again, is a matter of strict liability: *R v Harrison* [1996] 1 Cr App Rep 138, CA; *R v Jones* [1995] QB 235, CA (a firearm certificate does not constitute authority to carry in a public place).
11 Offences Against the Person Act 1861, s 18, as amended by the Criminal Law Act 1967, Sch 3, Pt III.
12 S Blocker, D Coln and J H T Chang 'Serious Air Rifle Injuries in Children' (1982) 69 Pediatrics 751.
13 Recently, shotguns have been made with rifled or partly rifled barrels through which single projectiles can be fired. Such weapons would be 'Section 1 firearms'.
14 These measurements can now be metricated (Gun Barrel Proof Act 1978, s 5).

from the shot by a wad or washer and the shot—which consists of spherical metal balls of diameters ranging from 2–9 mm[15]—was maintained in the cartridge by a distal wad. This format has been largely replaced by one in which the powder and the shot are contained in plastic cups which open out on discharge so as to form plastic sheets in the form of a George Cross.[16] The shot is propelled in a solid mass which begins to fan out as the compression by the wads is released. The propellant continues burning as the shot passes down the barrel and some powder always remains unburnt. The effective sporting range of a shotgun is approximately 50 metres. The shot is rapidly halted within the tissues of the target; this does not apply in the case of large shot which may be lethal at double the anticipated range.

The pathological evidence as to the distance from which the shot has been fired can be deduced from these principles, although it cannot be overstated that some variations occur in practice. A contact injury will show bruising and abrasion due to the recoil of the gun and a perfect representation of the single or twin barrels may be formed on the skin; the shot will enter the body as a solid mass so that the entry wound will approximate to the bore of the barrel; however, explosive gases will also enter the wound so that the external wound may be ragged—the skull, for example, may be literally blown apart; an exit wound may be seen, except in the very thick torso, because the shot in a contact wound is in a solid mass. Exit wounds are, however, not a feature of shotgun injuries other than in the contact situation. At very short range, the appearances described above will be modified by the differing effects of the gases of combustion—these will not be forced into the wound but may still cause some irregularity of the entry hole. Unburnt powder will be discharged into the surrounding skin, leading to what is known as 'tattooing'; soot is likely to be deposited. The hot gases will burn the skin or clothing, either of which may be charred; in both contact and close-range wounds, any carbon monoxide contained in the gases of combustion may form local carboxyhaemoglobin which can be recognised by its pink colour.

These effects diminish as the distance from muzzle to wound increases. The critical distance is at about 2 m as, at this distance, tattooing is scarcely visible and the wads fail to penetrate the wound; the modern plastic wads, however, become effective secondary missiles and may leave distinctive marks on the skin up to some 6 m. The shot now begins to fan out and creates a pattern of entry in the clothing and on the skin. Although the inclination of the body to the line of flight of the shot will alter the appearances, ideally the pattern will be circular. The size of this circle depends to some extent on the degree of 'choking' of the gun barrel, but British guns are sufficiently standardised to permit the use of a simple rule—the diameter of the shot pattern in centimetres is some two to three times the muzzle distance from the wound in metres (or the spread in inches is equivalent to the distance in yards). Small shot tends to disperse more rapidly than does larger when fired from the same gun; estimates derived from such a formula must be checked by test firing whenever possible. The interposition of solid matter between the gun and the skin leads to rapid dispersion of shot; thus, injury from a close-range discharge through a glass or wooden panel may give the

15 The number of shot in a cartridge varies from eight to as many as 700, the size and weight being chosen according to the main purpose for which the gun is to be used. Some cartridges contain mixed shot—an important matter, since the appearances may simulate a double shooting.

16 The cups for the smaller 0.410 ammunition have only three 'leaflets'.

impression of having been inflicted from a range of several yards. Fatal 12-bore shotgun injuries are unlikely at a range of over 20 m (or yards: see Figure 9.1). Unlawful shortening of the barrel (say, to about 25 cm—the typical 'sawn-off' shotgun) generally leads to a reduction in muzzle velocity of the shot of no more than 20%; the spread of the shot may be up to twice that produced by the normal full-length barrelled gun.

The majority of shotgun injuries are sustained at close range. The internal injuries are therefore due either to the violent expansion of gas within the body or to the penetrating effect of what is, essentially, a solid mass of lead more than 1.25 cm in diameter; the former effect is well seen in the head and the latter in the heart which can be torn apart by a shot fired from within a range of 2 m. Otherwise, the effects of a shotgun injury are variable and depend upon the ability of individual pellets to penetrate either the heart or individual blood vessels or other organs liable to severe bleeding; the surgery of such an injury may present a formidable problem.

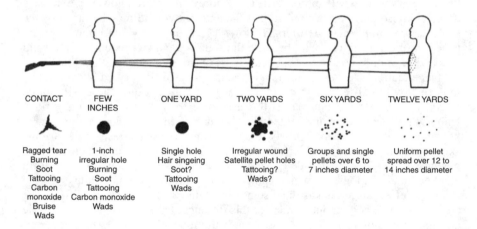

Figure 9.1 Effects of a shotgun injury related to distance. (Reproduced by permission of the author from B Knight *Legal Aspects of Medical Pratice* (5th edn, 1992) p 195 (Edinburgh, Churchill Livingston.)

Rifled weapons

The main diagnostic difference between wounds due to shotguns and those due to rifled weapons rests on the fact that, whereas shot will certainly be found in the body, a bullet is likely to have exited; contemporary entry and exit wounds are, therefore, a feature of the latter.

Contact and close-range entry wounds due to rifle bullets will have much the same characteristics as those of a shotgun injury—bruising, blast effects, soot deposition and tattooing will be present, the last being found up to a range of some 1.0–1.3 m; it is, however, to be remembered that the distance travelled by unburnt particles of gunpowder depends very much on the type of powder—

whether of flake or ball type, the latter marking the skin at greater distance than the former—and also on the calibre of the gun used.

If the range has not been so short as to cause explosive damage to the tissues, the characteristics of the entry wound will be governed by the gyroscopic stability of the bullet. In the early phase of its flight—up to some 50 m for a pistol or 150 m for a rifle—and towards the end of its effective range—of the order of 460 m for pistol and 2.4 km (1½ miles) for a rifle—there is considerable 'tail wag', which results in a relatively large and ragged entry wound. In the most efficient phase of flight, the bullet will enter the body neatly nose on and leave a regular, small hole which, because of the elasticity of the skin, may well not correspond exactly to the diameter of the missile and will generally be slightly smaller. The entry wound will show inverted edges and is characterised by an abrasion ring— where the bullet has abraded the skin—which is more prominent the more the skin can be depressed and which will be asymmetrical if the bullet has entered at an angle. The entry wound may demonstrate 'soiling' or 'bullet wipe'—that is, contamination of its edge by grease which the bullet has acquired in its passage down the barrel of the gun and which is wiped off either by the clothing or by the skin but it is found only uncommonly when the bullet has a hard metallic jacket.

As the bullet traverses the body, it may become deflected, it may be deformed or fragmented and it may take with it portions of tissue—particularly of bone— which can act as secondary missiles. The exit wound is therefore likely to be irregular, its edges will be everted and there will be no soiling—provided the bullet has remained intact, the exit wound cannot be smaller than the entry wound save at extremes of range. The modern, very high velocity rifle presents something of an exception. This weapon kills by virtue of the massive internal damage that results from the dissipation of large amounts of kinetic energy; the entry and exit wounds are, however, small and are of very similar size. The common tendency for the wound to enlarge from entry to exit is well shown in bone, particularly the bones of the skull, in which the penetrating wound bevels outwards so that it is of larger diameter on the exit side; this difference in size is useful in distinguishing a bullet wound from a surgical burr-hole in a skeletonised skull or fragment of skull bone presented for examination. Two variations on the pattern of exit wounds deserve special mention. The first is the so-called 'shored' wound which is seen when the skin at the point of exit is supported by a solid surface such as a door or wall; the everted skin then tends to become compressed with the formation of an apparent abrasion ring; the shored exit wound can thus closely resemble an entry wound, the main distinguishing features being that there will be no soiling and the 'abrasion ring' will tend to be irregular. Secondly, an exit wound arising, particularly, where the skin is folded may be linear and sharply edged; it is not difficult to confuse such an injury with a stab wound.

The pathologist is likely to be able to give a very good opinion as to the direction of an injury from a rifled weapon as compared with shotgun injuries but has less evidence on which to base an estimate of range. The recovery of a bullet from the body is, of course, of great importance to the investigation, as every weapon leaves a characteristic pattern of scoring on the surface of the bullet; test firing of suspected weapons may then result in a convincing identification by comparison. Equally good—if not better—comparative evidence can be derived from spent cartridges recovered at the scene of a shooting—marks of an individual nature are made by the firing pin and hammer, the ejection mechanism and during extraction; such methods of weapon identification are also open in the case of shotguns but all lie in the province of the ballistics expert.

Bullets may kill by virtue of penetrating the heart, a major vessel or a vital centre of the brain. The greatest damage is, however, caused, first, by the brute force of the bullet as it punches its way through the tissues and, secondly, by 'cavitation' in the track of the missile. The effect of the resultant stretching of the tissues depends upon their nature—the passage of a bullet through, for example, the liver will cause far more damage than will the same bullet passing through the bowel. The discharge of energy can tear vital tissues associated with, but removed from, the actual path of the bullet; widespread destruction may result from fragments of bullet and also of tissue which form 'secondary missiles'. Thus, the degree of injury is determined both by the speed of the bullet and its fate within the body. Delayed death is likely if a solid organ with a large blood supply is damaged; death from septic shock or simple sepsis may follow penetrating injuries of the bowel.

The nature of the wounding

The immediate need in any case of fatal firearm wounding is to distinguish between accident, suicide and homicide. The forensic doctor will often be able to give sound evidence as to the probability of suicide; the distinction between accident and homicide, is, however, a far more difficult problem. The medical evidence will rest upon both an examination of the locus and the post-mortem findings.

The scene of death will provide much evidence in relation to suicide. First, save in unusual circumstances, the weapon must be within reach and almost always will either be retained in the grasp or lie close to the hand of the dead person. A murderer may attempt to simulate suicide and it is most important that the doctor, called in to pronounce life extinct, takes full notes of the precise conditions. The observer might be fortunate enough to witness the rare phenomenon of cadaveric spasm; this is one post-mortem condition that cannot be produced artificially but few pathologists have seen it in this practical situation (see Chapter 4). Homicide is clearly indicated if the gun is found at the scene and is beyond reach of the deceased; the main exception rests in the possibility of a suicidal or accidental shot that is not immediately fatal—in which case, there may well be evidence of movement in the form of blood splashing and the like. Mention is generally made of suicide accomplished by means of a remote firing mechanism such as a pulley attached to the trigger; such contraptions are set for deep-seated psychological reasons, and not for the purpose of confusing the investigating officers—they rarely cause difficulty although, again, the possibility of an artefact rigged by an assailant has to be eliminated. The examining doctor should always confer with the police officer in charge as to the presence of spent cartridges; the firing of more than one shot is not unknown but is uncommon in suicide.

The post-mortem findings indicating suicide can be deduced from the previous pages. Findings indicative of a range within 1 m—in particular, the appearance of tattooing by unburnt powder—are clearly consistent with suicide, as this is the maximum distance it is possible to hold a pistol from the body; similarly, the absence of close-range characteristics in a shotgun or rifle wound will strongly militate against suicide, as the barrel length of the gun approximates to that of the arm. In practice, it is extremely uncommon for suicidal wounds to be other than of a contact nature. They will also almost always be in a 'site of election'; these vary according to the weapon. A suicidal pistol wound is generally inflicted in the right temple and an exit wound is usually close to the opposite temple; an alternative is the centre of the forehead—the precise symmetry is classic and of diagnostic importance—while the roof of the mouth may be chosen. Rifle wounds are, again, common in the centre of the forehead and in the mouth; in either case, massive tissue damage may result. The rifle suicide may lean on the gun with the muzzle on the brow or over the heart, a situation that is also not unusual with shotguns. The commonest suicidal shotgun wounds are, however, those in the roof of the mouth or in the centre of the forehead, just above the bridge of the nose; in either case, the head is torn asunder, often, again, in a characteristic, symmetrical fashion. The important general features of successful suicidal firearm wounds are that they are placed so as to minimise the possibility of failure, and that the entry point must be accessible. Other evidence of close contact with the gun, such as heat discoloration of the thighs where the barrel has been steadied, may also be present.

Accidental gunshot injuries may be 'self-inflicted', as in the classic 'cleaning the gun' situation, or involve a second party, as when a moving fellow hunter is mistaken for game. The former situation may closely simulate suicide, the essential differentiation being the asymmetry inherent in a random occurrence. The latter type of accidental injury, showing no more than the effect of a relatively long-range discharge, is indistinguishable from homicide on purely pathological grounds.

Certain features are strongly indicative of homicide—a single wound of contact or very close range type in an inaccessible position is an obvious example, the back, the nape of the neck or behind the ear being the commonest sites; similarly, the existence of more than one fatal injury will be very strong evidence against both suicide and accident—in circumstances of high emotional tension, such as marital brawls, a mixture of both non-fatal and fatal wounds may be found. The suspicion of homicide may, however, rest on the exclusion of suicide by the pathologist, coupled with the circumstantial evidence obtained by the police officers. Pathologists should be very wary of estimating the survival time following a fatal gunshot injury. The victim may be capable of considerable activity despite sustaining an injury which might well be judged likely to have caused immediate death and most people who have actually shot someone have been surprised at the apparently slight immediate effect.[17]

Examination of suspects

The medical examination of a suspected firearm assailant is directed, mainly, to the demonstration of firearm residues on his or her hands. Clearly visible soot

---

17 V Levy and V J Rao 'Survival Times in Gunshot and Stab Wound Victims' (1988) 9 Amer J Forens Med Pathol 215. Moreover, victims are not thrown over backwards as is so often seen in fictional motion pictures. Points such as these are important because judges and juries are likely to have watched numerous films and TV dramas in which gunshot wounding is portrayed. The contrast between fact and fiction is well laid out in P E Besant-Matthews 'Examination and interpretation of rifled firearm injuries' in J K Mason and B N Purdue (eds) *The Pathology of Trauma* (3rd edn, 2000) ch 4.

may be present; this derives from the burning—or destruction—of the gunpowder and, while it may indicate that the examinee has fired a gun, it provides comparatively little evidence as to the precise firearm used. Other residues may be invisible and yet provide something akin to a gun's 'signature'; a main function of the examining doctor will be to provide suitable specimens for analysis in the forensic science laboratory.

The older relevant tests were based on the assumption that residues of propellant will settle on the firing hand. Both gunpowder and modern smokeless powders contain nitrates which are readily detectable when present. It was the habit to remove skin-surface contaminants with paraffin and the test thus became incorrectly known as 'the paraffin test'. The identification of nitrates has since been regarded as non-specific and, in 1964, Interpol 'did not consider the traditional paraffin test to be of any value'.[18]

Modern work has concentrated on the identification on the hands of metallic residues derived from the primer mixture contained within the rim or the primer cap of the cartridge; compounds of mercury, antimony, barium and lead are present in varying proportions and can be quantified in this 'dermal residue' test. The residues are removed by swabbing with moistened filter paper. The test has several drawbacks—for example, the 'natural' or background residue is strongly dependent on occupation; moreover, the residues are easily removed by washing or even in the course of normal use of the hands. Residues are most likely to be found following the firing of a revolver, they are less common when a pistol has been used and they are relatively uncommon following the firing of a rifle or a shotgun; overall, only about half the known cases will test positive even in the best conditions. A positive test of this type is a useful indication that the subject has fired a gun; even so, it is not difficult to throw significant doubt on the specificity of the findings in the conditions of a criminal trial.

Injuries and death due to explosion

Injury and death due to explosion may occur industrially or in the home—as, for example, when gas filling a room is ignited. The resulting injuries will be due, first, to the air blast itself and, secondly, to random impacts as the body is hurled against other solid objects. If the blast is due to a bomb, there will be added damage from the splintered casing.

The effects of blast are due to a combination of positive pressure, the blast wave itself and the subsequent negative pressure. The effects, which are exaggerated in an enclosed space, are seen particularly in those organs capable of elastic recoil and containing multiple gas/fluid or fluid/solid interfaces. Thus, the lungs in particular are the subject of much disruption and haemorrhage; the ear-drums are also very sensitive to pressure changes. Blast effects are well transmitted in water; the hollow viscera are particularly vulnerable to underwater explosions and, since there are no injuries due to secondary impacts, those killed in these circumstances often present with little external but massive internal damage.

18 For review, see R Cornelis and J Timperman (1974) 14 Med Sci Law 98. At least one conviction deemed to have been unsafe in modern times has been based on such evidence.

Bomb injuries[19] may approximate to disintegration of the body; short of this, the wounds are characterised by their multiplicity and by their association with foreign particles not all of which necessarily derive from the bomb itself—many fragments of glass, brick dust or even pieces of furniture will contaminate the wounds and will give a distinctive pattern of 'peppering' of the body.

As in all types of wounding, death due to bomb explosions may be accidental, suicidal or homicidal. Accidental cases are of legitimate and illegitimate type. The former are confined to members of bomb disposal squads and to workers in authorised armouries—for example, in the armed forces. When the device involved is small, the track of metallic fragments can often be traced in the body so as to define the reconstruction of events with considerable accuracy. Accidental bomb injuries of an illegal character—eg occurring in those manufacturing bombs—are likely to be far more severe. Suicidal bomb injuries may be differentiated pathologically by the concentration of massive injuries in the abdominal region; the victims of random bomb attacks commonly show maximal injury in the legs.

Despite the fact that homicidal bombing in a civilian context occurs in very diverse circumstances, the pattern of injuries is surprisingly reproducible. It has been pointed out that, as compared with their military equivalent, terrorist bombs are relatively inefficient and that the severe damage they cause may be comparatively localised;[20] disintegration of the body is rare unless the victim is in direct contact with the device. Burns associated with bombs are of two types—the 'flash burn' affecting persons close to the explosion from which clothing provides good protection, and ordinary thermal burns resulting either from the clothes or from the building catching fire. The classic injury consists of the triad of punctate bruises, abrasions and small puncture lacerations—the last being less widespread than the others. If one adds the characteristic changes in the skin due to impaction of what is little more than dust, the picture is virtually diagnostic. The non-specific effects of falling masonry and the like may, of course, be superimposed.

In general, the radius of injury due to blast is less than that due to primary and secondary missile injury. The effects of pure blast are, therefore, unlikely to be seen unless the victim is protected from the latter by body armour—the resulting uncomplicated picture may be seen especially following the use of unsophisticated civilian terrorist bombs.[1] Powerful bombs will, however, produce blast effects beyond the range of missiles; at the end of the spectrum, therefore, pure blast is, a common cause of death following a nuclear explosion. The ear-drum is the organ most sensitive to blast and should always be examined in the relevant circumstances. Patchy pulmonary haemorrhage is as likely to be caused by direct trauma as by blast; the clearest sign which, when present, distinguishes the latter is that visible, sub-pleural haemorrhages often follow the line of the ribs.

The pathological diagnosis of death due to explosion is seldom in doubt. The cause of the *explosion*—eg bomb detonation or domestic gas ignition—may, however, be unknown and the pathologist has not discharged his responsibility by merely recording a relatively self-evident cause of death. Thus, the most

19 The offence of causing an explosion likely to endanger life or cause serious injury to property is defined in the Explosive Substances Act 1883, s 2, as amended by the Criminal Jurisdiction Act 1975, s 7.
20 J Crane 'Violence Associated with Civil Disturbance' in J K Mason and B N Purdue (eds) *The Pathology of Trauma* (3rd edn, 2000) ch 6.
 1 S G Mellor and G J Cooper 'Analysis of 828 Servicemen Killed or Injured by Explosion in Northern Ireland 1970–1984' (1990) 76 Brit J Surg 1006.

important evidence to be obtained from the post-mortem dissection lies in the search for and recovery of fragments of bomb casing, which will not only demonstrate the cause but, much as in the case of firearm wounds, will provide information of value to law enforcement; the importance of X-ray study as a means of localising such fragments cannot be overemphasised.

A major exception to the easy diagnosis of death due to detonation of a bomb lies in the deliberate destruction of a commercial aircraft in flight. This crime seems to have become less frequent than it was a decade ago when one could anticipate an occurrence on a world-wide basis as often as between once and twice a year; whether this is the result of reduced terrorist activity or of the great improvement in airport security has yet to be decided. The difficulty in making a diagnosis from the pathological findings lies in the unusual circumstances and the several mechanisms by which traumatic pathology can be generated. Thus, in addition to exposure to the bomb explosion itself, injury may result from explosive decompression per se, from turbulence within the aircraft and secondary missile production, from flailing during free-fall and from impact with ground or water; moreover, since many of these disasters occur over the sea, it may be that no typical 'target' bodies are recovered. In these last circumstances, it is likely that no wreckage will be available for examination and, paradoxically, the major part of the accident investigation will devolve on the pathologist; it may be very difficult for him or her to distinguish between simple structural failure and deliberate destruction of the aircraft—and the distinction may have far-reaching financial as well as criminal implications.[2] Success rests upon observations derived from a full examination of all the human wreckage recovered. The pattern of injuries throughout the dead may, when coupled with a knowledge of the seating plan, indicate a specific area of primary damage; search must be made for a 'target' who may present as an 'odd man out', by reason either of his position relative to the other passengers or of his injuries. Radiological examination of all human tissue is essential—and must nowadays be undertaken in all unexplained catastrophes occurring at altitude until a credible alternative to sabotage is agreed; finally, any metallic fragments other than those that are clearly part of the aircraft structure must be subjected to expert examination. The investigation of such a case is, inevitably, time consuming and extremely costly.[3]

The perpetrators of this form of mass murder have been found to be of various types—political motivation may be present but, possibly, the commonest reason in the past has been pecuniary and related to life insurance policies; suicides have been suspected and instances have been traced to motives of almost incredible frivolity, such as the removal of an unwanted girlfriend.

2   In the event of sabotage being shown as the cause of an aircraft accident, responsibility for insurance passes from the 'All Risks' insurers to those underwriting 'War Risks'—millions of pounds may be at stake. Perhaps the most vivid example in recent years in Britain involved the loss of the Air India aircraft in 1985.

3   Two early examples of the medical investigation of such cases are: (a) J R Dille and A H Hasbrook 'Injuries due to Explosion, Decompression and Impact of a Jet Transport' (1966) 37 Aerospace Med 5; and (b) J K Mason and S W Tarlton 'Medical Investigation of the Loss of the Comet 4B Aircraft, 1967' (1969) i Lancet 431. The more recent Air India disaster is referred to in P B Herdson and J K Mason 'The Role of Pathology in Major Disasters' in J K Mason and B N Purdue (eds) *The Pathology of Trauma* (3rd edn, 2000) ch 3. Pathological evidence as to the cause of the catastrophe was required only to a limited extent in the notorious explosion over Lockerbie in 1988—in respect of which, a trial for murder is ongoing at the time of writing.

Injury and death associated with breaches of human rights

Probably the most significant cultural change that has evolved since the last edition of this book has been the move towards the recognition of human rights as being fundamental to the global social system. Breach of these human rights is seldom seen in forensic medical or pathological terms but, at its extreme, it is manifested by torture, murder and, ultimately, genocide—all of which could be subsumed under crimes against humanity. Torture and killing while in custody are so rare in a country such as the United Kingdom as not to merit specific mention in a book of this sort. This is not to say that they can be dismissed out of hand as possibilities—indeed, such possibilities are likely to be raised whenever injury or death is associated with law enforcement.[4] The main forms of physical and fatal injury that might occur in such circumstances are described at various points in the text; only the locus distinguishes them as potentially public rather than private offences and, even then, the forensic physician or pathologist must be careful not to stray beyond his or her remit—the doctor may properly diagnose an abrasion as being due to the use of a baton (see page 110) but it is for the courts to say whether this was used lawfully or unlawfully.

United Kingdom pathologists and, indeed, lawyers are, however, becoming increasingly involved in the offences of war crimes and genocide.[5] This is for two main reasons. First, there is an increasing sense of international responsibility for maintaining human rights throughout the world,[6] which involves the use of international and independent experts; second, there may be many reasons why local pathologists should not want to exhibit a high profile in such cases or should be prevented from so doing.[7] The majority of deaths of this type are likely to be due to shooting, so this is not an illogical place to insert a short note.

The purpose of opening a mass grave may be simply to identify the remains and return them to their next-of-kin; more probably it will be in order to provide evidence for a criminal trial although, of course, the two objectives may be combined. The former may turn out to be a near impossible task—the bodies are likely to be severely decomposed, they will be unprotected by coffins and suitable comparative ante-mortem records are, for several reasons, likely to be scarce. The latter is, fundamentally, a matter of disclosing war crimes and/or genocide.[8]

In distinguishing victims of war crimes from battle casualties, much importance has been attached to the wounded:dead ratio. The former always exceed the latter

---

4   For particular reference to the subject, see P Vanezis 'Deaths in Custody' in J K Mason and B N Purdue (eds) *The Pathology of Trauma* (3rd edn, 2000) ch 8.

5   The United Nations Tribunal on Events in the former Yugoslavia addresses four potential crimes: grave breaches of the Geneva Convention of 1949, war crimes, genocide and crimes against humanity. For an analysis of these, see S C Neff 'Past and Future Lessons from the Ad Hoc Tribunals for the Former Yugoslavia and Rwanda' in P J Cullen and W C Gilmore (eds) *Crime sans Frontières* (1998).

6   Probably originated by the Universal Declaration on Human Rights adopted by the General Assembly of the United Nations, December 1948.

7   P Vanezis 'Investigation of Clandestine Graves Resulting from Human Rights Abuses' (1999) 6 J Clin Forens Med 238.

8   Genocide, in fact, comprises more than 'killing a race' and involves acts intended to destroy in whole or in part a national, ethnical, racial or religious group which include killing, causing severe bodily harm, enforcing intolerable living conditions, imposing methods designed to limit births and transferring children to another group: Genocide Act 1969, Schedule.

in the battle situation, whereas the reverse is true of war crimes.[9] It has also been noted that shooting of defenceless persons with automatic weapons tends to be concentrated on the head and central thorax. The pattern of injuries may be diagnostic. Thus, a large number of close range gunshot injuries to the head will strongly suggest a series of executions, as will death from head injuries other than by shooting—for example, by bludgeoning.

Genocide will be indicated if there is a gender mix, for as many women will be the target of 'ethnic cleansing' as will men. Similarly, absent the presence of multiple injuries attributable to indiscriminate shelling or bombing, the presence of children among the fatalities will militate against a claim that the mass casualties were the result of legitimate warfare. Otherwise, specific evidence of varied type— for example, the presence of injuries known to be associated with torture, evidence of fire and the like—must be sought and interpreted in conjunction with the circumstantial and historical evidence.

All who have been involved in this type of work remark on how difficult it is to remain neutral.[10] The pathologist may, of course, have been called in by any number of organisations from the United Nations, through the regional government, to semi-official bodies such as Amnesty International. Two caveats arise. First, it is essential that objectivity be maintained in very difficult circumstances and, second, that the pathologist should be at particular pains to establish his or her status and credentials. All governments have their rules as to disposal of and disturbance of the dead and these are likely to be vigorously enforced when questions as to the violation of human rights are in the balance.

---

9 R M Coupland and D R Meddings 'Mortality Associated with use of Weapons in Armed Conflicts, Wartime Atrocities, and Civilian Mass Shootings: Literature Review' (1999) 319 BMJ 407.
10 P Vanezis 'Forensic Pathology in a Troubled World' (1997) 37 Med Sci Law 277.

Accidental injury and death due to deceleration and acceleration[1]

Deaths due to accident provide a major part of the forensic pathologist's work-load; they come second in frequency only to sudden natural death in most medico-legal practices. They are of further, and particular, interest in that, almost uniquely, they offer the forensic pathologist an opportunity to contribute to the life-saving role of medicine. Finding the cause of an accident hopefully leads to elimination of that cause; elucidating the reasons for fatal injuries should transform similar future occurrences into non-fatal accidents. The accident autopsy can thus be seen as an aspect of preventive medicine. An immense amount of work has already been devoted to correlation of injuries with—and the consequent improvement of—the accident environment[2] and, to obtain maximum benefit, the pathologist should combine his autopsy with a visit to the locus or to the vehicle involved. Unfortunately, this is a counsel of perfection because, in current conditions, very few pathologists outside specialist units would be able to afford the time. The ideal should, however, be sought—certainly in any circumstances that are likely to lead to a public inquiry beyond that of the coroner's inquest.

The nature of the injuries

Accidents may occur in the home, at work or at play, and some of these situations are covered elsewhere in this book. Transportation accidents are, however, the most important single source of severe traumatic injury and death of young adults in the United Kingdom and, as a result, merit greatest attention.[3] The majority of significant injuries sustained in road-traffic accidents are of a decelerative or accelerative nature and the forces involved are applied in the horizontal plane. Injuries sustained in accidental falls essentially result from vertical deceleration.

1 'Deceleration' to the physiologists is a substitute term for 'negative acceleration'. But the word is used colloquially and it is in this sense that it is introduced here.
2 There is a very considerable literature, mainly devoted to transportation accidents. See M Mackay 'Engineering in Accidents: Vehicle Design and Injuries' (1994) 25 Injury 615.
3 Somewhat surprisingly, fatal accidents are approximately as frequent in the home as on the roads. The former, however, involve an older age group and are less important when measured in terms of lost life-years.

Aircraft accidents link these two conditions in that the injurious forces are a varying combination of the horizontal and the vertical.

Although a high proportion of accidental injuries might be thought to be non-specific, many abrasions and some bruises may be remarkably distinctive in both appearance and distribution. They may, therefore, provide important evidence in accident reconstruction and this is particularly well shown in the pedestrian road-traffic death.

Pedestrian injuries

The great majority of fatal pedestrian casualties derive from contact with a single vehicle and the source of any abrasions discovered may be obvious. Examples include the pattern imprinted by radiator grilles or by tyres; on occasion, this may be so individual as to provide corroboration of a cause-and-effect relationship with a particular vehicle. The importance of scaled photography of such abrasions, particularly in the hit-and-run type of accident, cannot be overemphasised as a means of preserving valuable evidence.

Useful pathological information can often be derived from an assessment of the sequence in which the injuries were sustained. Classically, these arise in three phases. Primary impact is with the front of the vehicle in some 70% of cases; secondary impact arises from rotation of the body and contact with the bonnet or windscreen surround; and tertiary impact injuries result from sliding or being dragged across the road surface or from crushing against a rigid structure. The time intervals are usually extremely short and an evaluation through appraisal of the degree of bruising or of vital reaction is often impossible. Nevertheless, an attempt to distinguish direct contact wounds from those of secondary or tertiary type—as shown by contained glass, paint or earth—may be of value both to the police and to other interested investigators. Whenever possible—which should mean in most cases—the autopsy should include an examination of the clothing in situ—the correlation of clothing damage and bodily injury is one of the most useful examinations in the pedestrian/vehicular accident.

Occupants of cars

Abrasions in the occupants of cars who are killed in an accident are of particular importance, not only in indicating the identity of the driver—through the characteristic 'steering wheel' abrasions so often imprinted on the chest with underlying fracture of the sternum—but also in relation to the use of seat belt restraint. This has important practical applications. The use of seat belts is now compulsory in the absence of a medical exemption.[4] Most insurance companies now tie the amount of indemnity to the use of or failure to use restraining harnesses, while judgments for damages for injuries sustained have taken this factor into account since 1975.[5] Damages awarded to plaintiff (or pursuer) as a result of a successful claim in negligence for personal injuries sustained in a motor vehicle accident will be reduced in part-proportion to the extent that his injuries were

4   Road Traffic Act 1988, s 14; Motor Vehicles (Wearing of Seat Belts) Regulations 1993, SI 1993/176 (adults). Road Traffic Act 1988, s 15; Motor Vehicles (Wearing of Seat Belts by Children) Regulations 1993, SI 1993/31 (children).
5   *Froom v Butcher* [1976] QB 286.

caused or aggravated by failure to use a seat belt.[6] Each case will be judged on its own merits—in *Owens v Brimmell*,[7] for example, the defendant failed to discharge the burden of proof that the plaintiff's failure to wear a harness contributed to his injuries;[8] the general tariff is, however, assessed as 25% for failure to wear any harness and, since it involves a statutory offence, a high limit is likely to be imposed rigorously.[9] The pathologist has, therefore, a considerable responsibility to seek evidence as to the wearing of a harness and must be prepared to give an opinion as to the excess of injury which could be attributed to failure to do so. Although there will often be no residual evidence even though the equipment was used, bruising may be found in accidents involving relatively low force; the shape may be specific to the belt but any fine pattern will be that of the clothing closest to the skin. In accidents of severer type, the abrasion is more likely to be of the parchmented pressure type without pattern or vital reaction. The relationship between belt restraint and more serious internal injuries is discussed on page 141.

Transportation injuries—general

Lacerations may have a 'general' specificity. Thus, notes should be available of damage to the legs of pedestrians that is characteristically caused by car bumpers and which may provide excellent evidence as to the positional relationship at the time of impact; very similar injuries are common in pedal cyclists knocked down by motor cars. Multiple lacerations due to fragmented glass are common in killed car occupants, particularly those in the front passenger seat; the distinction between those who have been so injured because they were not restrained by a seat belt and those who suffered injury when their belts failed can often be made by a simultaneous appraisal of abrasions in the harness area. On the other hand, lacerations may be very specific and diagnostic as to causation—this applies both in automobiles and in light aircraft. Particular attention should be paid to the hands. When they are present, lacerations of the palmar skin between thumb and index finger are almost diagnostic of having been caused on the steering wheel or control column at the time of impact; underlying fracture of the metacarpal or carpal bones may be present, particularly in the more severe aircraft accidents. It goes without saying that evidence as to who was controlling the vehicle at the time of the accident is of paramount significance both to the investigation and to subsequent litigation. The importance of photography in the accident autopsy is,

---

6   Law Reform (Contributory Negligence) Act 1945, s 1. It is worth remembering that a pedestrian involved in a traffic accident can also be liable in contributory negligence: *Fitzgerald v Lane* [1990] RTR 133; *McDonald v Chambers* 2000 SLT 454.

7   [1976] 3 All ER 765. Though contributory negligence due to accepting a lift from a driver known to be drunk was allowed.

8   In *Capps v Miller* [1989] 2 All ER 333 (a crash helmet case involving a faulty chin strap) the negligence was agreed to have been of relatively minor type and the award was reduced by only 10%. On the other side of the coin, the driver is under no obligation to point out the importance of using the restraint available—which should, by now, be apparent to everyone: *Eastman v South West Thames Regional Health Authority* [1991] RTR 389.

9   Although the percentage scale seems to have remained much the same and is now likely to be agreed. A 20% deduction was agreed in a case of severe brain damage: *Bogan's CB v Graham* 1992 SCLR 920. A reduction of 33% was ordered in another Scottish case, *Hill v Chivers* 1987 SCLR 452, but this was a cumulative total resulting from negligence in failure to wear a harness and driving with a person under the influence of alcohol.

again, emphasised; photographs serve not only as aides-mémoire but may also draw attention to a previously unnoted correlation between an injury and its cause. In addition, they greatly improve the quality of the evidence when it is given in the coroners' or civil courts.

Internal injury without external evidence

Severe or fatal deceleration injury may be transmitted to the internal organs without corresponding visible external damage. The two common circumstances are compression of the chest or abdomen and accelerative displacement of the viscera; damage to the spine is also important, particularly in survivors.

Compression of the chest may result from impaction against some object, such as the steering wheel of a car; superficial abrasive evidence may then be found and the breastbone (sternum) and ribs can be bruised or fractured. Alternatively, compression may be due simply to forceful flexion of the upper torso—the head and knees being thrown towards each other. This often occurs in motor cars when the occupant is restrained by a lap belt only; the legs and arms are flung forward with the body compressed into a shallow C-shape. The condition is even more apparent in aircraft accidents when the added component of vertical force exaggerates the deformity. The heart may burst like a blown-up paper bag if it is crushed between the breastbone and the spine. The weakest areas lie in the atria, especially at the entry points of the great veins,[10] but, often, the compression is such as to lacerate the muscular walls of the ventricles. There may be important residua if the forces have been severe yet insufficient to rupture the heart on impact. A lowering of the arterial blood pressure is an almost inevitable immediate physiological reaction to severe injury; areas of the heart that have been damaged in the accident may be unable to withstand the increase in pressure that accompanies the phase of recovery and delayed rupture of the heart may occur within minutes or hours. Additionally, the process of rupture, which often runs from within the heart to the outer surface, may cause laceration of only a partial thickness of the muscle; the wall in the area where the inner lining is thus damaged is weakened and may rupture some considerable time after the event; a cause-and-effect relationship may then be difficult to establish.

The heart will be squeezed downwards if the major compression between the sternum and spine occurs just above its case (or upper border); the aorta is, however, tethered to the tissues surrounding the spine and is unable to move. As a result, the heart is torn from its major blood vessel; the effect is similar to rupture of the heart itself. This sequence is even more probable if the heart is, itself, displaced downwards under the influence of a vertical force as occurs in falls or in aircraft accidents. The injury is common in both situations and, again, an incomplete laceration may result in delayed full-thickness rupture (see Figure 10.1). The likely modification of injuries sustained when using an air bag is reverted to below (page 141).

Injuries of broadly similar type may be inflicted on the organs in the abdomen. These, by virtue of the organs' functions, may be of less catastrophic nature and prompt surgical intervention may be life saving.

10 Damage at these points may also be due to sudden increase in pressure in the venous system due to compression of the legs or abdomen.

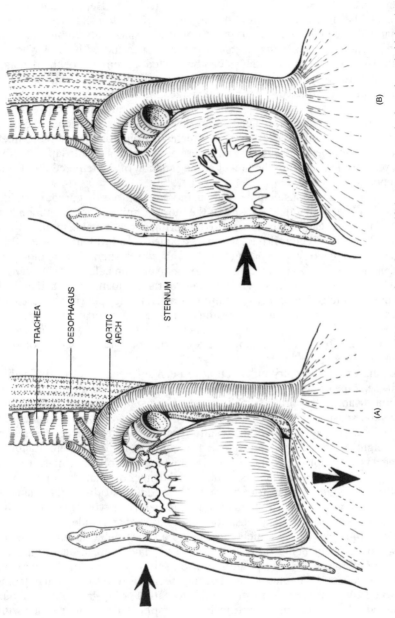

Figure 10.1 Major rupture of the cardiovascular system. (*a*) The heart will be torn from the aorta if the pressure on the breastbone is high. An alternative is when the force is vertical—as in a fall. The heart will then move downwards and be torn from the rigidly held aortic arch. (*b*) The heart will burst like a paper bag if the point of pressure is lower.

The great bulk of the liver renders it particularly susceptible to blunt injury. It is easily ruptured by bending and stretching of the upper surface during severe body flexion, while its solid structure is particularly vulnerable to the high-frequency oscillations that are set up in a severe accident. Hepatic damage may well be fatal because bleeding from the organ is hard to stop and the liver, being essential to life, cannot be removed in toto. The almost equally common rupture of the spleen—which is a disposable organ as far as the body as a whole is concerned—or of one of the kidneys can be treated by removal of the damaged part; the important feature is awareness of the possibility that such injuries can be present despite the absence of external damage. Although rupture of the bowel itself is comparatively rare, compressive damage to its nutrient blood vessels as they traverse the mesentery is not uncommon in car accidents and occurs frequently in aircraft accidents; it may result from violent flexion alone but is more likely when this is combined with sudden and severe pressure on a simple lap belt. Very severe pressure may rupture the bowel at the junction of the tethered duodenum and mobile jejunum.

The spine is under considerable strain in those conditions that produce sudden body flexion and, in practice, fracture of the thoracic spine is very common both in car and in aircraft accidents. There are two primarily vulnerable points; first in the cervico-thoracic region if the torso is restrained by a full harness—in which case the forces are likely to be beyond the tolerance of the body as a whole—and, second, in the lower thoracic area due to flexion over a lap belt. If severe vertical force is applied to the buttocks, as in a fall, an aircraft accident or, occasionally, in the unique situation of ejection from a military aircraft, the spine is weakest at the junction of the thoracic and lumbar portions. Very severe vertical force will cause fracture of the pelvis. The pelvis is also especially liable to damage from a direct lateral blow and fracture is common in pedestrian or cycling victims of road-traffic accidents.

The sum of bodily injury may well have been sufficient to cause immediate death if the spine or pelvis are severely damaged. Should there be recovery, the long-term disability resulting from fracture of the spine may be no more than stiffness and spasmodic pain of varying severity. If, however, the spinal cord is irrevocably injured, the extent of the resulting paralysis and anaesthesia is related to the 'height' of the injury in the spine. The common lower thoracic fracture is associated with paraplegia, that is paralysis of the legs and bladder; apart from the extremely severe disability, there is an increased danger of death due to infection, particularly infection of the urinary tract. The additional disability related to childbirth that may result from fracture of the pelvis in women also requires special consideration as to compensation accruing from an accident. Fracture in the cervico-thoracic region, which can also be a catastrophic feature of motor-cycle accidents or of being thrown from a car,[11] may result in quadriplegia or paralysis of all four limbs. Respiration is also compromised and may necessitate periods of mechanical ventilation; death from pneumonia is the common outcome.

Before leaving the spine, a word on the so-called 'whip-lash' injury should be inserted. Variations in definition have complicated the approach to this

---

11 In general, the injuries resulting from ejection from a car following an impact accident are greater than those sustained when retained by a harness. See G F McCoy, R A Johnstone, I W Nelson et al 'Incidence and Consequences of Ejection in Motor Vehicle Accidents' (1988) 297 BMJ 1244.

condition and the name has come in for some criticism. In this author's opinion, the cause of the condition is a true 'whip-lash' movement of the head as indicated in Figure 10.2; it is, therefore, typically due to a rear-ended impact and should, theoretically, be mitigated by an efficient head rest.[12] The signs of neck stiffness, pain and headache are due to injury to the neck ligaments and, in the acute stage generally respond well to treatment; occasionally, however, the onset of symptoms is delayed and, possibly due to involvement of the bony attachments, the injury gives rise to chronic disability. Since, by the nature of the accident, it is nearly always the result of another's fault, the whip-lash injury is a potent cause of litigation; the symptomatology may, in fact, result from a complex amalgam of physical and psychological factors.[13] It must be appreciated that 'neck sprain' can result from other types of accident and may, in fact, be exaggerated by the use of harness[14] (see below, page 141).

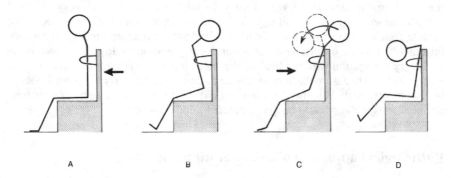

A   B   C   D

Figure 10.2 Mechanism of the specific whip-lash injury to the neck: (*a*) force is applied from the rear; (*b*) the body is accelerated against the harness but inertia leads to extension of the neck; (*c*) the vehicle and body are stopped but the head continues to accelerate, leading to a wide arc of unnatural forces on the neck, with the head finishing in forced flexion (*d*).

The condition of fat embolism

Fat embolism is a cause of death, nearly always associated with accidents, which is of sufficient medico-legal interest to deserve individual consideration. It is closely correlated with fractures of the long bones, spine or chest cage though, theoretically at least, it may result from severe injury to fatty tissue of any sort. Following fracture, there is a release of fat from the marrow cavity; this fat is passed into the venous system where, being particulate, it is caught up in the

12 D B Olney and A K Marsden 'The Effect of Head Restraints and Seat Belts on the Incidence of Neck Injury in Car Accidents' (1986) 17 Injury 365.
13 P K Newman 'Whiplash Injury' (1990) 301 BMJ 395.
14 G T Deans, J N Magalliard, M Kerr and W H Rutherford 'Neck Sprain—A Major Cause of Disability following Car Accidents' (1987) 18 Injury 10.

sieve of the pulmonary capillaries—the condition of pulmonary fat embolism is established. Pulmonary fat embolism is normally of no clinical significance; its main importance as a post-mortem finding is that it may be indicative of the time of survival between fracture and death (see page 149). It may, however, exacerbate the condition in those with pre-existing cardio-pulmonary disease; moreover, it appears that it may precipitate the adult respiratory distress syndrome when combined with generalised hypoxia. But in a proportion of fracture cases in previously healthy patients, the fat appears to pass through the lungs and lodges in the capillaries of the brain and kidneys; the potentially fatal condition of systemic fat embolism is established.[15] Some 24 hours after injury the patient's temperature rises and, in severe cases, fatal coma supervenes; treatment of the established fat embolism syndrome is unsatisfactory. It is only fair to say that this précis is a gross oversimplification, and the development of the clinical syndrome of systematic fat embolism probably depends on many interrelated factors including, particularly, the presence of surgical shock—which is, itself, associated with hypoxia. Whatever the precise mechanism may be, two considerations are unaffected. First, the condition is associated with injury in all but a handful of very unusual conditions; consequently, it always has medico-legal connotations. Secondly, despite a tendency to an association with manipulation of fractures under anaesthesia, fat embolism is an unfortunate but natural complication of injury. There is no necessary association with medical negligence although it is clear that care should always be taken to ensure that a patient with fracture—particularly of the leg bones—is fully oxygenated. Whether, and how, to transport a fracture case by commercial airline, for example, should be given careful prior consideration.[16]

Pathological appraisal of safety equipment

A correlation between the pathological findings and the safety equipment provided—whether the fatal accident results from the use of a vehicle or is of industrial type—is important for several reasons. First, there is the problem of the assessment of damages in car accidents which has been discussed above. Secondly, dependants of an employee killed at work are entitled to any evidence that indicates failure on the part of the management to provide an adequate safety environment; the employer must also be provided with any evidence that might limit his liability as to civil damages. Thirdly, as discussed in the introduction to this chapter, this aspect of the pathologist's work is rewarding preventive medicine. This is a main function of an inquiry under the Fatal Accidents and Sudden Deaths Inquiry (Scotland) Act 1976; it is a matter for regret that the corresponding function of the coroner has been markedly curtailed by the Coroners Rules 1984, r 36.

Pathological evidence on this score should be available both when safety equipment was provided and when it was not.

In the former case, the pathologist is certainly not the best person to evaluate the equipment because, by definition, he is dealing with a case in which it had

15 This seems to happen in up to 3% of cases overall—particularly when pressure is allowed to build up at the fracture site. For a recent review of the subject, which contains some controversial statements, see H J ten Duis 'The Fat Embolism Syndrome' (1997) 28 Injury 77.

16 Aircraft cabins are pressurised to 8,000 ft at which the partial pressure of arterial oxygen is about 60 mm Hg (10 kPa) (normal 100 mm Hg, 13.3 kPa).

failed in its purpose. The question often arises, however, as to whether the equipment actually contributed to death; an objective assessment, taking all the circumstances into account, is then essential. A number of road-traffic accident investigations describe 'seat belt syndromes' and there is no doubt that the seat belt, especially of the lap-strap-only type, can cause rupture of the mesentery, bowel or even major solid viscera.[17] But the alternative to such a syndrome is likely to be death, and an operable rupture of the bowel is a small price to pay for a life saved. Generally speaking, if the accident results in death from multiple injuries, the presence of lesions attributable to seat belts is no more than a part of the pattern of non-survivable loads on the body; but an isolated fatal injury positively associated with an intended safety device is of major concern. Thus, a number of fatalities have occurred in light aircraft due to the subject 'submarining' through the harness and sustaining injuries similar to those of the old judicial hanging—such accidents clearly indicate the need for incorporation of a crutch strap. Recently introduced equipment should be studied particularly carefully both by pathologists and clinicians; one such example lies in the now compulsory restraint available for children—correct selection and fitting of harnesses has been found to be essential if severe cervical spinal injury is to be avoided.[18]

It should be emphasised that no item of personal safety equipment can be expected to be effective in all possible circumstances. Its design is a matter of compromise—'child-proof' door locks on cars are, for example, potentially life saving in ordinary travel but may be positively detrimental to survival in the event of fire after a crash; it is a matter of calculating the risks involved and providing accordingly, the important feature being that a positive assessment has been made and a reasonable decision taken. Escape by traditional means from an aircraft in flight provides another good example of the dilemma—the provision of a bulky dinghy pack must complicate easy egress but survival after a descent into water is compromised without a dinghy; the decision to provide one would, therefore, depend upon whether the aircraft was operating predominantly over land or over water. With respect to the most commonly laid objection to the use of harnesses in cars, fire after motor-car accidents is in itself rare and the chances of dying from such incineration are in the region of 1 in 500 fatal accidents; the reduction in concussion, and its consequential failure to escape the fire environment, that is offered by restraining harnesses should be added to this assessment.[19]

Consideration of the injuries sustained using current safety equipment clearly suggests that many could be obviated by the use of air bags. It should be noted, however, that, at least in theory, the airbag will protect only against horizontal forces; thus, while the equipment may be of great value in cars, it would be less efficient, say, in passenger aircraft where many of the injuries following accidents derive from vertical forces. Air bags have scarcely passed the experimental phase in the United Kingdom and there are very few cases available for analysis. Fears

---

17 Eg Editorial Comment 'Seat Belt Injuries to the Colon' (1974) i BMJ 85. There is an almost inexhaustible number of papers describing 'one-off' injuries of various types.

18 G A Hoy and W G Cole 'The Paediatric Cervical Seat Belt Syndrome' (1993) 24 Injury 297. The relatively large head and laxity of the cervical spine in children may be predisposing factors.

19 The rather interesting arguments as to the compulsory use of helmets by pedal cyclists are referred to below at p 162.

as to premature inflation are almost certainly groundless. The force of the explosive opening is, however, considerable and superficial friction burns have been reported in the United Kingdom—once again, however, this is a small price to pay for a life saved. On the other hand, the possibility of suffocation of an incapacitated driver has to be considered but is, currently, compensated for by controlled rapid deflation of the bag. It is to be noted that the manufacturers insist that maximum safety from air bags is obtained only when they are used in *conjunction* with an adequate harness.[20]

If death occurred when no equipment was provided, the pathologist can only surmise as to the likely effect of the omission; an attempt must be made because important questions relating to liability may be raised. In cases in which the material was lost or damaged, it would also be important to seek pathological evidence as to whether equipment that had been provided was, in fact, used.

It is common sense to suppose that, were safety equipment to have any inherent danger, that danger would be exacerbated if the body part at risk were already diseased. The regulations governing the wearing of motor vehicle harnesses, therefore, include an exception in the event that a medical certificate identifies a contraindication to their use.[1] The general opinion is that conditions which fulfil such criteria are relatively few; if a person is fit to be in control of a vehicle, the probability is that he or she is fit to wear a seat belt.[2]

The most obvious question mark applies to the pregnant woman. There is no country in which pregnancy is an automatic ground for exemption from seat-harness law and it can be taken as a general rule that both maternal and fetal injuries are reduced by the use of restraint; if the forces are sufficient to cause fetal seat belt damage, it is well-nigh certain that the damage would have been as great or greater if the woman had been unrestrained.[3] This, however, presupposes that the harness is positioned correctly with the lap belt segment lying below the fetus and the diagonal being sited above it. The author has seen only one case in which fetal death could be positively attributed to restraint—death was due to severe linear haemorrhage in a placenta sited on the anterior uterine wall; pathological experience may, however, differ from that of clinicians.[4] The evaluation is of considerable importance in the event of fetal survival in a damaged condition. Intrauterine injuries sustained in a vehicular accident constitute the only circumstance in which a neonate can sue its mother for prenatal negligence.[5] Section 2 of the 1976 Act imposes a duty of care on a pregnant woman driver to her fetus similar to that owed to other people. So far as is known, what constitutes a duty of care in respect of seat belt use has never been tested in the courts; the first case will make interesting reading.

20 A news item of a few years ago reported that 27 children and 19 adults had been killed by air bags in the United States; it was said that no deaths had occurred in Britain: R Ramesh 'Airbag Injuries Force Design Change' *The Sunday Times*, 10 November 1996, p 1.10. For a good, early review, see A K Lund and S A Ferguson 'Driver Fatalities in 1985–1993 Cars with Airbags' (1995) 38 J Trauma 469.
 1 Road Traffic Act 1988, s 14(2)(b).
 2 M S Christian 'Exemption from Compulsory Wearing of Seat Belts—Medical Indications' (1979) i BMJ 1411. The evidence suggests that disabled drivers are more conscious of the need for restraint than are those without disability.
 3 M Pearce 'Seat Belts in Pregnancy' (1992) 304 BMJ 586.
 4 See, for example, G W Fakhoury and J R M Gibson 'Seat Belt Hazards in Pregnancy. Case reports' (1986) 93 Brit J Obstet Gynaecol 395.
 5 Congenital Disabilities (Civil Liability) Act 1976, s 2.

The interrelationship of disease and accidents

Natural disease may cause varying degrees of incapacitation in the operator of a vehicle and may thus precipitate an accident; by reason of the environment in which an emergency occurs, such disability is likely to have more serious consequence in solo pilots than in drivers of cars. Further, the driver or pilot may die from sudden natural causes while at the controls, and it is more than theoretically possible that a passenger might die in the same way while under the stress of an impending catastrophe. Thus, the precise relationship between discovered disease and a fatal accident is of medico-legal importance on two main counts—first, a suspicion of negligence may be raised either on the part of the operator, in that he was driving or piloting while he knew himself to be unfit, or on the part of those scheduling the task without apparently ensuring adequate medical supervision; secondly, questions may be raised as to the entitlement to indemnity under an insurance policy against accidental death.

Disease of any sort discovered after an accident may be causative of, contributory to, or merely incidental to that accident. The distinction is often difficult to make. This is for two main reasons which are particularly well illustrated by coronary disease (see page 101). First, there is the simple 'population' problem illustrated in Table 10.1; a random search of persons killed accidentally will demonstrate a high proportion with potentially lethal disease of the coronary arteries yet in few, if any, of the cases could there have been more than an incidental association. Secondly, there is the technical problem arising from the fact that the disease process may need to do no more than cause symptoms—eg angina—for it to precipitate a crash; death is then due to injuries and the pathologist is confronted with appearances in the heart that will have been stopped short of those that are seen in natural death. The interpretation of events then rests on a personal opinion as to cause and effect—and this has to be given with what must sometimes seem to be undue reservation. There is often less difficulty in automobile cases in which the findings may well be those that are normally accepted as good evidence of a coronary 'heart attack'; these will still have to be distinguished from the effects of direct trauma to the heart—a problem that is also relevant to aircraft accidents.

Table 10.1 Prevalence of coronary artery disease in UK aviators. Results are given as numbers of cases, with percentage of group in parenthesis.*

Grade of disease	Military	Civilian	Total
0	114 (40)	38 (34)	152 (38)
I	103 (36)	48 (43)	151 (38)
II	46 (16)	16 (14)	62 (15.5)
III	23 (8)	10 (9)	33 (8.5)
Mean age (years)	27.6	34.9	29.7

* In the UK, almost a quarter of persons subject to relatively strict medical surveillance show restriction of 50% or more of the lumen of a main coronary vessel without accompanying symptoms (Grades II and III).

In making his assessment, the pathologist must consider, on the one hand, the special quality of his autopsy findings that might distinguish significant from asymptomatic disease [6] and, on the other, the circumstantial details of the accident. He must also know the extent of the disease in the particular group of persons concerned—eg drivers or pilots. Having all this information, he can ascribe the accident to disease in the operator on the basis of probability ranging from, say, a significant association that is just possible (+) to a very probable association (+ + + +). It is doubtful, however, if he should often be more definite. A classic account of how these problems of interpretation can be argued was given at the inquiry into the accident at Staines involving a Trident aircraft in 1972.[7]

The practical extent of the problem of disease as a cause of accidents deserves careful evaluation. The threat is clearly very real in the case of aircraft pilots who, accordingly, are stringently screened for fitness—screening includes, in particular, periodic electrocardiography (ECG). But, by and large, disease of the coronary arteries and experience go hand in hand. In the long run, therefore, greater safety may be achieved by 'double crewing' than by intensive medical selection. Similarly, the potential danger to the public dictates that drivers of public services vehicles should be subject to medical examination but, in practice, serious motor-vehicle accidents of any sort due to disease in the driver are rare—there is a 'fail-safe' mechanism as the foot comes off the accelerator and, before this, most drivers will be able to pull into the side on feeling the premonitory symptoms which accompany most potentially fatal conditions. Thus, while some 75% of deaths at the wheel are due to coronary heart disease, the condition is responsible for only 15% of accidents due to disease. Cerebral diseases which manifest no prodromal symptoms are more important in relation to *fatal accidents* and, of these, epilepsy is by far the most significant. The difficulty, as with all medical conditions, is to adjust the regulations so as to balance the safety of the public against unnecessary disadvantage to the disabled.[8] Currently, prohibitions as to epilepsy are relatively lax as to obtaining an ordinary driving licence in the United Kingdom—the main precaution being that an applicant with epilepsy must have been free from epileptic attacks in the previous year; for obvious reasons, the restrictions on a vocational licence are far more severe and demand freedom from an attack or treatment for ten years.[9] More argument surrounds the problem of the insulin-dependent diabetic—although most diabetics are well trained in appreciating anticipatory symptoms, coma of either hyperglycaemic or hypoglycaemic type can come on without warning. There is no intention that insulin dependent diabetics should be barred from driving, but the current limitations on the *size* of vehicle[10] that can be driven by such persons seems illogical—what matters is the *purpose* for which he or she is driving. Since, in general, an autopsy diagnosis can be made neither

6 In the case of coronary disease, these include evidence of previous damage to the heart muscle (fibrosis), calcification of the coronary vessels and evidence of activity of the disease in the form of infiltration of the vessel's coat by white blood cells (adventitial lymphocytosis).

7 *Report of the Public Inquiry into the Causes and Circumstances of the Accident near Staines on 18 June 1972.* Civil Aircraft Accident Report 4/73, London, HMSO.

8 Motor Vehicles (Driving Licences) Regulations 1999, SI 1999/2864, regs 70–75.

9 Motor Vehicles (Driving Licences) Regulations 1999, SI 1999/2864, reg 73 (8). See S Shorvon 'Epilepsy and Driving' (1995) 310 BMJ 885: Persons who knowlingly drive with potentially dangerous medical conditions can be guilty of dangerous driving: *R v Lowe* [1997] 2 Cr App Rep (S) 324, *R v Marison* [1997] RTR 457.

10 Motor Vehicles (Driving Licences) Regulations 1999, SI 1999/2864, regs 73 (6) and (9). See also European Council Directive on driving licences (91/439/EEC), Annex III.

of epilepsy nor of diabetic coma,[11] the pathologist must depend on awareness and the circumstantial evidence when reaching a conclusion as to the cause of death.

Diseases likely to lead to accidental death in pedestrians are of a different type and, again, are scarcely amenable to detection at autopsy—in particular, diseases of the locomotor system or of the special senses. Fatal accidents in the home are especially common in the elderly and, as a logical corollary, are very largely associated with degenerative disease, much of it having a causative or contributory role.

Toxicological factors in vehicular accidents

Toxic substances contributing to vehicular accidents may be deliberately ingested or accidentally inhaled. Alcohol is the outstanding example of the first category and is discussed in detail in Chapter 24. Other drugs do play a part but the extent of their contribution is difficult to determine. To be a significant cause of accidents, a drug must be readily available, it must be used generally for the treatment of common ailments, and it must have a deleterious effect on concentration and performance; the antihistamines—widely used as cold cures—fulfil this specification outstandingly. Most of these drugs are available as pharmacy-sale drugs (see Chapter 22) but, when they are sold, their labels must indicate not only that they may cause drowsiness but must also include warnings not to drive, operate machinery or consume alcohol. Amphetamines used to be a potential cause of accidents, particularly when used to excess in night driving or as weight controllers without appreciation of their effect on function; this group is, however, now controlled under the Misuse of Drugs Act 1971. Other commonly prescribed drugs, eg of the tranquilliser groups, may cause accidents by virtue of the taker being unaware of their intrinsic effect on driving or, more commonly, of the potentiating effect of combinations of drugs, particularly with those that include alcohol.[12]

There are two major difficulties in assessing the role of such drugs in accident causation. First, there is the technical problem of random searching *post mortem* for the presence of substances in near therapeutic concentrations; to do so is generally beyond the laboratory's resources in manpower and finance—and it is unlikely that the medico-legal authorities would support such analyses on a routine basis. Secondly, there is again the problem of interpretation. Who, for example, is to say that a light-aircraft pilot is any less safe when on a recognised dose of antinauseants than is the same pilot suffering from air sickness? And if traces of the drug are found at autopsy, how is one to distinguish with certainty between a causal and an incidental association with the accident? It could be that, in an ideal world, no one would drive a car while under medication; in practice, such counsel is of unattainable perfection.

Barbiturates are no longer a potent cause of accidents per se. Their presence may, however, be a significant indicator of psychiatric or other nervous disease

---

11 Post-mortem changes in blood glucose are so variable as to make their interpretation very suspect. Examination of the vitreous humour of the eye may be helpful in hyperglycaemic states but is unpredictable in the diagnosis of insulin overdose.

12 Benzodiazepines are Class C controlled drugs but are, nevertheless, very widely available: Misuse of Drugs Regulations 1985, SI 1985/2066.

that is not demonstrable by standard post-mortem techniques—the prime example being epilepsy. Notification of epilepsy to the Driving and Vehicle Licensing Authority is the personal responsibility of the subject and it is not difficult for the regulations to be bypassed. A search for barbiturates or anticonvulsants might, therefore, be expected to yield useful clues in indicating the basic cause of an apparently inexplicable accident. In practice, however, the value of such investigations is limited by the fact that it is the *undersuppressed* epileptic who is at risk of a fit.

It will be seen that it is not easy to attribute any fatal accident to the therapeutic use of drugs—nor is it easy to show that a person is unfit to drive by reason of being under the influence of drugs.[13] He or she may *appear* to be intoxicated but the charge is difficult to substantiate if the tissue concentration of the drug is within therapeutic limits. Effectively, either the level discovered must be in the toxic range or the 'drug' must be one with no therapeutic use; in this connection, it is to be noted that a solvent is classified legally as a drug.[14]

Of the gaseous toxic factors in vehicular accident causation, only carbon monoxide deserves emphasis. Being a natural product of the internal combustion engine, it may leak into the cabin of the car through a faulty exhaust system or into an aircraft cockpit via a defective cockpit heater; carbon monoxide may also be drawn in from the exhausts of other cars if a car heater fan is operated in heavy traffic conditions.

Fatal levels of carbon monoxide in the blood are unlikely to be discovered in accidental deaths involving cars or aeroplanes; only a level sufficient to cause lack of concentration is required to cause a fatal accident. Levels of 20–30% carboxyhaemoglobin[15] are commonly associated with symptoms of dizziness and headache, but there are two reasons why even lower levels may be of significance in drivers and pilots. First, fine judgment is certainly affected at much lower levels. Secondly, a synergistic effect may result from the interaction of carbon monoxide, alcohol, fatigue or hunger while, in aviation, the effect of even slight oxygen lack due to altitude may be compounded to produce a most dangerous situation.

True intoxication of the operator is not the only possible cause of a raised carboxyhaemoglobin level discovered in the blood after a fatal vehicular accident. Survival in a fire after the crash is by far the commonest cause (see page 199).[16] Low levels, particularly in aircraft, may indicate an engine defect rather than an effect on the pilot, while the 'natural background' of carboxyhaemoglobin—which may reach 8% in heavy smokers—must be considered in the interpretation of results.

Ideally, an analysis for carboxyhaemoglobin should be an integral part of the investigation of any vehicular death but, since levels of less than 20% saturation may be of significance in an accident, the methodology must be adequate for the purpose. The methodology should, indeed, be considered whenever a scientific result is quoted for medico-legal purposes. The technical method used must be shown to have adequate sensitivity and specificity at the range of levels required

13 Road Traffic Act 1988, s 4. It is to be noted that a specimen of blood for the purposes of drug analysis can only be taken at a police station on the advice of a medical practitioner (1988 Act, s 7).
14 *Bradford v Wilson* [1983] Crim LR 482; *Duffy v Tudhope* 1983 SCCR 440.
15 That is, 20–30% of the normal respiratory haemoglobin of the blood is combined with carbon monoxide and is not available for the transport of oxygen.
16 See D P Wirthwein and J E Pless 'Carboxyhemoglobin Levels in a Series of Automobile Fires' (1996) 17 Amer J Forens Med Pathol 117.

and the method must also be related both to the quantity of the specimen and to its quality—a method useful for examining good samples of blood taken from a living person may be quite inadequate when applied to a partially decomposed post-mortem specimen. The laboratory must be able to state its range of normal values when these factors are taken into consideration. These aspects are discussed further in Chapter 25.

Accidents as a cause of disease

Although discussion has thus far centred on disease as a cause of accidents, the converse proposition is also of medico-legal importance.

Much of the debate on this subject has centred on the induction of cancer by injury; there is no doubt that this can occur, the most obvious examples being the growth of a tumour in scar tissue—especially in scars resulting from burning. Skin cancer is relatively obvious and its topographical associations are clear. The attribution of cancer of the deep tissues to previous trauma is a far less certain matter due, in the main, to the time lapse between any precipitating injury and the clinical recognition of the tumour. Most interest has lain in the possible association of tumours of the brain with head injury, although cancer of other tissues—for example, the breast—might well be related to injury. But accidental injury, albeit slight, to the head is commonplace while brain tumours are rare; moreover, even were it suggested that *all* such tumours were precipitated by injury—and it most certainly is not—the time interval would be such as to make it very difficult to decide which particular traumatic incident during that time represented the trigger mechanism. It is now generally agreed that, before a tumour can be reasonably attributed to injury:

* There must be evidence of previous normality of the part.
* The injury must have been substantial.
* The interval during which the tumour matured must have been of reasonable length.
* The tumour must have developed at the site of injury.

Even accepting these premises, the attribution of a tumour to a previous traumatic incident is a matter of probability and there may be room for appreciable divergence of expert opinion.[17]

Similar reasoning can be applied to other types of disease that may be associated with trauma. Very often, there is little ground for disagreement. Thus, it would not be disputed that acute inflammation can be set up in a broken bone if virulent bacteria are present in the bloodstream at the time of injury. Or, if a man's pelvis were fractured in a car accident and his bladder was repeatedly catheterised, subsequent damage to the kidneys due to ascending infection would clearly bear a cause-and-effect relationship with the accident.

More difficulty arises in relation to the repair of injury—scar tissue is inherently weak and the effect of its substitution for normal connective or muscle tissue in an

17 As an example, see *Barty-King v Ministry of Defence* [1979] 2 All ER 80, where death in 1967 from cancer developing in a wound sustained in 1944 was held to be attributable to war service—a matter of great importance in relation to estate duty.

organ may appear only some considerable time after the original incident. It has been noted above that the inner lining and associated muscle of the heart or aorta may be lacerated during a severe fall or vehicular accident; in the event of survival, such areas must be permanently weakened and liable to rupture. Similarly, bruising and local damage to the muscle fibres of the heart may be caused by direct injury to the chest wall—the area when repaired is likely to be of less than normal strength. The same type of blunt injury causes haemorrhage into the wall of, or into the tissues surrounding, the coronary arteries. In either case, the reparative fibrosis may cause restriction of the blood flow and a coronary 'heart attack' at an unpredictable point in the future. Relationships of this type are very much open to argument, though few would deny the possibility of such sequences of events occurring.

Simultaneous death

Prior to the late nineteenth century, the establishment of the precise order of death and the consequent disposal of estates seldom gave rise to difficulty. The advent of the steamship, the train and the increasing risk of major conflagrations then exaggerated the problem; the solution of *commorientes* is now a problem that is virtually confined to fatal transportation accidents with occasional cases arising from hotel fires.

The legal solutions to simultaneous death are, basically, of two types. That operating in England and Wales states in general that, in the event of two (or more) persons dying in circumstances that make the order of death uncertain, the younger will be presumed to have survived the older.[18] In the United States and in most central European and Scandinavian countries, it is presumed that neither survived the other. France and Belgium include clauses in their codes to allow for extremes of age and for the legalistic nicety that, in similar adversity, the female is weaker than the male.[19] It is clear that the English system introduces the possibility that a finding of uncertainty as to whether the husband or the wife survived the other may result in their estates being distributed in a way that was not anticipated. This is because the test in deciding if s 184 of the 1925 Act applies is not whether there *was* a simultaneous death, but whether there was uncertainty as to which of two or more persons survived the others; the courts appear to take the view that simultaneous death cannot be proved pathologically.[20] A 'survivorship clause' is, therefore, a near essential to an English will. Scots law has recognised this imperfection and, while generally following that of England, has excluded 'spouse commorientes' from the general rule.[1] In fact, it seems that, whenever possible, opportunity has been taken to adopt the American system—if, in England, one of the commorientes is intestate, then the estates devolve as if neither had survived the other.[2] It is possible that the rejection of the English system by New Zealand in 1958[3] was precipitated when the law's manifest unfairness was demonstrated after the disastrous eruption of Mount Ruapehu the year before.

18 Law of Property Act 1925, s 184.
19 *Code Civil*, arts 720–722.
20 *Hickman v Peacey* [1945] AC 304, HL. But see the common sense approach adopted in *Re Pringle, Baker v Matheson* [1946] Ch 124 at 129–131 per Cohen J.
 1 Succession (Scotland) Act 1964, s 31.
 2 Intestates' Estates Act 1952, s 1(4).
 3 Simultaneous Deaths Act 1958.

From the forensic pathologist's point of view, however, it is not the differences in the systems that matter so much as that all have it in common that the presumption of simultaneous death is rebuttable by the evidence and that evidence of survival will be taken into consideration by the courts; such evidence must be mainly medical and the difficulties are compounded by the fact that no limit of time is set—survival for seconds is as significant in law as is survival for days.

Taking the commercial-aircraft accident as a typical example, the useful pathological evidence may be of several types and of varying sophistication. First, there is the precise cause of death. Thus it could well be assumed that a person who had survived the crash only to die from burning would have survived longer than another who had sustained a rupture of the cardiovascular system. Such evidence should not, however, be accepted uncritically. As we have seen, delayed rupture of the cardiovascular system—particularly of the atria or of the aorta—is a well accepted phenomenon. Moreover, the modes of death must be markedly dissimilar to be of good evidential value; thus, while the example above might well be valid, it would not be reasonable to suppose that a person with severe head injury had survived for a longer or shorter period than one with severe heart damage in the absence of other corroboration. Nor would it be right to assume that a person who had a greater overall degree of injury had necessarily predeceased someone with a single fatal injury.

The finding of carbon monoxide in the blood is objective evidence of an asphyxial death due to burning. A raised carboxyhaemoglobin in X compared with a negative result in Y could be taken to imply that X sustained a longer agonal period than did Y; but it would be wrong to reach the same conclusion if both showed raised values but X's level of carboxyhaemoglobin was higher than that of Y—such a difference could be related to the precise environment in which each died and to the air intake of each, which could be affected by disease, by activity and by other factors.

Further evidence of survival for a limited time may be found in persons with fractured bones in the form of microscopic particles of fat or of bone marrow in the lungs (see page 140); bone marrow particles provide the more unequivocal evidence because their structure indicates their origin beyond dispute. None the less, bone marrow emboli are often difficult to find, and a negative result might mean no more than that fragments were present but were not detected by the pathologist. Only a positive finding in indicating a definite time interval between injury and death is of true evidential value. Moreover, the *degree* of involvement of the lung in two persons cannot be used comparatively to assess the length of the survival period and anomalous cases, of both positive and negative type, occur. The author's own studies indicate that what appeared to be something of a breakthrough in forensic pathology is, in fact, of doubtful value.[4] These results derived, however, from a series of unrelated small accidents; the experience of others suggests that the method may be more useful in the more uniform conditions, say, of a major disaster.[5]

Pathological observations designed to distinguish in time between apparent simultaneous accidental deaths thus require very careful analysis. But they cannot be interpreted unless they are sought; this implies the need for post-mortem

4   D Buchanan and J K Mason 'Occurrence of Pulmonary Fat and Bone Marrow Embolism' (1982) 3 Amer J Forens Med Pathol 73.
5   A R Bierre and T D Koelmeyer 'Pulmonary Fat and Bone Marrow Embolism in Aircraft Accident Victims' (1983) 15 Pathology 131.

dissection and for time-consuming and technically difficult follow-up investigations in the toxicological and microscopic fields—a daunting prospect with up to 150 families possibly involved in a single incident. Opposing results as to the likelihood of relative survival may be obtained depending on the diligence and motivation of individual medical examiners. If justice is to be even in this sphere, the standards of autopsy must also be even—and this is unlikely to be so, particularly on an international scale. The disposal of a family estate may depend to a large extent on the precise geography of death; the routine use of 'survival' clauses in wills is therefore particularly important for those who travel frequently by air.

The special problems of commorientes when both parties are maintained on artificial life support are considered at page 168.

Novus actus interveniens

It is a clear legal principle that a person is responsible not only for his actions but also for the logical consequences of those actions. This applies in both aggravated assault and accidental injury. It is logical to assume that competent medical treatment will be available, if sought, for any injuries sustained. Should such treatment—or lack of it—be negligent and should that negligence result in a deviation from the logical sequence of events, then the responsibility for the subsequent disability or death may pass from the original incident to the later negligent action—this by virtue of novus actus interveniens (an unrelated action intervening). The majority of such interventions will be of a medical nature and the pathologist must provide evidence on this point in relevant cases.

The possible variations on novus actus interveniens are legion and no purpose would be served in listing potential causes—some may be obvious as, for example, the leaving of a surgical instrument in the abdomen after the repair of a treatable internal injury, while some may be more subtle. The most vivid example in the author's experience was the accidental substitution of poisonous potassium chloride for the innocuous sodium chloride during treatment by the artificial kidney of a man injured in a road-traffic accident.

An element of negligence is essential to a plea of novus actus; a foreseeable complication or a failure of a recognised form of treatment could not be so categorised. On the other hand, the mere fact that there *was* negligence does not automatically infer a break in the chain of causation.[6] Novus actus often presents a difficult pathological problem and differences in expert opinion may be well held on such questions as the proportionate contribution to death of the original and the new events, or as to whether an admitted error in treatment did, in fact, affect an inevitable outcome. In practice, the plea of novus actus is rarely accepted by the courts—at least in cases of homicide;[7] the medical evidence must show, as a minimum, that the intervention was the cause of death and that the original injury was no longer operative at the time of death.

6   *R v Smith* [1959] 2 QB 35; *R v Cheshire* [1991] 3 All ER 193.
7   In fact, the only officially reported case appears to be *R v Jordan* (1956) 40 Cr App Rep 152—and this is regarded as a suspect precedent. *R v Vickers* (1981) Daily Telegraph, 9 October, p 3, in which a man was acquitted of manslaughter on the basis of a faulty anaesthetic having been given to the victim, was a newspaper report only. The paucity of material in the civil field may well result from the most blatant cases being settled out of court.

11

Head injury

The mechanics of head injury

The common head injuries may all occur either singly or in combination. Superficial lesions include bruising, abrasion or laceration of the scalp. Fractures of the skull—or cranium—must be divided into those involving the vault, which covers the upper and outer surfaces of the brain, or the base, on which the brain rests and through which the cranial nerves and the spinal cord pass. Intracranial haemorrhage may be extradural, subdural or subarachnoid (see page 14). Deep lesions include laceration of the brain and intracerebral haemorrhage. These injuries may be produced by sharp weapons or by blunt force; they may be homicidal, suicidal or accidental in origin. For practical purposes, suicidal head injuries, which will generally result from falls from a height, will be similar in nature to those of accidental origin, although the author has seen bizarre examples of suicide, for example, by the use of an axe—in which case the distinction from homicide may not be easy. Homicidal head injuries have only a few characteristics that distinguish them from such wounds elsewhere and will be discussed first; the bulk of this section will be concerned with accidental injuries.

The tissues of the scalp are comparatively dense and are lined internally by firm but vascular fibrous tissue. Direct violence to the scalp, which lies on the rigid vault of the skull, results in a unique form of crushing between two hard objects. If the crush is of minor nature, a contusion or bruise will be produced; tracking of blood is likely to be slight in the dense connective tissue and, although bruising will usually be evident on both the outer and inner surfaces, it will commonly be more apparent on the deep aspect of the scalp. At the same time, since the scalp is held firmly over the skull, it is not unusual for its outer surface to reproduce the pattern of the weapon or object responsible for the violence. The skin will split when the compressive force is greater—the scalp is the classic site for lacerated wounds produced by blunt force (see page 112); because the skull is convex, such lacerations may well be of linear type even when the object with which contact was made—for example, the roadway—was flat.

The underlying skull may fracture if greater force is applied. The skull is not uniformly solid but is composed of two layers or tables of bone separated by spongy tissue. The skull will deform when it is struck and the extent of the deformation depends largely upon its age. A child's skull will bend before breaking but, since blood vessels will be torn in the process, head injury in children often shows a surprising degree of haemorrhage when compared with the relative lack of damage to the skull—it is, indeed, quite common for a child to sustain severe brain damage in the absence of fracture. Once the bounds of moulding are passed, the bone will break. In the adult, direct trauma could theoretically break only the outer table and, in these circumstances, a relatively perfect impression of the striking object would be reproduced; such a condition is very rare in practice. More usually, lines of stress fracture radiate from the point of contact while that part of the skull struck is depressed—a situation almost exactly comparable with striking the shell of a hard-boiled egg. These radiating fractures may damage blood vessels over a wide area, thus explaining those deaths which result from what seemed to be a relatively mild impact injury.

The membranes of the brain, with their accompanying blood vessels, may be crushed or torn beneath a depressed fracture; more seriously, the brain itself may be lacerated either by the instrument causing the external injury or by the fragments of bone that are forced inwards.

The above description encompasses the characteristics of homicidal head injuries which are, essentially, of *contact* type. They may be modified by the type of weapon used—for instance, as between a cleaver and a baseball bat—and they may well be multiple, a factor that clearly provides evidence as to intent. Essentially, the injuries are local and result from a blow to the static head, they are related to the shape and size of the weapon and they are not difficult to understand.

Head injury predominantly related to accident

Fracture of the base of the skull is particularly dangerous not only because dissipation of the force needed to cause such an injury produces general effects on the brain but also because of local and indirect damage done to the blood vessels as they pass through the bone on their way to the vital centres controlling the life processes; these vessels are concentrated close to the tentorium and to the foramen magnum—the apertures through which the hindbrain and the spinal cord pass. Several cranial nerves pass through the base and the very important pituitary gland is lodged in its fossa which, in turn, lies along the main 'fault line' of the base of the skull.

Fractures of the base may be continuous with those originating in and radiating from the vault of the skull. Thus, a blow to the front of the head, such as that sustained by an unrestrained front-seat passenger in a car crash, may fracture the frontal bones and radiate into the anterior fossae—this is a specially dangerous injury because, by breaking into the frontal air sinuses, direct communication is established between the brain coverings and the outside environment (see below). A blow to the side of the head, fracturing the temporal bone, is likely to radiate into the middle fossa of the base—and, again, allowing outside contact and the possibility of infection through the middle ear; a blow to the back of the head, as sustained in falling or being pushed over backwards, may produce a fracture that radiates into the posterior fossa and involves the foramen magnum. These fractures may be multiple and cause extensive 'comminution' or fragmentation of the bone.

Accidental force can be transmitted to the base of the skull by way of two main mechanisms. The commonest is that transmitted through the spine when the body falls heavily on the feet or buttocks; a fracture may be formed that surrounds the foramen magnum in a 'ring' and, in very severe cases, the spine may be driven into the skull cavity. The vault of the skull may then be burst open, giving the impression of an original massive fracture in that area. The distinction of this type of injury is of importance in forensic medicine, as a similar ring fracture of the base can be caused by a severe blow to the vertex—in this case, however, the accompanying fracture of the vault will be depressed rather than of 'explosive' type. The second important transmitted fracture stems from the point of the chin—force is applied through the lower jaw to the base of the skull in the region of each ear and the middle fossae of the base shatter. Such an injury rarely results from a fist blow—unless 'knuckledusters' are involved—but is common when, say, a person falls on the chin in the roadway or when the chin is impacted on the instrument fascia of a car or light aircraft. The essential determinant is the hardness of the object struck, which influences the 'jolt' or the rate of application of force.

Diffuse axonal injury

Head injury of more than minor severity will commonly be associated with loss of consciousness—in its simplest, short-lived, recoverable form this is known as concussion, a condition that is generally more severe when damage is caused to the moving head (ie decelerative injury) rather than when it results from blows to the skull. In addition to losing consciousness, the patient enters a state of surgical shock (see page 488), the severity of which greatly influences the rate of, or failure of, recovery. The precise cause of concussion is still disputed but is generally attributed to 'diffuse axonal injury' which is the underlying cause of states of unconsciousness ranging from minor concussion to the persistent vegetative state. Diffuse axonal injury is commonly associated with angular accelerations of the head and is characteristic of head injury due to road traffic accidents. Well recognised microscopic, and macroscopic, changes in the form of midline haemorrhages within the brain substance have now been demonstrated, and the severity of these correlates with the severity of the trauma sustained;[1] the casualty must, however, survive for at least several hours before microscopic changes become recognisable. The damage that has been done accounts for the late ill-effects of post-traumatic unconsciousness from which an apparent recovery has been made.

Concussion has several important medico-legal connotations. In the first place, it commonly produces a genuine state of retrograde amnesia for events immediately before injury—a concussed person is likely to be an unsatisfactory witness. Secondly, the sufferer may be left with sequelae of varying severity which will be mentioned later. Perhaps of greatest immediate importance, concussion is a signal of potentially severe intracranial injury—it is an indication for examining the skull by X-ray and for retaining the patient under observation lest he develop an intracranial haemorrhage.[2]

1   D A Crookes 'The Pathological Concept of Diffuse Axonal Injury: Its Pathogenesis and Assessment of Severity' (1991) 165 J Pathol 5.
2   But, overall, a fracture is present in only some 30% of cases of concussion. X-ray examination, particularly in mild cases, might well be regarded as a form of insurance rather than as good medical economics. The consensus is, however, that an X-ray is indicated whenever there is loss of consciousness: M J Powers and N H Harris *Medical Negligence* (1990) paras 21.45, 34.4.

Intracranial haemorrhage (see Figure 11.1)

Intracranial haemorrhage can be divided into surface contusion of the brain and haemorrhage of extradural, subdural, subarachnoid and intracerebral types. The loss of blood is insignificant per se. What matters is the effect of the resultant raised pressure on the brain itself; this can act directly or indirectly and may result in extensive destruction of tissue. The quantity and the type of bleeding—arterial or venous—are of major importance to the outcome.

Contusion of the brain

Contusion of the brain is found in the great majority of fatal cases of head injury. Occasionally, contusion by itself may be sufficient to produce a fatal increase in intracranial pressure. From the forensic pathologist's point of view, however, the importance of contusions lies in their position and causation. Thus, contusions may be of *coup* or contact type underlying a fracture or the point of impact with a blunt object. But brain damage as a whole—and particularly that resulting from vehicular accidents—requires a more subtle explanation. This depends on the fact that, when the skull is accelerated or decelerated, the contained brain tends to move in relation to the skull itself; since its vascular attachments will, thereby, be torn, the superficial brain tissue will be damaged elsewhere than where the external force is applied. Thus, cerebral contusion associated with linear deceleration will appear not only at the point of impact but, characteristically, at a site precisely opposite to that of primary impact; this is known as *contrecoup* haemorrhage.[3] A man falling on the back of his head may show local contusion of the brain; characteristically, however, his brain will be contused—often markedly more so than at the point of contact—at the tips of the frontal and temporal lobes; less frequently, a man falling on his face will demonstrate contrecoup bruising at the tips of the occipital lobes. The important diagnostic feature is that the finding of internal bruising remote from the primary external injury clearly indicates *motion* of the head at the time it was sustained. This observation may be of great importance in trials for homicide in which the distinction between head injury due a fall and that due to being struck, say by a baseball bat, is often hotly disputed.

Extradural haemorrhage

Extradural or epidural haemorrhage refers to bleeding between the skull itself and the outer covering of the brain. It is associated with fracture of the skull in some 90% of cases. Venous extradural haemorrhage may be due to disruption of small veins and, occasionally, one of the large sinuses may give way. Tearing of a meningeal artery is, however, by far the commonest cause of this type of bleeding. About half the cases are complicated by intracerebral bleeding which is often of contrecoup type; this reflects the frequent aetiological factor of a fall. Extradural haemorrhage is of particular medico-legal importance in two respects. First, it is reasonably easy to treat and deaths from this cause should be rare. Secondly, there may be an interval between injury and the onset of symptoms during which the

---

3   Well discussed in D I Graham and T A Gennarelli 'Trauma' in D I Graham and P L Lantos (eds) *Greenfield's Neuropathology* (6th edn, 1997) pp 197 et seq.

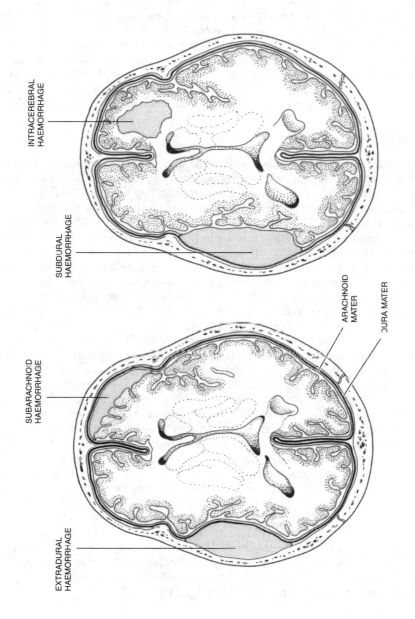
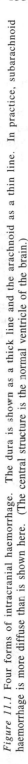

INTRACEREBRAL HAEMORRHAGE

SUBDURAL HAEMORRHAGE

SUBARACHNOID HAEMORRHAGE

EXTRADURAL HAEMORRHAGE

ARACHNOID MATER

DURA MATER

Figure 11.1 Four forms of intracranial haemorrhage. The dura is shown as a thick line and the arachnoid as a thin line. In practice, subarachnoid haemorrhage is more diffuse than is shown here. (The central structure is the normal ventricle of the brain.)

patient, after an initial period of concussion, is perfectly normal; there is, therefore, a tendency for patients to be discharged to home and for the onset of symptoms there to be unappreciated—it may be 12 hours before the injured person is returned to hospital, by which time severe cerebral compression and brain damage may have occurred.[4] The importance of observing a patient who has been concussed is again stressed, as is the strong indication for the need of a CT scan of the brain in all cases involving fracture of the skull. The frequent concurrence of this type of head injury with alcoholic intoxication—or the mimicry of the latter by the former—is also to be noted; the death of such a case in a police cell is a tragedy that occurs not infrequently. Recovery may be complicated by emotional and intellectual disability if operative treatment of extradural haemorrhage is delayed.

Subdural haemorrhage

Subdural haemorrhage is found in the space between the dural and the arachnoid membranes. A large venous sinus may occasionally be lacerated but, commonly, the vessels torn are 'bridging' veins that are so small that no main bleeding point can be discovered either at operation or at post-mortem. This type of bleeding is not necessarily associated with fracture and results particularly from the shearing forces set up by movement of the brain in relation to bone and to the relatively fixed dura matter. Thus, subdural bleeding often accompanies the violent head movements involved in the 'whip-lash' injury to the neck; it is also characteristic of shaking of the young child.[5] Subdural haemorrhage is usually associated with more force than is required to produce extradural haemorrhage and is often accompanied by severe cerebral contusion; the resulting so-called 'burst lobe' injury carries a poor prognosis.

By the nature of the relatively wide and open subdural space, bleeding into it will take some time to produce symptoms; generally this is a matter of hours, but the effect of bleeding is aggravated by concurrent respiratory embarrassment and the consequent hypoxia. This 'latent interval' may be of very great importance in the assessment of non-accidental head injury in children; at post-mortem in such cases, it is often clear that blood has been collecting over a long period. Subdural bleeding is also a common accompaniment of birth injury (see Chapter 19).

A chronic form of subdural haemorrhage may occur, particularly in children and the aged. Although these cases may represent the long-term effects of trauma, evidence of previous injury is lacking in the majority. Bleeding from small veins is slow and the body manages to contain the extravasations, which then become fixed to the underside of the dura by granulation and fibrous tissue. The lesions are very often symptomless or do no more than cause a general confusion of the intellect which is attributable to 'being a bit slow' or 'getting on in years'—and, even then, the haemorrhage may be the result of primary shrinkage of the brain rather than the cause of the symptoms. Haemorrhage may, however, continue intermittently and severe symptoms may result from compression of the brain. It may then be difficult to decide what is the cause-and-effect relationship in respect of an injury that may have been sustained a long time past.

---

4   Although this is generally described as 'typical', it is now considered that a lucid interval occurs in a minority of those who develop intracranial haemorrhages: D I Graham 'Closed Head Injury' in J K Mason and B N Purdue (eds) *The Pathology of Trauma* (3rd edn, 2000) p 195.
5   J Caffey 'The Whiplash Shaken Infant Syndrome' (1974) 54 Pediatrics 396.

It goes without saying that, in both extra- and subdural haemorrhage, death is due to raised intracranial pressure and not to blood loss. Brain tissue is forced downwards and impacts either in the opening in the dura which separates the cerebrum from the cerebellum (*tentorial herniation*) or in the foramen magnum at the base of the skull. The resultant damage to and distortion of the brain may be lethal in itself; alternatively, the vital centres are destroyed by intracerebral haemorrhage which arises secondary to the displacement of the tissues. The problem is discussed further below under the heading of 'cerebral oedema'.

Subarachnoid haemorrhage

We have already noted subarachnoid haemorrhage as being a fairly common form of sudden natural death (Chapter 7); it is also a frequent sequel to injury and some degree of haemorrhage is an invariable accompaniment of cerebral contusion. Subarachnoid haemorrhage occurring alone must be suspected of being due to spontaneous rupture of a congenital aneurysm, or of having been caused by injury to a vessel that was already weakened by aneurysmal changes. The possible association of natural disease and violence—that is, the increased likelihood of a pre-existing aneurysm bursting during, say, an altercation—has been mentioned in Chapter 7.

True 'traumatic subarachnoid haemorrhage', however, has a rather different aetiology and results from damage to the vertebral artery as it passes from the spinal column to the base of the brain. The lesion is, therefore, one of a group of cerebral injuries which originate in damage to the neck.[6] The typical history is of a blow with a relatively hard object that is of such a shape as to impact in the cavity behind the ear and mastoid process; the autopsy clue to the condition is the finding of bruising in the muscles of the area.[7] A fracture of the first cervical (*atlas*) bone is found in about half the cases but is little more than confirmatory of trauma in the area; the fractures are generally visible only after cleaning of the bone and are best demonstrated by X-ray. It is technically difficult to demonstrate the bleeding point and, ideally, this should be done using radio-opaque injections in situ; this, however, implies the availability of a radiologist with the necessary equipment and, also, some foresight on the part of the pathologist. An association with drunkenness has been noted in these cases[8] but this may be no more than a reflection of the environment in which such injuries are sustained. Death may be very rapid and may be complicated by inhalation of vomit.

Subarachnoid haemorrhage is seen after injury in combination with bleeding in other sites. Aside from that associated with contusion of the brain, more generalised haemorrhage is due to local rupture of small vessels. Alternatively, massive subarachnoid haemorrhage may be no more than an extension of a severe intracerebral haemorrhage which bursts into either the cerebral ventricles or the external subarachnoid space.

---

6   The others involve trauma to the carotid artery which may precipitate a dissecting aneurysm of the vessel (see p 100) or which may establish a carotid thrombosis and the potential hazard of cerebral embolism.

7   For good reviews of the condition, see W A Harland, J F Pitts and A A Watson 'Subarachnoid Haemorrhage due to Upper Cervical Trauma' (1983) 36 J Clin Path 1335. And, more recently, J T Gray, S M Puetz, S L Jackson and M A Green 'Traumatic Subarachnoid Haemorrhage: A 10-year Case Study and Review' (1999) 105 Forens Sci Internat 13.

8   J Simonsen 'Massive Subarachnoid Haemorrhage and Fracture of the Transverse Process of the Atlas' (1976) 16 Med Sci Law 13.

Intracerebral haemorrhage

Haemorrhage within the brain tissue may be of several types. The first, as we have seen, is represented by contusion or bruising of the superficial areas of the brain, the position of which depends on movement of the head. If the acceleration is rotational, sheer forces will be set up; if deceleration is linear, 'cavitation' will occur behind the still accelerating brain. Either may result in laceration of the brain and consequent extravasation of blood into its deeper parts at a distance from the point of impact.

Deep intracerebral haemorrhage is also caused by tearing of the deep arterioles under tension or torsion; its occurrence in the absence of severe external damage is particularly common in young persons. Because weaker vessels will give way to both trauma and disease, this tends to occur at sites that are commonly involved in haemorrhage due to natural disease; the distinction between haemorrhage that *results* from an accident and that which *causes* an accident may be difficult to make (see Chapter 10). The incompressible brain resists the extension of such haemorrhages, and relatively unexpected death may be delayed until several days after the incident—but consciousness is not regained as so often occurs when extracerebral haemorrhage follows head injury. It will be apparent that death in these circumstances can raise a number of medico-legal problems.

Intracerebral haemorrhage of macroscopic proportions is always serious but is almost inevitably fatal when it occurs in the brain stem, the site of the centres vital to life. Brain-stem haemorrhage may be primary—that is, caused during the traumatic event; it may also be secondary to raised intracranial pressure and often underlies delayed death after head injury. Primary brain-stem haemorrhage may give rise to some of the most tragic neurological conditions such as the 'locked-in syndrome' where an active brain survives in the presence of total motor failure.[9]

Petechial haemorrhage

A word should be said about *petechial haemorrhage*, despite the fact that it differs conceptually from the foregoing. Petechial haemorrhage implies bleeding from the pre-capillaries; it therefore results from generalised dysfunction at the cellular level rather than from local trauma. The appearances are those of pin-head spots of bleeding widely distributed throughout the cerebral substance although being often more prominent in the white matter. Hypoxia is the most common cause of breakdown of the capillary membranes. In theory, petechial haemorrhage should be seen in any condition of which hypoxia is a component part—including natural death; in practice, their appearance is erratic unless there is a triggering factor. The most important of these is raised intracapillary pressure (cf Chapter 13—asphyxia). Others are more subtle; thus cerebral petechiae are common in deaths from barotrauma and are often reported as being present in deaths from cerebral fat embolism—both these conditions are associated with abnormal particles within the blood which may be significant 'triggers'. A specific form of widespread cerebral petechial haemorrhage, now described as 'diffuse vascular injury of the brain', can be found in persons—particularly children or young adults— who die at the time of or shortly after severe head injury. The lesion probably results from severe shearing forces involving the small blood

9 C M C Allen 'Conscious but Paralysed: Releasing the Locked-in' (1993) 342 Lancet 130.

vessels but it may represent no more than a severe form of diffuse axonal injury.[10] By and large, however, mention of 'cerebral petechiae' in an autopsy report adds very little to the understanding of the overall picture.

Cerebral laceration

Cerebral laceration may be caused directly, either by an object that penetrates the skull or by fragments of bone that are driven inwards. Widely radiating fractures with extensive isolation of skull fragments may be associated with equivalent tears in the superficial substance of the brain.

Alternatively, severe contrecoup forces may cause laceration opposite the point of impact while rotational forces may drive the brain substance into the natural ridges that are found in the base of the skull. There is less restraint on the movement of the brain if the skull is fractured and, in these circumstances, the cerebrum or cerebellum may be torn from the brain stem.

The effect of cerebral laceration must vary with its location. In practice, lacerations are commonest in the frontal and temporal lobes. Comparatively major damage in the frontal area may provoke no serious sequelae in the absence of haemorrhage; by contrast, a small laceration in the brain stem may well be fatal. It is worth emphasising that the outcome of a head injury depends on the effect that injury has on the brain. Death, for example, is not due to 'fracture of the skull'; it is due to the consequent cerebral damage.

Cerebral swelling

After trauma to the head, the patient very often falls into progressively deeper coma despite the fact that no localised haemorrhage is present; the condition of cerebral swelling is established. This may be due to an increase in the blood volume within the skull or of the water content of the brain—in which case it is known as cerebral oedema.

The precise cause of the latter condition—which is particularly common in children—is uncertain.[11] The effect is that the veins, rather than the arteries, are first compressed as the size of the brain increases while the circulation of cerebrospinal fluid is also compromised—the condition is therefore self-perpetuating and can cause death in its own right in the absence of any other apparent injury. It also occurs as a result of cerebral hypoxia due to any cause—including, for example, severe poisoning by respiratory depressants.

The pathological evidence of such swelling will often be referred to in the post-mortem report as 'herniation of brain substance'. As occurs in the presence of a space occupying lesion such as haemorrhage described above, the resulting increase in pressure within the skull may force the undersurface of the temporal lobe through the tentorial opening at each side of the midbrain (*tentorial* or *uncal herniation*), or the cerebellum may be pushed through the foramen magnum (*tonsillar herniation*). A further form of herniation that may be described in the pathologist's report results from escape of brain tissue through burr holes made in the skull in an attempt to relieve the condition.

10 See D I Graham 'Closed Head Injury' in J K Mason and B N Purdue (eds) *The Pathology of Trauma* (3rd edn, 2000) p 205.
11 D I Graham, I Ford, J H Adams et al 'Fatal Head Injury in Children' (1989) 42 J Clin Path 18.

One of the main dangers of cerebral oedema lies in the secondary effects of brain-stem compression associated with tentorial herniation. The interference with the local blood flow that results may cause complications in the form of haemorrhage into the brain stem or damage due to obliteration of the arterial supply to the area—a process known as *infarction*. This is a common mode of death following closed head injury; equally importantly, any damage done is irrecoverable and the patient who survives may be left with particularly severe disability.

Diffuse ischaemic brain damage—resulting from oxygen deprivation of the whole brain—can occur after head injury and may lead to irreversible brain damage of varying severity, culminating in the permanent vegetative state. There are, however, many other more important causes of this very serious condition; since the common feature of all is lack of oxygen, the subject is, perhaps, best considered in Chapter 13.

Long-term effects of head injury

If a portion of brain is damaged by injury there will be localised effects of varying severity and expression which depend upon the precise area involved. A detailed description of potential disabilities cannot be undertaken here—the problems are covered in textbooks of neurology.

Some mention must be made of the generalised pathological conditions or symptoms that may properly be attributed to injury. Sepsis may be introduced through an open wound of the skull—especially one involving the nose. The origin of this may be obvious if the open fracture involves the vault of the skull. Fracture of the base of the skull, which may communicate with the outside through either the nose or ear, is less easy to detect and is certainly harder to repair. Generalised infection or overt abscess formation attributable to such injuries may be delayed for days or weeks. Even in the absence of infection, a distressing leak of cerebral spinal fluid may persist for some time.

Neuropsychiatric sequelae are considered in more detail in Chapter 27. After head injury, many persons suffer from chronic headache, loss of concentration, unexplained attacks of giddiness and memory deficit; these may be the result of sub-clinical contusions. Post-traumatic epileptic seizures occur after head injury without fracture in some 3% of cases and follow 16% of severe head injuries. They can manifest themselves shortly after recovery or be delayed in onset for a few months; late epilepsy of this type, which is more common in adults than in children, is particularly associated with severer injuries involving local compression of the brain tissue—as by a depressed fracture or an extradural haemorrhage.

It is to be noted that some extra-cerebral conditions are typically associated with severe brain damage. Those under prolonged treatment are often affected by pulmonary oedema which may be fatal. Erosion and ulceration of the stomach occurs in a way similar to that following severe burning. An association with acute pancreatitis has also been reported.

The prevention of head injury

The prevention of head injury is of major concern in mining, in the construction industries in general and, of greatest general importance, in vehicular transportation.

Different forms of head protection have been developed for these various situations. Because they have to protect against impacts of very varying intensity and direction, the helmets used in aircraft and on motor cycles are the most sophisticated. The major design feature involves the separation of the skull from the hard shell by the use of a suspension harness. A good fit is important, as is the provision of ear flaps to prevent injuries originating in the temporal region. Opportunity has been taken in helmets designed for motor cyclists to incorporate protection against the weather such as face shields and the incorporation of eye guards is now universal.[12] Inevitably, arguments persist as to whether the advantages of helmets in preventing fatal accidents are outweighed by their disadvantages, in that they may increase the number of accidents—for example, by limiting the field of vision. But, as has been discussed above (see page 141), all safety equipment involves an element of compromise and there is abundant evidence that the prevention of fatal head injury is the most important factor in motor-cycling safety.[13]

It is compulsory in the United Kingdom—and in at least half the United States—for persons riding on motor cycles, excluding those in side-cars, to wear protective headgear.[14] The courts will take the same attitude to contributory negligence in regard to the wearing of helmets as they do to the use of harnesses in motor cars.[15] The use of helmets by motor cyclists is far more strictly observed than is that of seat belts in cars; this is more likely to be due to the near certainty of detection of non-use of the former rather than to any variation in the arguments based on individual liberty in respect of self-protection.

It would be too much to expect the ordinary driver or front-seat passenger in a family motor car to wear protective headgear—although some lives would certainly be saved thereby—but there is undoubtedly a case for their use in open sports cars. This is because, in addition to windshield contact injuries—the prevention of which is largely a matter of shoulder harness (see Chapter 10)—preventable skull injury in road-traffic accidents stems from secondary impact with the roadway after ejection from the vehicle. Interest now centres on the extension of compulsory head protection to pedal cyclists. Again, the argument is keen and, in this case, is heightened by the fact that pedal cyclists cannot be expected to wear the expensive and heavy equipment recommended for those travelling at high speed; by and large, current pedal cyclists' helmets will provide significant protection only in the solo accident situation.[16] Within this parameter, however, the evidence indicates that cycle helmets are valuable, particularly when worn by children.[17] Many more cyclists are wearing

---

12 Motor Cycles (Eye Protectors) Regulations 1999, SI 1999/535.
13 Editorial Comment 'A Grim Experiment' (1980) 281 BMJ 406; D Gloag 'Crash Helmets for California' (1991) 302 BMJ 1487.
14 Motor Cycles (Protective Helmets) Regulations 1998, SI 1998/1807. The exemption for Sikhs wearing turbans is retained (Road Traffic Act 1988, s 16(2)). Interestingly, however, this exemption does not hold where an employer regards it as necessary for the employee's safety: *Singh v British Rail Engineering Ltd* [1986] ICR 22.
15 *O'Connell v Jackson* [1972] 1 QB 270; *Capps v Miller* [1989] 2 All ER 333.
16 N J Mills 'Protective Capabilities of Bicycle Helmets' (1990) 24 Brit J Sports Med 55.
17 H R Trippe 'Helmets for Pedal Cyclists' (1992) 305 BMJ 843; S Thomas, C Acton, J Nixon et al 'Effectiveness of Bicycle Helmets in Preventing Head Injury in Children: Case-control Study' (1994) 308 BMJ 173. An interesting argument has developed in relation to adults which suggests that compulsory use of expensive helmets would deter people from riding bicycles and that this would have a negative effect on health in general: D Carnall 'Cycle Helmets should not be Compulsory' (1999) 318 BMJ 1505.

helmets and conditions are comparable to those pertaining to seat belts in cars before legislation was introduced. At that time, it was said:

> 'Everyone knows, or ought to know, that when he goes out in a car he should fasten the seat belt. It is so well known that it goes without saying.'[18]

It will be interesting to see the courts' attitude should an apposite case come up in respect of a pedal cyclist.[19]

18 *Froom v Butcher* [1975] RTR 518 at 527 per Lord Denning.
19 See L Evans 'Cycle Helmets and the Law' (1994) 308 BMJ 1521.

12

The transplantation of organs

Although it might seem unusual to introduce this subject so early in this book, the reader will see that cerebral disaster, whether that be of natural or traumatic origin, is a major source of transplantable organs; it, therefore, seems appropriate to conjoin transplantation with Chapter 11.

The processes involved in transplantation

In essence, the human body dies naturally in one of two ways. Either it 'wears out'—generally by way of its cerebral or cardiovascular system—or a single, vital organ system fails within an otherwise healthy body; death will then be averted if a substitute for that organ can be found. Mechanical organ substitutes—as, for example, the artificial kidney—are often bulky, they restrict the lifestyle of the user and may even dictate where he or she lives, they may break down, and ultimately some form of incompatibility arises between patient and machine. The concept of transplantation of substituted biological organs is, therefore, extremely attractive.

The major difficulty in such a procedure, apart from the required technical expertise, lies in the rejection by the body of foreign substances (or antigens), a principle which has been discussed in Chapter 1. The more 'foreign' the substance, the more rapid and inevitable will be the body's resistance to the implant. In the present state of knowledge, transplantation of organs from animals to man— xenografting or xenotransplantation—is impossible save as a 'stop-gap' measure, although modern genetic engineering methods are closing the gap.[1] Even were it otherwise, there is still a major risk of transferring animal pathogenic organisms— particularly viruses—to man and many would question the morality of using animals in this way.[2]

---

1   D White and J Wallwork 'Xenografting: Probability, Possibility or Pipe Dream?' (1993) 342 Lancet 879. Currently, there is a moratorium on such operations in the UK.
2   For major reviews, see Nuffield Council on Bioethics *Animal-to-Human Transplants: The Ethics of Xenotransplantation* (1996); the Department of Health Advisory Group on the Ethics of Xenotransplantation *Animal Tissue into Humans* (1997); M Fox and J McHale 'Xenotransplantation: The Ethical and Legal Ramifications' (1998) 6 Med L Rev 442.

For the time being, all organs designated for long-term transplantation into human recipients must be obtained from human donors. The closer the antigenic similarity between recipient and donor, the more likely is the acceptance of the transplant but, apart from identical twins, the chances of finding two persons completely 'graft compatible' are negligible; at best, some—for example, siblings or parents versus children—are less incompatible than others. Techniques designed to limit the body's immunological response have improved beyond recognition in recent years. Nevertheless, a relatively close antigenic match is always desirable and this is a far more complex task than is needed in, say, blood transfusion (see Chapter 31). As a result:

- transplantation must be accompanied by efforts to reduce the instinct of the recipient to reject the donated organ (immunosuppression);
- immunosuppression in humans cannot, as yet, be selective. The defences of the body against invasion are, therefore, reduced overall—eg against bacterial infection;
- the body will still reject the graft when, ultimately, its power to do so exceeds the available immunosuppressive methods.

Moreover, any transplant must be effective in its own right if it is to be useful. It must be obtained from a 'healthy' donor—that is, from a person not suffering from a generalised disease which affects the organ—and it must remain healthy during the period between becoming available and implantation. A donation from a living person is more likely to succeed than is one from a dead donor and, in the latter case, success will be inversely proportional to the length of time between death and donation—and the importance of this will depend on which particular organ is being harvested. It is convenient to discuss the legal and ethical issues related to live and cadaver transplants separately.

Living donation

The propriety of live donation of organs for transplantation depends on three main factors. First, there should be a reasonable prospect of the transplant being successful; it might be legal for a man to consent, but it would certainly be unethical for a physician to encourage him to do so if there was a high chance that the organ would be rejected by the recipient's body. Secondly, the benefit to the recipient must far outweigh the likely detriment to the donor. Potential donations are of three types:

1. of tissues that are readily replaceable, blood being the most obvious example, which cause no difficulty;
2. at the other extreme, of organs that are essential to the life of the donor (since consent is no defence to a charge of a serious assault[3]—and especially of homicide—removal of such organs in life is illegal);
3. of one of paired organs, the remaining one of which would be capable of maintaining life so long as it were healthy or of part of an organ which can be removed safely and the residue of which will function adequately.

3   *A-G's Reference (No 6 of 1980)* [1981] QB 715.

The scope for donations of the last type is increasing along with surgical expertise. At one time they could be said to be limited to the provision of a kidney; now they would include portions of the pancreas, lobes of the lung and parts of the liver—indeed, this last technique may well be the optimal treatment for liver failure in infancy.

In any event, the donor must be capable of consent as described in Chapter 30. The major problem specific to the present discussion is whether parents or guardians can give consent for a minor to undergo a surgical procedure that can be of no benefit to him or her. It is doubtful whether such a practice would be wholly desirable because it is unlikely that a child would fully understand a complex subject and because the possibility of a child subsequently needing his or her own donated organ may be greater than would be so in the case of an adult. It is, in practice, unlikely that a British surgeon would accept a minor as a live donor[4] and in many jurisdictions—eg in some of the Australian States—it is illegal to do so.

The ultimate success of an organ transplant rests on the quality of the donated organ; this, in turn, depends largely upon the 'warm anoxic' time to which it is subjected—ie the time between cessation of its arterial oxygen supply and refrigeration of the isolated organ. Living donation therefore offers two major advantages. First, time is available for a full appraisal of the case, and, secondly, the warm anoxic time can be reduced almost to zero.[5] It is, in many ways, surprising that the proportion of live kidney donations in the United Kingdom is only some 5–10% of the total and that it has fallen in the last decade; in Japan, by contrast, live donation is the preferred method—although this is largely because the concept of brain-stem death (see below) is unacceptable in that culture.

The overall legal position as to live organ donation in the United Kingdom has now been largely codified in the Human Organ Transplants Act 1989.[6] The main purpose of this legislation was to criminalise the sale and purchase of organs of either the living or the dead. For present purposes, however, its most important function was to establish the Unrelated Live Transplant Regulatory Authority (ULTRA), as a result of which it is now illegal to perform a live transplant unless either the recipient and donor are related[7] or the operation has been authorised by ULTRA.

4   See J K Mason 'Contemporary Issues in Organ Transplantation' in S A M McLean (ed) *Contemporary Medico-legal Issues* (1995). The position as to the mature minor's rights in this area, both as to statute and at common law, were addressed by the Master of the Rolls in *Re W (a minor)(medical treatment)* [1992] 4 All ER 627 at 635, 639. The courts' attitude to the incompetent adult can, however, be said to be pragmatic: see *Re Y (mental patient) (bone marrow donation)* [1997] Fam 110, in which donation of, admittedly, bone marrow by a woman who could not consent was authorised.

5   And, as a consequence, the 'half life' of a kidney transplanted from a living donor is about twice that of one from a cadaver (about eight years). See M L Nicholson and J A Bradley 'Renal Transplantation from Living Donors' (1999) 318 BMJ 409.

6   An organ is defined in s 7 as 'any part of the human body consisting of a structured arrangement of tissues which, *if wholly removed*, cannot be replicated by the body' (my emphasis). Thus, bone marrow donation is excluded, although it is a relatively serious procedure for the donor. Interestingly, it would seem not to include a lobe of a liver, as the liver can grow again.

7   Human Organ Transplants (Establishment of Relationship) Regulations 1998, SI 1998/1428. The accepted relationships, which include uncles and aunts of the half blood, are, however, so wide, as to throw doubt on the immunological basis of the regulations. Note that inter-spouse donations must be referred to ULTRA; the results of such unrelated live kidney donations are still better than those from relatively well-matched cadaver donations.

Cadaver donation

In the case of a cadaver donation, the kidneys must be removed from the dead body within 30–60 minutes of circulatory failure and, in general, can be stored for no longer than 12 hours. The intervals are even shorter in relation to liver and heart transplants. It will be seen, therefore, that reliance on failure of the cardio-respiratory system as an indicator of death—which is the normal practice in everyday medicine—will result either in the loss of a number of potential donations or the use of organs which are in a less than ideal state.[8] The dramatic improvement in the results of transplantation surgery that has evolved over the years has been largely due to the approximation of the cadaver to the living donor through the medium of the 'beating-heart donor'—a concept that was originally directed to the management of patients in the neurosurgical wards but is now essential to the understanding of modern transplant surgery.

Beating heart donation

The cells of the brain will die if they are subjected to anoxia or hypoxia—an absolute or relative lack of arterial oxygen. The hypoxic insult may have many causes and, as we have seen in the preceding chapter, accidental injury to the head is high on the list; even so, a significant proportion of cerebral deaths will be due to natural disease such as brain tumour or subarachnoid haemorrhage. Simplistically, one can speak of functional regions within the brain that vary in their resistance to oxygen deprivation (see Chapter 1). The most sensitive is the cortex, broadly responsible for the intellect or humanising functions of the brain; this is followed by the thalamic region which is, in general, responsible for our animal behaviour; and, finally, there is the brain-stem which regulates the basic functions of the body and, in particular, respiration. Thus, varying degrees of oxygen lack will lead to varying degrees of 'brain death', the evidence of which may range from intellectual deterioration, through the condition that is known as the 'permanent vegetative state' (for which, see page 189), to death resulting from destruction of the respiratory centre that lies within the brain stem. Thus, the brain stem is not only the controller of 'life' but is also that part of the brain which is most resistant to hypoxia. As a consequence, we can not only say that, when the brain stem is dead, the whole brain is dead but also that the patient so affected is incapable of an existence independent of the ventilator and he is 'brain-stem dead'.

The standard cardio-respiratory methods of diagnosing death cannot be applied in the context of ventilator support but, since the brain stem controls the lungs and, therefore, the heart (Figure 12.1), we can certify death of the individual by diagnosing death of the brain stem and this can be done while the mechanically oxygenated heart is still beating independently. Stringent criteria are laid down.[9] These include the exclusion of drug overdose, hypothermia or metabolic disorder as a cause of deep coma; establishing that the reason for the coma is irremediable structural brain damage; testing to establish that all brain-stem reflexes are absent;

---

8   There is a modern movement to circumvent this by way of in situ cooling of the organs which can be done while the legal formalities are being observed. See K Varty, K S Veitch, J D T Morgan et al 'Response to Organ Shortage: Kidney Retrieval Programme Using Non-heart Beating Donors' (1994) 308 BMJ 575.
9   Conference of Medical Royal Colleges and their Faculties in the UK ' Diagnosis of Brain Death' (1976) ii BMJ 1187.

and in particular, establishing, under very standardised conditions, that no respiratory movements occur when the patient is disconnected from the ventilator. It is recommended that the tests be repeated, the interval between investigations depending upon the nature of the primary condition and the clinical course of the disease. It is standard practice for the diagnosis to be made by two doctors, and it is axiomatic that they should be independent of any transplant team concerned with the case.[10]   More elaborate tests, including the use of the electroencephalograph (EEG) are not considered necessary to establish a diagnosis of brain-stem death.[11] It has further been agreed in the United Kingdom that the establishment of brain-stem death means that the patient is dead.[12] There is some evidence that the heart will cease to beat even with continued ventilator support within a few days of brain-stem death having occurred.

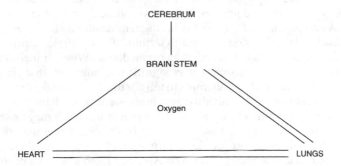

Figure 12.1 The process of dying. Both the heart and lungs are functionless without the other and both can be overridden mechanically. The brain will die without circulated oxygen, but the lungs cannot function without the brain stem. Since the brain stem is irreplaceable, it is reasonable to regard it as the seat of life and the measure of death.

The patient is available as an organ donor once the diagnosis of brain-stem death has been made. Maintenance of a brain-stem dead cadaver in a suitable state for beating heart donation is, however, a complex and time-consuming task which must be eased as far as is possible. Administrative arrangements for both donor and recipient operations are now in the hands of transplant co-ordinators, whose expertise is especially needed when donation of multiple organs to several recipients is undertaken.

It is essential to the understanding of beating heart donation to appreciate that it is discussed under the major heading of 'cadaver donation'. It cannot be over-emphasised that death is an absolute concept. There is no room—particularly in the field of transplantation—for equivocations such as 'as good as dead' or 'at death's door'. The success of the transplantation programme, and its legality, depend upon the rigid acceptance of this rule. Otherwise praiseworthy attempts

10 For the accepted guidelines, see Working Party on behalf of the Health Departments of Great Britain and Northern Ireland *Cadaveric Organs for Transplantation: A Code of Practice including the Diagnosis of Brain Death* (1983).
11 For a very early but still easy analysis of the problem, see C Pallis *ABC of Brain Stem Death* (1983).
12 Conference of Medical Royal Colleges and their Faculties in the UK 'Diagnosis of Death' (1979) i BMJ 332.

to improve the supply and the quality of transplantable organs by transferring moribund patients to intensive care for the express purpose of preserving their organs have, correctly in this writer's view, been held to be unlawful.[13]

Patients are admitted to intensive care for many reasons, including for diagnosis, assessment and treatment. It is a fundamental tenet of medical ethics that the health carer's actions must be taken in the best interests of *the patient*—looked at in this way, the consequent availability of beating heart donors is no more than a collateral benefit. But every patient must ultimately be withdrawn from the ventilator. In some, the criteria of brain-stem death may not have been met yet the patient's condition is such that further mechanical support is pointless, offensive or both.[14] A proportion of such patients will then breathe spontaneously. Others will be unable to maintain their respiration and will die. In either circumstance, the decision to withdraw support must be made by the physicians on the basis of clinical judgment and, in doing so, the doctor attracts no criminal sanction.[15] There is now no problem of any sort if brain-stem death has been declared; the patient is dead and the decision whether to terminate or continue ventilation rests upon whether the corpse is to be used as an organ donor. Whether there should be a law defining death is arguable;[16] it is significant, however, that no existing legislation in other jurisdictions attempts to tell doctors *how* to make the diagnosis.

While the problems of criminality and brain-stem death have been settled, there have been no cases to clarify some of the problems which may arise in civil litigation, particularly as to the time of death. Brain-stem death may occur at a given point, but this is imperceptible; the time at which the actual diagnosis is made is to some extent arbitrary and is retrospective to an unknown degree. One can thus conceive, for example, of problems arising in relation to the currency of life insurance policies. There is also the real dilemma in applying the criteria of brain-stem death to the solution of commorientes—a dilemma that seems to the author to be insoluble, save in a negative sense.[17]

The law and cadaver transplantation

Under anglophone common law, the deceased has very limited rights as to the disposal of his body and, in the event of conflict, the wishes of the executors

1 3   H Riad and A Nicholls 'Elective Ventilation of Potential Organ Donors' (1995) 310 BMJ 714 and related papers. S Ramsay 'UK Organ-retrieval Scheme Deemed Illegal' (1994) 344 Lancet 1081.

1 4   For the doctor's discretion to withhold futile treatment, see Lord Donaldson in *Re J (a minor) (wardship: medical treatment)* [1993] Fam 15 at 26.

1 5   First in Scotland—*Finlayson v H M Advocate* 1979 JC 33—and then in England—*R v Malcherek, R v Steel* [1981] 2 All ER 422—appeals against conviction for unlawful killing were based on the argument that switching off the machine broke the chain of causation. In neither instance did the judges consider specifically the question of death; in both, the appeals were dismissed on the grounds that the doctors had followed good medical practice. The classic paper on the subject remains I M Kennedy 'Switching Off Life Support Machines: The Legal Implications' [1977] Crim LR 443.

1 6   There is in many places. See, for example: Uniform Determination of Death Act 1980 (US); Human Tissue Act 1982, s 41 (Victoria); Human Tissue Act 1983, s 33 (NSW).

1 7   For example, if tests indicate that two persons are 'brain-stem dead', the time at which the tests were done *cannot* be used as evidence of relative survival and *ought* not to be certified as the time of death—though, perforce, it often is.

would normally be supported rather than those of the dead person, irrespective of how the latter had expressed his or her intentions. In the United Kingdom, however, the common law position is modified by two major statutes—the Human Tissue Act 1961 and the Anatomy Act 1984.[18] Here, we are concerned only with the former.

The Human Tissue Act 1961

Section 1(1) of the 1961 Act deals, first, with the situation when the deceased has asked during his life that his body should be used for medical education or research or for therapeutic purposes—the last, of course, includes organ donation. Then, the 'person lawfully in possession of the dead body' may authorise the removal of any part of his body for use as requested. In the absence of a specific request, s 1(2) empowers the 'person lawfully in possession' of the body to authorise removal of organs—

> 'if, having made such reasonable enquiry as may be practicable, he has no reason to believe (a) that the deceased had expressed an objection to his body being so dealt with after his death and had not withdrawn it; or (b) that the surviving spouse or any surviving relative of the deceased objects to the body being so dealt with.'

Thus, it will be seen that, under s 1(1), the donor 'contracts into' the system; under s 1(2), the relatives of the deceased have the opportunity to 'contract out'.

As has already been discussed, violent deaths will provide a major source of donations. Other than those professionally concerned with the transplant procedure, there are thus two groups of persons who have primary control of the provision of cadaver organs—the medico-legal authorities, represented by the coroner or the procurator fiscal, and those 'lawfully in possession' of the dead body.

Lawful possession

The main problem related to those 'in lawful possession of the body' lies in the fact that the term is undefined. Thus, it has to be decided whether the Act is speaking of those 'in possession' of the body—who are clearly the hospital authorities—or of those 'with the ultimate right to possession'—who are the executors. This writer believes that there is now no doubt that authority is vested in the hospital authority.[19] The Act itself infers that this is the correct view—in s 1(6), undertakers are specifically excluded as being in possession of the body for the purpose of authorising organ donation while, in s 1(7), allowance is made for the delegation of authority within the hospital. If there is no authority, how can this be delegated? Section 1(7) is, in fact, of practical importance in so far as it allows for delegation of powers to the transplant co-ordinator.

On the face of things, the right of a person to 'contract in' to the system and to proceed to donation after death is secured by the Act. Two hurdles, however,

---

18 The Anatomy Act 1984 deals specifically with the donation of the body for anatomical dissection in teaching units. The conditions as to consent are essentially the same in both Acts (see ch 5).

19 This still begs the question of the person who dies at home where, by analogy, the person in lawful possession would be the householder or, if that were the deceased, his or her executors—but this is supposition. In practice, the chances of such a person being suitable for organ donation are minimal.

stand in the way. First, the onus on the person in possession of the body is discretionary rather than obligatory even in respect of s 1(1). The second is a more practical matter. Very few transplant units would, nowadays, act on the written instructions of a deceased—for example, in the form of an organ donation card—were the next-of-kin to object. This may be pragmatic humanity but it is clearly against the spirit of the Act. The reasons for what is almost universal practice may be varied and understandable; even so, it is difficult to explain why the deceased's autonomous and inalienable right to treat his body as he wishes should be ignored simply because he is dead.

'Reasonable enquiry'

The meaning of 'reasonable enquiry' must also be questioned. Authoritative opinion suggests that this must be interpreted in relation to the time available; it must be *unreasonable* to carry inquiries beyond the point in time after which an effective transplant would be unlikely. In practice, most suitable donors will be maintained on a ventilator and timeous difficulties related to consultation now occur only rarely—especially as a close relative who can speak for the family will almost certainly be in attendance. Nevertheless, it would be valuable to have a list of relatives who could be contacted in order of seniority, the most senior available being empowered to take responsibility—such a system operates in Australia.[20]

Medico-legal authorities

All of the above considerations are, of course, subject to the authority of the coroner or the fiscal. They will be responsible for disposal of the body in a majority of instances, although it has to be remembered that the mere fact that a patient is to be removed from intensive care is no reason, of itself, for involving the medico-legal authorities—that is dictated by the reason for *admission* to the ventilator. It is axiomatic that there must be no interference with a body so constrained unless specific permission is granted—unauthorised removal of tissue is expressly prohibited under s 1(5) and (9) of the 1961 Act. No authority wishes to obstruct unreasonably a potentially life-saving measure and most coroners and fiscals agree to prior discussion of cases and the consequent immediate waiving of objection to organ donation in the event of death. Previous inquiry will dispose of the possibility that the removed organ may have been of importance to the medico-legal investigation—in ordinary practice, this will only be of major concern in heart transplantation. Some medico-legal authorities may take the view that a patient whose death is likely to be the subject of criminal proceedings should not be used as a transplant donor and this is understandable; a possible compromise is that the coroner's or fiscal's pathologist attends the donor operation, which then becomes part of the autopsy.

It is worth noting that the medico-legal authority is in *control* of the body until it is released but is not in *possession*. The coroner or fiscal cannot authorise donation; all he or she can do in this respect is not object to the removal of organs.

---

20 Eg Human Tissue Act 1983, s 4 (NSW). There is no reason why a hierarchy similar to that available in the Mental Health (Scotland) Act 1984, s 53 could not be incorporated in the Act.

The donor operation

The 1961 Act states, at s 1(4), that no removal shall be effected except by a registered medical practitioner, who must have satisfied himself by personal examination of the body that life is extinct. The requirement for medical registration is now waived in the case of donation of the cornea.[1] The problem of 'personal examination', however, remains one of some difficulty. The fact that the Act means precisely what it says is clear form the wording of s 1(4A)(b)(ii), inserted by the Corneal Tissue Act 1986, which specifically validates a statement by another practitioner as to life being extinct in the case of corneal grafting. But is it possible in the ordinary case for the surgeon to conform? Current guidelines clearly dictate that those who certify brain-stem death must function apart from those who are concerned with organ transplant therapy. The surgeon confronted with a donor who is still breathing artificially and whose heart is still beating cannot *know* that his patient is dead. Some will disconnect the ventilator and will not operate until the electrocardiogram is flat—but imposing a warm hypoxic period will vitiate one of the main practical advantages of beating heart donation, particularly, for example, in the event of a cardiac transplant. The vast majority of surgeons will depend upon a reading of the hospital notes—and this scarcely satisfies the wording of the Act. The surgeon—and, indeed, the public—might be reassured if a death certificate were always completed before the donor operation, but, at present, there is no such obligation.

The shortage of organ donations

There is no doubt that, in common with all other developed countries, the demand for donated organs in Great Britain exceeds the current supply. But, before accepting this as a misfortune, it is well to remember that transplant therapy is not an unmitigated blessing—one person's future health is gained only at the expense of another's death, often in especially distressing circumstances. The improved logistics of transplantation allow for multi-organ donation, by which some five lives can be salvaged from one death; this may assist in breaking down any popular antipathy and, thus, improve the consent rate among the next-of-kin involved. Many administrative ploys to increase the harvest of available organs have been suggested but the one which is most commonly advocated—and which appears to have succeeded in those countries in which it has been introduced[2]— is to change from a 'contracting in' system to one based on 'contracting out', in which consent to donation is assumed unless the deceased has left positive instructions to the contrary. This is no place for a full discussion of the issues involved.[3] It is, perhaps, sufficient to quote a spokesman for the government at the time:

> 'We must accept that nobody has a right to anybody else's organs. If something untoward happens, our organs may be of value to someone else but that should be the

1   Corneal Tissue Act 1986.
2   In particular, Belgium and Austria.
3   For full review of the various options, see B New, M Soloman, R Dingwall and J McHale *A Question of Give and Take* (1994).

result of an altruistic decision about how we want our bodies to be used when we die. It should not be as a result of a right of the recipient . . . It is the responsibility of the living whose organs may be of use to someone else; it is not anyone else's job to claim the organs.'[4]

and one suspects that that would be the policy of any government within the reasonable future.[5]

Donation of ovarian tissue

Special medico-legal considerations surround the donation of ovarian tissue for the treatment of infertility—something which may, at the moment, lie in the realms of science fiction but which, at the same time, is being seriously considered. It could, conceivably, be effected by both living and cadaver routes. In either event, there is a different quality to consent to donation in that genetic material is being handed on—perhaps indefinitely; moreover, the donor's parents arguably have an interest in the process. It seems certain, at least, that authority for donation should not be vested in the hospital management and that the Human Tissue Act 1961, s 1(2) and (3) should be amended in this respect. In the event, the Human Fertilisation and Embryology Authority is prepared to sanction the use of donated ovarian tissue for therapeutic purposes only from living persons over the age of 18; it may reconsider the use of adult cadaver tissue for this purpose in the light of further studies. The use of any tissue donated by an adult for research purposes is acceptable provided that adequate consent has been obtained.[6]

Donation of neonatal tissues

There is an ever-increasing need for paediatric transplant therapy. The potential donor supply is, however, very limited[7]—happily, very few infants are killed accidentally, while the tissues of neonates dying, for example, during childbirth, are unlikely to be in a condition fit for implantation. In ordinary circumstances, the provisions of the Human Tissue Act 1961, s 1(2) will apply; the case of the anencephalic neonate, however, raises specific practical and ethico-legal problems.

The essential dilemma stems from the fact that the anencephalic is close to death but, as in the case of the patient in the permanent vegetative state, cannot be described as dead. Tests for brain-stem death may be impossible and the diagnosis of death rests on the cessation of spontaneous respiration.[8] Neonatal tissues are particularly sensitive to oxygen lack while, even in the best circumstances, tissues from anencephalics do not function as well as those derived from anatomically normal neonates; the impulse to cut short the diagnostic period of respiratory

---

4   188 HC Official Reports (6th series) col 1142, 28 March 1991, per Stephen Dorrell.
5   The Organ Transplants (Presumed Consent) Bill 2000 is currently before Parliament but is unlikely to succeed.
6   Human Fertilisation and Embryology Authority *Donated Ovarian Tissue in Embryo Research and Assisted Conception: Report* (1994).
7   Although lobes from a living adult liver can be used; there is no reason other than conditional why adult cadaver liver tissue should not also be used.
8   *Report of the Working Party of the Conference of Royal Colleges and their Faculties in the United Kingdom on Organ Transplantation in Neonates* (1988).

failure before reconnection to ventilator support is, therefore, very strong. The use of anencephalic neonates as tissue donors is not unlawful but the practice involves a high moral cost.

The use of fetal tissues

Fetal tissues are immature and the constituent cells are primed to replicate; moreover, they are, in general, poorly antigenic and, thus, are less subject to rejection than are those of the adult. Fetal cells are, therefore, attractive as replacement tissues—and this is particularly so when the cells secrete a substance which the recipient lacks. This is the basis of replacement therapy for the treatment of Parkinson's disease, which is a degenerative condition of the ageing brain.

Aside from the very considerable doubts as to its efficacy, the problems surrounding such treatment are ethical rather than legal.[9] The fetal tissues to be used must be immature—at around ten weeks' gestation. The laws relating to the disposal of stillbirths do not, therefore, apply; moreover, the fetus, never having had a legal personality, is not subject to the Human Tissue Act 1961. Guidelines for the use of fetal tissues, which it would be unwise for the practitioner to ignore, have, however, been laid down;[10] prominent among the recommendations is that the mother's consent must be obtained before fetal tissues—whether derived from spontaneous or therapeutic abortion—are used for either research or treatment.[11] The ethical objections include the general concern that the treatment is inevitably tied to abortion and the more particular doubts as to the propriety of using the fetus as a form of 'pharmaceutical preparation' with which to treat the elderly. These are subjective problems. The more objective problem rests on the inescapable fact that the fetal brain cells must be viable; the fetus is, therefore, not 'brain dead' when its tissues are used. The obvious riposte is that the 10–12 week fetus was never alive—but this has a ring of sophistry. There can be little surprise that fetal brain tissue implantation has been subject to political control in the United States and the programme is currently in abeyance in the United Kingdom.

A more recent controversy now surrounds the use of fetal ovarian tissue and ova for research purposes and for the treatment of infertility in women. The opposition to this is largely of an intuitive nature, the main objective concern being that we do not know whether ova in the naturally maturing ovary are subject to natural selection—it could be that abnormal ova were used in vitro which would not have survived in vivo until the woman's puberty. Any arguments are, for the moment, sterile, as the use of fetal ova or of embryos derived from their use has been declared unlawful by reason of a hastily debated clause in an otherwise unrelated parliamentary bill.[12]

It is apparent that much of the legislation surrounding transplantation therapy is unsatisfactory. It is fragmented, the basic law is both outdated and uncertain

9 A very useful modern study, albeit with a trans-Atlantic emphasis, is to be found in N M C Bell 'Regulating Transfer and Use of Fetal Tissue in Transplantation Procedures: The Ethical Dimensions' (1994) 20 Amer J Law Med 277. For a brief report, see R Gillon 'Ethics of Fetal Brain Cell Transplants' (1988) 296 BMJ 1212.

10 *Review of the Guidance on the Research Use of Fetuses and Fetal Material* (Cmd 762, 1989) (The Polkinghorne Committee).

11 Cmd 762, para 3.10.

12 Criminal Justice and Public Order Act 1994, s 156.

and much of the more recent legislation has been introduced by way of 'panic' measures. There is little expectation, however, that it will be modernised and consolidated in the foreseeable future.

Property in body parts

The Human Tissue Act 1961 and the Human Organ Transplants Act 1989, in particular, raise problems as to the ownership of the body and body parts—a problem that is accentuated in modern times by the enormous potential for commercialisation of human tissues by the biotechnical industry. A brief note on the current status of the law is needed, despite the fact that very little of it can be described as definitive.

The 1961 and 1989 Acts clearly indicate that a person has some control of his or her body and its parts—but control is not the same as ownership and, while it is possible for body materials to be regarded as property,[13] both the courts and Parliament fight shy of the issue. Undoubtedly, a major reason for this lies in a deep-seated fear that to acknowledge a property right in one's bodily parts would lead to a trade in human tissue and, consequently, to exploitation of the vulnerable. The law is, thus, forced into what might be described as 'knee-jerk' responses of which the Human Organ Transplants Act 1989 is a classic example.[14]

The effect of the 1989 Act is to criminalise any activity associated with the sale or purchase of a human organ (s 1(1)) or to advertise to that end (s 1(2)). The ban covers organs taken from both the living and the dead, it applies whether it is intended to operate in Great Britain or elsewhere and the principals—the donor and the recipient—themselves commit an offence by participating. All of which is, no doubt, unexceptional at the instinctive level but there are strong arguments that suggest that the legislation is flawed on both practical and theoretical grounds.[15] As to the latter, it is questionable whether such overt paternalism, which allows for no special pleading, is acceptable in the current medico-legal ethical environment. As to the former, there can be little doubt that the supply of organs would improve if some form of regulated reward, even if only in kind, were introduced.[16] None the less, the law is clear and is unlikely to be amended.

Such matters are concerned with personal relationships. Thus far, neither the British legislature nor the courts have been concerned with the commercial connotations of the ownership of body parts. A foretaste of the difficulties to come is provided by the American case *Moore v Regents of the University of*

---

13 There are a number of old and very tenuous cases in the criminal law indicating that hair, blood and urine might be seen as property in certain circumstances, but the writer sees little precedental value in them in the conditions envisaged here. *R v Rothery* [1976] RTR 550 is an example relating to a specimen of blood.

14 There is a similar ambivalence in the Human Fertilisation and Embryology Act 1990, Sch 3, where control of gametes and embryos in vitro is vested in consent as to their use but the question of ownership is avoided. That aspect is, however, beyond the scope of this book.

15 See J Radcliffe-Richards, A S Daar, R D Guttman et al 'The Case for Allowing Kidney Sales' (1998) 351 Lancet 1950.

16 For trenchant support of these views, see J Harris *Wonderwoman and Superman* (1992) ch 6. Similar objections could be taken to the soon to be de jure ban which operates to prevent donors putting conditions on their 'altruism': L Beecham 'Donors and Relatives Must Place No Conditions on Organ Use' (2000) 320 BMJ 534.

California,[17] in which a doctor developed a cell line from a patient's spleen that had been removed at operation and, later, sold his patent for $15m. The patient brought an action for conversion of his 'property rights' and also for breach of the doctor's fiduciary duty to inform him of the full implications of the operation. After a long trail through the courts, the Supreme Court of California allowed the latter claim but refused the former—and this largely on the grounds that to do otherwise would jeopardise the commercial interest in biomedical research. In short, it seems that the American courts will not recognise an individual's property rights in parts of his or her body that have been removed but will accept that third parties may legitimately acquire and protect such an interest.[18]

There is some evidence that the British courts incline to such a line, albeit only in part. The case of *R v Kelly*[19] concerned the supposed theft of a number of specimens from a medical museum. Given the long-standing rule that there is no property in a dead body or dead parts of a body,[20] it was contended that there could be no theft. The Court of Appeal, however, held that this applied only to the body in its natural state; the body could 'acquire different attributes by virtue of the application of skill such as dissection or preservation techniques, for exhibition or teaching purposes'.[1] This clearly included the mounting of museum specimens which is, therefore, in an infinitely smaller way, equivalent to the development of Mr Moore's cell line in the laboratory. The Court of Appeal thus consolidated an earlier ruling[2] and, in doing so, established that 'ownership' was then vested in the party that performed the work that altered the status of the specimen. This does not, however, address the problem of the 'operation specimen'—who, if anyone, 'owns' a stone-filled gall bladder or, more importantly, a ruptured spleen? The Nuffield Council has recommended that such tissues be regarded as abandoned material.[3] This, however, would leave them to the next person to whom they came to hand and who could use them properly—that is, the medical authorities. On all counts, therefore, the stage is set for a British *Moore* and the court in *Kelly* was clearly of the opinion that the topic should be considered by the legislature.

The subject has, in fact, surfaced dramatically at the time of writing—albeit in the form of autopsy, rather than operation, specimens. It transpired that a large number of children's hearts had been retained in the pathology department of a major hospital without the knowledge or consent of the parents.[4] An inquiry was

17 793 P 2d 479 (Cal, 1990).
18 G T Laurie 'The Body as Property' in J K Mason and R A McCall Smith (eds) *Law and Medical Ethics* (5th edn, 1999) ch 20.
19 [1998] 3 All ER 741.
20 For discussion, see P D G Skegg 'Medical Uses of Corpses and the 'No Property' Rule' (1992) 32 Med Sci Law 311.
 1 [1998] 3 All ER 741 at 749.
 2 *Dobson v North Tyneside Health Authority* [1996] 4 All ER 474. This is an unsatisfactory case on its own, particularly from the medical angle.
 3 Nuffield Council on Bioethics *Human Tissue: Ethical and Legal Issues* (1995) para 9.14. While recognising the serious difficulties involved, the writer believes that patients should, at least, have a right to return of their specimen should they so wish.
 4 In fact, such practice is fairly widespread and at least two other major examples are being investigated officially: R Woodman 'Storage of Organs Prompts Three Inquiries' (2000) 320 BMJ 77. The whole issue is complicated by the fact that the great majority of autopsies are carried out on behalf of the coroner, for which consent is not required. Otherwise, consent to autopsy by the surviving relatives is required by the Human Tissue Act 1961, s 2(2).

set up under the chairmanship of Professor Kennedy and an interim report was severely critical of the laboratory's conduct.[5] The circumstances at this particular hospital were especially disturbing; there can be no doubt that the parents concerned suffered considerable distress. The problem is to decide whether this was due to unethical or unlawful behaviour and the relevant law merits consideration.

On the face of things, a combination of ss 1(2)and 2(2) indicates that the retention of organs without consent from the surviving relatives constitutes a breach of the Human Tissue Act 1961. Having said which, in the absence of any firm statement within the statute, it is difficult to see that this constitutes a criminal offence, other than, possibly, one of an obscure nature.[6] Moreover, the organs have certainly been the object of skilled dissection and they have been preserved for teaching purposes; it is, therefore, arguable that they have become the property of the pathologist in *Kelly* terms. The Coroners Act 1988 is, perhaps, more explicit. Undoubtedly, the pathologist undertaking a coronial autopsy is entitled to retain specimens[7] but this is subject to restrictions—retention must be motivated by its bearing on the cause of death and is valid only for so long as the coroner sees fit.[8] Outside these terms, retention of tissue is governed by the 1961 Act and is a matter for discussion between the pathologist and the relatives—and this applies even, say, if the problem is related to possible civil litigation in the future. But it is still difficult to see what offence has been committed by the pathologist who ignores the relatives' wishes and this may be a suitable subject for future legislation.

Most would agree that, in the circumstances envisaged, the precise legal position of the pathologist is less important than is his or her ethical relationship with the surviving relatives and the Royal College of Pathologists has recently published guidelines designed to improve the latter.[9] Guidelines such as this have no force of law but few doctors would wish to be involved in the civil courts or to come before the General Medical Council for having ignored them.

5   *The Inquiry into the Management of the Care of Children receiving Complex Heart Surgery at the Bristol Royal Infirmary* (I Kennedy, chairman), Interim Report *Removal and Retention of Human Material* (2000) makes 69 recommendations, most importantly directed to the need to obtain the consent of parents and agreement of the hospital Ethics Committee before tissue is retained for purposes other than, in the case of a coroner's autopsy, establishing the cause of death. Changes in the law are also proposed. The report has the broad support of the BMA: C Dyer 'Consent Needed for Organ Retention, BMA Says' (2000) 321 BMJ 1098.

6   The situation is well argued by P D G Skegg 'Liability for the Unauthorized Removal of Cadaveric Transplant Material' (1974) 14 Med Sci Law 53 and I M Kennedy 'Further Thoughts on Liability for Non-observance of the Provisions of the Human Tissue Act 1961' (1976) 16 Med Sci Law 49. See also P D G Skegg 'Liability for Unauthorised Removal of Cadaveric Transplant Material: Some Further Comments' (1977) 17 Med Sci Law 123.

7   And, indeed, sometimes s/he must do so. The examination of the brain, for example, is generally inadequate without prolonged fixation in formalin. It is to be noted that the *police* are instructed to retain relevant evidence for three years after a conviction or a plea of not guilty and at least until after an appeal has been heard: Criminal Procedure and Investigation Act 1996, Code of Practice.

8   Coroners Rules 1984, SI 1984/552, r 9.

9   Royal College of Pathologists *Guidelines for the Retention of Tissues and Organs at Post-mortem Examination* (2000).

13

Asphyxia and allied conditions

Asphyxia is here defined as the result of interference with the oxygenation of the red blood cells. There are, however, a number of conditions that do not fit comfortably into such a definition, yet which are so closely associated with the concept of asphyxia that they must be discussed as part of the general picture—foremost among these is neurogenic inhibition of cardiac function. On the other hand, tissue hypoxia due to anaemia, which is a deficiency of the red blood cells themselves, is excluded from discussion.

Asphyxia is of five main types (see Figure 1.2, page 11 above):

1. *Mechanical*—in which the airways are blocked in an unnatural fashion.
2. *Pathological*—where the transfer of oxygen to the lungs is prevented by disease of the upper air passage or of the lungs themselves.
3. *Toxic*—when poisonous substances prevent the uptake of oxygen.
4. *Environmental*—or an insufficiency of oxygen in the inspired air.
5. *Iatrogenic*—or caused by the medical profession and mainly associated with anaesthesia.

Mechanical asphyxia

Atmospheric oxygen may be excluded from the lungs at various anatomical levels.

First, the nose and mouth may be obstructed—the process of *suffocation* or *smothering*.[1] Secondly, the glottis—or upper portal of entry to the air passages—may be blocked as in *choking* due to impaction of food or of a gag. The most important level of occlusion in the context of forensic medicine is at the larynx, where the process is generally described as *strangulation*. If this is accomplished by hand alone it is manual strangulation or *throttling*; strangulation by ligature or cord may also be performed manually, the most specific example being *garrotting*, or it may result from suspension, ie *hanging*. Still lower in the air passages, the whole trachea or a main bronchus may be blocked after *inhalation* of foreign bodies or of stomach contents. Finally, the muscles of respiration may

---

1   Total occlusion of the nose and mouth by liquid—that is, drowning—is described separately in Chapter 14. Although suffocation also results from burial in trenches following land falls etc, the results are those described later under 'traumatic asphyxia'.

themselves be immobilised, for example, by crushing; the condition known as *traumatic asphyxia* results.

Suffocation

Unnatural suffocation or smothering in infancy presents one of the most difficult problems in forensic pathology. It is a simple matter to place a pillow over a baby's face, leaving, as likely as not, no evidence of external pressure. The only signs demonstrable at autopsy will then be those of anoxia in general, which can be summarised as:

1. *Cyanosis*. In the absence of oxygen, most of the oxyhaemoglobin will be converted to and remain in its reduced form; the colour of this is of dark plums which will be seen in the skin. This sign is of little medico-legal value because death itself is a matter of permanent tissue anoxia; some degree of cyanosis is therefore found in most natural deaths and may be very marked in those due to cardiac failure.
2. *Venous congestion*. Failure of the right side of the heart, with stagnation of blood in the veins, is an accompaniment of all asphyxial deaths save those that terminate immediately or very suddenly. Congestion of the lungs is most common but, as this is a frequent finding in natural heart failure, its significance is slight; acceptable diagnostic importance is confined to systemic congestion—that is, congestion of the skin and of the organs other than the lungs. A main result of raised venous pressure is rupture of capillaries or of postcapillary venules and the consequent formation of *petechial haemorrhages* which are often found in asphyxial deaths[2]—and in live persons who have survived an asphyxial episode. The distribution of these haemorrhages is important and is greatly influenced by:
    (i)   *Impairment of the venous exit from the capillaries*. Thus, pressure on the veins of the neck while the heart continues to beat, as in strangulation, will cause local pressure in the capillaries of the head—petechiae will, therefore, be pronounced in the eyes and on the face.
    (ii) *The nature of the tissue*. The capillaries will give way more readily where they are least supported—thus, petechiae will appear to be more concentrated in fatty fibrous tissue such as the eyelids.
    (iii) *General visibility*. Other than on the skin, petechiae will be most readily visible when confined by a transparent membrane. Internally, therefore, they are seen most often on the lungs beneath the pleura or on the heart beneath the pericardium. In infancy, they are often obvious beneath the covering of the thymus gland and, in severe asphyxia, they will be seen underneath the inner covering (mucosa) of the pharynx, larynx and other hollow organs—but whether or not these are truly evidence of asphyxia is controversial.
    (iv) *Intensity of congestion*. The intensity of congestion may cause the petechiae to coalesce into larger haemorrhage; if the pressure builds up still further, the covering material may rupture and frank bleeding will occur.

2   This 'evidence' of asphyxia was first described in infant suffocation by a French police surgeon; as a result, the haemorrhages are often referred to as 'Tardieu spots'. In point of fact, Tardieu was describing specific petechiae on the surface of the lungs; with hindsight, it is fair to say that he was probably describing the findings in the sudden infant death syndrome—the eponym should be relegated to forensic history.

Since venous back pressure is a major factor causing the petechiae, it is quite certain is that they can result—both in life and in the dead body—from any form of raised pressure within the thorax, eg in a severe asthmatic attack or during childbirth. However, as noted below, a deficiency of oxygen alone will damage the structure of the smallest blood vessels; since such a deficiency must occur during any process of dying, the question arises as to whether petechiae can be found following other forms of natural death. There is certainly no shortage of written authority to the effect that they *can* be and virtually every textbook on forensic medicine emphasises the possibility. In these circumstances, the 'spots' are usually confined to the pleural surface of the lungs, most often between the lobes; they are also found in the posterior pharynx following death from coronary disease. Iconoclasm is an essential part of academic analysis[3] but, while such possibilities must be acknowledged, a distinction between 'natural' petechiae and those resulting from mechanical asphyxia is very often a matter of quantitation or, even more importantly, of their distribution (see 'strangulation' below); 'natural' petechiae are generally few in number and must be sought with determination. Moreover, it is the *overall* picture that matters—the diagnosis of an asphyxial death on the basis of a single feature is fraught with danger.[4]

3. *Oedema.* Hypoxic damage to the capillaries will, of itself, result in increased permeability of their walls which will allow the passage of fluid plasma rather than of particulate red blood cells; oedema (or 'water in the tissues') will accompany asphyxia provided the hypoxic stimulus is relatively long lasting. The process is generally best demonstrated in the lungs. Again, the distribution of oedema may be important, as its production will be exaggerated by concurrently raised intravascular pressure—thus, oedema of the face, tongue and pharynx is a frequent feature of strangulation.

The suffocated infant, therefore, may well show no more than generalised congestion with, perhaps, the formation of petechial haemorrhage on the surface of the lungs, heart and thymus; the changes are certainly not specific to suffocation and their interpretation must depend largely on the circumstantial evidence. Suffocation with the hand may leave identifiable evidence because the generalised congestion of asphyxia will not develop at the points of pressure; areas of pallor recognisable as the imprint of the palm or fingers may be seen together with small finger-nail abrasions around the angle of the jaw. There may be similar findings on the back of the head if the baby's face has been forced into a pillow, but it is evident that the interpretation of such findings is highly subjective. The main difficulty is to distinguish the appearances from those due to hypostasis; hypostasis normally shows areas of pallor where the head has rested on the pillow and this is a prominent feature in 'cot deaths' (see page 276). In the latter case, the child will almost certainly have been moved by distraught parents, the consequent anomalous position of these areas may cause some confusion and, in the final analysis, a great deal will depend on the history of the discovery.

---

3   One of the most eloquent iconoclasts is B Knight *Forensic Pathology* (2nd edn, 1996) ch 14.
4   Bleeding from the ends of congested small vessels that are cut at autopsy can give an impression of petechiae, especially within a homogeneous tissue. Thus, the pathologist should speak of 'congestion of the vessels of the brain' rather than 'petechial haemorrhages within the brain'.

Can suffocation of accidental type occur in infancy? Most authorities would agree that it is improbable because a baby suffocating with its face in a pillow will move reflexly so as to breathe; but there may be cases when, because of entanglement in a harness or bedclothes, movement is impossible and true accidental suffocation can result. Suffocation by overlaying, essentially a matter of overcrowding, is now rare; occasional instances are associated with drugs and drunkenness. The condition may never have been as common as tradition supposes; many deaths so diagnosed must have been unrecognised examples of the sudden infant death syndrome[5] (see Chapter 19).

Accidental asphyxia in older children focuses attention on the specific hazards of 'plastic bags'. Numerous tragedies have occurred due to such activities as 'playing spacemen' when a 'helmet' of polythene, attracted to the nose and mouth both by respiration and natural adhesion, becomes moulded firmly to the shape of the face. The airway occlusion is often sudden; death may be rapid and signs of asphyxia are often absent. The great majority of plastic bags are now either marked as 'dangerous' or are perforated when their intended use permits.[6] A more sinister form of plastic bag asphyxia in children is associated with 'glue sniffing', where a bag is used to concentrate the volatile substance; although the majority of deaths are due to the toxicity of the substances inhaled, some result from asphyxia as above.[7]

It should be mentioned that adult suicide is not uncommonly accomplished by the use of plastic bags. Pathological findings are, then, remarkable for their absence. The appearances are those of a peaceful death and it is general experience that it would be difficult to identify an unnatural death if the bag was removed before the examination of the body.[8]

The sexual asphyxias

Plastic bags also play a part in the interesting group of conditions known as sexual asphyxias; these may also include features of strangulation.

These deaths are characterised by a strongly male distribution and by an equally common association with transvestism together with the use of some asphyxial mechanism, such as a plastic or other bag; a masochistic tendency is often shown by tying the hands or binding the torso and by the superimposition of some form of suspension by a neck ligature. The sexual nature of the condition may be emphasised by a display of pornographic literature.

These features taken together virtually eliminate the involvement of another party, particularly when, as is usual, the victim has taken precautions to preserve his solitude. Occasionally, however, the possibility that the dead man was the victim of a sadomasochistic partnership needs to be excluded—death may be very rapid in any highly emotional state, particularly when the neck is involved and, should it occur, any others involved are likely to leave the scene. The common problem in

5   Even so, suffocation in bed of an infant by a person over the age of 16 while under the influence of drink remains a specified offence under the Children and Young Persons Act 1933, s 1(2)(b), as amended by the Children Act 1989, Schs 12 and 13.
6   Special regulations are in force for items specifically directed to children: Toys (Safety) Regulations 1995, SI 1995/204, Sch 2(II)(1)(e).
7   In general, see J M Watson 'Morbidity and Mortality Statistics on Solvent Abuse' (1979) 19 Med Sci Law 246 and, more recently, P McBride and A Busuttil 'A New Trend in Solvent Abuse Deaths?' (1990) 30 Med Sci Law 207.
8   T L Haddix et al 'Asphyxial Suicides Using Plastic Bags' (1996) 17 Amer J Forens Med Pathol 308.

the classic sexual asphyxial death is, however, to distinguish between accident and suicide. A proportion are probably correctly categorisable as 'reckless risk-taking' but, unless there is specific evidence to the contrary, such deaths should generally be regarded as accidental, caused either by unexpectedly rapid loss of consciousness or by failure to escape from the manufactured conditions. Not only does this seem kinder to the relatives but, since there is an in-built reluctance to invoke the verdict of suicide, most coroners would be happy to grasp the opportunity when it is available.[9] The motivation in cases involving females may be different and they are, perhaps, not as rare as most practitioners would believe.[10]

Obstruction at the mouth and laryngeal opening

Gagging is seldom intentionally homicidal. More commonly, death occurs accidentally when the mouth has been stuffed with material to stifle calls for help—this may have been premeditated, as when immobilising a night watchman, or done on impulse, for example, during the course of a sexual assault. Suicidal gagging must be very rare and is likely to be found only in those who are mentally disturbed. Death in such circumstances may be of an asphyxial type but sudden death due to reflex neural inhibition of the heart is a strong possibility.

Accidental gagging—or *choking*—can also follow impaction of a bolus of food in the larynx. This may be associated with drunkenness but is most commonly seen in elderly persons who bolt their food as a symptom of senile dementia—the process of mental ageing—or who cannot masticate efficiently without teeth. Paradoxically, it is also a feature of the 'executive lunch'—so much so that the condition was once known as the 'café coronary syndrome'. As this last title indicates, death is almost always sudden and is due to reflex stimulation of the parasympathetic nervous system. An asphyxial type of death may follow if the food passes the larynx and lodges in the trachea; impaction of something smaller—for example, a nut—in a main bronchus may result in death of almost any degree of suddenness, ranging from reflex cardiac inhibition to death far removed in time due to bronchopneumonia or lung abscess. This type of death needs to be distinguished from that due to aspiration of regurgitated stomach contents—discussed later in the chapter—which is far less satisfactorily defined.

Strangulation

Strangulation is that aspect of asphyxia that most often results in serious criminal charges. It is, therefore, considered here in some detail.

Manual strangulation

Except in unusual circumstances—for example, in retributive gang warfare—it is doubtful if throttling is often the result of deep premeditation; far more frequently, exasperation or fear provokes a murderous impulse which, in the absence of any weapon, is satisfied by 'wringing his or her neck'. The circumstances surrounding

---

9 The author regards the sexual asphyxias as the classic example for preferring the Scottish confidential investigation of unnatural deaths to the publicity attached to the coroner's inquest.

10 R W Byard, S J Hucker and R R Hazelwood 'Fatal and Near-fatal Asphyxial Episodes in Women. Characteristic Features Based on a Review of Nine Cases' (1993) 14 Amer J Forens Med Pathol 70.

the crime and the precise type of a strangling are, therefore, of great importance in assessing the mind of the assailant at the time. Much may be reflected in the mode of death, and the pathological evidence may be of particular significance in the final evaluation.

Throttling can be accomplished single-handedly, in which case the thumb of a right-handed assailant is pressed into the right-hand side of the victim's neck close to the angle of the jaw, or bimanually, when each thumb is used to exert pressure; in an attack from behind, the fingers of each hand act as the main constricting agent. The local signs of throttling may consist, therefore, of bruising or superficial abrasion of the neck corresponding to a number of thumb or finger-pads. Both structures involved—the neck and the fingers—are relatively soft and resultant bruises, although sometimes obvious, may have indefinite edges; the appearances may well be clearer some hours after death when the process of blood stasis has produced a general pallor of the surrounding area. The edges of the bruises may show elliptical abrasions caused by the finger-nails of the assailant. It is important to remember that the presence of bruising is evidence of sustained pressure; bruising cannot occur in the absence of a heart beat and its presence vitiates the defence of sudden, unexpected neurogenic cardiac collapse (see below).

Thus, the signs of death from throttling depend upon the precise mode of death; this also applies in other types of violence to the neck. There are, essentially, four mechanisms:

1. *The windpipe is occluded.* In this case, the changes will be those of generalised oxygen deficiency and, because of the associated struggling, petechial haemorrhages are likely to be prominent. Pulmonary oedema will have been provoked if the anoxia has been prolonged and may show itself as froth at the nose and mouth if the pressure has been intermittent. This finding is not specific and occurs in prolonged hypoxia of many other types. Occlusion of the wind-pipe is the deliberate result of the neck hold popularly known as the 'choke hold', in which the victim is attacked from behind and the forearm is placed as a bar across the front of the neck; pressure is applied by pulling on the wrist with the free hand (see Figure 13.1). Choking as a result of the tongue being forced backwards into the pharynx is a rather more common result of this form of attack than is anoxia due to actual compression of the wind-pipe.

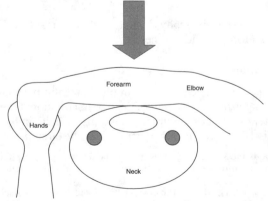

Figure 13.1 Choke hold—force applied across the front of the neck compressing the airway.

2. *The venous return is obstructed.* Anoxia in the brain results from stagnation of the blood and, because this is a gradual process, the cumulative effects of local oxygen lack will be prominent—thus, suffusion of the face with many petechial haemorrhages will be found; but generalised signs of asphyxia will be slight because the rest of the body is adequately oxygenated. There is some division of opinion amongst authorities as to how long is the agonal period in such cases. Some believe that, in throttling with the hands, the pressure must be applied for two minutes or more to cause death. Such estimates cannot be based on experiment and there is no doubt that two minutes is a lengthy period for sustained activity.[11] Others hold that most stranglings are over within half a minute—irrespective of the intervention of factors discussed below in (3) and (4). This latter estimate has been borne out in studies of accidental strangling and would seem to be the more reasonable.

3. *The blood supply to the brain is cut off by pressure on the carotid vessels.* This is an unlikely mechanism in manual strangulation. First, it is mechanically difficult to achieve the necessary compression through the tissues; secondly, the pressure is localised and difficult to maintain; and, thirdly because of this, the alternative blood supply to the brain through the arteries of the vertebral column remains available. These conditions do not apply in the case of strangulation by suspension (see below). Occlusion of the arterial blood supply to the brain is the object of using the neck hold known as 'the carotid sleeper'. Here, the neck is caught from behind in the crook of the elbow, additional pressure being, again, applied with the free hand. Thus, the anterolateral structures of the neck, including the carotid arteries are compressed (see Figure 13.2). Moreover, since the pressure is applied low down in the neck, the vertebral arterial supply may also be compromised—unconsciousness is likely in about six seconds. Pressure on the carotid arteries by the fingers or thumbs is more likely to cause:

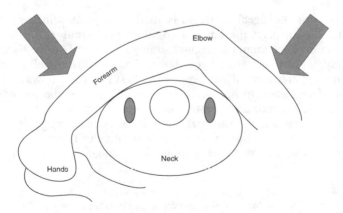

Figure 13.2 Carotid sleeper—direction of force on neck aimed at compressing the carotid arteries.

11 For recent discussion, see A M Anscombe and B Knight 'Case Report. Delayed Death after Pressure on the Neck: Possible Causal Mechanisms and Implications for Mode of Death in Manual Strangulation Discussed' (1996) 78 Forens Sci Internat 193.

4. *Death from neurogenic (or vagal) inhibition of the heart.* As described in Chapter 1, a sudden unexpected and, particularly, abnormal sensory stimulation of the sympathetic nervous system may result in an equally sudden and abnormal reflex through the motor component of the vagus nerve; the heart is arrested and death occurs with great suddenness. The carotid plexus in the neck is particularly sensitive and pressure at this point may well be the predominant cause of this type of sudden death; alternatively, fracture of the laryngeal cartilages may provide the main reflex stimulus. It is, however, fair to say that sympathetic stimulation may, itself, provide the primary stimulus, in which case, death will be equally rapid but, in this scenario, will be due to ventricular fibrillation or abnormal speeding up of the heart beat. Medico-legally speaking, the implications are the same irrespective of which mechanism operates.[12]

The significance of this form of death will be clear to the reader. The defence that 'I only tweaked her neck in play and she collapsed' is very common and, given the absence of vital changes, the pathologist would find it very difficult to deny the possibility. As discussed in deaths associated with anaesthesia (Chapter 31), autonomic reflexes are likely to be less inhibited when the higher control centres are functionally depressed and, for many years, it has been observed that death due to activity of the autonomic nervous system is most common following strangulation when the victim is moderately to severely affected by alcohol— often of the order of 200 mg alcohol per 100 ml blood.[13]

Injuries to the tissues of the throat and larynx provide the most important findings in the post-mortem dissection after manual strangulation. Bruising is the most constant of these and is found at all depths corresponding, in the main, to the pressure marks under the fingers; posterior bruising of the larynx may be caused by pressure against the spine and the base of the tongue may be affected by traction as much as by direct pressure. The thyroid gland may, itself, show bruising.

Fracture of the laryngeal cartilages is another diagnostic finding. The most frequent fracture involves the superior cornu of the thyroid cartilage, since the natural position of the thumb in manual strangulation rests on the ligament that joins the thyroid cartilage to the hyoid bone. The hyoid is, therefore, also often involved, due either to upward displacement by the thumb or to downward traction as the point of attachment to the thyroid is broken. Fracture of the cricoid cartilage is rare and, when found, is suggestive of pressure from the thumbs during an attack from the front; it is also said to result from the classical mugging manoeuvre of the 'choke hold' described above. The association of haemorrhage with any fractures is a most important post-mortem observation. This is the acid test of

12 An innovative approach to these problems is to be found in B N Purdue 'Asphyxial and Related Deaths' in J K Mason and B N Purdue (eds) *The Pathology of Trauma* (3rd edn, 2000) where the descriptive terms 'remotely stimulated cardiac dysfunction' and 'instantaneous neurogenic cardiac arrest' are introduced.

13 See, for example, K Simpson (ed) *Taylor's Principles and Practice of Medical Jurisprudence* (12th edn, 1965): 'States of narcosis and drunkenness may considerably shorten the period [of time taken to die from asphyxiation]' (p 359); T A Gonzales et al *Legal Medicine* (2nd edn, 1954): 'Alcoholic individuals may be asphyxiated easily by manual compression of the neck and succumb without revealing any demonstrable signs of violence at autopsy' (p 472). The author's own experience fully supports these classic views.

injury associated with a finite period of survival; subject to the caveat below as to pre-existing injury, the finding of a fractured laryngeal cartilage without bruising would be consistent with death due to neurogenic cardiac arrest—this, indeed is the modus operandi of the fatal karate chop. It is, however, wise to question the significance of haemorrhages in the mucous membrane of the larynx as, in rather similar fashion to petechial haemorrhages, these are not specific to mechanical asphyxiation and may even be found following natural death. It is also well established that bruising can occur as a result of the dissection itself—particularly around the neck structures. For this reason, it has been suggested that the cranial cavity should be dissected first in any case of suspected throttling; the potential for artefact is thus reduced by releasing the pressure in the engorged veins. The laryngeal cartilages can also be broken during removal of the neck organs but this should not occur other than in unskilled hands. Finally, the possibility that an injury discovered derived from a previous episode far removed in time cannot always be entirely discounted; such a fracture will, of course, be bloodless.

The pathologist is almost always asked for his opinion on the force required to cause a fracture of the larynx. Such an assessment is bound to be subjective and must, in any case, be related to the physical status of the victim. However, damage to the larynx beyond fracture of the cornua of the thyroid and hyoid—for example, fracture of the main wings of the thyroid—will imply 'considerable force', whether this be sustained or applied in the manner of the martial arts. Cartilages that are calcified are certainly easier to fracture than are those that are young and supple— but this is a comparative estimate only, which still fails to answer the question of how much force was applied in the individual case. In order to improve the objectivity of the assessment, it is advised that the larynx be X-rayed in every case in which apparent fracture is discovered. But it must be remembered that the muscles and ligaments will tend to realign any broken ossicles. A fracture may well be present but may not be visible in the X-ray because of this tendency to a normal position and because of variable calcification in the area; by the same token, the normal articulations present in the young cartilages must not be mistaken for fractures.

Strangulation by ligature

Strangulation by ligature without suspension is not uncommon as a form of homicide. Apart from the classic premeditated crime of *garrotting* (or, it is understood, the one-time lawful method of execution in some jurisdictions)—in which the assailants used their own prepared form of ligature—the material used to strangle is usually that which happens to be near at hand; because of the close association with sexual assaults and of the rarity of an original intention to strangle, nylon stockings or pantihose are most frequently found in adult cases; the victim's own scarf is also often used.

The ligature may or may not be knotted in homicidal strangling; although the former is more common, the assailant sometimes depends upon his own strength to maintain the pressure on the neck. This must involve pressure on the veins and is usually sufficient to cause actual obstruction of the windpipe and of the arterial circulation. The time to death, therefore, and the findings at autopsy, depend very much on the efficiency of the ligature.

Death may be rapid and would certainly be expected to be faster than in manual strangulation. Consequently, signs of asphyxia may run from nil to those of generalised anoxia with exaggerated appearances in the head and a well-established 'tide mark' formed by the ligature. The ligature causes a mark which is characteristically horizontal and of regular depth; it nearly always passes in front of the neck across the membrane connecting the hyoid and thyroid cartilages, which are fractured far less commonly than in manual strangulation. Very little external evidence of the presence of a ligature may remain if it is composed of soft material and is removed immediately after death. Cord or rope may, however, leave a distinctive pattern, while irregular finger-nail scratches, inflicted by the victim in an attempt to loosen the constriction, are highly suggestive of homicidal strangling.

Suicidal strangulation by ligature is uncommon but certainly occurs. It is generally associated either with an intricate system of tourniquet application or with the use of elastic material which will spring back to give powerful constriction after having been knotted—nylon stockings behave effectively in this way. At the same time, this effect may be accidental rather than suicidal—self-strangulation is sometimes used as a form of exhibitionism with no intention of a fatal outcome. Accidental strangulation is not all that rare—particularly in infants who can become entangled with their harnesses; somewhat similar deaths are found in geriatric patients who are restrained to stop them falling out of bed.

The umbilical cord is occasionally used to strangle a newborn infant—the question then arises as to whether the cord can encircle the neck so as to cause fatal accidental strangulation either in utero or during the act of birth. Few would dogmatise that either cannot happen and, in cases of precipitate labour, the cord may be markedly tightened. Such cases must arouse suspicion but, no matter how great this may be, the onus is still with the prosecution to prove the *fact* of a separate existence before a charge can be upheld. A separate existence will scarcely ever be possible in accidental strangulation by the cord, but proof *may* be forthcoming in cases of infanticide or child murder; the problem is discussed in Chapter 18.

Strangulation by suspension

Judicial hanging has now been wholly abolished in the United Kingdom.[14] It was said that it gave rise not to an asphyxial death but to disruption of the cervical spinal cord due to a separation fracture of the neck induced by the massive jolt following a drop of some 2.2 m; the most common fracture site was at the level C2-3.[15] It is known that the heart could continue to beat for several minutes following hanging and it is to be hoped that the jolt also caused severe diffuse cerebral axonal injury or reflex cardiac arrest—otherwise, modern concepts of brain death suggest that there may have been a significant period of consciousness before the onset of cerebral anoxia. Nowadays, death by hanging is almost entirely suicidal, with a small accidental element.

14 Crime and Disorder Act 1998, s 36.
15 Recent research indicates that these estimates were horrifyingly wrong. Fracture of the neck occurred in a minority of cases and death was anoxic in at least 10%: R James and R Nasmyth-Jones 'The Occurrence of Cervical Fractures in Judicial Hanging' (1992) 54 Forens Sci Internat 81. For confirmation, see D T Reay, W Cohen and S Ames 'Injuries Produced by Judicial Hanging' (1994) 15 Amer J Forens Med Pathol 183—even so, the heart stopped beating within one minute.

The suicidal nature of the case is nearly always apparent from the circumstances—although attempts to disguise a homicide as a suicidal hanging are not unknown.[16] Arrangements involving some elaboration are often made and steps are usually taken to offset the possibility of detection before death; consequently, it is not unusual for suicidal hangings to have been dead for some days before discovery.

The post-mortem findings depend, again, on the degree of vascular occlusion which, in turn, depends on the efficiency of the hanging. Thus, the circular pressure exerted by the noose is fully sufficient to occlude the carotid arteries when the body is completely suspended; unconsciousness and death will, then, be rapid and congestion of the tissue above the ligature may be minimal. Cerebral hypoxia will be induced even if the feet are on the ground; unconsciousness may then, again, come on rapidly but death will be delayed and there will be a varying degree of facial congestion. Characteristically, there will be severe hypostatic changes in the legs and forearms. The ligature mark in the neck is deep and is maximal opposite the point of suspension; it often passes between hyoid and thyroid cartilages in front, rising to the point of an inverted V, corresponding to the knot of the noose, either in the midline posteriorly or behind one ear. The internal appearances may be those of generalised anoxia but, even if death has resulted rapidly from neurogenic cardiac failure, the effects of blood pooling in a vertical position will still be visible externally. Anomalies of hypostatic staining may indicate the possibility of simulation but it has to be remembered that the ligature may be so firm and death be so rapid that vital reaction is absent; a false impression of hanging may be gained post-mortem. Fractures of the laryngeal cartilages may occur in hanging but are by no means invariable; much depends upon the age of the subject.

Accidental death from hanging is generally sexually orientated and is associated with the sexual asphyxias previously discussed; simple exhibitionism may, however, end disastrously. It is the speed with which unconsciousness supervenes that explains the 'success' of many suicides in situations that appear easily recoverable. It is, in fact, surprising how often this happens in conditions that eliminate the possibility of homicide; although relatives may often find it difficult to accept, hanging even in a semi-kneeling position is compatible with suicide.

Other forms of accidental hangings scarcely need special mention, though many need careful differentiation from homicide—the baby strangled in its restraining harness is one example already mentioned. Industrial accidents of many types can be imagined. A somewhat bizarre form of accidental hanging may occur in sport or military parachuting when the neck becomes entangled with the shroud lines; the severe jolt often imparted gives rise to intimal laceration of the carotid arteries—an autopsy sign that is useful in strongly indicating a sudden stretching of the neck in hanging incidents of all types.

Obstruction in the lower air passages

Drowning, discussed in Chapter 14, is an obvious form of obstruction involving the lower respiratory tract. But it is also possible effectively to 'drown' in one's

---

16 The classic case was *R v Emmett-Dunne*, 1954 General Court Martial, Dusseldorf, which was surprisingly poorly reported. A soldier killed his wife with a karate blow and suspended her body. The cause of death was undiscovered until a second autopsy was performed.

own body fluids—the accumulation of fluid in the lungs is known as pulmonary oedema, which forms part of the syndrome of hypoxia described above.

Pulmonary oedema is not specific to mechanical asphyxia. It occurs in all forms of hypoxic death, including those of central origin such as barbiturate poisoning, and following any trauma to the air passages themselves—such as exposure to fire or to irritant gases. It is also a natural result of heart failure—an ineffective left ventricle is unable to clear the blood returning from the lungs; severe pulmonary oedema is commonly present in deaths due to coronary insufficiency. Oedema will also result when the volume of the circulating blood is increased beyond the capacity of the left ventricle; this occurs when fluids are transfused over-liberally into the body and is a form of iatrogenic asphyxia which is discussed in Chapter 31. Pulmonary oedema commences within the alveoli but it may be so intense that the bronchioles and bronchi are filled with fluid. Irritant gases produce the extreme of the condition—and it is worth remembering that even the comparatively innocuous tear gas may provoke severe pulmonary reaction in high concentration.

The interpretation of obstruction of the lower airways by inhaled stomach contents presents a practical problem in forensic pathology. This is certainly a common post-mortem finding which is particularly frequent in hypoxic deaths. Although it is easy to presume a cause-and-effect relationship, a diagnosis of asphyxia due to inhalation of stomach contents may well be a misconception; it is widely held that vomitus in the air passages is usually there because of, rather than as the cause of, tissue anoxia.[17] To complicate matters further, the act of vomiting itself may cause the appearance of petechiae by suddenly raising the venous pressure. In practical terms, the presence of inhaled material from the stomach should not be accepted as the precise cause of death unless products of digestion can be demonstrated microscopically in the small air passages. Despite the opposition to the concept, the present author, at least, believes that a valid diagnosis of death due to inhalation of gastric contents is acceptable when the appearances are compatible with more than artefact and the circumstances are reasonable; these will include, especially, when death is associated with conditions that depress the reflex ability to expel foreign material from the lungs—head injury and intoxication due to drugs or alcohol are frequent causes, as is anaesthesia given without adequate pre-operative preparation.

Restriction of chest movement

Pressure on the chest sufficient to inhibit respiratory movement will cause asphyxia. There are two major variants which may, according to the circumstances, merge into one another.

The first is *postural asphyxia*, which can occur when the victim finds him- or herself in a position where chest movement is compromised; very often there is a predisposing factor which inhibits the normal righting reflexes—such as alcoholism or drug intoxication. The condition is of particular medico-legal importance because of its frequent association with police custody of violent detainees. The attribution of death to position or posture may be relatively easy in, for example, the case of the trapped tunneller. By contrast, it is often difficult

---

17 B Knight 'The Significance of the Postmortem Discovery of Gastric Contents in the Air Passages' (1975) 6 Forens Sci 229.

in the more common situations due to the interplay of many factors. There is no doubt that it is a valid diagnosis—albeit one that should be made with considerable care.[18]

The second condition is commonly known as *traumatic asphyxia*, which is an unfortunate term, as 'trauma' should include all forms of violence; the better term is *crush asphyxia*—when the circumstances likely to produce the effect become self-evident. They include crushing under rock falls, burial in a collapsing trench or in a silo, pinning in a vehicular accident—including pinning against the garage wall—and crushing in a crowd, particularly if the crowd collapses; the most recent and vivid example in the United Kingdom of this last possibility was the disaster at Hillsborough Football Stadium in 1989. The pathological findings are characteristic—there is intense congestion with widespread formation of petechiae in the tissues, especially in those of the upper thorax and neck; occasionally, there is little or nothing to be seen externally. Crush asphyxia could just possibly be induced homicidally by the assailant sitting on the victim's chest—some such method, coupled with manual suffocation, was admitted by Burke and Hare, hence the descriptive title of 'burking'. The more important medico-legal connotation is that the great majority of cases, other than those which constitute a major disaster, are likely to be associated with occupation and, thus, liable to investigation by the Health and Safety Executive followed, perhaps, by criminal proceedings.

Crushing of the body in this way may have serious long-term effects in the event of survival. In the first place, injury to the muscles leads to the very serious condition of the crush injury syndrome, the most potentially lethal aspect of which is acute renal failure (see page 19); indeed, practical experience indicates that, in the conditions of an earthquake, the most important medical requirement is for simple and widely available facilities of the artificial kidney.[19] Secondly, crushing that compromises breathing must also compromise the brain; varying degrees of brain damage are, therefore, to be expected in those who survive the experience.

The permanent vegetative state

This, then, coupled with the mention of the Hillsborough disaster,[20] provides a suitable point at which to discuss the medico-legally very important condition of the permanent vegetative state. We have seen that death as a result of asphyxia is essentially a matter of death of the brain due to anoxia. However, as we have also seen (see page 166), the various components of the brain show a varying sensitivity to *hypoxia*. Thus, given a shortage or arterial oxygen, the cells of the cortex will die before those of the thalamus which, in turn, will die before those of the brain stem. Brain cells that have died as a result of hypoxia cannot regenerate. Further death can, however, be prevented by reoxygenation, in which case, we will be left with a brain that is *partially* dead. The worst possible scenario results when only

---

18 E A Laposta 'Positional Asphyxia during Law Enforcement Transport' (1993) 14 Amer J Forens Med Pathol 86.
19 J E Tattersall, N T Richards, M McCann et al 'Haemodialysis during the Armenian Earthquake Disaster' (1990) 21 Injury 25.
20 The English law relating to the management of the permanent vegetative state was built around a victim of that incident: *Airedale NHS Trust v Bland* [1993] AC 789. The Scottish equivalent is *Law Hospital NHS Trust v Lord Advocate* 1996 SC 301.

the brain stem is alive; since the brain stem is responsible for our vegetative functions, we can then say that the patient is in a permanent vegetative state (PVS)—the permanence being decided on the basis of clinical experience and diagnosis. The patient is then in a wholly insensate state and has lost all relationship with his or her environment. None the less, the patient will instinctively sleep, can digest food if it is provided artificially and, most importantly, he or she has a beating heart and can breathe spontaneously.

It follows that the patient in PVS is not dead and, given intensive nursing care, can exist in that state for many years. Yet, to bring about that person's death could be manslaughter or, possibly, murder. It is important to appreciate that the permanent vegetative state can arise whenever the brain is subjected to the requisite hypoxic insult, irrespective of the origin of that insult. Thus, cases will arise not only as a result of crush asphyxia but also by way of conditions such as drug overdose, environmental deprivation of oxygen, poorly administered anaesthesia, resuscitation following a period of respiratory failure and a host of other conditions. As a result, the condition is by no means rare and its management poses a dilemma.

This is no place in which to delve deeply into the intense moral and legal arguments involved.[1] Suffice it to say that the House of Lords in Mr Bland's case decided that it was not in the best interests of the PVS patient to be treated indefinitely, that artificial feeding was included in treatment and that, accordingly, it is not unlawful to withdraw alimentation and hydration from such patients—despite the fact that this will, inevitably, result in their deaths. At present, however, each case must be judged in the courts on its individual merits.[2]

Pathological conditions

Any pathological condition of the lungs that interferes with the free interchange of gases across the alveolar capillary membrane will cause some degree of tissue hypoxia. Bronchitis, emphysema and pulmonary fibrosis are the main conditions but, although they are a major cause of mortality in the general population, they have only limited medico-legal significance.

Many significant pathological pulmonary conditions are intimately associated with work and are likely to be the subject of compensation for industrial injury. They are discussed in some detail in Chapter 15. The presence of lung disease may result in severe strain on the right side of the heart—that side which is responsible for pumping blood into and through the lungs; a failing heart in this situation is known as *cor pulmonale*. While most sufferers exist in a state of chronic ill health, an acute exacerbation may be a cause of sudden death resulting in a coroner's or fiscal's inquiry—most likely to be directed at the provision of medical aid.

The presence of a condition predisposing to tissue anoxia will compound the effects of any other asphyxial mechanism; the pre-existing condition of the victim's lungs may, therefore, have considerable bearing on the evaluation of a case of,

---

1   The interested reader is directed, amidst a mass of relevant literature, to J K Mason and G T Laurie 'The Management of the Persistent Vegetative State in the British Isles' [1996] Juridical Rev 263.

2   *Practice Note* [1996] 4 All ER 766.

say, manual strangulation. This concept of synergism holds for all the main categories of asphyxia discussed.

Paralysis of the respiratory muscles may result from disease—the most well-known example being acute anterior poliomyelitis or 'infantile paralysis'. While poliomyelitis has been virtually eliminated by way of immunisation, there remain a group of progressive neurological diseases—of which, perhaps, the most important are motor neurone disease and the most serious instances of the Guillain-Barré syndrome—which are coming more to the forefront as it becomes more usual for sufferers to survive intercurrent infection. Rather in the same way as those of PVS, these cases raise serious questions related to the morality and legality of withdrawal of treatment, in this instance by assisted ventilation. A full discussion would, again, be out of place in this book but it is to be noted that cases within the Commonwealth jurisdictions have already been decided—generally, though not always, in favour of the ending of an intolerable existence.[3]

Toxic asphyxia

Toxic asphyxia is of two main types. Either the capacity of the haemoglobin to bind oxygen is impaired, or the enzymatic processes whereby the oxygen in the blood is utilised by the tissues are blocked.

Conversion of haemoglobin to the compound methaemoglobin is effected by many industrial poisons (see Chapter 21). This change produces more frightening signs than genuine pathological effects and the only haemoglobin derivative that is of major practical medico-legal importance is carboxyhaemoglobin—formed by the combination of haemoglobin with inspired carbon monoxide. Cyanides are outstanding examples of enzymatic poisons. These two substances will, therefore, be treated individually.

Carbon monoxide poisoning

The most readily available source of this asphyxiant was once the domestic gas supply which contained some 5–15% of carbon monoxide (CO); this supply is now provided by natural gas which, although asphyxiant in that it is irrespirable, has no positive toxic qualities. Consequently, the number of cases of suicidal poisoning due to domestic gases in the United Kingdom is now negligible. Most CO with which the public comes in contact nowadays derives from the combustion of carbon-containing material; carbon dioxide (CO_2) is the end product of ideal combustion but, since very few flames are totally efficient, all gas produced by fire contains some carbon monoxide. CO_2 is relatively unimportant, as its physiological effects can be compensated save in an enclosed environment (see page 194); the affinity of haemoglobin for CO is, however, some 300 times that of its affinity for oxygen. The formation of carboxyhaemoglobin (COHb) is, therefore, cumulative and a potentially fatal proportion of respirably inert COHb in the blood can derive from only a small concentration of CO in the inspired air.

3 Two important cases that have been included in the British reports are: *Nancy B v Hôtel-Dieu de Québec* (1992) 15 BMLR 95 (Canada—decided on the right of the patient to refuse treatment) and *Auckland Area Health Board v A-G* [1993] 4 Med LR 239 (New Zealand—decided on the basis of good medical practice).

In practice, therefore, two factors are needed to endanger life through carbon monoxide poisoning—first, there must be combustion and, secondly, the removal of the products of combustion must be inefficient.

The most common sources of poisoning include:

- Solid-fuel, gas or oil fires fitted with inadequate flues or used in rooms without sufficient ventilation. Oil heaters in bedrooms (including caravans) or geysers in bathrooms are obvious examples. Note that, although domestic gas now contains no CO, the toxic gas can still be generated through inadequate combustion.
- Internal combustion engines having defective exhaust systems—or operating within closed garages.
- Mines—where the perpetual minor fires leave pockets of contamination.

Death from CO poisoning may be homicidal, suicidal or accidental.

Homicidal poisoning must be extremely rare, not only because of its uncertainty of success, but also because the possibility of a toxic supply being deliberately opened in the presence of a sleeping or otherwise unconscious victim is not now available; the same is true of the one-time, and less unlikely, attempts at infanticide combined with suicide.

The motor-car exhaust is now the most frequent source of the poison for suicidal purposes. The true nature of a suicidal CO poisoning is likely to be shown by the intricate arrangements made—not only to ensure a concentrated delivery of the gas but, often, for the comfort of the subject. Additional suicidal agents—such as drugs—may well have been used. Car exhaust gas, which contains about 6% CO, can kill in a matter of minutes but this time will be greatly influenced by variations in the efficiency of delivery and ventilation.[4]

Several other factors affect the individual's susceptibility to CO. As with all poisons, the elderly are likely to be killed more easily than the young and the presence of disease that, of itself, contributes to or kills through tissue hypoxia must be taken into account—coronary insufficiency is an obvious example. Similarly, an anaemic person will succumb more quickly than will the normal, as it is the sum of hypoxic factors that matters. It follows that the symptoms of CO poisoning will also depend on the physical state of the individual. Thus, it is generally stated that conversion of 30% of the haemoglobin to COHb results in dizziness and headache, inco-ordination appears at 50% saturation, unconsciousness at 60% and death at 70–80%; but these are proportions relative to the total oxyhaemoglobin available and it is this total that conditions symptoms. Moreover, the more rapid and deep is the respiration, the more contaminated air will be inspired and the faster will be the accumulation of COHb. From the purely legal aspect, all these factors will be relevant when problems of survival arise, as they may well do if members of a family are found dead in a room or caravan; they also greatly influence the medical assessment of accidental CO poisoning.

Accidental intoxication by CO is of interest on two counts—first, it may of itself be the cause of death and, secondly, it may be the cause of a vehicular accident and, indirectly, of death from trauma.

4   An extraordinary self-recorded case has been reported in which death occurred in 20 minutes; the critical point of poisoning appeared to be at 6–7 minutes (N G Flanagan et al (1978) 18 Med Sci Law 117).

All sources of CO are associated with accidental poisoning. An inefficient coal or gas fire or a gas-fired hob can produce sufficient CO to be lethal in a confined space. Fumes from the exhaust of stationary cars contaminate the passenger compartment either through a faulty exhaust or heater system or as a result of escape into the air of a closed garage. Coal mining accidents can occur but, thanks to safety measures taken, are now rare—as is mining itself. Death is almost invariably associated with a degree of unawareness—senility, sleep, alcoholism or preoccupation with other matters are obvious examples. Accidents connected with senility are, now, generally associated with financial economy— for example, running heating appliances at what is, in fact, reduced efficiency. Accidents occurring while asleep are usually associated with open-flame heating apparatus—in particular, oil burners. It must be remembered that individuals may react differently, that CO tends to layer and that concentrations in a room will vary greatly according to the positions of draughty windows and doors. The maximum concentration of CO in the air of a room will not be very great and the effects are spread over a relatively long period; alterations in the environment will exaggerate differences in clinical response and, when there are several persons in a room, it may well be that some will wake up or be roused when others are already dead—such a result by no means rules out accident. Alcoholism may be a particular feature predisposing to death amongst the homeless who are huddled around inefficient braziers or boilers, especially if these have inadequate flues. Preoccupation may be a feature of deaths in garages while making car repairs. The combination of preoccupation and exercise leads to sudden deaths during sexual activity—often in cars in which the heater is left running; the importance of the respiratory rate on the build-up of carboxyhaemoglobin is, then, surprisingly frequently demonstrated by survival of the female partner and death of the male. Perhaps the bathroom geyser is the only apparatus likely to be lethal to a person normally aware and occupied. The usual small size of the room exaggerates the danger of failing to turn off the flame before entering the bath but, even so, the improved construction of modern gas heaters serves to minimise what was once a real hazard.

CO is a potential—and actual—cause of death due to traumatic injury in motor cars and in aircraft; the problem is discussed in Chapter 10. For the present, it is necessary merely to emphasise that only low levels of COHb—sufficient to cause no more than distraction or disorientation—are needed to cause a vehicular accident and, further, that there will be a marked synergistic relationship with other adverse physiological factors such as fatigue. The forensic pathologist and toxicologist will, therefore, be dealing with concentrations of COHb that are only slightly raised and which must be interpreted with care and in relation to the accident as a whole.

Cyanide

Poisoning by cyanide is uncommon but has historical interest; it is also the most significant example of histotoxic asphyxia—tissue enzymes are blocked by the process known as molecular substitution and are unable to transfer the oxygen in the blood. Death is essentially due to poisoning of the respiratory centre which is especially sensitive to hypoxia. If death is not sudden—and it often is—the high proportion of oxyhaemoglobin in the venous blood may show itself through the bright pink colour of the skin and internal organs; the colour must be distinguished from that of COHb and from the effects of cold, including post-mortem refrigeration. Delayed death only occurs in cases of ingestion of cyanide salts; hydrocyanic acid itself is one of the most rapidly fatal poisons known.

The use of hydrocyanic acid as a gaseous fungicide or, more commonly, rodentricide is specifically controlled.[5] Cyanide salts are used in the steel industry and in other industrial processes; they are common laboratory chemicals and are widely used in photography. Natural sources of cyanide include bitter almonds, the kernels of many fruit-stones and the leaves and fruit of some plants.

Death from cyanide poisoning is now rare. Homicidal poisoning seems to be a matter of history only—including its use for the genocidal killings of the 1940s. Accidental poisoning occurs mainly in industry and in laboratories. The sale of cyanide salts is unlawful save as provided by the Poisons Act 1972, s 4; suicide by cyanide is now virtually confined to those who require the poison for their trade or business—eg chemists and photographers—or their close associates.

Environmental asphyxia

Reduction in the available oxygen to a level inconsistent with life arises as a medico-legal problem most commonly in relation to enclosed spaces—too many people may be closeted in too small a space or the space may be too small to support a single human life. The former may be murderous in intent—the 'Black Hole of Calcutta' is history's most vivid example—or a matter of reckless indifference;[6] occasionally, overcrowding in small, cold rooms may cause the accidental death of whole families living in ghetto conditions. The second category is commoner and is typified by a child being trapped inside a disused refrigerator or trunk;[7] it is generally clear that such instances are accidental—although the precise nature of the accident, particularly of the part played by other children, may be in doubt—and the pathologist has to be aware of the possibility of the disposal of a child dead from other causes. Adults can also be locked in containers—eg safes—accidentally though such circumstances would almost always be highly suspicious as it would, otherwise, normally involve failure of the alarm system. An interesting variation on this theme involves the use of sprays—eg insecticides—within a small space such as a bunk bed; when used to excess, the heavy carrier gas replaces the normal atmosphere and asphyxia results. Accidents of industrial type may also result in anoxic deaths—mining and submarine disasters are obvious examples.

There is often some difficulty in deciding whether to attribute a death of this type to oxygen deficiency or to poisoning by excess CO_2; the author believes that the former is correct unless CO_2 is introduced into the environment in some way other than as a product of normal respiration. However, both physiological mechanisms operate and the process of asphyxiation in an enclosed environment is self-accelerating. As oxygen is utilised the concentration of CO_2 builds up; an increase in CO_2 reflexly increases the respiratory activity which, in turn, accelerates

5   Control of Substances Hazardous to Health Regulations 1994, SI 1994/3246, reg 13, as amended by Control of Substances Hazardous to Health (Amendment) Regulations 1996, SI 1996/3138.
6   A contemporary equivalent is the crowding of illegal refugees into confined spaces in lorries.
7   The disposal of containers which cannot be opened from the inside is controlled.

the depletion of oxygen; a rapidly fatal vicious circle is established, gross biochemical changes being added to lack of oxygen. Persons entering an irrespirable environment—eg the contaminated hold of a ship—without warning tend to die suddenly; the mechanism must be of a reflex nature, possibly triggered through the respiratory centre.

Environmental asphyxia due to altitude must be mentioned although, as its unnatural occurrence is virtually confined to aviation, it has only slight medico-legal implications. Death truly due to high-altitude hypoxia is rare. Mountaineers and those living at heights are able to adapt to the conditions; balloonists were early historic casualties but are scarcely a large group now; emergency oxygen is available to airline passengers and, so far as is known, has never failed when required.

Hypoxia at altitude is of greater importance in two other respects. In the first place, a person who is particularly susceptible to oxygen lack is at increased risk as ascent is made. The normal pressure of oxygen in the arterial blood is about 100 mm Hg (13.3 kPa); this falls to about 60 mm Hg (10 kPA) at 2,400 m (8,000 ft) which is the cabin altitude in most commercial aircraft. While this is quite safe for normal fit persons, it may precipitate fatal myocardial ischaemia in the presence of an already inadequate coronary circulation; similar altitudes could precipitate a crisis in a person with sickle-cell disease.[8] The ability of hypoxia to cause an aircraft accident is even more significant. Precision performance falls off rapidly with decreasing oxygen pressure, and it is generally accepted that 3,300 m (11,000 ft)—at which point, the partial pressure of environmental oxygen falls below the critical level of 100 mm Hg (13 kPa)—is the effective upper limit at which a man can operate an intricate machine without supplemental oxygen; above 10,000 m (33,000 ft), the total atmospheric pressure falls to about 150 mmHg (20 kPa) and the supplemental oxygen must be provided under positive pressure. The effects of hypobaric hypoxia are quite insidious, the victim being wholly unaware of his decreasing efficiency; it follows that failure of the oxygen supply to a military aviator or undiscovered loss of pressure in cabin-type aircraft[9] are potential causes of accidents. Sudden loss of pressure ('explosive decompression') in a large aircraft—such as might be caused by the detonation of a bomb or by major structural failure—is a complex pathological problem; death and injury may result from turbulence in the cabin, anoxia, the effects of low pressure and of cold, ejection from the aircraft and, of course, from the likely crash.

Iatrogenic asphyxia

Some degree of hypoxia may occur whenever a general inhalation anaesthetic is administered, the relative avoidance of this being a measure of the anaesthetist's vigilance and skill. Since oxygen lack in these circumstances is often imposed upon patients who are particularly susceptible by reason of disease, there is a real possibility of death due to hypoxia under anaesthesia. The medico-legal importance of the subject is great and is treated separately in Chapter 31.

8   See, in general, Aerospace Medical Association 'Medical Guidelines for Air Travel' (1996) 67 Aviat Space Environ Med B1.
9   This is, of course, a virtual impossibility in major commercial aircraft which have multiple means of detection available.

14

Fire, water, heat, cold and neglect

This chapter deals with a number of conditions which, while being related to asphyxia, have a wider interest than the simple production of tissue hypoxia. Those that are not so associated are logically related through at least one line of interest.

Injury and death from burning

Legally, burns include the destruction of tissue through the application of any form of heat or of any chemical substance. There is no distinction in law as to the degree of burning—to burn someone in any way is a serious assault and the use of corrosive substances is a specific aggravation in Scots law.

Burns may be natural—as in exposure to non-ionising solar radiation or due to lightning; they may be due to dry heat—generally from open fires but also from such articles as hot-plates, hot-water bottles, etc; burns due to moist heat are commonly known as scalds; corrosive substances have their own individual pathologies, and burns due to electricity and X-rays should be included in this classification—the common factor is the transfer of energy to the skin.

The distribution of burns varies with age. Under the age of three years, a high proportion are due to scalding; scalding also occurs in later childhood but accidental setting light to clothes is more important in this age group and is the most significant source of burning in old age; in normal adult life the great majority of accidental burns stem from industry, which provides examples of dry, wet and corrosive burning. However, with the exception of those due to lightning and man-made electricity (see below), the local medical effects of all burns are similar; this section will deal with burns due to fire as being the most typical, the most common and, medico-legally, the most important form of thermal injuries.

Burning in the human varies from simple reddening and blistering of the skin to severe charring and destruction of deeper parts of the body; the author was once involved in the investigation of one aircraft disaster in which no fewer than 23 bodies remained unaccounted for—it could only be assumed that they had been effectively cremated. It was at one time customary to classify burns according to their appearance; it is more rational to speak in terms of depth—eg:

(a) Partial thickness skin loss:
  (i) superficial;
  (ii) deep;
(b) Full-thickness skin loss;
(c) Deep burning.

Partial thickness loss of the skin should be self-healing as epithelial elements derived from the hair follicles and sweat glands will, eventually, replace the epidermis that has been destroyed; the deeper the partial loss, the greater will be the resultant scarring and the greater the need for urgent treatment. Full-thickness loss will require skin grafting if severe deformity due to scarring is to be avoided. Very deep burning will inevitably cause some loss of function or lead even to amputation (see Figure 14.1). This classification, essentially related to treatment, is also helpful in assessing the hurt and inconvenience sustained. The immediate prognosis of a burn depends to a great extent on susceptibility to pain—paradoxically, the superficial burn, in which sensory nerve endings are left exposed, is far more painful than is the deep partial-thickness burn in which the nerve endings are destroyed. Once over the initial impact, the outcome of a burn involving loss of skin is largely dictated, first, by age and, secondly by the extent of the loss of body fluids, the severity of which correlates, within limits, with the area rather than the depth of burning. There is a massive loss of water, protein and electrolytes from the raw areas and severe surgical shock arises if treatment is inadequate. Later still, the results of a burn are dictated by the risk of overwhelming infection—and the infection may well come from the patient himself rather than be introduced from outside.[1] Burn infection is particularly difficult to control because it is biphasic—the

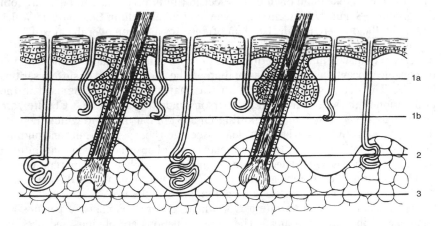

Figure 14.1 Diagram showing the microstructure of the skin and its relationship to the different levels of burning. Levels 1a and 1b are both superficial partial-thickness burns capable of healing spontaneously with no true scarring. A burn at level 1a can heal in 1 week; at 1b it is likely to take 2–3 weeks. Level 2, a deep partial-thickness burn, can heal spontaneously but may produce dense scarring. Level 3 passes deep to all epithelial structures, is full-thickness skin loss and can only heal by scar formation or skin grafting. (Reproduced with permission from J K Mason and B N Purdue (eds) *The Pathology of Trauma* (3rd edn, 2000).)

1   E A Deitch 'Intestinal Permeability is Increased in Burn Patients shortly after Injury' (1990) 107 Surgery 411.

streptococci, or organisms that commonly cause sore throats, are particularly destructive of the superficial layers of skin while the *bacilli*, or organisms which predominantly exist in the bowel, penetrate and invade the deeper tissues. Children and the elderly are more susceptible to secondary infection and septicaemia than are young adults. The general rule is that burning that destroys more than 70% of the skin is likely to be fatal irrespective of the treatment; an elderly person may not survive a 20% burn (see Figure 14.2).

Severe burns due to fire may be accidental, suicidal or homicidal. The first is by far the commonest and is a particular hazard of childhood and of old age;

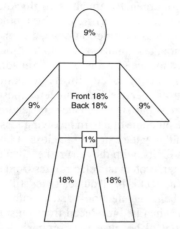

Figure 14.2 The area of burning is generally assessed using the 'Rule of Nine'; the percentage of the whole body area of the various components is as shown. (From R F Brown 'Injury by Burning' in J K Mason (ed) *The Pathology of Trauma* (2nd edn, 1993) by permission of the author.)

catching the clothes in an open or an electric fire is very liable to occur in both age groups.[2] Statutory protection is given to children both in England and Wales and in Scotland where it is declared an offence for a person over the age of 16 to expose a child under the age of 12 (age 7 in Scotland) in his or her care to the dangers of contact with an open fire grate or any heating appliance without taking reasonable precautions and, by reason thereof, the child is killed or suffers serious injury.[3] The dangers of 'playing with fire' have also been recognised in the prohibition of the sale of fireworks to persons under the age of 18.[4] Children are notoriously prone to scalding by boiling fat and similar things to which they are drawn by inquisitiveness. There is a clear association between infirmity and burning in the aged; frank illness may lead to a sequence of collapse, concussion and burning while in the unconscious state. Acute alcoholism also plays an important part in accidental burning; the combination of intoxication and smoking in bed is extremely dangerous and the latter practice is illegal in hotels in the USA.

Mass accidental burnings are a risk whenever large numbers of persons are congregated in a confined area. The likely situations are obvious and need no

2   Current regulations require that a guard be fitted to all domestic heating appliances whether they be coal, gas, electric or oil fires (Heating Appliances (Fireguards) (Safety) Regulations 1991, SI 1991/2693 and Gas Appliances (Safety) Regulations 1995, SI 1995/1629). See also Nightwear (Safety) Regulations 1985, SI 1985/2043, as amended by Nightwear (Safety) (Amendment) Regulations 1987, SI 1987/286.
3   Children and Young Persons Act 1933, s 11, as amended by Children and Young Persons (Amendment) Act 1952, s 8 and Children Act 1989, Sch 13; Children and Young Persons (Scotland) Act 1937, s 22.
4   Fireworks (Safety) Regulations 1997, SI 1997/2294.

detailed discussion; tenements, hotels, dance halls, theatres etc provide the common examples. Prevention of disaster is a matter of rigid application of building regulations, of ensuring a competent fire-fighting capacity and of provision of adequate escape facilities.[5] The disastrous fire at Bradford Football Stadium in 1985 was largely responsible for extensive legislation in respect of sports grounds.[6]

Burning in transport accidents must be mentioned. It is far less common than might be expected in automobile accidents—largely because there are generally a number of potential rescuers at the scene. It is by no means rare in aircraft accidents, although these do not constitute a numerically important cause of unnatural death; it is noteworthy that the outcome of an aircraft accident that is 'survivable' in terms of crash forces is determined almost entirely by whether or not fire breaks out.[7] The classic example is the accident at Manchester in 1985[8] involving little more than an aborted take-off. It was shown that the rate at which people became incapacitated through the effects of fire was greater than had been thought and that there is clear room for improvement in the design of seats, exits and emergency escape procedures in commercial aircraft.

Suicidal burning is not all that uncommon. It may be committed when maximum publicity is sought—igniting one's own kerosene-drenched body became something of an extreme form of political protest in the middle of the twentieth century. Otherwise, this form of suicide must generally be associated with severe mental derangement; the author has experience of one case where the subject, in addition to soaking her clothes, also drank over a pint of paraffin, presumably in the hope of dying by explosion. The practice of suttee—or ritual suicide by a Hindu widow on her husband's death—has long been abandoned but has been replaced by extensive 'dowry deaths', where the distinction between suicide, murder and accident has become a major forensic problem in India.[9]

Other than in that unusual situation, homicide by burning must be very exceptional owing to the uncertainty of success. But murder by fire after having immobilised the subject—for example, by injury or by drugs—or, more probably, attempted concealment of a murder through post-mortem incineration—are not at all unlikely; many of the classic examples of inspired forensic pathology have derived from such attempts.[10]

The distinction of ante-mortem from post-mortem burning is, therefore, essential. The demonstration of 'vital reaction' (see Chapter 4) around a burn is of minimal value in this context, as the body will almost always be severely charred. Major importance attaches to the demonstration of products of combustion either in the form of soot in the air passages or upper gastrointestinal tract or as COHb in the blood—values of 20–50% are common. The two parameters do not always

5 Fire Precautions Act 1971, as amended.
6 Fire Safety and Safety of Places of Sport Act 1987. For description of the incident from the aspect of forensic medicine, see S Sivaloganathan and M A Green 'The Bradford Fire Disaster' (1989) 29 Med Sci Law 279.
7 A comparison of two almost identical accidents at Stockport in 1967 and Kegworth in 1989 makes interesting reading: P B Herdson and J K Mason 'The Role of Pathology in Major Disasters' in J K Mason and B N Purdue (eds) *The Pathology of Trauma* (3rd edn, 2000).
8 Air Accidents Investigation Branch *Report on the Accident to Boeing 737-236, Series I, G-BGJL at Manchester International Airport on 22 August 1985* (1988).
9 See J R Gaur 'Forensic Examinations in Two Cases of Alleged Dowry Deaths' (1993) 33 Med Sci Law 269; K S Latha and R Narendra 'Dowry Death: Implications of Law' (1998) 38 Med Sci Law 153.
10 For example, *R v Rouse* (1931) Northampton Assizes; *R v Dobkin* (1943) CCC.

follow one another logically and the reasons for this are not easy to establish; it is often a matter of choosing what one regards as the 'best' evidence. In the event of fractures having been found, the discovery of bone-marrow or fat emboli in the lungs (see Chapter 10) would strongly suggest that the bony injuries were sustained in life; it has been claimed that burning by itself will cause fat embolism but the author has not been able to substantiate this observation—in fact, the demonstration of bone-marrow emboli would provide more objective evidence. The most certain evidence of a cause of death other than burning would be a finding positively indicating that cause—such as the discovery of a bullet or of evidence of manual strangulation. It must, however, be remembered that the bony tissues become very friable on exposure to intense heat and the possibility of post-mortem artefact must always be borne in mind (see below).

The unlawful disposal of bodies by burning is something of a vexed subject.[11] Practices differ in crematoria, but a reasonable programme for the reduction of a body to ashes involves exposure to a temperature of 600°C for at least one hour. Such a temperature would be unlikely to be achieved in normal domestic conditions. It might be possible to destroy portions of the cadaver after disarticulation—in itself, a fairly complex task—in a domestic stove but it would be a very prolonged process. It is doubtful if it can be done on an average bonfire and, in practice, attempts to promote a more spectacular fire are commonly thwarted by neighbours reporting the matter to the fire brigade.

Burning of itself causes artefacts that must be distinguished from ante-mortem injury; the lawyer should have some knowledge of them as they may appear as unqualified factual statements in post-mortem reports. The most common of these are muscle contractures which often result in the so-called 'pugilistic attitude'; this is simply due to heat coagulation of protein which has greater effect in the flexor than in the extensor muscles and is not evidence of a defence reaction. Contraction of the skin may lead to splits which are very like incised wounds. Boiling of body fluids in enclosed spaces may lead to apparent intravital haemorrhage; the most common type presents as a false extradural haemorrhage. Burning may of itself cause bony fractures; these are common in the bones of the arms and legs but are also seen in the skull, where they may result in severe loss of bone. The combination of artefactual haemorrhage and fracture can pose a most difficult pathological problem which can often be solved only by reference to the totality of evidence.

Death from burning may be immediate—the intense pain may cause reflex inhibition of the heart or the thermal injury may simply be so severe as to be incompatible with life. Alternatively, death may be asphyxial in type; fire victims seldom die from carbon monoxide poisoning per se—the discovery of COHb is a measure of survival in a fire environment rather than an expression of the cause of death. Early stupefaction can occur but this is probably due to the inhalation of other poisonous substances—eg cyanides—which are combustion products of many man-made materials.[12] The distinction of the mode of death is of more than academic interest; it may be important evidence in the application of the laws of succession (see Chapter 10). At the same time, a lack of uniformity in the precise

11 Irrespective of the cause of death, burning of a body other than in a certified crematorium is always unlawful (Cremation Act 1952, s 1).
12 For discussion, and consideration of the thermodynamics, see I R Hill 'Immediate Causes of Death in Fires' (1989) 29 Med Sci Law 287.

terms of the death certificates supplied tends to complicate an analysis of the mortality from burning.

Delayed death from burning is commonly due either to surgical shock—the particular conditions of a burns wound lead to a massive loss of body fluid that is, to an extent, self perpetuating—or to infection spreading from the damaged areas;[13] even if the problems of fluid loss and toxaemia are overcome, acute renal failure may have occurred and the response to dialysis is universally bad when this condition follows burning. This poor prognosis is probably due to the fact that renal failure is but one facet of what is known as the multiple organ failure syndrome, in which all the organs of the body are compromised to a greater or lesser extent. The syndrome has apparently only come to light following the increasingly successful support of single organ failure in intensive care units.[14] It is particularly common after burning and may be mainly associated with sepsis arising from a damaged bowel. Death more remote in time may result from pneumonia due to enforced and prolonged immobilisation, and it is possible— though not everywhere agreed—that the effects of prolonged stress may exhaust the capacity of the adrenal glands to sustain life.

It scarcely needs emphasis that the long-term results of survival from severe burning may be disfiguring and disabling and that such features must be very prominent in assessing damages when the injuries result from negligence. The most disturbing complications, which can arise following impeccable treatment, are hypertrophic and keloid scar formation. The latter is distinguished from the former in that it is progressive and never shows evidence of remission; its occurrence is also probably genetically determined. Some effects may not be immediately apparent—blindness, for example, may be threatened not only by the immediate fire but by an increasing inability to close the eyes or blink as the injured tissues contract. The tendency to malignant transformation in burn scar tissue has been mentioned at page 147. Overall, accidental burning results in a substantial reduction in the efficiency of the young and active population, not the least of which is due to psychiatric reaction to disfigurement; post-traumatic stress disorder is a very real complication of injury by burning. There is also a risk that the lung damage consequent upon inhalation of fire and smoke may lead to widespread fibrosis and the serious clinical state known as the adult respiratory distress syndrome.

Death from electricity

Electricity is used on a vast scale even by persons with negligible understanding of its behaviour. The fact that it causes so few deaths is a tribute to the safety engineering that has accompanied the development and regulation of the electrical components industry.[15]

The outcome of an electric shock depends upon physical factors in the discharge and on the physiological state of the subject.

13 In addition, the condition known as the toxic shock syndrome—characterised by vomiting, pyrexia and a rash—may occur a few days after burning, especially in children. It appears to be due to colonisation of the wound by a particular organism—the *staphylococcus*.
14 T E Oh 'Multiple Organ Failure' in T E Oh (ed) *Intensive Care Manual* (1990) ch 83.
15 Electrical Equipment (Safety) Regulations 1994, SI 1994/3260; Plugs and Sockets etc (Safety) Regulations 1994, SI 1994/1768.

The determinants in the discharge are the current (measured in ampères), the voltage (or electromotive force of the current, measured in volts), the time over which the discharge is passed (ampères x seconds = coulombs) and the type of current—whether direct or alternating. The major factors in the subject include his resistance to an electrical discharge, his body weight—children are more susceptible than are adults—his earthing and his degree of preparedness.

The relative importance of the discharge factors depends significantly upon the period of application. Ultra-short exposures are unpredictable in their effects, which depend upon the precise state of excitability of the heart when the shock is received. If the electric current is passed for less than three seconds, the danger is related both to the magnitude of the current and to the duration of the shock. Applications of longer than three seconds depend almost entirely on the amperage for their lethal effect; amperage to some extent dictates duration, as a high current (15–20 mA AC) initiates muscle spasm—the subject is unable to release the conductor until he or she becomes unconscious and long exposure results. Direct current is less hazardous to life than is alternating. The danger of the latter increases with the frequency and probably reaches its peak at the frequency of the public supply—50 hertz (cycles per second) in Britain and Europe and 60 Hz in the USA. Alternating current becomes less dangerous once the power frequency range of 1 kHz is passed, ultra-high frequencies being only a source of intense heat.

The voltage of the discharge is important when related to the resistance of the subject. The latter is almost entirely a matter of skin moisture; a completely dry person would have an exceptionally high resistance—some 1,000 times that of wet skin—and might well tolerate voltages of the order of those used in supply systems. The skin is, however, generally of such conductivity that voltages above 200V are likely to be fatal due to the limb-to-limb passage of a current of over 50 mA. Efficient movement of current depends, in ordinary circumstances, on the efficiency of earthing—a subject standing on wet ground is at far greater risk than is one on a dry surface. In the worst conditions, an alternating current at 25 V and 50 Hz has been fatal. Short-duration impulse shocks are used in agricultural electric fences; pulses of the order one tenth of a second in each second are usually considered non-lethal, but children of small body weight have been killed in exceptional circuit conditions. All workers with electricity will testify to the protective effect of preparedness for a shock; this is scarcely surprising since death from electric shock involves a considerable element of reflex nervous activity.

Suicidal electrocution is uncommon despite the ready availability of the method; the diagnosis can seldom be in doubt owing to the complexity of the arrangements made—one electrode is commonly attached, say, to a wristwatch and the underlying patterned burn with vital reaction testifies against a post-mortem attempt to mask death from another cause. Homicide by electricity must be equally rare save, perhaps, in the context of the 'battered baby' (see Chapter 19). It must be admitted, however, that homicide or fabrication may be suspected in an apparent suicide *without* elaborate preparations. The difficulty lies in proof. The same applies to the distinction between accident and homicide, particularly in cases of death in the bathroom; there have been several reports of electric apparatus falling into the bath water—proof that this was done deliberately may depend on an expert examination of the apparatus.[16] Judicial electrocution—which involves the passage of at least two currents of very high voltage —is used in a number of

16 As in the case described by B Knight *Forensic Pathology* (2nd edn, 1996) p 328.

those United States which currently retain the death penalty and a doctor is required to certify death in 23 of these.[17]

Accidents are overwhelmingly responsible for death due to electricity and are of several types.

Industrial accidents are kept to a minimum by stringent safety precautions but nevertheless continue to occur as a result of genuine mishap or flouting of the regulations due to overconfidence. Direct contact may not be necessary if very high tension cables are involved as arcing may occur at a considerable distance depending on the voltage—the figure of 2–3 cm for every 10,000 V is quoted and the zone of danger may be very much wider when the air is damp.[18]

Domiciliary accidents are more common and are of three main types: the apparatus may be defective, due often to fraying of insulation; attempts may be made to repair equipment without disconnecting it from the mains supply while using makeshift tools; or apparatus may be dangerously used—the most common example involves the use of electric equipment in the bathroom, where conditions for electrical conduction are optimal. Neutral fusing, which can give a false indication that the apparatus is 'dead', is a hazard peculiar to older apparatus of British manufacture.

Iatrogenic accidents are of major medico-legal importance, as they will almost invariably lead to actions for negligence. Electroconvulsive therapy, in which convulsions are deliberately precipitated by electrical stimulation of the brain, is occasionally used in the treatment of mental disorder; traumatic injury may be sustained during the convulsion and deaths have been reported due to the electric shock itself.[19] The hazards associated with 'invasive' diagnostic or therapeutic techniques ie those that involve penetration of the skin or of a mucous membrane—deserve special mention; since the resistance of the skin is eliminated and blood is an excellent conductor, death may be caused by misapplication of very low intensity currents. Other dangers of electricity in the operating theatre are mentioned in Chapter 31.

The use of electricity as an *autoerotic stimulant* deserves special mention. The author has seen one case in which a penile vibrator was connected to a mains plug; when the dead body was discovered the plug was not in the socket and no marks were found on the penis—the cause of death could not, therefore, be attributed to electricity with certainty.

The diagnosis of death due to electric shock may, in fact, be difficult—especially if there are no localised points of entry and exit of the current; in such circumstances, electric marking may well not be present. Characteristically, however, there is a mark which shows a central area of necrosis surrounded by a

17 The doctor may have to decide whether further lethal action, including further shocks where applicable, is required. Physician-involvement in the death penalty is a matter of intense ethical debate: Editorial Comment 'Doctors and Death Row' (1993) 341 Lancet 209; 'US Physicians and the Death Penalty' (1994) 343 Lancet 743, although this is clearly of more significance when death is induced by lethal injections.

18 J A D Settle 'Burns' in J K Mason and B N Purdue (eds) *The Pathology of Trauma* (3rd edn, 2000) ch 14.

19 What is arguably the most consequential English medico-legal case stemmed from just such an action: *Bolam v Friern Hospital Management Committee* [1957] 2 All ER 118.

white zone which is, in turn, encircled by a blush of dilated vessels. Contact with a flat electrode leaves a circular blister; sometimes, the electrode responsible leaves a replica of itself; an electric arcing entry burn is characteristically small and circular but may be associated with particularly severe resulting injury. A true burn of parchmented or charred type may result if the current has been prolonged. An 'exit' mark may also be present and may take on the shape of the exit contact. All of these marks may be faint and a determined search may be needed for their demonstration. A rare form of multiple flash burning spread over a wide area results from long distance arcing from a very high voltage source; the appearances are known as 'crocodile skin'. Microscopically, the electric burn shows 'bubbling' of the keratin layer due to the liberation of steam together with 'streaming' of the basal nuclei; the appearances are typical of electricity only in that they result from intense localised heat—there is no reason why similar changes should not follow heat of any type which was delivered in similar fashion.

Death is predominantly physiological when due to the electric shock itself; the post-mortem findings are, accordingly, often slight and generally non-specific. Three modes of death are described. In the least common, the current passes through the head and the respiratory centre of the brain is directly affected; a variant hypothesis is that stimulation of the autonomic nervous system causes cardiac arrest. Alternatively, the entire musculature may be involved in the spasmodic contracture described above; death is then akin to that in crush asphyxia (see page 189) and this accounts for those cases of electrocution that show the post-mortem changes usually associated with mechanical hypoxia. The most common cause of death is said to be ventricular fibrillation—that state in which the ventricles of the heart beat so rapidly as to be ineffective pumps. Interestingly, the current passing must be of fairly critical intensity to produce this effect—the deliberate application of a high-intensity current is used medically as a *treatment* of ventricular fibrillation. This may account for some remarkable survivals that are reported after very high intensity electric shocks, as any counter-shock, including painful injury, can act as a defibrillator. There are two major points of medico-legal interest associated with death from fibrillation. First, it has been reported that death may not be immediate and can be preceded by volitional movement—the effect on the heart is, for uncertain reason, delayed; movement of the body during this phase may give rise to a suspicion of homicide. Secondly, and of far greater importance, cardiac function may be restored; prompt resuscitative measures are therefore essential and artificial respiration can be successful even after having been applied for a long time.[20]

Finally, death may be caused by, but not be due to, electrocution. Thus the fatal outcome may be due to burning if the clothes are set alight; alternatively, death may result from traumatic injury if a high-intensity shock precipitates the subject, for example, from a high ladder. And the possibility of multi-organ failure as a result of the primary insult remains.

Lightning as a source of electrocution

A lightning flash incorporates several physical features. These include the application of an electric current of extremely high intensity, the effects of primary 'flash' and secondary thermal burning and the pressure effects of a high-intensity

20 But the associated risk of recovery in a severely brain damaged state must also be considered.

blast wave (see page 128). The subject struck may, therefore, sustain injuries of traumatic type—including fractures—and the clothes may be torn; the appearances must be distinguished from those due to assault. Superficial skin burns of a leafy or arborescent type are characteristic, when present, of lightning strike—it is said to be present in some 30% of cases,[1] although this author has never seen the sign. Beyond this aspect of differential diagnosis, lightning strikes are of no medico-legal importance since they are always occurrences of unpredictable, accidental type. Despite the apparent ferocity of lightning strike, it is noteworthy that death occurs in less than half the subjects who are treated promptly.[2]

Death from hyperthermia

Although it has little medico-legal significance, a note on hyperthermic death is added for the sake of completeness. The human body is fairly well adapted to hot climates; sweating is the main protective mechanism and severe effects may follow abnormalities of this function.

Direct effects of heat on the brain may lead to heat stroke. The thermoregulating mechanism of the body is affected and the body temperature rises precipitously in association with a failure to sweat. The condition is essentially due to exposure of the head to direct heat, usually in an arid climate. This type of death could be criminally associated with deliberate exposure of soldiers or prisoners; some cases were the subject of war crimes. Death may be due to the condition known as disseminated intravascular coagulation—a form of shock in which multiple thrombi form in the small blood vessels.[3] The malignant hyperthermia of anaesthesia (see Chapter 31) probably kills in much the same way.

Heat exhaustion is a different condition and arises in two forms. Anhidrotic heat exhaustion—that is, heat exhaustion due to failure of sweating—is secondary to a form of skin disease that occurs in hot, damp climates and is of no concern in the present context. Hyperhidrotic heat exhaustion, due to excessive sweating, could well form the subject of a medico-legal inquiry. In this condition, sweat flows so freely that enough sodium chloride is lost to provoke severe physiological effects unless it is purposefully replaced. This is the characteristic exhaustion of the long-distance runner or of the soldier on forced march, but the pure condition is not often seen in outdoor activity—a highly dangerous situation arises when heat stroke is superimposed. Heat exhaustion has considerable importance in industry and is a hazard to stokers in ships etc, where the effects have been declared industrial accidents in the distant past.[4]

Death due to drowning

Although closely related to asphyxia, death from drowning is not a simple matter of oxygen lack. This certainly occurs but an additional, and perhaps the main,

1 C V Wetli 'Keraunopathology' (1996) 17 Amer J Forens Med Pathol 89.
2 Settle, fn 18 above, believes that lightning itself so alters cellular activity that the dangers of a prolonged anoxic period are minimised.
3 T C Chao, R Sinniah and J E Pakiam 'Acute Heat Stroke Deaths' (1981) 13 Pathology 145.
4 *Dover Navigation Co Ltd v Craig* [1940] AC 190 is an example.

effect of water inhaled in the lungs is to alter the biochemical balance of the blood; how this occurs depends upon the medium of immersion.

Drowning in salt water is closest to a true asphyxial death and, generally, there is ample evidence of a struggle to breathe; petechiae, however, rarely form in the lungs due, possibly, to the mechanical pressure of the inhaled water upon the capillaries. During the death throes, water not only passes into the lungs but is gulped into the stomach and is forced into the middle ear. Death may result from total immersion for some 5–8 minutes.

The mechanism differs in fresh water which is removed from the lungs and transferred to the bloodstream far more quickly than is sea water. During this process, which, by raising the blood volume, is dangerous in itself, the protective covering of the alveoli—so called 'surfactant'—is removed and this, among other results, causes the classic frothing at the mouth. Such frothing is not specific to drowning—it occurs in burning and in virtually any condition associated with pulmonary oedema—but it is very good evidence of death having been due to drowning when found in a body removed from the water. The fresh water passing into the pulmonary capillaries dilutes the plasma and an osmotic differential is built up between the plasma and the interior of the red blood cells. Water than passes into the cells which burst, liberating large quantities of intracellular potassium; a state of *hyperkalaemia* results which poisons the heart. Death from drowning in fresh water is, therefore, predominantly cardiac rather than asphyxial in nature and, consequently, is more rapid (of the order of three minutes). It is fair to add that not all authorities are convinced that this sequence, which was elaborated in experimental animals, occurs in the human; none the less, the autopsy appearances in salt- and fresh-water drowning are generally sufficiently distinct to support the hypothesis.

The nasopharynx and larynx are particularly sensitive to unusual stimuli; the sudden impact of cold fresh or salt water on the back of the throat is a classic potential cause of reflex cardiac arrest. Those who have fallen out of boats, slipped into canals and the like may, therefore, show none of the standard signs of drowning and often present a difficult pathological problem. Persons who slip in the bath, particularly children, may die in this way; indeed, a *normal* type of drowning of a child in the bath would, in itself, be a suspicious circumstance and should stimulate a specific search for additional signs, such as finger-tip bruising where the victim has been held.[5]

Death from drowning may, as ever, be accidental, suicidal or homicidal. Accidental drowning is commonly associated with steep-sided water courses, whether natural or unnatural, or containers. Thus, children tend to drown in water tanks and the domestic swimming pool takes a severe toll, particularly in the USA and Australia, in the absence of safety fencing etc; brewery workers may drown in the vats and adults falling into canals are less able to extricate themselves than are those who fall into rivers. Alcohol is a very important factor in the last example—not only as a cause of the fall but because the associated depression of cerebral function predisposes to death from reflex cardiac arrest. Ill health may also contribute to accidental drowning; something of the order of 4% of drownings are epileptic in origin, and epileptics may drown face down in only inches of

5   But this need not always be so. George Smith, who drowned his 'brides in the bath' is, nevertheless, thought to have done so through the medium of reflex cardiac arrest—the method being to immerse the woman's head suddenly by lifting her feet.

water. Unconsciousness from any cause will produce the same effect and a person falling into a dock may sustain concussive head injury in the process; the importance—and difficulty—of distinguishing such an injury from one due to an assault needs no emphasis.

Suicidal drowning is surprisingly common, even in conditions which must give ample scope for reconsideration—thus, every work on forensic medicine will feature an example of suicide by putting one's head in a bucket, and suicidal drowning in the bath, which has a remarkable female distribution, is not uncommon.[6] Walking out to sea provokes the same surprise but certainly occurs. The placing of weights in the pockets or the tying of legs may be indications of suicide but such methods will also be adopted in criminal activity—including an attempt to hide a dead body. The distinction of suicide from either homicide or accident must depend largely on the circumstantial evidence. In this connection, the disposal of belongings or clothing may provide significant distinguishing features.

There are many variations in homicidal drowning. The possibilities of immersion or electrocution in the bath have already been discussed—and it is to be noted that there is a close association of drugs and/or alcohol with drowning in the bath irrespective of its cause. Pushing a non-swimmer into inshore water would scarcely be an elective method of murder due to the likelihood of rescue; such cases are more likely to be in the nature of manslaughter—the drowning resulting from a brawl on land. On the other hand, even the best of swimmers will die if thrown from a boat on the open sea; a conclusive distinction between murder and accident might well be impossible on pathological grounds but a charge of murder may still be brought in the absence of a cadaver.[7] However, the most likely association between criminality and 'drowning' is the disposal in the water of a body already dead; as in incineration, the pathological problem is to distinguish between ante-mortem and post-mortem immersion.

This is often complicated by severe putrefaction following failure to recover bodies from the water for relatively long periods. Not only do the pathological findings change—fluid, for example, passes from the lungs into the pleural spaces—but, during the period of immersion, there is opportunity for destruction of tissue by fish and crustaceans. Additionally, artefacts simulating ante-mortem injury can be produced by contact with rocks, ships' propellers and the like. The rare condition of cadaveric spasm is probably most often found in drowning; almost certainly the casualty was alive on entering the water if weeds or flotsam are discovered firmly clenched in the hands. However, the finding of mud or weeds in the upper air passages has been criticised as providing good evidence of respiratory movements while under water. It has been stated that such foreign bodies can enter a dead body; it is difficult to generalise on this—the interpretation depends on the amount of foreign material and the depth of its penetration. Two further approaches to the diagnosis of inhalation of water are theoretically available. First, there is the biochemical concept that a high concentration of electrolytes entering the lungs from sea water will be reflected in a higher chloride content in the blood of the left side of the heart than in that of the right; the converse should hold if the pulmonary blood is diluted by fresh water. The test is,

6   C Devos, J Timperman and M Piette 'Deaths in the Bath' (1985) 25 Med Sci Law 189.
7   *R v Onufrejczyk* [1955] 1 QB 388; *Blanco v HM Advocate* (1991) Times, 13 December.

however, relatively insensitive—a difference of at least 25 mg chloride/100 ml blood must be demonstrated—and becomes non-specific with the onset of putrefaction. It generally gives a good result when the diagnosis of death from drowning is obvious; it fails in just those instances where help is needed. The demonstration of other mainly sea-water constituents—for example, magnesium—may be of more value, while others have drawn attention to the low specific gravity of the blood in the left side of the heart that is found in deaths from drowning irrespective of the type of water. The second test of inhalation depends on the demonstration of diatoms within the body. These are silica-covered organisms of minute size which are found to a varying extent in both salt and fresh water—the precise type of diatoms discovered in the cadaver has been used as an indication of the exact place of death. Most diatoms will be found in the lungs but post-mortem diffusion cannot be ruled out as the cause. It is, therefore, generally held that organisms must be discovered in the systemic circulation—for example, in the bone marrow—to give proof of inhalation in the presence of a beating heart. The test has also been criticised on the grounds that airborne diatoms are widespread in some districts and that these could be present not only in the lungs but also in the tissues. The problem is essentially one of quantification—the finding of many diatoms is good evidence of drowning, but if only a few are discovered the result must be considered equivocal. The extreme resistance of the organisms to all forms of digestion makes the test especially valuable in the face of severe putrefaction. The technique is not easy and it hardly needs emphasis that a failure to find diatoms does not *exclude* drowning as the cause of death.[8]

Drowning is associated with one specific form of delayed death—post-immersion pneumonitis. This inflammatory condition is the result of the structural damage inflicted on the lungs by inhaled water. It may come on only hours after an apparently successful rescue and has a high mortality.

Death from hypothermia

Hypothermic deaths of medico-legal importance fall into two major groups—first, those associated with fit persons exposed to the cold, as an example of which immersion in water forms a logical link with the preceding section; secondly, there are the cases involving elderly, unfit persons who die in conditions associated with subnutrition.

In contrast to its relatively good defences against a hot environment, the human body adapts very poorly to cold; the protective mechanism of shivering operates only when the body temperature has actually fallen. The warmest clothing compatible with function, and not artificially heated, will fail to protect a man at rest from a fall in body temperature when that of the ambient temperature is -20°C; it will not keep him in comfort at an ambient temperature of 0°C or less. The subject is at grave risk when the body temperature falls to 30°C, evidence of life is difficult to detect at 27°C and recovery from a fall in temperature to 24°C is unlikely. Shivering ceases when the body temperature has fallen to 33°C and,

8   For review, albeit rather dated, see A J Peabody 'Diatoms and Drowning—A Review' (1980) 20 Med Sci Law 254.

after that, the only defence open to the body is one involving shifts of blood from the periphery to the deep core. This causes profound physiological changes to which the body may be unable to adapt—they may, indeed, account for the surprising number of cases on land in which the casualty has removed his clothes. Concurrent alcoholism accelerates death probably by interfering with these protective vascular responses.

The body temperature falls with surprising speed. It is doubtful if many persons could survive for more than 15 minutes in the North Sea in winter. Clothing may postpone the end and fat persons will survive longer than thin. The author has seen one case in which three partially clothed children equipped with life-jackets were precipitated into the Bristol Channel in very cold weather; there was no evidence of drowning and death was estimated to have occurred in about ten minutes. A moribund condition of persons removed from the water may be due either to drowning or to hypothermia but the treatment of the one condition is likely to be dangerous in the other. The diagnostic dilemma confronting the attending physician may be very complex.

As metabolism approaches zero, so do the body's requirements for oxygen; sufficient quantities of the gas may, in fact, be dissolved in the plasma. States of 'suspended animation' can, therefore, occur. The most outstanding example reported is that of a young boy who travelled for nine hours in the unpressurised nosewheel compartment of an aircraft at 8,800m (29,000 ft).[9] Death in these circumstances would be expected either from hypoxia or from hypothermia; occurring together, they resulted in unconsciousness which was rapidly reversed in hospital. Any condition greatly reducing the body's need for oxygen—for example, narcotic poisoning—coupled, perhaps, with a low atmospheric temperature as in extreme poverty, might simulate death so closely as to deceive the examining physician; conditions in the mortuary refrigerator might conceivably perpetuate the simulation and cases have occurred when life has been discovered on the autopsy table. Hypothermic deaths do, therefore, require very careful certification and this applies particularly to the classic case of the elderly person living alone in poor conditions.

The post-mortem diagnosis of death due to hypothermia is largely circumstantial and a matter of exclusion. The circulation of blood is affected and leads to the development of surgical shock characteristically associated with widespread clotting of the blood in the small vessels, the condition of disseminated intravascular coagulation. There is a strong tendency for discoloration of a violet hue to affect the skin around the joints or other bony prominences; swelling of the hands and feet is often seen. Ulceration and punctate haemorrhage into the mucosa of the stomach is common and acute inflammation without bacterial invasion of the pancreas is found in a proportion of cases, the underlying mechanism being the generalised microthrombosis. The most characteristic lesions are said to be microscopic areas of degeneration and reaction in the heart muscle.[10] Very likely, however, nothing specific will be found. The most typical deaths of this type in

9 J Pejares and F Merayo 'Unique Clinical Case, Both of Hypoxia and Hypothermia Studied in a 18-year-old Aerial Stowaway' (1970) 41 Aerospace Med 1416. A rather similar set of circumstances resulted in the survival of a child submerged in icy water for over an hour: R S Bolte, P S Black, P S Bowers et al 'The Use of Extracorporeal Rewarming in a Child Submerged for 66 Minutes' (1988) 260 J Amer Med Ass 377.

10 For a very good description, see J Hirvonen 'Necropsy Findings in Fatal Hypothermia Cases' (1976) 8 Forensic Sci 155.

the United Kingdom are likely to be confined to hill climbers and fell walkers. Otherwise, cases will be associated with serious sociological deprivation and, here, the autopsy findings will be confused by those of neglect and of disease.

Death due to neglect

Neglect is, in practice, divisible into two categories—self-neglect and neglect by those with a legal or moral duty of care; the latter will, in general, concern the care of old people and of children. While skin ulcers, parasitic infestation and the like are an integral part of neglect, it is the accompanying starvation that is the most important factor contributing to death. 'Starvation' consists of subnutrition—which is the intake of an insufficient quantity of food—and malnutrition—which is feeding of inadequate quality. Malnutrition can and does occur as a separate entity; subnutrition must always include some degree of malnutrition. Total starvation is fatal in some two weeks, but life may be prolonged for up to ten weeks so long as fluid is available. In the typical case of fatal neglect, starvation is an unlikely cause of death per se; but the accompanying malnutrition will reduce the body's defences so as to make the neglected person particularly vulnerable to intercurrent infection.

The usual case of neglect, therefore, presents as an emaciated body that shows multiple trophic ulcers, is verminous and shows evidence of severe vitamin deficiency. The inevitable weakening of the body may open the way to wide dissemination of natural disease but disease may, of course, be the primary cause of the marasmic state; this distinction between cause and effect is of great importance in the event of criminal charges being pressed.

Self-neglect commonly represents a failure of society itself, often abetted by the individual's ignorance or fault—alcoholism being a frequent precipitating factor. Other cases of self-neglect have a psychiatric background; certainly not all elderly persons suffering from malnutrition are impoverished, although the fear of impending poverty may motivate the condition. Statutory powers are available to remove aged people from their homes who are, inter alia, living in insanitary conditions and who cannot give themselves proper care and attention.[11] These powers are rarely used, although they can be invoked not only in the individual's interests but also to prevent injury or serious nuisance to others. Thus, death from self-neglect is commonly a matter of ignorance on the part of others—the conditions under which the old person was living are simply unknown until she is discovered dead from infection or, equally possibly, from hypothermia. All cases of apparent self-neglect deserve intensive forensic study because this is an area of community preventive medicine in which the medical and social services can be properly and usefully integrated.

The hunger strike by a detainee is one unusual aspect of self-neglect—virtually suicidal in nature—that may return to public interest through its use by asylum seekers. The situation raises fascinating problems in criminological and medical ethics; the point at which a doctor should actively engage in saving life against

11 National Assistance Act 1948, s 47 as amended. The Act confers powers on the medical officer of health who is now designated for this purpose as the 'proper officer' (Local Government Act 1972, Sch 29). The comparable person in Scotland is known as the 'designated medical officer' (National Health Service (Scotland) Act 1972, Sch 6, para 83(a)).

the wishes of the subject, thereby committing an assault and often apparently associating himself with a political bias, is one that needs careful assessment. Current policy is that the doctor's role is to advise the prisoner of the dangers of starvation, to have treatment and hospital space available but, otherwise, to refrain from interference.[12] While this policy accords with the Declaration of Tokyo,[13] the physician must at times be concerned as to whether the prisoner can, in truth, form an 'unimpaired and rational judgment'.[14] Voluntary starvation leads to severe metabolic dysfunction and, from the aspect of potential litigation, it should be noted that, once the watershed of some 21 days is passed, refeeding carries a serious risk of cardiac failure.[15]

Greater general forensic concern relates to the neglected old person who is, nominally, being cared for—the possibility of criminal charges will then arise in the event of death. For this to happen there has to be more than simple neglect—there must be evidence of deliberate intent to cause harm or of a reckless indifference to the well-being of a person in the charge of the accused. Moreover, it may be difficult to establish a legal duty of care. For these reasons, charges of manslaughter by neglect are very rare.[16] The forensic evidence may well be of added importance in that active neglect in the form of physical abuse will, of course, alter the complexion of the case—there may be great difficulty in assessing the cause of bruising and the like in emaciated bodies.

Child neglect is, perhaps, the more important aspect of the subject—although there is little doubt that the extent of neglect and other abuse of the elderly is greatly underestimated. Undoubtedly, some parents are so ignorant as to be incapable of adequately caring for their children but, in many cases, child neglect must have criminal undertones. In the event of death, charges of manslaughter could be brought, and succeed,[17] though this would depend upon a 'wilful' element to the neglect.[18] Aside, however, from any common law principles, a statutory obligation is placed upon a parent, or other person legally liable to maintain a child, to provide adequate food and clothing, to obtain medical care and to provide housing—or, in the event of these being impossible, to take steps to procure such advantages—throughout the United Kingdom[19] and charges can be brought under that heading in the event of the child's death.

---

12 *Secretary of State for the Home Department v Robb* [1995] Fam 127.

13 *Guidelines Concerning Torture and Other Cruel, Inhuman or Degrading Treatment or Punishment in Relation to Detention and Imprisonment* (1975). The complete text is reproduced in J K Mason and R A McCall Smith *Law and Medical Ethics* (5th edn, 1999) Appendix D.

14 The courts seem happy to shelter under the umbrella of the Mental Health Acts and to regard forced feeding as treatment for the underlying mental disorder; the case of the notorious murderer Ian Brady is apposite but does not seem to have been reported: see C Dyer 'Force Feeding of Ian Brady Declared Lawful' (2000) 320 BMJ 731. They will also do so outwith the criminal justice system: *B v Croydon Health Authority* [1995] Fam 133.

15 M Peel 'Hunger Strikes' (1997) 315 BMJ 829.

16 The classic case is *R v Stone, R v Dobinson* [1977] QB 354, in which two elderly and inadequate carers were convicted of manslaughter; it is a very unsatisfactory precedent from many aspects.

17 *R v Senior* [1899] 1 QB 283; *HM Advocate v Clarks* 1968 JC 53.

18 A charge of murder could succeed if the wilfulness were of sufficient severity: *R v Gibbins and Proctor* (1918) 13 Cr App Rep 134.

19 Children and Young Persons Act 1933, s 1(2); Children and Young Persons (Scotland) Act 1937, s 12(2). But the offence does not attract strict liability: *R v Sheppard* [1980] 3 All ER 899, HL.

The pathologist has often a difficult task in the interpretation of a death due apparently to child neglect. The mere discovery of subnutrition or malnutrition is not evidence of criminal neglect, while, as in the case of the adult, the role of intercurrent disease may be very difficult to assess; much will depend upon the ancillary evidence—often this will be in the form of unusually severe skin disease. Infant death due to neglect must, of its nature, raise questions of culpability, as efficient social services are widely available to arrange for adequate care and protection while recovery is still possible. The subject of child maltreatment is discussed further in Chapter 19.

Child neglect includes abandonment or exposure which, in the event of death, could amount to infanticide (or child murder), manslaughter (or culpable homicide) or even murder. The pathological contribution will be likely, in these cases, to be equivocal as the findings will not be those of neglect but rather those of simple hypothermia. Infants are more susceptible to the cold than are adults, but the post-mortem diagnosis can seldom be made other than on the basis of exclusion.

In a very different context, the concept of what might be termed *iatrogenic neglect* must be considered. In certain circumstances, doctors may, as a clinical decision, withhold treatment from neonates and infants whose quality of life will be abysmal in the event of it being maintained. The question is, perhaps, one of medical ethics rather than of forensic medicine and cannot be considered in detail here. It should, however, be noted that there is abundant evidence that the law accepts the principle of selective non-treatment of severely physically defective infants.[20] The same is not true of neonates that are mentally handicapped and who may, for that reason, be rejected by their parents. Dr Arthur was, certainly, acquitted of attempted murder when he authorised 'nursing care only' for an apparently physically normal baby suffering from Down's syndrome[1] but that was a jury decision and the law undoubtedly lies in *Re B*.[2] In that case it was held that a Down's syndrome infant was to be treated as any other infant and 'be given a chance to live'. The autopsy difficulties and the trial of Dr Arthur should, even at a distance of 20 years, serve as a potent reminder of the pathologist's important role in this area of medical practice. The subject is considered further on page 469.

20 *Re C (a minor) (wardship: medical treatment)* [1990] Fam 26, CA; *Re J (a minor) (wardship: medical treatment)* [1990] 3 All ER 930, CA.
 1 *R v Arthur* (1981) 12 BMLR 1.
 2 *Re B (a minor) (wardship: medical treatment)* [1981] 1 WLR 1421, CA.

15

Industrial injury and disease

Definitions and administration

It is axiomatic in a developed society that persons should be compensated for disability attributable to their working conditions. Ideally, such compensation should be payable irrespective of contributory fault and, while not excluding the possibility, should be free from the uncertainties of litigation on the bases of negligence or of contributory negligence. Such a system has been in operation in the United Kingdom since 1948, when the original National Insurance (Industrial Injuries) Act became operative. The relevant legislation for Great Britain is now consolidated in the Social Security Contributions and Benefits Act 1992 (hereafter the 1992 Act).[1]

All persons employed in an insurable occupation are automatically insured—through contributions from employees and employers—against disablement, incapacity or death resulting from an injury by accident arising out of and in the course of employment.[2] The definition of injury is wide, including any physiological injury or change for the worse, and that of accident is equally embracing, being 'an unlooked-for-mishap or an untoward event which is not expected or designed'.[3] The course of work need not be the proper course—for example, failure to take such safety measures as have been ordered has no effect on the payment of benefits (s 98). Accidents due to misconduct by another also attract benefit (s 101).

There are, however, limits to which an insurance fund can stretch and disputes as to definition[4] are bound to occur and may be decided with apparent inconsistency; nor is industrial disease an entirely straightforward subject.

1 Northern Ireland has its own Act (Social Security Contributions and Benefits (Northern Ireland) Act 1992).
2 A two-stage test is explained in *Chief Adjudication Officer v Rhodes* [1999] ICR 178, CA—what are the employee's work duties and was the employee discharging a duty at the time of the accident?
3 *Fenton v J Thorley & Co* [1903] AC 443 at 448, per Lord Macnaghten. Inevitably, this formula is open to interpretation and has been criticised and extended in practice—CI/15589/1996 (starred decision 5/98); cf *Chief Adjudication Officer v Faulds* [2000] 2 All ER 961, HL for its application.
4 Examples being the definition of 'place of work' in relation to transport and physical boundaries. A person is generally held to be at his place of work if he is in transport provided by his employers (positively enacted, s 99) but not when in his own or public transport; an accident occurring in the grounds of a factory would also probably qualify for compensation, provided the area was one from which the ordinary public was excluded.

Injuries that are self-evident—that is, those that involve external mutilation—will not be discussed here; not only are these beyond dispute but they are so various that a detailed description would be impossible. But the term 'accident' also includes injuries sustained in circumstances that are accidental merely by virtue of being unexpected. These circumstances need not be exceptional; an unexpected event may be brought about by the routine engagement in work and it is immaterial that the work did no more than exacerbate known pre-existing disease.[5] A person more prone to accident than normal is still covered by the Act.[6]

Disease contracted at work is dealt with in two main categories. There is, first, a disease that results from a single occurrence at work—and this is clearly an accident. The precise moment of injury need not be defined in all circumstances; a nurse contracting tuberculosis was clearly infected at a certain time although the precise exposure that was responsible for infection cannot be ascertained—given that the condition was the result of a series of events, the earliest probable time of being injured will be accepted as 'the accident'.[7] In certain circumstances, however, there is continuing exposure to a work hazard and a disease contracted as a result is a matter of process rather than of accident.[8] To qualify for insurance benefits, the second category of disease must be prescribed by regulations (s 108). These diseases are loosely defined as those that can be attributed with reasonable certainty to the occupation and that do not constitute a risk to the whole population;[9] sufferers from such diseases are treated for insurance purposes as if they had sustained an accidental injury. A list of prescribed diseases is given in Appendix L.[10]

Industrial injuries benefits are payable when an employed earner suffers personal injury by an accident arising out of and in the course of his employment. How these benefits are paid is of little concern in the present context. Suffice it to say that they have now been consolidated and, effectively, they are available by way of disability benefit or disability pension so long as the disablement loss amounts to not less than 14%.[11] They can be supplemented by an allowance for constant attendance and for exceptionally severe disablement.

Problems as to whether an injury is to be regarded as industrial[12] are decided by the Secretary of State[13] who can revise or supersede his earlier decisions (1998

---

5 *Clover, Clayton & Co Ltd v Hughes* [1910] AC 242; *Oates v Earl Fitzwilliam's Collieries Co* [1939] 2 All ER 498.
6 R(I) 6/91. But the employer's liability is not open-ended: see *Whitfield v H & R Johnson (Tiles) Ltd* [1990] 3 All ER 426.
7 *Chief Adjudication Officer v Faulds* [2000] 2 All ER 961, HL. A distinction is to be drawn between the interpretation of the old legislation and of the Social Security Contributions and Benefits Act 1992, s 94(1).
8 For the concept of progression, see *Roberts v Dorothea Slate Quarries* [1948] 2 All ER 201.
9 1992 Act, s 108(2).
10 Social Security (Industrial Injuries) (Prescribed Diseases) Regulations 1985, SI 1985/967, Sch 1, Pt 1, as amended by Social Security (Industrial Injuries and Diseases) (Miscellaneous Amendments) Regulations 1996, SI 1996/425 and Social Security (Industrial Injuries) (Miscellaneous Amendments) Regulations 1997, SI 1997/810.
11 1992 Act, Sch 6, para 6(3). But this is reduced to 1% in the case of pneumoconiosis (s 110(3)). Death benefit was removed as being superfluous after April 1988 in the 1992 Act, s 94(2) and Sch 7.
12 It is the Secretary of State who is charged with the duty of deciding whether the *occupation* was insurable under the 1992 Act (s 95); Social Security (Employed Earners' Employments for Industrial Injuries Purposes) Regulations 1975, SI 1975/467, as amended.
13 Social Security Act 1998 (hereafter the 1998 Act), s 29.

Act, ss 9 and 10). An appeal is available to an Appeal Tribunal which may consist of 1–3 persons of which one must be legally qualified (ss 12 and 13). There is a further right of appeal to a Commissioner which is limited to questions of law (s 14). The Commissioner's decision is binding, subject to appeal direct to the Court of Appeal or Court of Session or to the Secretary of State (s 15). The degree of disablement is, however, decided by an adjudicating medical authority, who is normally a medical practitioner appointed by the Secretary of State;[14] a medical board consisting of either two or three members may be set up to consider mobility allowance claims. Appeals from their decisions are made to the Appeal Tribunal (ss 5–7). Both the adjudicating medical authority and the Appeal Tribunal may reverse their assessments if there are reasonable grounds for so doing; they cannot, however, reverse the Secretary of State's decision that a condition did result from industrial injury.

Specific regulations are made as to prescribed diseases. Questions are referred to and determined by a specially qualified adjudicating medical practitioner or to a medical board if the Secretary of State so requires.[15] Provisions are made in regard to the pneumoconioses that cover initial and periodic medical examinations and also allow for suspension or non-employment of persons found to be suffering from pneumoconiosis. Attendance at, and provision of facilities for, such examinations are compulsory. A list of occupations for which pneumoconiosis is prescribed is given in Appendix M.[16]

Decisions, unless setting a precedent, will largely depend upon previous rulings which can be studied under the heading of 'Commissioners' Decisions'. The list of conditions that have been held to be industrial accidents is steadily lengthening—some of the more extreme examples including a nervous shock resulting from watching a fatal accident that involved a workmate; a 'drop foot' sustained as a result of continual kneeling (this being something of an extension of accident as opposed to process) and coronary thrombosis arising during the act of tightening a nut.

However, nothing in the social security regulations prevents a worker who sustains loss, personal injury or damage suing his employer in tort or delict; both the solicitor and the advocate may, therefore, be further involved in civil litigation. Here, the normal requirements as to the duty of care, causation and actual loss will apply and, in a proportion of cases, any damages awarded may fall to be reduced on account of the contributory negligence of the injured party himself.[17] Thus, the issues will be keenly fought and expert medical evidence will be required by both parties. While there have been a significant number of successful actions for negligence against employers by workers who have been injured or who have contracted prescribed diseases, there is no certainty that this will always be so.[18] Thus, although industrial benefit—and civil damages—have been awarded for, say, nervous shock, others may fail on

---

14 Social Security (Adjudications) Regulations 1995, SI 1995/1801, as amended by Social Security (Industrial Injuries) (Miscellaneous Amendments) Regulations 1997, SI 1997/810.
15 Social Security (Adjudications) Regulations 1995, SI 1995/1801, reg 36.
16 See fn 10 above.
17 Law Reform (Contributory Negligence) Act 1945, s 1.
18 Most successful cases appear to be settled out of court and are therefore unreported, but damages of £7,500 (at the values prevailing in 1970) have been awarded to a man with coal miners' pneumoconiosis: *The Sunday Times,* 1 February 1970.

grounds of causation or even of policy.[19] Decisions may be contradictory as has been evidenced over claims for repetitive strain injury. Here substantial damages were awarded against British Telecom in 1991,[20] and the Inland Revenue made a large out-of-court settlement in 1994,[1] in the meantime, a High Court judge said: '[I agree that] repetitive strain injury is in reality meaningless in that it has no pathology . . . [and] no place in the medical textbooks . . . Its use by doctors can only serve to confuse.'[2] Such disputes are likely to multiply in the future.

In the event of death believed to be due to industrial accident or disease, the cause must be founded on sound medical evidence. Ideally, all deaths occurring at the place of work should be reported to the coroner and, although the registrar is obliged to notify the coroner only in the event that death 'appeared to be due to industrial disease or industrial poisoning',[3] coroners will, in practice, require doctors to notify them if the death could be in any way related to the deceased's employment (Appendix C); moreover, the English certificate of death requires an opinion on the point from the certifying doctor.[4] Any death of a person while at work in Scotland must be reported to the procurator fiscal and will be the subject of a Fatal Accident Inquiry.

The medical nature of conventional 'accidents' at work is generally readily understandable and the logical sequence implied in disease contracted as a result of an accident is also normally clear. The nature—and rationale—of the prescribed diseases may not, however, be common knowledge in legal circles and a brief description is apposite.

The pneumoconioses

Pneumoconiosis is defined as fibrosis of the lung due to silica dust, asbestos dust or other dust and includes the condition of the lungs known as 'dust-reticulation'.

Fibrogenic dust may be mineral or vegetable in nature. The former is by far the more important and, while all occupations associated with mineral dust carry some risk, three conditions are outstanding—coal miners' pneumoconiosis because of its incidence in the United Kingdom,[5] silicosis because it is, perhaps, the underlying basis for the clinical manifestations of the majority of mineral dust diseases, and asbestosis because of its severe effects and because it is a particularly good example of how workers other than miners—even the general population— may be affected by dust.

---

19 *Robertson v Forth Bridge Joint Board* 1995 SCLR 466—the fact that a man was an employee does not affect his position as a mere bystander. Cf *Wigg v British Railways Board* [1986] NLJ Rep 446n, where the action of a train driver who cared for a passenger killed by the guard's negligence succeeded—he was clearly involved in the affair.
20 In an apparently unreported case: D Brahams 'Keyboard Operators' Repetitive Strain Injury' (1992) 339 Lancet 237.
1 'Revenue to Pay £79,000 to RSI Victim' *The Scotsman*, 19 January 1994, p 5.
2 *Mughal v Reuters Ltd* (1993) 16 BMLR 127 at 140, per Prosser J. This view was generally supported in the House of Lords: *Pickford v Imperial Chemical Industries plc* [1998] 3 All ER 462.
3 Registration of Births and Deaths Regulations 1987, SI 1987/2088, reg 41.
4 Resulting from the Industrial Diseases (Notification) Act 1981.
5 Though the interest is now mainly historic due to the closure of the majority of the coal-mining industry. Even so, new cases continue to be reported.

Coal miners' pneumoconiosis

Although coal workers' pneumoconiosis was at one time very common in the United Kingdom—and constituted over 85% of all cases of pneumoconiosis—it was decreasing among young miners even before the run-down of the coal mining industry. Historically, it represents a condition full of paradoxes and one which was always difficult to understand fully.[6] The problems posed are still worth recapitulation.

The pulmonary changes in the condition are often originally symptomless and are gauged radiologically. The disease is divided into simple and complicated forms and, in view of the difficulties of clinical assessment, the former is empirically quantified on the radiological appearances. The lesions seen in the X-ray are known as nodules and these are classified according to size (Group p nodules are up to 1.5 mm in diameter, Group m from 1.5 to 3.0 mm and Group n between 3.0 and 10.0 mm). The severity of the disease is further classified by its distribution, Category 1 diseases being limited to defined portions of the lungs while Category 3 denotes affection of the whole or both lungs; Category 2 is intermediate.

Complicated pneumoconiosis is alternatively known as progressive massive fibrosis (PMF). Nodules larger than 10 mm in diameter appear and coalesce to produce extensive destruction of the lung with severe symptoms of respiratory distress. The incidence of PMF rises with the extent of the simple disease but, while the two must be in some way connected, the relationship is by no means a simple one. The effects of any coincident tuberculosis are treated as though they were the effects of pneumoconiosis;[7] emphysema and bronchitis are treated similarly but only if the resultant disability would be assessed as not less than 50%.[8]

Simple pneumoconiosis is not itself a cause of disability and does not reduce the expectation of life; the interrelationship of pneumoconiosis and other respiratory disease is, however, complex and, sometimes, contradictory. Because of the clinical difficulties involved, compensation is largely based on 'rule of thumb' observations. The suspected case is examined by two members of the special medical panel and the subject is certified as suffering from pneumoconiosis if they agree that Category 2 disease is present—Category 1 disease is sometimes accepted if the subject is young. Any degree of disability is assessed on the basis of the vital capacity of the lungs—which is a measure of the amount of oxygen the lungs can make available to the body—and on the forced expiratory volume of the breath—which is a measure of the effectiveness or impairment of the elasticity and, hence, efficient function of the lungs. No appeal is normally available against the decision of the special medical panel but rejection of a claim does not prohibit repeated applications.

This valiant attempt to ensure a uniform procedure, the rationale of which is readily demonstrable, causes some problems which are particularly related to the difficulties of correlating clinical symptoms—which may have several different origins—with the radiological appearances, which are related to a single causative factor. It is often difficult for a legal adviser to understand how one man with

---

6 Other lung diseases, such as bronchitis and emphysema, are also attributable to coal dust and can be the subject of a claim in negligence: C Dyer 'Miners Win Historic Battle for Compensation' (1998) 316 BMJ 331. The author is currently unable to trace the apparently seminal case referred to in the article.

7 1992 Act, s 110(1).

8 1992 Act, s 110(2).

apparently appreciable respiratory distress can be denied benefit while a much fitter colleague is a certified pneumoconiotic; yet it can and does occur.

Further causes of confusion may attend the result of post-mortem dissection. The Registrar of Deaths is obliged to report to the procurator fiscal or to the coroner any deaths due to or arising from industrial disease or poisoning (see Chapter 2). The coroner must also notify the pneumoconiosis panel (or special medical board) of the date and place of the post-mortem examination and the board may be represented there; no such obligation rests on either the procurator fiscal or the registrar in Scotland. The rules prevent a coroner asking a member of the special medical board to carry out the dissection;[9] it also seems that the throracic organs will not be available to the board unless the coroner requires clarification of the diagnosis. Thus the coroner's certificate of death—whether it be by virtue of his own Form B or of a Certificate after Inquest—may conflict with the previous opinion of the special medical board. These considerations have lost much of their urgency since the abolition of the industrial death benefit but they may still introduce an element of confusion in the event of civil actions being brought against the employers. The importance of post-mortem dissection and of the availability of the evidence to the equitable settling of cases is obvious.

Silicosis

Silica in its large particulate form causes no more than a harmless reaction to a foreign body. But when the size of particles is small, the cellular defences of the lungs are poisoned and a fibrotic reaction is set up which has profound pulmonary effects. Silica is, in essence, the primary source of the pneumoconioses, and is likely to be dispersed whenever rock is drilled or sand is particalised as in the cleaning of blast furnaces, building in sandstone, grinding and the like. Coal dust as such is relatively innocuous in the absence of silica; true silicosis in coal miners generally occurs only in those confronted with the harder seams—that is, in anthracite miners and in the 'hard headers' who drive the tunnels to reach the face. Gold mining is particularly dangerous as a source of the disease.

The lesion in silicosis is that of formation of fibrotic nodules due to the locally poisonous properties of silica when dissolved—possibly in the form of silicic acid. The process is self-perpetuating, the amount of fibrosis is disproportionate to the quantity of dust and the end result is massive destruction of lung tissue with death from a combination of cardiac and respiratory failure. In the process, the originally isolated nodules coalesce to form what is known as massive conglomerate nodular silicosis; alternatively, a form of progressive massive fibrosis, not unlike that seen in coal miners' pneumoconiosis, may arise.

Silicosis is clearly associated with tuberculosis and potentiates the virulence of the organism causing the latter disease. There is, however, no fully acceptable evidence that silica stimulates the formation of cancer.[10] Thus, silicosis differs markedly from the third of the most important dust diseases—asbestosis.

---

9 Coroners' Rules 1984, SI 1984/552, r 6(1)(d).
10 Two haematite mines in Cumbria, separated by only 48 km (30 miles), showed a marked difference in the incidence of lung cancer. In the mine associated with soft clay substrate, cancer was not an occupational hazard; the incidence of cancer among workers in the hard-rock mines was some 70% above the general level. The difference, however, might well have been due to radioactivity—cf the iron-ore miners in Czechoslovakia.

Asbestosis

Asbestos occurs in two main types—chrysotile and amphiboles. There are three varieties of amphiboles: crocidolite, amosite and anthophyllite. The fibres of chrysotile are long and are used mainly for the preparation of asbestos clothing; those of amphiboles are shaped like needles and are used to make roofing, tiles and insulating material.

As with all dust disease, asbestosis consists of fibrosis of the lung tissue which can be finely nodular or dense and massive. Since asbestos is virtually indestructible, its effects on the lung are progressive even after the removal from the dusty environment. Fibrosis of the lung does occur in asbestos miners but, because the main offending condition is the 'asbestos cloud', those who are exposed to asbestos in its purified—or purifying—form are at greatest risk. Asbestos is used in very many industrial processes but maximum exposure outside the factories concerned with preparation occurs in the building trade; in shipbuilding, where it is used mainly as a thermal insulator; and in the manufacture of brakes, clutches and the like. The danger is particularly great during the destruction of asbestos products when masses of very dry dust are dispersed in relatively uncontrolled conditions.[11] There is, therefore, a potential hazard to the public in the vicinity of large reconstruction projects, which is now limited by very strict controls.[12]

Although simple asbestosis may cause lethal dysfunction of the lungs, it is distinguished from almost all other forms of pneumoconiosis by its incontrovertible association with malignant tumours of the lungs—at least 60% of workers who are accepted as disabled by pneumoconiosis due to asbestos subsequently develop lung cancer; the death rate in asbestos workers from the common form of lung cancer, bronchogenic carcinoma, is some ten times that of the general population. The increase is largely taken up with an association with smoking although the risks are also substantial for a heavily exposed non-smoker. Bronchogenic carcinoma is probably associated with all types of asbestos and with a relatively long exposure, but one particular form of cancer—mesothelioma—is particularly associated with exposure to crocidolite or 'blue asbestos'.[13] It is very rarely associated with chrysotile and never with anthophyllite. There is some evidence that mesothelioma occurring in miners results from exposure to an asbestos/manganese complex, but it is workers in an atmosphere laden with the dust from prepared asbestos products who are at greatest risk;[14] the exposure to blue asbestos need only be short and, of major medico-legal significance, there is always a long incubation period—the condition may not

---

11 Although the courts are prepared to accept that injury can result from mere exposure to damaged lagging to the extent of £1.15m in damages: C Dyer 'Surgeon Dies from Hospital Exposure to Asbestos' (2000) 320 BMJ 1358.
12 Control of Asbestos in the Air Regulations 1990, SI 1990/556. The Commission of the European Communities (*Public Health Risks of Exposure to Asbestos* (1977)) argued that simple ambient exposure to asbestos carries no definite risk but that too many uncertainties exist to deny such a risk. Liability for injury to other workers in the vicinity of asbestos processing has been accepted: *Bryce v Swan Hunter Group plc* [1988] 1 All ER 659.
13 Under the Asbestos (Prohibition) Regulations 1992, SI 1992/3067, as amended by the Asbestos (Prohibition) (Amendment) Regulations 1999, SI 1999/2373, the importation of crude amphiboles is prohibited under reg 3 and the use of chrysotile under reg 7.
14 For control, see Control of Asbestos at Work Regulations 1987, SI 1987/2115, as amended by Control of Asbestos at Work (Amendment) Regulations 1998, SI 1998/3235.

manifest itself for some 20–40 years after exposure. A cause-and-effect association may be difficult to prove—or defend—at such a distance in time, particularly as mesothelioma may occur without any other features of asbestosis; the provisions of the Limitation Act 1980, which extend the period in which an action for personal damages can be brought in the event of there being no symptoms for some time after an untoward event, must be invoked in any suit for negligence.

Other prescribed diseases

The pneumoconioses are so distinct and so important that they have been given particular prominence. Other prescribed diseases are of such diversity as to preclude a full description outside a work confined to industrial medicine.[15] The reader will be able to understand the great majority from a view of Appendix L; some specific aspects of poisoning are, however, considered in Chapter 21.

Safety at work

The subject of safety at work is dominated by the Health and Safety at Work, etc Act 1974, which attempts to provide a comprehensive system of law designed to integrate the safety and health of work people and of the public. In the words of s 1(2):

> 'the making of health and safety regulations and the preparation and approval of codes of practice shall in particular have effect with a view to enabling specified enactments and the regulations . . . in force under those enactments to be progressively replaced by a system [operating under this Act] and designed to improve the standards . . . established under those enactments.'

Thus, the 1974 Act does not repeal but rather integrates all previous legislation devoted to specific industries or aspects of working conditions.[16]

Part 1 of the Act imposes strict obligations on employers—in particular, the duty to establish 'safety committees'[17]—and sets up a Health and Safety Commission and Health and Safety Executive. The commission, consisting of representatives of employers, employees and local authorities, is charged with effecting the purposes of the Act and with arranging research, training and provision of information relevant to safety at work. The executive, a triumvirate, gives effect to the decisions of the commission, enforcing these through appointed inspectors who are given wide powers of entry, investigation, interrogation and discovery, although answers given to the inspector carrying out his duties cannot be used in evidence in any proceedings taken against the person answering.

---

15 The importance of—and the description of the qualifying occupations for—occupational asthma is certainly increasing.

16 Schedule 1 specifies 31 statutes, of which the following are representative and especially important: The Alkali, &c. Works Regulation Act 1906; Employment of Women, Young Persons and Children Act 1920; Petroleum (Consolidation) Act 1928; Mines and Quarries Act 1954; Agriculture (Safety, Health and Welfare Provisions) Act 1956; Factories Act 1961; Offices, Shops and Railway Premises Act 1963; Nuclear Installations Act 1965; Employment Medical Advisory Service Act 1972.

17 Safety Representatives and Safety Committees Regulations 1977, SI 1977/500.

Inspectors may serve 'improvement' or 'prohibition' notices on persons in control of activities who then have the right of appeal to an industrial tribunal at which they may be represented by legal advisers. A number of offences concerned with obstructing or disobeying the executive are specified, and proceedings may be taken against the person as a result of a coroner's inquest or a public inquiry under the Fatal Accidents and Sudden Deaths Inquiry (Scotland) Act 1976. No public inquiry under this Act is held if an investigation is already being undertaken by the Health and Safety Executive.

A very large number of consequential regulations have been issued under the Act which have had a profound effect on those areas of employment not covered by the previous essentially 'industrial' legislation, including hospitals, laboratories and the police force.[18] Many of the regulations are of a consolidating type, an important example being the Reporting of Injuries, Diseases and Dangerous Occurrences Regulations 1995.[19] An accident is notifiable to the enforcing authority—that is, the executive or, by agreement, the local authority— if it involves the death of any person or injury to an employee resulting in more than three days' absence from work; in the latter case, a consequent death occurring within one year must also be notified. Seventeen examples of dangerous occurrences that are notifiable wherever they occur are specified, and there are additional notifications in the cases of mines, quarries, railways and off-shore workplaces.[20]

Certain industrial poisonings must also be notified by a doctor to the executive; these are listed in Appendix N. A number of other diseases, which also correspond closely to the more important conditions prescribed as industrial diseases (Appendix L), must also be notified under this head.[1]

The Employment Medical Advisory Service was established by the Secretary of State under the Employment Medical Advisory Service Act 1972 and must now be maintained under the Health and Safety at Work, etc Act 1974.[2] This replaced appointed factory doctors by employment medical advisers, who now form the medical wing of the Health and Safety Executive; the medical advisers are granted the full powers of an inspector and they may investigate the cause of death, injury, disease or poisoning resulting from employment.

In England and Wales and in Scotland, the minister may direct that a full investigation be held into the causes and circumstances of any accident occurring or of any disease acquired in a factory—it is not uncommon for a legal man to be appointed as the assessor and lawyers will be involved on behalf of the parties concerned.

Deaths resulting from a notifiable disease or accident must be reported to the coroner or to the procurator fiscal. The former is obliged to hold an inquest with a jury at which any interested party may be legally represented. In Scotland, the same situation is covered by the inquiry that must be held under the Fatal Accidents

---

18 For example, the Control of Substances Hazardous to Health Regulations 1999, SI 1999/437 and the Genetic Manipulation Regulations 1989, SI 1989/1810. For the police, see Police (Health and Safety) Act 1997.
19 SI 1995/3163.
20 The list is not exhaustive as other accidents or occurrences must be notified under other regulations—eg the Civil Aviation (Investigation of Air Accidents and Incidents) Regulations 1996, SI 1996/2798.
1 SI 1995/3163.
2 Of which, ss 55 and 60 specify the functions and responsibilities of the service.

and Sudden Deaths Inquiry (Scotland) Act 1976, s 1(1)(a)(i) if it appears that death was due to an accident at work; but, as already noted, such an inquiry will not normally be held if an inquiry is being undertaken by the Health and Safety Executive—nor will it be held if a Ministerial Public Inquiry has been ordered.

16

Medico-legal aspects of sport

Generally speaking, medico-legal aspects of sport are governed by the doctrine of *volenti non fit injuria*. However, this cannot always hold. There are several interests involved in organised sport—including those of the participants, the promoters and the public. So much is now materially at stake in what once were games that the law must become involved; injury and death at sport are now integral parts of forensic medicine.

Comparing the dangers of particular sports is a difficult exercise. Mere statistics can be very misleading in that they fail, very often, to distinguish between deaths or injuries that were *due* to the sport from those which occurred *during* sporting activity. By the same token, the age of the persons involved must be taken into consideration. Thus, the mortality of golf is very high—but this only reflects the number of elderly men involved in an exercise loaded with high emotions. Similarly, more severe head injuries derive from golf than from other sports.

There is no intention here to consider all potential injuries that can arise in risk sports; most are relatively obvious, and few—other than accidental gunshot wounds which are discussed in Chapter 9—have particular medico-legal significance other than in respect of standards of professional medical care; negligent treatment of a knee injury occurring in a man who made his living from football would be likely to attract greater damages than would be the case in similar circumstances involving an elderly bank clerk.[1] But those sports that are, in effect, legalised assaults require separate consideration and there are other, more general, aspects of forensic medicine that can conveniently be discussed under this chapter heading.

Boxing and wrestling

Springing from its roots in illegal prize-fighting and being most obviously associated with 'intent to inflict bodily injury', boxing has inevitably attracted the greatest forensic attention among sports.[2]

---

1   *Girvan v Inverness Farmers Dairy (No 2)* 1998 SC (HL) 1.
2   For the legality of boxing, see *A-G's Reference (No 6 of 1980)* [1981] QB 715.

Attitudes to boxing have altered dramatically in a lifetime. In the amateur sphere, the annual school boxing tournament has fallen so far from its position as the event of the year that the Royal College of Physicians has concluded 'it must be generally questioned whether there is any justification for including boxing as a school sport'.[3] It is fair to point out that, against this view, there are many who regard organised boxing as a controlled method of unleashing a normal predisposition to violence and, consequently, as a positive contribution to the reduction of violent crime. On the professional side, there is no doubt that stricter controls introduced since the Second World War have transformed the image of boxing. Perhaps the administrative changes have been accelerated by the campaign against the sport which has been based to a small extent on its mortality but, more importantly, on the associated long-term morbidity.

There are, in fact, surprisingly few acute fatalities in boxing. It is claimed that there have been fewer than 25 deaths from boxing since 1945—and none in amateur boxing since records were kept. When it occurs, death is most commonly due to intracranial haemorrhage. Intracerebral bleeding into the midbrain is the injury said to be the most specific to boxing, but subdural bleeding with its attendant latent period, is, in practice, less uncommon and may be cumulative as a result of repeated sheering forces being applied to the brain (see Chapter 11); the importance of limiting the length of the bout is, thereby, emphasised. Subdural haemorrhage may be followed by progressive cerebral oedema and the mortality is said to exceed 45% even in the face of efficient treatment.[4] Abnormal stimulation of the autonomic nervous system, as by blows to the neck or to the solar plexus, are occasional causes of sudden death.

Far greater interest centres on the long-term effects of boxing—traumatic encephalopathy or 'punch drunkenness'. There is no doubt as to the reality of this syndrome although its prevalence may have been exaggerated. The precise mechanism is unknown but it probably results from a succession of attacks of 'diffuse axonal injury' such as have been described in Chapter 11 as the cause of concussion. The subtle pathological changes are very similar to those seen in Alzheimer's disease which has led to the suggestion that the latter may also be associated in some way with trauma to the head.[5] Traumatic encephalopathy, which is characterised by defects of memory, slurring of speech, unsteadiness of gait and clumsy movements, appears related to persistent repetition of severe injury to the head[6]—it is, therefore, one that occurs in poor-quality boxers forced by economic necessity into frequent bouts beyond their capability and who consequently receive more than average punishment; there is also some evidence that punch drunkenness is associated with the length of each bout—while the brain can recover from five contests of three rounds each, it has no interval in which to do so during 12–15 consecutive rounds. The *Report on the Medical Aspects of Boxing*[7] concluded that, while the likelihood of severe disablement due to

3   Royal College of Physicians *Report on the Medical Aspects of Boxing* (1969).
4   N Cater and M A Green 'Injury and Death in Sport and Recreational Activities' in J K Mason and B N Purdue (eds) *The Pathology of Trauma* (3rd edn, 2000) ch 18.
5   G W Roberts, D Allsop and C J Bruton 'The Occult Aftermath of Boxing' (1990) 53 J Neurol, Neurosurg Psychiat 373.
6   For review, see J A N Corsellis 'Boxing and the Brain' (1989) 298 BMJ 105. Protective headgear must now be worn in amateur boxing at the highest level.
7   Royal College of Physicians (1969).

brain damage was rare in boxers, there was evidence of a lesser degree of damage in a high proportion of persons who had boxed professionally for over ten years.

This being so, the effects of boxing should be preventable by regulation and, certainly, much effort is put into this aspect of the spectacle. A strict medical code has been enforced in British professional boxing since 1953 and includes general annual examinations of licensed boxers as well as immediate pre-fight medical check-ups. The number of bouts is controlled by the Medical Commission of the British Boxing Board of Control, which also has the power to withdraw a man's licence on the grounds of ill health. Appointed doctors are present at the ringside to advise on fitness to continue the fight and to assess the injury in the event of a knock-out; a boxer who has been knocked out or who has been stopped by the referee must be suspended until he is declared fit for another bout—and, in the case of professionals, the medical examination must include an electroencephalogram and a CT scan. In addition, an investigation is mounted if a boxer loses four fights in succession.

In view of all these precautions, a death in the ring can scarcely be regarded as anything other than accidental; this, however, depends upon the regulations being observed.[8] Death resulting from a deliberate mismatch could certainly attract a charge of culpable homicide as would one that could be attributed to premeditated failure to stop a fight that was clearly leading to severe injury. Disability sustained because of inadequate pre-fight medical examination could be construed as being attributable to medical negligence.

Wrestling as a sport is to be distinguished from the popular 'all in' wrestling which is probably better described as a spectacle; considering the nature of the action and the absence of restriction on holds or blows, there is a surprising dearth of morbidity and mortality. Several styles of 'controlled' wrestling are practised, each being overseen by a controlling body and each incorporating limitations as to holds in the interests of safety. Special rules are enforced to avoid injury to the cervical spine, which is at particular risk in wrestling. As a result, deaths during supervised sporting wrestling are virtually unknown in the United Kingdom but the same may not be true where the rules are more liberal—it is said, for example, that there is a considerable morbidity, and mortality, in Eastern Europe where wrestling is especially popular.

Having said which, it has to be noted that, even in the United Kingdom, there is a growing commerce in relatively uncontrolled exhibitions such as 'total fighting' which, from what little has been seen or read about, appear, at least to this author, to be little other than attempts to inflict grievous bodily harm for the benefit of the public. Since such bouts must be licensed by a local authority, they must be lawful. None the less, it is difficult to see them as being covered by, at least the spirit of, the *A-G's Reference (No 6 of 1980)*;[9] so far as is known, there have been no deaths from such displays but the legal reaction to one, should it occur, will be interesting.

8   The British Boxing Board of Control has a legal duty to establish adequate safety arrangements for bouts arranged under its aegis: *Watson v British Boxing Board of Control Ltd* [2000] ECC 141.

9   [1981] QB 715. 'Chain wrestling' may be a case in point although, here, the chain may be used to inflict injury: Parliamentary Report (1985) *The Times*, 12 July, p 4.

Contact sports

Perhaps the majority of team sports involve some form of body contact ranging from the near-gladiatorial encounters of American football to basketball in which contact is reduced to a minimum. Very large numbers of relatively minor injuries are inevitable and will not be discussed here. Death due to trauma on the sports field must, however, involve the lawyer and merits a brief note.

Rugby union football is probably the most dangerous 'popular' sport in the United Kingdom[10]—and the dangers increase in parallel with the widespread professionalism of what was developed as a purely amateur activity.[11] The most typical severe injury in rugby union was once fracture of the cervical spine and this was more or less equally attributable to the scrum and the tackle.[12] The incidence within the former can be markedly reduced by legislation through the Rugby Football Unions;[13] the latter is also amenable to strict enforcement of the rules in so far as a high proportion of severe injuries derive from foul tackles that are subject to the deterrent of 'sending off'. Association football also takes a considerable toll in the form of non-fatal injuries.[14]

The legal relationship of players in contact sports is complex. On the one hand, the participants have accepted the risks which are inherent in those sports; on the other, they still owe a duty of care to one another. That duty is not necessarily synonymous with obeying the rules; a player can fail in that duty even within the rules but, depending on the facts, may still not be acting unreasonably in infringing those rules.[15] Depending on the severity of the lapse, a player can be guilty of either civil[16] or criminal negligence.[17] The Law Commission has considered the

10 Sports Council *Injuries in Sport and Exercise* (1993). But the risk of death when riding a horse is twice that of playing a game of rugby.
11 This is, however, not to say that it is a specially dangerous game when the standards of coaching and refereeing are maintained: *Van Oppen v Trustees of the Bedford Charity* [1989] 3 All ER 389 at 415, per Croom-Johnson LJ. But, note that the referee can be guilty of negligence: *Smoldon v Whitworth* [1997] ELR 249, CA. It will be interesting to see if *Smoldon* will be extended to other sports—eg aimed at the umpire who allows too many short pitched balls at cricket: S Greenfield and G Osborn 'Aesthetics, Injury and Liability in Cricket' (1997) 13 PN 9.
12 H C Burry and C J Calciani 'The Need to Make Rugby Safer' (1988) 296 BMJ 149.
13 Although the true effect of legislation is still unclear—T Noakes and I Jakoet 'Spinal Cord Injuries in Rugby Union Players' (1995) 310 BMJ 1345; M Garraway and D Macleod 'Epidemiology of Rugby Football Injuries' (1995) 345 Lancet 1485.
14 Sport accounts for some 22% of fractures of the tibia going through major hospital departments and about 80% of these derive from association football: P A Templeton, M J Farrar, H R Williams et al 'Complications of Tibial Shaft Soccer Fractures' (2000) 31 Injury 415. For an overview, see J P Nicholl, P Coleman and B T Williams 'The Epidemiology of Sports and Exercise-related Injury in the United Kingdom' (1995) 29 Brit J Sports Med 232.
15 *Rootes v Shelton* [1968] ALR 33, per Barwick CJ at 34, Kitto J at 37. Quoted by Sir John Donaldson MR in *Condon v Basi* [1985] 2 All ER 453. As an international player said: 'In the modern game of rugby, punching is the rule rather than the exception' (in *R v Billinghurst* [1978] Crim LR 553). But the rules have been strengthened considerably since then.
16 Eg *Condon v Basi*, [1985] 2 All ER 453—a case in which damages were awarded for injuries following a foul tackle (in association football) where the defendant showed a reckless disregard for the plaintiff's safety; *McCord v Swansea City AFC Ltd* (1997) Times, 11 February—a tackle in association football 'inconsistent with taking reasonable care'.
17 *R v Lloyd (Steven)* [1989] Crim LR 513, CA—in which a sentence of 18 months' imprisonment was imposed for deliberately kicking an opponent outwith the playing pattern of the game.

problems of the latter;[18] it is leaning away from considerations of consent to injury by the players and towards the adoption of objective criteria which will include not only the nature of the suspect action but also the conditions under which the game in question is played.[19] The essential distinction to be made is that between, on the one hand, dangerous play and, on the other, conduct which is motivated by retaliation and which is intended to cause harm.

Sudden death in non-contact sports

Occasional deaths occur in apparently healthy young adults engaged in strenuous exercise such as long-distance running, protracted swimming or severe marching. Sometimes the environmental conditions are obviously extreme and can be held responsible for the death—eg in severe heat, death may be due to heat stroke or heat exhaustion (see Chapter 14) or, at the other end of the spectrum, an enforced stop may lead to death from exposure; many deaths of this type result from ignoring authoritative advice or from inadequate planning.

Very often, however, the cause of death is obscure and may only be presumed after a diligent search has revealed some unusual abnormality which is then assumed to have a causal relationship to the death; it must, however, be appreciated that this is by no means certain; in fact, coincidence is often just as likely. Very often, however, no potential cause may be discovered and the death is, in effect, physiological; the possibility of a 'sudden death in young adults syndrome' has been mooted already (see Chapter 7 for a fuller discussion). Anatomic attention is generally focused on any conditions discovered that might be expected to leave the heart dangerously short of oxygen during excessive demand—in particular, developmental abnormalities of the coronary circulation or an unusual degree of atheroma. The importance of these conditions in a medico-legal context is twofold—first, they would not have been recognisable by routine medical tests for fitness and, as a corollary, no blame for the death can reasonably be attached to the organisers of the activity. A number of such deaths have been attributed to blood disorders that are sensitive to hypoxia; sickle-cell disease has been cited and other unusual conditions[20] may cause collapse and dangerous sequelae even if not sudden death. Selection both for employment and for recreation on the basis of possessing the sickle-cell trait is seldom practicable in the absence of symptoms;[1] at least, however, persons known to have the trait should be warned of the possible dangers and doctors responsible for certifying fitness should obtain written acknowledgement that appropriate advice has been given. Some form of abnormal reflex nervous stimulation—or, equally nebulously, an acute failure of

---

18 *Criminal Law: Consent and Offences against the Person* (1994) Law Com Paper no 134.
19 Discussed in detail by S Gardiner 'The Law and the Sports Field' [1994] Crim LR 513. The author quotes five convictions for inflicting injury in rugby union and four in association football.
20 For example, the condition known as 'march haemoglobinuria' in which the red blood cells break down in the particular circumstances of strenuous exercise. The main danger lies in associated acute renal failure.
 1 A major difficulty is that many of these genetically controlled conditions are markedly associated with ethnicity. Selection, say, for employment would, therefore offend against the Race Relations Act 1976 by way of indirect discrimination unless the prospective employer could demonstrate medical unsuitability for the appointment.

an essential endocrine gland such as the adrenal—must be supposed in those cases in which no cause of death can be discovered; the present author has been impressed by the number of these deaths that appear to be associated with very full stomachs—this suggests the former possibility, but such diagnoses are rarely satisfying. There remains the possibility of post-viral debility but, again, this is often no more than a diagnosis of last resort.

Sport and steroids

Competition in any walk of life leads to the search for advantages of doubtful morality. International sport is no exception and much attention has focused on the use of a group of hormones known as *anabolic steroids* as intended aids to the improvement of physical performance.

The total muscle mass is undoubtedly increased by their use but it may well be that this is achieved through water retention rather than by an increase in the size and number of fibres;[2] much of the physical result attributed to steroids has been ascribed to psychological effects, including a euphoric attitude to hard training. The balance of evidence seems, however, to indicate that, provided the subjects are already highly trained, steroids can significantly improve performance—and this applies particularly in power events. It has been pointed out that standards in women's field sports improved very rapidly from 1968 and it could well be that this coincided with the general introduction of steroids—there is little doubt that the habit of steroid medication is now fairly widespread among high-grade athletes.

The probable benefits of steroids must be balanced against their potential ill-effects, particularly as there is a strong probability that some self-medicators will inevitably overprescribe, especially if there has been a good response to small doses. The side effects involve hirsutism, spotty skin (acne), prostatic enlargement and, of greater importance, some degree of liver damage including carcinogenesis. There is loss of libido and, perhaps, loss of fertility. Many of these effects, which may also include increased aggressiveness, are due to the associated androgen (or 'maleness-producing') effects of the steroids.[3] More serious effects on growth etc may, therefore, result from the use of these hormones in high dosage in prepubertal subjects. As with any substances used, essentially, to alter the physiology of the body, withdrawal should be gradual lest a sudden imbalance be precipitated.

Laboratory tests for anabolic steroids are available, but are expensive and require considerable expertise; control of their abuse in sport is, therefore, difficult—prohibition without detection is an unsatisfactory state of affairs. The Technical Commission of the International Federation of Sports Medicine firmly condemned the use of steroids by healthy sportspeople, but the onus of discovery and elimination rests on the governing bodies of the sports concerned.[4] The anabolic and androgenic steroids are now Class C controlled drugs and are subject

---

2   A distinction that is of no consequence in 'body building' competitions; steroid adjuvants are permitted by the organisers of these events.
3   R E Ferner and M D Rawlins 'Anabolic Steroids: The Power and the Glory?' (1988) 297 BMJ 877; B Dixon 'The Modern Olympic Ideal' (1988) 297 BMJ 926.
4   (1975) 9 Brit J Sports Med 111. Punishment is also a matter for individual Federations: *Edwards v British Athletic Federation* [1998] CMLR 363.

to the legislation as to production, supply, possession and export that applies to such drugs (see Chapter 22).[5]

Other forms of 'doping' have been—and may well still be—used in competitive sports; the amphetamines, for example, had a vogue as stimulants. The amphetamines, in particular, are unlikely to pose any problem in British athletics, since they are Class B controlled drugs[6]—they are also readily demonstrable in body fluids. The difficulties in screening for known drugs that are excreted in the urine or saliva are not, in fact, so much technical as emotional and political; very adequate control can be exercised over racehorses. Against this, it has to be said that several drugs that are 'illegal' in the sporting world could be used legitimately for therapeutic purposes; in the absence of a strict liability arrangement, there is, therefore, always room for discussion as to intention in the event of a positive test.[7]

Sex and sport

Problems in the differentiation of sex are discussed in relation to marriage in Chapter 17. Comparable problems have often arisen in competitive international sport where intimate medical examinations of competitors as a routine would be unacceptable. This is, therefore, an appropriate place to draw attention to some of the unexceptional methods available for the determination of the genetic sex on a screening basis; such methods depend upon the positive demonstration of either the Y chromosome or of what may be the XX agglomerate.

The latter process is that most commonly used and depends upon the fact that a high proportion of female cell nuclei show one or two dots of chromatin, easily visible under the microscope, beneath the nuclear membrane—the so-called 'Barr bodies'. These bodies are well seen in the skin or smooth muscle when a surgical biopsy is taken but this is, of course, impossible for routine use. Screening on a large scale is facilitated by the use of the surface cells of the mucosa of the mouth which are a good source of diagnostic Barr bodies. It is quite practical to rub the inside of the cheek with a blunt edge, to transfer the cells removed to a slide and to stain them. The proportion of cells showing Barr bodies is not high. One must find them in at least two nuclei out of every 100 cells examined to make a firm diagnosis of femininity.

A variation on this theme is the demonstration of sex chromatin or 'Davidson' bodies in the polymorphonuclear white cells of the blood. These appear as drumstick appendages to the multilobular nuclei. They are not easy to distinguish with certainty from other nuclear excrescences which occur independently of XX chromosomes and they are, again, by no means universal in the cells. The classic test for femininity involves discovery of six drumsticks. If these are found in less than 300 consecutive polymorph cells then the subject is regarded as 'chromatin positive'—this being a properly purist way of expressing 'femininity' through the finding of chromatin bodies. It will, however, be noted that the demonstration

5 Misuse of Drugs Act 1971 (Modification) Order 1996, SI 1996/1300.
6 Misuse of Drugs Act 1971 (see Chapter 22).
7 J Collier 'Drugs in Sport: A Counsel of Perfection Thwarted by Reality' (1988) 296 BMJ 520. For a more recent review, see D MacAuley 'Drugs in Sport' (1996) 313 BMJ 211.

of Davidson bodies depends upon the provision of a blood sample which, again, may not be politically acceptable.

The only advantage to be gained in sport from a sex transfer is for a chromosomal male to masquerade as a female—the deception need not be deliberate and may be due to genuine error. The tests described above therefore suffer from being of a negative nature. It is the *failure* to demonstrate chromatin bodies that indicates a deception. It would be preferable to demonstrate the Y chromosome positively and this can be done using, again, either desquamated cells from the inside of the mouth or white blood corpuscles; a positive result depends on the ability of the Y chromosome to fluoresce when treated with the dye quinacrine. The technique is considerably more complex than is that involved in searching for female chromatin masses. The portion of cells that are clearly 'Y positive' varies from 15% to 80% with different observers; a very occasional cell that is apparently male may be found in normal females. The technique is sufficiently perfected to be regarded as acceptable in routine diagnosis.

Problems of false sex are of decreasing importance in sport largely due to their increasing ease of discovery. Sexing by cells is, however, widely used in population studies and in the investigation of infants of doubtful genital sex—the chromatin bodies are developed in utero and much subsequent psychological difficulty can be avoided by an early diagnosis. In circumstances involving no urgency, however, cells can be cultured and their precise chromatin pattern—or *karyotype*—can then be demonstrated.

Death and injury in the crowd

The extent of violence in a crowd depends on two main characteristics—the quality of the crowd and its quantity as related to available space.

As to quality, it is a matter of common observation that the corporate nature of crowds at sporting events has changed dramatically in the last 30 years, so much so that a proportion of spectators at some events appear to attend with the express intention of being violent and others must take steps to defend themselves.[8] Despite intensive police action, offensive weapons find their way into stadia and injuries ranging from those due to kicking to those involving the use of razors and knives can never be eliminated entirely. Violence may, of course, be continued after the event itself. Inevitably, there is a close association between fighting and alcohol; Scotland took the lead with legislation to prevent drunkenness at major sporting events[9] and similar legislation has been operating in England and Wales since 1985.[10] There has undoubtedly been a major improvement at domestic games in the last decade—although the same cannot be said about the international ambience; even so, such injuries as are inflicted, which include stab wounds, do not differ materially from those that are described elsewhere and they need no further consideration here. Some forms of traumatic injury and death that are

---

8 The Football Spectators Act 1989 represented a legislative attempt to improve the situation through such devices as registration of spectators. The 1989 Act has been strengthened by the Football (Offences and Disorder) Act 1999 and the Football Disorder Act 2000. In Scotland, most football-associated offences are dealt with as breaches of the peace at common law.
9 Criminal Law (Consolidation) (Scotland) Act 1995, Pt II.
10 Sporting Events (Control of Alcohol etc) Act 1985.

related to the number and density of persons are, however, typified by sports crowds and can conveniently be discussed in this section.

A human being can tolerate considerable crowding in normal circumstances and in a normal atmosphere. Minor physiological disturbances such as fainting or collapse due to heat exhaustion occur frequently but, provided the subject can be removed from the crowd, no lasting injury results. Danger is associated with loss of 'herd' control which may be accidental or impulsive. The former is exemplified by the collapse of a stand or of crowd-control barriers and the latter by a crowd's reaction when attempting to move in difficulty or under threat of danger—the most remarkable example being the disaster at Hillsborough Stadium in 1989 when 94 died and more than 200 were seriously injured, some to die later.

In the event of crowd collapse, death may result from crush—or traumatic— asphyxia. This has already been mentioned in Chapter 13. The sheer weight of bodies—the condition is very rare except on inclined terraces or when the subjects are supine—prevents the use of the thoracic and abdominal muscles of respiration. An element of suffocation by occlusion of the nose and mouth may be added. A feature of this type of death is that the major blood vessels are also compressed; the classic appearances of asphyxia—congestion and petechial haemorrhage— are characteristically grossly exaggerated in crush asphyxia.

When a person has been crushed, death may be delayed for some days and be ultimately due to the 'crush syndrome'. This condition, which is certainly not confined to crowds,[11] results essentially from the crushing of the muscle masses and the consequent release of degeneration products which poison the kidneys. Death is due to acute renal failure but, in practice, recovery is the rule in those who survive the initial trauma and who can be maintained by dialysis until the kidney function returns. Finally, it must be mentioned—and will probably never be forgotten—that the intense hypoxia of crush asphyxia is likely to affect the brain; recovery may, therefore, result in the persistent vegetative state with its associated medical horrors and legal complexities.[12]

Somewhat similar conditions arise if the crowd piles up at an exit, particularly when the route funnels downwards. The conditions are self-generating, as those who find themselves obstructed by others in front attempt to escape the crush of those behind. Panic ensues and injuries due to trampling may well predominate; the extreme of such a situation is seen when a pressing danger such as fire is propelling the crowd forward.

At one time, the responsibility of the owners of a stadium for the safety of spectators was governed only by liability in tort or delict; heavy damages were, for example, awarded to the estates of those killed at Ibrox Park, Glasgow in 1971, when a crush barrier collapsed following an unexpected goal-score. Legislation had been introduced as a direct result of that disaster but was lost twice on procedural grounds; it was not until 1975 that safety standards were regulated by statute.[13] Safety certificates are required for sports grounds accommodating more than 10,000 persons, stipulating the number who can be admitted to various parts of the ground, the number of entrances and exits and the number of crush barriers

11 The crush syndrome is seen mainly in persons buried under falling rocks or masonry. It is common following garage accidents when the subject is impacted between two vehicles. Train accidents provide a number of cases due to the often lengthy process of extricating survivors.

12 See *Airedale National Health Service Trust v Bland* [1993] AC 789.

13 Safety of Sports Grounds Act 1975.

required. Records of attendance and maintenance must be kept. Before issuing a certificate, the local authority must confer with the local police, fire and community health officers.[14] The inadequacy of the controls was, however, demonstrated at Bradford, where 56 persons died from fire in a stand in 1985—the clear indication being that the danger lies in the stand rather than in the total capacity of the ground. The Fire Safety and Safety of Places of Sport Act 1987 resulted from the inquiry into the Bradford catastrophe; as a consequence, certification is now required for any covered stand which can accommodate more than 500 persons.[15]

The hazards of diving

An appreciable number of recreational divers die each year—22 persons died in the United Kingdom in the year 1997–98—and the depth to which amateur divers can descend is increasing with the use of improved equipment. The diver is essentially at risk on four counts—the properties of the external environment, the effect of pressure, the need for an artificial respiratory environment and the dangers from marine wild-life.

The pressure increases by 101 kPa (1 atmosphere) with every 10 m (33 ft) of depth. A great excess of air is therefore needed to fill the lungs and this expands during ascent; the same principles apply to gases dissolved in the body fluids— which may lead to decompression sickness—and to the gas containing body cavities such as the ear. Interference with the free egress of air may then lead to the condition known as barotrauma.

While breathing air at depth, the diver may suffer from either nitrogen narcosis—a condition that has been likened to acute alcoholism—or acute oxygen poisoning which can occur when this essential gas is inhaled under pressure (over 200 kPa) and causes epileptiform convulsions of central cerebral origin. In either case, the diver may die from the direct effects, he may become inco-ordinated and mismanage his task or his apparatus, he may drown or he may ascend precipitously.

Rapid ascent leads to massive expansion of the lungs and to release of bubbles of gas—nitrogen being especially significant—from the body fluids. Pulmonary distension is of no consequence provided that the airways are opened; failure to exhale during ascent, which is a common error among sports divers, may, however, lead to rupture of the alveoli and blood vessels—the condition of pulmonary barotrauma is established and, in severe cases, death may result from cerebral arterial gas embolism (CAGE). CAGE is not the same as central nervous system decompression sickness, although the two conditions may well co-exist. Decompression sickness is due to the release of gas from the blood and other tissue fluids. This causes severe pain in the joints ('the bends'), difficulty in breathing ('the chokes') or, most seriously, widespread blockage of the vessels supplying the spinal cord and brain. The greater the number of exposures, the greater the risk of developing cavitation of, and permanent damage to, the central nervous system and the bones. Decompression sickness is a hazard of all work undertaken at pressure and is a prescribed occupational disease (Appendix L). Serious neurological complications in the form of the high pressure nervous

14 See, now, Safety of Sports Grounds Regulations 1987, SI 1987/1941.
15 Safety of Places of Sport Regulations 1988, SI 1988/1807. It could be that the stringent regulations go beyond the financial capacity of some smaller clubs.

syndrome—producing tremors, convulsions and even death—were thought to be beyond the reach of the recreational diver; however, the introduction of so-called 'technical diving', in which varying gas mixtures are either carried or stashed along the route, has greatly increased the hazards to which he or she can be exposed.[16]

These may be increased by anxiety (overbreathing) or by hypothermia (see page 208), either of which may be fatal in their own right. Overbreathing endangers life by reducing the respiratory centre's sensitivity to oxygen lack; the diver may simply lapse into hypoxic unconsciousness and drown. Fatalities of this type have been recorded even during underwater exercise in swimming pools. The prevention of diving fatalities rests on good training, maintenance of apparatus, adjustment of the artificial atmosphere—for example, by the substitution of helium for nitrogen—the correlation of depth of dive with the apparatus available and on the rigid application of decompression schedules; the deeper the dive, the longer the time that must be allowed for ascent. Sports divers should always conform to the advice of a body such as the British Sub-aqua Club.

Somewhat similar, though generally far less severe, exposures to the hazards of decompression result from ascent in unpressurised high-altitude machines. Serious effects, which include some unique and baffling delayed deaths due to post-descent shock, are limited to professional aviators and astronauts; prevention rests on pressurisation either of the cabin environment or of the man by a pressure suit. The effects of high and low pressure may, however, be summative; occasional holidays have ended tragically through taking a 'last quick scuba dive' soon before the aircraft, the cabin pressure of which is equivalent to a height of some 2,400 m (8,000 ft), leaves for home—diving should not be practised within 24 hours of an intended flight.

Dangerous animals

The sea has its share of dangerous animals. Many have poison apparatus in tentacles, gills or fins and are most dangerous at spawning time. Marine venoms are generally toxic to the central nervous system and, while most 'stings' cause little more than local pain, others may be rapidly fatal; highly poisonous fish are virtually limited to tropical waters. As with all poisons, the effect is to some extent dependent upon body weight and children are, therefore, more susceptible than adults.

Fish are carnivores and some may attack man; of these, the shark is pre-eminent but, even so, is probably unfairly maligned. The size and aggressiveness of sharks, of which there are many varieties, is very roughly proportional to water temperature. Their teeth cause extensive laceration and death from shark-bite can result rapidly from haemorrhage; occasionally, drowning may be precipitated by panic. The moods of sharks are unpredictable; adults have died from shark-bite sustained while paddling. Shark netting or shark patrols are essential where bathing occurs in infested tropical or subtropical waters. It is worth remembering that, despite the foregoing, sharks are not confined to warm waters—the author has seen many cadavers mutilated by sharks in the Irish Sea; it is, however, very unlikely that such species would penetrate shallow waters—thus, they constitute no practical threat to those living in Northern Europe.

16 This is an inadequate summary of a very complex subject. A good modern update is to be found in J A S Ross and J H K Grieve 'Underwater Diving' in J K Mason and B N Purdue (eds) *The Pathology of Trauma* (3rd edn, 2000) ch 22.

17

Medico-legal aspects of marriage and pregnancy

A number of legal problems that are of immediate concern to the medical profession, or that can be resolved only on the basis of medical opinion, surround the state of matrimony. The subject is important in forensic medicine, although cases for decision are relatively rare.

Disputed sex

Marriage is defined as the union of a man and a woman and, on occasion, the definition of sex may be difficult. A marriage would be declared void if it were shown that the sex of one spouse was not that supposed.[1]

The sex of a person can be judged on various criteria.[2] First, there is the chromosomal or genetic make-up. As has been discussed elsewhere (see page 4), the possession of a Y chromosome in the cell nucleus determines maleness.[3] If the Y chromosome is discovered on testing, it is reasonable to assume that the person is a male. Even so, the situation is not without difficulty as the sex chromosomes tend to split abnormally and a person may have a karyotype of, say, XXY (Kleinfelter's syndrome) or, even, XXXY; while such persons are usually clearly males—albeit sterile—they occasionally have a preponderance of female characteristics. Mosaicism, or the presence in one body of both male and female cell populations, may produce complex anatomic anomalies.

Secondly, the sex may be indicated by the gonads—basically, whether there are testes or ovaries. In practice, this is a poor indicator of sex as the female ovaries cannot be visualised and non-descent of the male testes is not uncommon.

---

1 Matrimonial Causes Act 1973 (s 11(c)). Under the Marriage (Scotland) Act 1977, s 5(4)(e) the fact that both parties were of the same sex would constitute a retrospective legal impediment to marriage which would, thus, be void.
2 The classic medico-legal analysis is that of R Ormrod 'The Medico-legal Aspects of Sex Determination' (1972) 40 Med Leg J 78.
3 By contrast with the determination of sex in sport (see p 229 above), there would be no objection to relatively invasive techniques being used in these circumstances. Cells would be cultured and the precise chromosomal make-up could be established.

Thirdly, there is the appearance of the external genitalia and here there may be very great difficulties. The commonest abnormalities include failure of the development of the normal male genitalia when a gross degree of *hypospadias* may leave the genitalia closely resembling those of a female. Alternatively, there may be excessive secretion by the adrenal gland in a female which leads to hypertrophy of the female genitalia and to a spurious appearances of maleness (the adrenogenital syndrome). Cases of either type may be mistaken at birth[4] but are usually discovered during childhood and puberty; they are of little significance in the context of marriage but they may be of considerable psychiatric importance as the subject may have been reared incorrectly for some years. A far more important variation is to be found in the testicular feminisation syndrome where the testes do not descend and the genitalia fail to respond to the male hormones. The result is a typical female body with female external genitalia but no uterus and a vestigial vagina; the subject has undescended testes and an XY chromosomal constitution. The full extent of the abnormality is often undiscovered until marriage.

Fourthly, there is the person's own psychological assessment of his or her sex which may be contrary to all the other evidence; in its most intractable form, this state is known as transsexualism or the gender dysphoria syndrome.[5] The medico-legal importance of this abnormal state lies in the fact that surgical intervention is considered a legitimate form of treatment despite its grossly mutilating nature. Generally, this involves removal of the male genitalia and then fashioning others simulating those of the female; the breasts are implanted and femaleness is maintained by treatment with the female sex hormone (oestrogen). A similar approach is adopted in female to male conversion but, for obvious reasons, the physiological result cannot be as satisfactory.[6] A person's sex has very little effect within the civil law of the United Kingdom[7] but major problems arise if a converted transsexual wishes to marry in his or her new sex. The British courts have firmly closed the door on 'sex change' as a legal construct ever since the seminal case of *Corbett v Corbett*.[8] In that case, a marriage between a man and a converted male-to-female transsexual was declared void on the grounds that both persons were male, the respondent having at all times been a biological male notwithstanding operative intervention; it was also held that, even if the marriage had been valid, normal intercourse—which means intercourse per vaginam and not through an artificial vaginal passage—could not have occurred. The decision in *Corbett* has been widely criticised but has, nevertheless, been followed consistently in England as

4   There is provision for the correction of registration as to sex: Births and Deaths Registration Act 1953, s 29; Registration of Births, Deaths and Marriages (Scotland) Act 1965, s 42. The name may also be changed; registration is, however, a matter of historic fact and the only legal basis for correction is a genuine error at the time (see *X Petitioner* 1957 SLT (Sh Ct) 61).
5   Transsexuals are not necessarily homosexual. They firmly believe that they are imprisoned in the 'wrong' body type.
6   The validity of the operation and its availability within the National Health Service has been confirmed in *North West Lancashire Health Authority v A, D and G* [1999] Lloyd's Rep Med 399, CA. For a description of the surgical techniques see J J Hage 'Medical Requirements and Consequences of Sex Reassignment Therapy' (1995) 35 Med Sci Law 17.
7   In *White v British Sugar Corpn* [1997] IRLR 121, a woman was treated as a 'man' for national insurance purposes but as a woman as regards the Sex Discrimination Act 1975. Persons can, for example, obtain a passport or a driving licence in whichever sex they chose.
8   [1971] P 83.

to marriage and has been extended into the criminal field.[9] The principle has, however, been seriously challenged in the European Courts. In *Rees v United Kingdom*,[10] it was very clearly held that United Kingdom law did not transgress the rights of a citizen to privacy and to marriage; four years later, however, a similar case was, again, decided in favour of the United Kingdom but by a narrow majority only.[11] An anticipated verdict against the United Kingdom did not, however, materialise in 1998.[12] The decisions in favour of the defendants were related, at least in part, to the generally otherwise lax attitude to gender in the United Kingdom; in *B v France*[13] for example, the plaintiff's right to a change of sex was firmly upheld. In this last case, the European Court of Human Rights also took into account the improved medical and scientific knowledge of genetic disease and sexual orientation; the court's sympathetic attitude to the United Kingdom is confined to marriage—failure to recognise a transsexual's altered state offends against the EEC Council Directive 76/207, which deals with equality of treatment for men and women at the workplace.[14] It is to be noted that no case involving the testicular feminisation syndrome, which would be the ultimate test of the *Corbett* philosophy, has reached the United Kingdom courts.[15] Meantime, we are left in the rather bizarre situation where homosexual marriage is impossible but an *apparent* homosexual marriage involving a converted transsexual is perfectly legal.

Other reasons for nullity of marriage

A distinction must be recognised between void and voidable marriages. The former never were marriages and, in addition to those between persons of the same sex, include ceremonies undertaken when either party was below the age of 16, when one was already lawfully married, when they were within the prohibited degrees of relationship or in the case of a polygamous marriage when one of the parties was domiciled in England or Wales.[16] Voidable marriages, however, are valid until they are annulled. The list of voidable marriages in England and

---

 9 In *R v Tan* [1983] QB 1053, for example, a converted transsexual was considered still to be a man for the purposes of the Sexual Offences Act 1956, s 30.
10 [1987] 2 FLR 111, (1987) 9 EHRR 56.
11 *Cossey v United Kingdom* [1991] 2 FLR 492, (1991) 13 EHRR 622. Admittedly, *Rees* concerned a female-male reassignment which the courts are less inclined to accept in several jurisdictions. In the United States, compare *MT v JT* 355 A 204 (NJ, 1976) (male to female, marriage allowed) and *B v B* 355 NYS 2d 712 (1974) (female to male, marriage disallowed).
12 *Sheffield v United Kingdom* [1998] 2 FLR 928, (1999) 27 EHRR 163. Although the UK was criticised for its intractable attitude.
13 [1992] 2 FLR 249, (1993) 16 EHRR 1.
14 *P v S and Cornwall County Council* [1996] All ER (EC) 397. See now, Sex Discrimination (Gender Reassignment) Regulations, SI 1999/1102. For a discussion of this and other cases, see J K Mason 'United Kingdom v Europe: Current Attitudes to Transsexualism' (1998) 2 ELR 107. The Sex Discrimination Act 1975 must now be interpreted in accordance with *P v S: Chessington World of Adventures Ltd v Reed* [1998] ICR 97.
15 In fact, many of the early cases dealing with non-consummation of marriage almost certainly involved instances of the testicular feminisation syndrome which was not identified at the time. See, in particular, *SY v SY* [1963] P 37.
16 The conditions are very similar in Scotland but comprise 'marriages' which are specifically void by virtue of the Marriage (Scotland) Act 1977, ss 1 and 2 and those to which there is a legal impediment (which may operate prospectively or retrospectively) (s 5(4)).

Wales is long but includes non-consummation—due either to incapacity or to refusal—marriage without valid consent, and mental disorder, venereal disease or pregnancy by another man at the time of the ceremony. In Scotland, impotency constitutes the only ground for a voidable marriage, although most of the other English conditions would constitute either a legal impediment to marriage or grounds for divorce.

Sexual intercourse is a most important factor in a functioning marriage; it must be of 'normal' type and must be potentially satisfying to be acceptable in civil law as true intercourse.[17] Incapacity on the part of either spouse to consummate the marriage in this way enables the court, on the appropriate proceedings being taken, to declare a marriage null and void provided that the incapacity is incurable. The incapacity is still so regarded if the spouse refuses a remedial operation and the same is true if the proposed operation is likely to be dangerous or is unlikely to succeed. Consummation of marriage depends on successful coitus; sterility or failure of emission is immaterial.[18] The procreation of children is not, in law, a principal intention of marriage and, therefore, neither the use of contraceptives nor the practice of coitus interruptus constitutes grounds for a declaration of nullity.[19]

The court must, in practice, base its decision on medical evidence and, in England, appoints its own medical examiners to whom both parties must submit for examination. In Scotland, however, it is for the pursuer to lead what evidence he or she can; the courts will not normally order a defender to undergo an examination. Obvious defects may be apparent externally, the extreme being sufficient to induce a genuine error as to sex although, as described above, such cases are unlikely to persist until marriage. Even so, a true penis may be of such small size as to be incapable of penetration and a vagina may be so rudimentary as to inhibit entry of a normal male organ.

Most often, however, the allegation will be based on impotence in the male. There is now no lower or upper age limit beyond which there is a presumption of impotence in either England or Scotland.[20] Impotence may be physical in origin—it is a frequent, though not invariable, accompaniment of paraplegia—or it may have apparently no more than a psychological basis. Demonstration of the former may be easy for the doctor but, in the presence of normal genitalia, the latter may be hard to prove in the face of a resolute defence. Impotence in the female in the sense of failure to have orgasm is clearly not grounds for annulment but frigidity—or hatred of intercourse—to the extent that the vagina was thereby stimulated to a state of persistent spasm would be competent grounds, were it possible to prove its existence. Occasionally, women reach the same condition by reason of the pain experienced in sexual intercourse. Physical disease other than malformation in women is an uncommon cause of impotence.

Impotence arising from any cause after the marriage has been consummated cannot be grounds for a declaration of nullity. There is, however, a famous case in which a declaration was made despite the fact that there was a child who was the

17 *W (otherwise K) v W* [1967] 1 WLR 1554.
18 *R v R* [1952] 1 All ER 1194.
19 *Baxter v Baxter* [1948] AC 274; *White v White* [1948] P 330—but they could result in a divorce decree being granted since such behaviour might be held to be unendurable.
20 In England, this brings the criminal and civil law into line. For discussion, see *L v K* [1985] 1 All ER 961. The presumption in criminal law that a boy under 14 cannot penetrate was abolished in the Sexual Offences Act 1993.

undisputed offspring of the couple concerned.[1] It was held that entry of the sperm and fertilisation of the ovum could occur without legal penetration; medically speaking this is so, though it must be a fortunately rare occurrence.

Medical evidence may, but is unlikely to, be called in relation to the other statutory bases for nullity. Certain degrees of consanguinity and affinity are a lawful impediment whether the relationships exist in the legitimate or illegitimate state[2] and scientific evidence, at least, might be called for in such circumstances (see page 242); a marriage can be annulled if, at the time of the marriage, one party was suffering from mental disorder of such a kind or to such an extent as to render him or her unfitted to marriage—clearly a matter of medical assessment; there are grounds for annulment in England and Wales when one partner was suffering from venereal (or sexually transmitted) disease at the time of marriage—provided that the petitioner was unaware of the situation when the marriage took place.[3] Pregnancy by another man at the time of marriage, unsuspected by the petitioner, is grounds for annulment in England and Wales but not in Scotland—contrariwise, a false threat of pregnancy as a spur to wedlock does not constitute grounds for nullity.

Pregnancy

Aside from these considerations, and the criminal connotations that are discussed in Chapter 18, pregnancy is of obvious medico-legal importance in civil litigation involving problems such as divorce and succession. The question of paternity will loom large in these issues; the legal and scientific bases for its settlement are addressed briefly at page 240 below. For present purposes, it is intended only to recapitulate the circumstantial evidence that bears on the probability of conception being as averred by one or other party.

Certain presumptions as to age and pregnancy are made—at least in relation to perpetuity law. These include, first, that a young woman is capable of conceiving a child in her 13th year and, secondly, that an old woman is past childbearing in her 56th year.[4] As to the lower age limit, the most extreme case reported is that of a Peruvian girl who is said to have given birth at the age of 5¾ but, if it is true, it and others like it must be regarded as freak occurrence; it would be reasonable to accept the 13th year as the practical lower limit for young birth, with the 12th year as the earliest at which conception is possible. At the upper end, it is generally

1   *Clarke v Clarke* [1943] 2 All ER 540.
2   Nine relationships are absolutely prohibited in England (Marriage Act 1949, Sch 1). A man cannot marry (and the reverse applies for women) his mother, adoptive mother or former adoptive mother, daughter, adopted daughter or former adopted daughter, grandmother, granddaughter, sister, aunt, niece. A number of more distant relations by affinity are restricted in particular ways. The list in Scotland is even longer (Marriage (Scotland) Act 1977, Sch 1) where, as in the case of incest, the possibility of an association between more distant generations is taken into account. Marriage between cousins is permissible, as is marriage to a former wife's sister, aunt or niece.
3   It can only be assumed that this would include HIV infection, although it is arguable that, as this could well be contracted other than by sexual intercourse, it does not qualify as a sexually transmitted disease.
4   Perpetuities and Accumulations Act 1964, s 2 (subject to a medical opinion in the case of the living). There are no such general presumptions in Scots law.

agreed that impregnation is unusual after the age of 45 but that exceptions here are more numerous and more acceptable; each case must be considered individually as to probability. It has certainly been held that inability to bear children after the age of 53 was a rebuttable presumption.[5]

The duration of pregnancy is of greater medico-legal significance. The normal average gestation period is regarded as 280 days, but this depends on numerous factors, including the length of the menstrual cycle, which may vary quite markedly from the norm of 28 days. Additionally, allowance must be made for the possibility that fertilisation of the ovum does not occur immediately after coitus; although spermatozoa lose their viability rapidly in the vagina (see Chapter 20), they can survive for some 48 hours in the receptive environment of the uterus and, exceptionally, have been demonstrated as fecund five days after injection—natural fertilisation occurs most commonly in the fallopian tube.

Such physiological variations will account for divergences from the normal of at most ten days; there is no doubt, however, that less explicable cases do occur, and the courts are prepared to accept wider limits in reaching decisions as to paternity when the length of a pregnancy is the main or only evidence. What is, perhaps, the extreme decision held that a husband was not entitled to a divorce on the grounds of adultery simply because a child was born 349 days after the last intramarital coitus.[6] A similar claim involving a gestation of 360 days was, however, upheld.[7] Extended gestation periods may be examples of superfetation. This condition arises from the fertilisation of ova liberated from the ovaries at different monthly ovulations. Even if it is accepted that a second ovulation can occur in the presence of a normal fetus, it is generally believed that this must be incredibly rare; it is possible, however, that a fetus could die in utero and a second impregnation occur before the onset of a menstrual period—the appearances would therefore be of a grossly prolonged gestation period. Superfecundation is a different and well-accepted concept whereby two ova released at the same ovulation are fertilised by two different acts of coitus; such an event would be distinguishable from the bearing of binovular twins only in exceptional circumstances.

There can be no comparable concept of the minimum length of a pregnancy as all pregnancies may terminate either as miscarriages, stillbirths or premature births—medical viability in the last category depending largely on the efficiency of the obstetric services available. Viability (see Chapter 18) is not, however, a legal concept in the United Kingdom; the preferred term is 'capable of being born alive'. A fetus can be so described if it is capable of breathing and oxygenating its tissues through the use of its own lungs—with or without the use of a ventilator.[8] There is a statutory presumption that a fetus of 28 weeks' gestation is capable of being born alive[9] but there is no comparable legal presumption as to incapacity though the physiological barrier imposed by the immaturity of the lungs persists

5   These cases are all very old and it might be better, today, to speak in terms of ability or inability to conceive. Elderly women can *carry* children resulting from in vitro fertilisation.
6   *Hadlum v Hadlum* [1948] 2 All ER 412.
7   *Preston-Jones v Preston-Jones* [1951] 1 All ER 124.
8   *C v S* [1988] QB 135.
9   Infant Life (Preservation) Act 1929. It is unaffected by the Still-Birth (Definition) Act 1992 under which the 24th week of gestation distinguishes a miscarriage from a stillbirth. The 1929 Act does not run to Scotland.

until 22–23 weeks. The precise age of a newborn infant, whether alive or dead, may be of considerable medico-legal importance in both the civil and the criminal law; the process whereby it is assessed is discussed in Chapter 18.

Testing for parentage

Very occasionally, an allegation may be made that a child has been wrongly identified in the maternity crèche, while extraordinary instances of fabricated pregnancy followed by appropriation of an infant have been reported; there can be few other occasions in which the identity of a mother is in doubt and, for practical purposes, testing for parentage is a matter of paternity testing; it is in this context that the subject will be discussed.[10] The principal circumstances in which paternity tests are called for are in divorce proceedings and in the adjudication of affiliation orders.

In either case, the putative father is denying responsibility for a child and, prior to the introduction of DNA profiling, the main function of the laboratory was to exclude paternity in a man unjustly accused. Since standard blood group genetic studies could not prove paternity *conclusively*, it used to be said that paternity testing was unfair in that, while the man had little to lose and perhaps everything to gain from blood testing, the mother of the child had, by contrast, comparatively little expectation of advantage. That aphorism no longer holds because DNA techniques, which it is not proposed to discuss in detail, can now identify a father positively.

The law relating to parentage testing in England and Wales lies in the Family Law Reform Act 1969, as anticipated in the Family Law Reform Act 1987.[11] Under s 20(1), the courts may give a direction for the use of scientific tests to be made on bodily samples to ascertain whether a party to the proceedings is or is not the father or mother of the child.[12] The direction may be made on application from any party to the proceedings or the court may so direct of its own motion; in practice, tests are generally agreed between the parties and court orders are seldom required. Consent is necessary, the age of consent being 16 (s 21) but, under s 23(1), the court may draw inferences from the fact that a person has failed to take steps as directed.[13] A pattern of judicial decisions appears to be developing in this context

10 The complications introduced by modern reproductive techniques involving ovum donation, womb-leasing and the like are referred to on p 246. It is to be noted that a woman who has carried the child, and no other woman, is to be regarded in law as the mother of the child and this presumption is irrebuttable (Human Fertilisation and Embryology Act 1990, s 27). Any exclusion of parentage is subject to the 1990 Act, ss 27–29 (Family Law Reform Act 1969, s 25, as amended).

11 Strangely, s 23 of the 1987 Act is still not in force. The author has, however, used the substituted text on the assumption that it will become operative.

12 Civil Procedure Rules 1998, SI 1998/3132. But the court cannot *order* blood or tissue samples for paternity purposes: *Re O and J (children) (blood tests: constraint)* [2000] 2 All ER 29. In this case, Wall J drew attention to the fact that the Family Law Reform Act 1969, s 21(1) and (3), from which this principle derives, may not be compliant with the Human Rights Act 1998.

13 And the court's powers are wide enough to include drawing an inference as to the child's actual paternity: *Re W v G (paternity), Re A (a minor)* (1994) Times, 18 May; *F v Child Support Agency* [1999] 2 FLR 244.

in that refusal by a person already having care of a child will not, on the grounds of the best interests of the child, be accepted as indicating an adverse inference; adverse inferences will, however, be drawn where a person is seeking to avoid responsibility of a child.[14]   The pattern may, however, be broken—depending largely on how the court views the importance to the child of a stable family life as against a knowledge of his or her true paternity.[15]

The history of paternity testing has been stormy in Scotland, where great store has been laid on the unfairness of forcing a person to submit to an invasive examination which was being undertaken for the benefit of his adversary[16]—and this position was still being sustained as recently as 1990, when it was said that:

> 'the fact that a conclusive test such as DNA fingerprinting is now available makes no difference to the principle set out in *Whitehall* [that it was not in the interests of justice to make such evidence available].'[17]

The Scottish courts have also traditionally been unwilling to allow a child to be subjected to a course of action that might have a serious effect on its primary interests;[18] as something of a corollary to this, the court invoked the best interests of the child in one of the very few reported instances of the courts supporting a blood test investigation.[19]

The situation has, however, changed dramatically, starting with the passage of the Law Reform (Parent and Child) (Scotland) Act 1986. Section 6 of the Act established that consent to the taking of a sample from a [now][20] child under the age of 16 could be given by his [now] guardian or by any person having custody or care and control of him; in the absence of such persons, the court could give consent (s 6(3)). The section has been greatly amended and substituted by the Law Reform (Miscellaneous Provisions) (Scotland) Act 1990, s 70. This provides for the court to request the parties to a dispute to donate samples on its own motion, whether or not an application has been made; it substitutes the words 'samples of blood or other body fluid or of body tissues' for 'blood samples' wherever appropriate; and, most importantly, it allows for an adverse inference to be drawn in the event of a refusal of such a request. Although this appears to be following English law, Scots law has, in fact, taken the lead in so far as the provisions of the 1990 Act are already in force. Case law has gone even further than might have been expected. In *Mackay v Murphy*[1] the court found itself able to request a sample from the mother of a deceased putative father on the grounds that she was his executrix and, accordingly, a party to the action. The same court quoted with approval the English view that the truth ought to prevail—'. . . there is nothing more shocking than that injustice should be done on the basis of a

---

14 For the former, see *Re F (a minor) (blood tests: parental rights)* [1993] QB 314; *K v M (paternity: contact)* [1996] 1 FLR 312. For the latter, *Re A (A Minor) (Paternity: Refusal of Blood Test)* [1994] 2 FLR 463 and the cases in fn 13 above.
15 *Re H (Paternity: Blood Test)* [1996] 2 FLR 65.
16 The leading authority is the old case of *Whitehall v Whitehall* 1958 SC 252.
17 *Torrie v Turner* 1990 SLT 718 at 720, per Lord Mayfield.
18 See Lord President Clyde in *Imrie v Mitchell* 1958 SC 439 at 466.
19 *Docherty v McGlynn* 1985 SLT 237. The case was unusual, however, in that a man was *claiming* to be the child's father.
20 Substituted by virtue of the Age of Legal Capacity (Scotland) Act 1991.
1 1995 SLT (Sh Ct) 30.

legal presumption when justice can be done on the basis of fact'.[2] On the other hand, another court would not take an adverse inference from the refusal to provide a sample by a woman who was having sexual relations with both her husband and the putative father; it was thought that there was, as a result, insufficient evidence on which to overturn the deeply held presumption that the husband is the father of a child born in wedlock.[3] It is clear that the courts have considerable discretion in both jurisdictions. There is no doubt that the child's interests are very persuasive when reaching decisions, although it is sometimes difficult to see precisely where those interests lie.

Certain essentials must be met before the results of the tests can be admitted as evidence in England and Wales. First, specimens must be obtained as a minimum from the mother, the child and any putative father. Secondly, the specimen must be suitably identified by the parties concerned and by their legal advisers. Thirdly, declarations of consent and agreement as to the validity of the specimens must be signed. Verified photographs of the principals are essential if a doctor not attached to a testing centre is asked to take the samples.

DNA profiling and paternity

As already noted, paternity testing is now almost entirely a matter of demonstrating DNA polymorphisms—or variations at the same genetic locus—as described in Chapter 1. The number of 'bands' that can be visualised are inherited in such a way that about half the bands of the genetic profile—or 'bar code'—are derived from each parent. Given that one can characterise a child and its mother, it is possible to compare the two autoradiographs and to establish which bands in the child are of maternal origin. The remaining bands must come from the father and paternity can be positively confirmed, or excluded, by, again, matching the child's against the putative father's profile. The odds against a match occurring by chance alone—or, put another way, the probability of the matching man being the actual father—increase with the number of bands that can be visualised and compared and this depends, to an extent, on the methodology. Arguments as to the statistical reliability of DNA profiling are referred to briefly in respect of criminal offences in Chapter 20. The problems are, perhaps, less urgent in the civil law context of paternity testing, where many factors will contribute to establishing a balance of probabilities—the threshold required to dismiss the possibility of a chance match is considerably lower and is well within the probability figures generally accepted for DNA comparisons. In practice, the chances of two persons having a similar profile when obtained by modern techniques can be narrowed down to one in several million.[4]

DNA 'bar codes' are classically produced by using what are known as multi-locus probes, which demonstrate so-called variable number tandem repeats. The techniques are, however, improving steadily. One alternative form of investigation involves the use of the single locus probe, which concentrates on a specific portion of the DNA molecule. In this method only two bands are demonstrated which are

---

2   *Holmes v Holmes* [1966] 1 WLR 187 at 188, per Ormrod J.
3   Law Reform (Parent and Child) (Scotland) Act 1986, s 5(1)(a). The presumption holds in the case of void, voidable and irregular marriages.
4   The subject is described in simple terms by P J Lincoln 'From ABO to DNA . . .' (2000) 40 Med Sci Law 3.

usually well-formed.[5] These bands are inherited from one's parents after the manner of blood groups. The use of single locus probes at several sites and, thereby, obtaining multiple independent matches, increases the probability of paternity to near absolute certainty.

The necessary technology is now readily available and the process is fully computerised. Suitable test material can be obtained by the non-invasive method of taking smears from the inside of the mouth. Even so, analysis of the results is a matter for scientific experts and lists of those qualified to do so are in process of preparation.

Assisted reproduction

It is said that some 10% of married couples who wish to have children are unable to do so and that the causes of childlessness are split equally between husband and wife. In the event that surgery or hormone treatments are inappropriate, recourse may be had to gamete replacement therapy. This will take the form or artificial insemination when the childlessness is attributable to abnormalities in the male or of some form of embryo transfer when the abnormality lies in the female. The legal complications—though not the moral problems—of assisted reproduction have been largely resolved by the Human Fertilisation and Embryology Act 1990. The general effect of the Act is to render unlawful the manipulation of an embryo outside the body of a woman unless the procedure is carried out at a place and by a person licensed to do so by the Human Fertilisation and Embryology Authority (s 12); donor insemination is also tightly controlled but is not, of itself, illegal when performed outside a licensed clinic.

Artificial insemination

Artificial insemination may be accomplished by the use of the husband's semen (AIH) in the case of failure to penetrate or of donor semen (AID)[6] in the event of primary male infertility. The seed is introduced into the cervical canal by means of a syringe and a surprising number of insertions may be needed to achieve success.

Artificial insemination with the semen of the husband poses few problems. The effect on a plea of nullity on the grounds of incapacity to consummate has been mixed;[7] there are no modern precedents but it is suspected that the courts would regard the conditions as representing approbation of the marriage. The effect of the posthumous use of a husband's semen is now dealt with in statute; the dead husband is not to be regarded as the father of the child in such circumstances.[8]

---

5   Because the single locus probe is some 50 times more sensitive than the multi-locus probe.
6   There is a movement to refer to donor insemination (DI) rather than AID to avoid confusion of the latter with the acquired immune deficiency syndrome. The old terminology is preferred here.
7   The question of whether the wife had accepted the conditions of an abnormal marriage having become pregnant by AIH was addressed in *L v L* [1949] 1 All ER 141. By implication, the court did not consider the marriage to have been consummated thereby. Similar conduct was adjudged to have approbated the marriage in the Scottish case of *A B v C B* 1961 SC 347 (*G v G* 1961 SLT 324).
8   Human Fertilisation and Embryology Act 1990, s 28(6)(b). The problems of death and 'effective' consent were paramount in *R v Human Fertilisation and Embryology Authority, ex p Blood* [1999] Fam 151. The problem of non-paternity will, however, be voided if the Human Fertilisation and Embryology (Amendment) Bill 2000 becomes law.

The legal status of artificial insemination by donor—which used to be loaded with forensic imponderables—has now been largely clarified. Perhaps the most important consideration from the aspect of forensic medicine is that the doctor concerned with the arrangements is liable in negligence not only to the mother of the resultant child and her husband but also to the child itself;[9] the liability relates to a disability arising as a result of negligent selection or keeping or use outside the body of the gametes or embryo carried by the mother.

The remainder of the easements provided by statute depend very much on consent. Thus, the woman's husband—or bona fide partner[10]—will be treated as the father of the child unless it can be shown that he did not consent to the insemination—or to the placing of an embryo in her (1990 Act, s 28(2) and (3)). Similarly, the sperm donor who has given the required consent to its use[11] is not to be treated as the father of the child for any purpose (1990 Act, ss 28(4) and (6), 29(2)). Theoretically, therefore, the woman's husband could disclaim parental responsibility by proving he did not consent; however, s 28(5) retains the common law rule of *pater est quem nuptiae demonstrant*—as a result he might also have to prove non-paternity by conventional means (see page 242 above). The 1990 Act makes no direct mention of the vexing problem of birth certification. However, under s 29(1), the consenting husband or partner is to be regarded as the father of the child for all purposes—which must, presumably, include so stating on the child's birth certificate. There are difficulties in accepting a statute condoning what is a palpable misrepresentation and a major purpose of the birth certificate is to provide a record of the person's heredity—the interests of the child are, however, accepted as being overriding. There is a further problem in that the presence of a single donor in a district could lead to consanguineous marriages in the future; again, the Act is silent but the accompanying Code of Practice recommends that not more than ten inseminations should be provided by a single donor. This is one reason why records of donations are to be kept. Tight controls on confidentiality are enjoined[12] but, even so, the availability of information gives rise to some concern—there is no reason why future legislation should not allow for retrospective disclosure. Currently, a person who, having reached the age of 18, has reason to doubt his paternity or maternity may apply to the Authority for limited information as to his or her parentage but this cannot extend to information which would lead to the identification of a gamete donor (1990 Act, s 31(5)). In the event of prospective marriage, a person over the age of 16 can obtain similar information together with information as to a possible genetic relationship.

The relationships between husband and wife in the AID situation are now relatively clear. It is certain that AID, even without the consent of the husband,

---

9 Congenital Disabilities (Civil Liability) Act 1976, s 1A. There is no liability if, at the time of the insemination, either the woman or her husband knew of the risk which materialised.

10 In this case, only so long as the insemination is carried out in a licensed clinic. But paternity will not be acknowledged when the 'male' partner is a converted transsexual: *X, Y and Z v United Kingdom* [1997] 2 FLR 892, (1997) 24 EHRR 143. Note that the word 'partner' is not used in the Act and there is no indication as to how long a relationship must have lasted in order to 'qualify'. One major firm set the watershed for its own purposes at two years: *Grant v South West Trains Ltd* [1998] All ER (EC) 193.

11 The requirements for consent—and to procedures involving embryo transfer—are set out in the Human Fertilisation and Embryology Act 1990, Sch 3.

12 And had to be relaxed: Human Fertilisation and Embryology (Disclosure of Information) Act 1992.

does not constitute adultery—this being on the grounds that adultery involves coitus.[13] Nevertheless, to attempt to conceive in this way without the husband's consent would almost certainly be considered conduct such as to cause breakdown of a marriage and would constitute grounds for divorce. It has been suggested that the donor's spouse might have grounds for divorce if it were known he were the father of other women's children; it is doubtful if this could constitute grounds for 'irretrievable breakdown of marriage' by virtue of intolerable behaviour. It is reasonable to expect that consent to his role should be obtained from the donor's wife—but there is no statutory requirement to do so.

Embryo transfer methods

The general term embryo 'transfer' is used here in the sense that the methods described have it in common that, at some point, the embryo must be manipulated from the in vitro to the in vivo environment. Since this involves the creation of an embryo outside the body of a woman, all are subject to the controls imposed by the Human Fertilisation and Embryology Act 1990.

Abnormalities leading to sterility or childlessness in the female result, in almost equal proportion, from failure of ovulation or from inability of the ovum to reach the uterus. We are concerned here only with those cases which cannot be treated successfully by surgery or hormone therapy. Failure of ovulation is, then, treatable by ovum donation, which is the female equivalent of artificial insemination by donor. Ova for donation are, however, very difficult to acquire— and doing so may carry some hazards for the donor; this is at least part of the reason why the most common procedure involving embryo transfer relates to blockage of the fallopian tubes.[14] In this, the woman donates her own ova which are fertilised in vitro by her husband's sperm; the resulting embryo is then implanted in her uterus. The process is generally known as in vitro fertilisation (IVF) and corresponds to AIH described above. There are thus no direct medico-legal problems associated with IVF; numerous moral and legal difficulties, however, arise indirectly.

These follow, first, from the fact that more ova must be obtained and more must be fertilised than will be used for treatment. Whether the resultant eggs and embryos are destroyed, stored, donated or used for research purposes depends on the provision of a licence by the licence committee of the Human Fertilisation and Embryology Authority (1990 Act, Sch 2)[15]and on consent. The 1990 Act holds that consent must come from both gamete donors (1990 Act, Sch 3, para 6); disagreement as to disposal has led to bitter private litigation, especially in the United States.[16] The main public concern in the United Kingdom lies in consent to research on surplus embryos and whether it should be allowed. The argument sharpens when it is extended to the creation of embryos for the express purpose of using them for research. While many would make a moral distinction between the

---

13 *MacLennan v MacLennan* 1958 SC 105.
14 Many jurisdictions then prefer 'egg sharing'—ie the woman who is being treated will donate the surplus eggs that are always produced.
15 No licence may be given, inter alia, for keeping or using the embryo after the appearance of the primitive streak—or 14 days after its creation (1990 Act, s 3(3)). This excludes any time during which the embryo is stored.
16 Eg *Davis v Davis* 842 SW 2d 588 (Tenn, 1992).

two processes, the United Kingdom is, perhaps, unique among Western nations in allowing the formation of embryos which were never intended for therapeutic use.[17]

Secondly, the best results are obtained when more embryos are transferred to the uterus than it will be desirable to carry to full term. Although good practice limits the number of embryos inserted to three,[18] the need for the reduction of multifetal pregnancy[19] may yet arise. Any legal doubts have now been erased and the procedure is lawful provided the terms of the Abortion Act 1967 are fulfilled[20]—not a difficult task in the circumstances.

Childlessness due to non-ovulation can be managed by way of ovum donation—subject to the considerable difficulty in obtaining ova. The procedure as a whole is technically complex but the legal difficulties are of the same order as those involved in AID, with maternity substituted for paternity. In this respect, the 1990 Act is unequivocal in holding that the woman who is carrying or who has carried a child, and no other woman, is to be treated as the mother of the child (s 27(1)). In a surprising number of cases, childlessness is due to gamete inadequacy in both husband and wife. The technique of embryo donation can then be employed using embryos created in vitro from both sperm and ovum donors. The same rules as to paternity and maternity will then apply, although the resultant child has no greater genetic affinity to its 'parents' than does the adopted child.

It is to be appreciated that, although the techniques involving embryo transfer have advanced rapidly in the last decades, the 'take-home baby' rate remains low at about 20% of treatment cycles in the best hands; moreover the treatments are expensive. Their provision under the National Health Service is far from universal and individual health authorities can apply their own conditions based on clinical experience.[1]

In certain circumstances, the treatment known as gamete intra-fallopian transfer (GIFT) can be used in preference to in vitro fertilisation. In this procedure, the gametes are transferred to the woman's fallopian tube rather than handled in the laboratory petri dish. Since no embryo is created outside the body, the conditions of the Human Fertilisation and Embryology Act 1990 do not, strictly speaking, apply so long as only husband and wife are involved; however, since a licence is required to practice GIFT using gamete donors, there is little doubt that the Authority exercises a de facto if not de jure control over the practice in general. Increasingly complex technologies—such as ICSI (intra-cytoplasmic sperm injection)—are being introduced steadily and are, of course, subject to licensing by the Authority.

Surrogate motherhood

Surrogate motherhood offers an alternative to both reimplantation and adoption. From a series of cases occurring closely in the late 1980s, the procedure has

---

17 1990 Act, Sch 2, para 3. But note that this can only be done, at present, in support of five specific research objectives: infertility, congenital disease, miscarriages, contraception and the pre-implantation detection of genetic and chromosomal disease.
18 Human Fertilisation and Embryology Authority *Code of Practice* (4th edn, 1998) para 7.9.
19 Sometimes known as selective reduction of pregnancy—but, strictly speaking, this should be limited to the elimination of one or more specific fetuses known to be defective.
20 1990 Act, s 37(5).
 1 Eg as to the age of the patient: *R v Sheffield Health Authority, ex p Seale* (1994) 25 BMLR 1.

progressed from being a media specialty to one which is now practised fairly widely in the United Kingdom without comment. There are two main techniques. The first involves artificial insemination of another woman with the sperm of an infertile woman's husband; the infant is passed to its biological father and his wife at birth. This is more correctly known as partial surrogacy but is, none the less, the process which most people equate with surrogate motherhood. In the second, a husband and wife create an embryo in vitro which is then implanted in a surrogate, and the resultant child is then returned to its genetic parents; this is known as full surrogacy, although the term 'womb-leasing' is perhaps satisfactorily descriptive. The rapid habilitation of surrogacy since 1978—when a surrogacy arrangement was dismissed as 'pernicious and void'[2]—probably stems from the realisation that, if it is acceptable to employ assisted methods of reproduction when a woman has, say, no ovaries, it is unreasonable to deny such services to one who has no uterus or who cannot gestate. It is to be noted that, although 'womb-leasing' appears to be open to abuse—for example, on the grounds of convenience—there are far more pathological conditions in which 'womb leasing' would be the option of choice than there are in favour of partial surrogacy. The practical differences lie in the difficulty and relative lack of success of the former process and in the fact that it can only be carried out under licence from the Authority.

The legality—and limitation—of surrogacy has developed almost entirely through case law. In 1985, an American couple who had entered into a surrogacy arrangement were given care and custody of the child and were allowed to remove it to the USA on the grounds that this was in the child's best interests; the judge specifically repelled the suggestion that they were unfit parents by virtue of having arranged the surrogacy.[3] Two years later, a couple who had received a surrogate baby two and a half years previously, applied for its adoption. The question arose as to whether the payment of money to the surrogate vitiated an adoption. It was held that this was not so, provided that the payments did no more than compensate for the inconvenience of pregnancy.[4] There was complete agreement between the commissioning couple and the surrogate in these cases. By contrast, in *Re P (minors)*[5] the surrogate refused to hand over the twins to which she had given birth. The children were made wards of court and custody was given to the gestational mother on the grounds that it was in their interests to preserve the link with the mother to whom they were bonded.

Statute has intervened in the main to counteract the influence of commercialism which has been such a feature of the American scene. Thus, the Surrogacy Arrangements Act 1985 criminalises a third party who engages in surrogacy for financial gain while, at the same time, freeing the principals from criminal liability (s 2(2)). Payments made to and by way of expenses for the surrogate are not regarded as being made on a commercial basis.[6] There is nothing to prevent the

---

2   *A v C* (1978) 8 Fam Law 170.
3   *Re C (a minor)* [1985] FLR 846.
4   *Re an adoption application (surrogacy)* [1987] Fam 81.
5   [1987] 2 FLR 421.
6   A fairly liberal view is being taken. The complex interplay between adoption and issue of a parental order (see fn 8 below) is also partly based on the 'expenses' issue. See, in England, *Re Q (a minor) (Parental Order)* [1996] 1 FLR 369 and, in Scotland, *C v S* 1996 SCLR 837, IH.

striking of a surrogacy arrangement but any contract implied thereby is unenforceable.[7] A major concession has been made in that, subject to stringent conditions, including that the principals are married, the court may make a parental order providing for the child to be treated in law as the child of the commissioning couple if the gametes of the husband or the wife or both were used to bring about the creation of the embryo;[8] the manifest absurdity of a couple being required to adopt their own genetic child is thus avoided. The Human Fertilisation and Embryology Authority has no direct responsibility for surrogacy but maintains an indirect interest in that artificial insemination or embryo donation are most commonly involved.[9] It is to be noted, however, that the artificial inseminator who works on a 'do-it-yourself' basis is not breaking the law in so far as he or she is not 'providing services for the public or a section of the public'[10] and it is said that the majority of surrogacies are managed privately

The legal position in the United Kingdom can, therefore, be summed up: surrogacy is not unlawful and no criticism is levelled at those who enter into a surrogacy arrangement; a surrogacy arrangement is no bar to adoption provided there has been no element of financial gain but, in any event, a parental order may be available; the courts, when they become involved, will settle any issues on the basis of the best interests of the child and this will depend, in some measure, on the degree of agreement between the parties; and, finally, while there is no bar to a surrogacy arrangement, the terms of that arrangement are unenforceable—the very unsatisfactory situation remains that either side can back out of the agreement without penalty.

Sterilisation

A woman may be surgically sterilised—that is, rendered incapable of having children by natural means—by removal of the ovaries, by section, ligation or diathermy of the fallopian tubes or by removal of the uterus. Similarly, a man may be rendered unable to procreate by removal of the testes or by section of the vas deferens on each side. Removal of the ovaries or testes, which is castration, may cause considerable hormonal upset and is undertaken only in exceptional circumstances.

Medico-legal problems associated with sterilisation relate, essentially, to the validity of consent. This will vary, first, according to whether sterilisation is the primary object of, or merely incidental to, the operation and, secondly, on the competence of the person consenting.

As to the first, while a man may have both testes removed because they contain tumours, by far the commonest form of unavoidable sterilisation is associated

---

7   Human Fertilisation and Embryology Act 1990, s 36.
8   Human Fertilisation and Embryology Act 1990, s 30. In *Re W (minors) (surrogacy)* [1991] 1 FLR 385 an order was made pending the introduction of regulations. See now Parental Orders (Gamete Donors) Regulations 1994, SI 1994/2767.
9   The wording of the 1990 Act suggests that it would not be possible to give a parental order if the surrogate was impregnated by natural means—but the courts would scarcely want to make such a distinction in view of the needs of the child.
10 1990 Act, s 2(1)—but this author, at least, wishes that the draftsman could have been more explicit in several areas. See the problems of Johnson J in *Re Q (a minor) (Parental Order)* [1996] 1 FLR 369. Unregulated surrogacies were a source of major concern to the Review Team (M Brazier, Chairman) *Surrogacy: Review for Health Ministers of Current Arrangements for Payments and Regulation* (1998).

with the removal of the female uterus—either for the eradication of a tumour or as a relief of problems in menstruation. There is no serious medico-legal difficulty associated with sterilisation which is imposed as a price for treatment of such a condition.[11] A competent adult woman is entitled to consent to or dissent from medical treatment for herself whether she is married or not. This implies fully informed consent by the patient (see page 473 below); ideally this might include consent by the husband after the patient has given permission for him to be brought into discussion but there is no legal requirement for his involvement and he has no right of veto. No surgeon can be compelled to operate against his conscience but he would be open to an accusation of negligence were he to refuse to do so and not make alternative arrangements for the patient.

Primary sterilisation is a different matter. Sterilisation may be performed, among other reasons, as a punitive measure, on eugenic grounds or as a form of birth control. The first two are so foreign to British thought as to need no consideration. The ethical issues relating to sterilisation as a form of birth control have long been settled so far as the competent adult is concerned. Some doubt perhaps still remains as to the need for spousal consent to sterilisation as a way of family planning, although the legality of the operation backed by consent of the patient alone is not in dispute—the courts would never grant an injunction to stop sterilisation in either the male or the female.[12] There is, however, a possibility that a 'unilateral decision' to be sterilised might constitute intolerable spousal behaviour and be grounds for divorce;[13] the doctor might well not wish to run the risk of involvement in the proceedings.

The question of incompetence—whether by reason of immaturity or of mental incapacity—and sterilisation is a matter of intense debate, full review of which is beyond the scope of this chapter.[14] Difficulty arises along two, albeit interwoven, lines—first as to what constitutes the incompetent's 'best interests' and, second, as to what distinction, if any, is to be made between his or her therapeutic and social needs. The former is exemplified by the contrast between the classic English case of *Re D (a minor) (wardship: sterilisation)*, in which prophylactic sterilisation was refused[15] and two major cases which came before the House of Lords and in which authority to sterilise was granted on the basis of the patient's best interests.[16]

---

11 Nor is there in respect of the incompetent: *Re E (a minor) (medical treatment)* [1991] 2 FLR 585; *Re GF* [1992] 1 FLR 293.

12 *Paton v British Pregnancy Advisory Service Trustees* [1979] QB 276 at 280, per Sir George Baker P.

13 This was accepted in *Bravery v Bravery* [1954] 3 All ER 59 but a controversial case of half a century ago is a more than doubtful authority. It should be noted that sterilisation before marriage is not grounds for a declarator of nullity.

14 There is a vast literature on the subject. An adequate, short exposition is to be found in J K Mason and R A McCall Smith *Law and Medical Ethics* (5th edn, 1999) ch 4.

15 [1976] Fam 185. The local authority made an application for wardship in order to prevent the sterilisation of a girl who was aged 11 and suffering from severe behaviour problems. This was granted on the grounds that the proposed operation was one that deprived a woman of her basic human right to reproduce; an operation without her valid consent would be a violation of that human right and not solely within the clinical judgment of a doctor.

16 *Re B (a minor) (wardship: sterilisation)* [1988] AC 199. Compare the view with that in *Re D (a minor) (Wardship: sterilisation)* [1976] Fam 185: 'To talk of the 'basic right' to reproduce of an individual who is not capable of knowing the causal connection between intercourse and childbirth . . . appears to me wholly to part company with reality' (per Lord Hailsham LC at 204). *Re F (mental patient: sterilisation)* [1990] 2 AC 1 (concerned with an adult patient). There have been several other comparable cases in the lower courts.

Major controversy surrounded these decisions although the present author feels that insufficient weight was given to the difference in the *degree* of disability in the individual cases.

Nevertheless, despite the fact that Lord Oliver in *Re B*[17] could see no logic in excluding preventive medicine from therapy directed to the incompetent's interests, there *is* a distinction to be drawn between that and sterilisation purely for the convenience of others. Certainly, any case falling in the latter category would have to be brought before the court which, it is to be noted, cannot *consent* to treatment of the incompetent adult;[18] what the court *can* do is to declare the procedure to be not unlawful. In the current climate, it is most likely that the courts will follow the closely reasoned Canadian case of *Re Eve*—in which it was held that 'it can never safely be determined that [non-therapeutic sterilisation] is in the best interests of the person'.[19] It is, in fact, fair to say that some recent decisions indicate a hardening of the courts' attitudes to sterilisation, often, and somewhat ironically, because the carer is providing an exceptionally good environment; there are, accordingly, no 'best interests' to be served.[20]

There remains the problem of civil liability in the event of failure of sterilisation; this is probably the most important medico-legal hazard associated with sterilisation as a method of contraception. Sterilising operations cannot always guarantee infertility. Some techniques are more efficient than others but, in general, the certainty of success is related proportionately to the extent of mutilation. The ethical problem thus resolves itself into balancing the immediate effect against the possibility of a later wish to reverse the procedure—say, on remarriage or on the death of an existing child. This poses a real dilemma. The success rate for reversal of sterilisation by vasectomy in the male is unlikely to be better than 25% and many surgeons would decline to perform an operation that was specifically limited by the patient to one that could be undone. Reversal in the female is likely to be more successful—up to about 75%—but the original operation must have been of limited extent; sterilisation techniques that eliminate the possibility of failure must be regarded as irreversible.

It is the word 'irreversible' that has, in fact, been at the root of many actions in tort or delict that have followed pregnancies after operations for sterilisation—patients who were told the operation was irreversible have contended that this meant they could never have any more children while surgeons maintain that it refers only to the surgical possibilities.[1] There is, in fact, always a small risk that nature will circumvent the operation and re-establish a path for the gametes.

17 *Re B (a minor) (Wardship: sterilisation)* [1988] AC 199.
18 Due to the loss of the parens patriae jurisdiction in England and Wales, despite its persistence in Scotland: see G T Laurie 'Parens Patriae in the Medico-legal Context: The Vagaries of Judicial Activism' (1993) 3 ELR 96. For the avoidance of doubt, nor can the next-of-kin consent as the law currently stands. But, for the innovative approach in Scotland, see Adults with Incapacity (Scotland) Act 2000, Pt 5, discussed in G T Laurie and J K Mason 'Negative Treatment of Vulnerable Patients: Euthanasia by any Other Name?' [2000] JR 159.
19 (1986) 31 DLR (4th) 1 at 32, per La Forest J. Although some cases decided at first instance have come close to taking the opposing view: *Re M (a minor) (wardship: sterilisation)* [1988] 2 FLR 497; *Re P (a minor) (wardship: sterilisation)* [1989] 1 FLR 182.
20 *Re S (medical treatment: adult sterilization)* [1998] 1 FLR 944; *Re A (mental patient: sterilization)* [2000] Lloyd's Rep Med 87 (a very unusual case of a male patient); *Re S (adult patient: sterilization)* (2000) Times, 26 May, CA.
 1 See, in particular, *Thake v Maurice* [1986] QB 644. To be contrasted with *Eyre v Measday* [1986] 1 All ER 488 or *Gold v Haringey Health Authority* [1988] QB 481.

Hence the majority of claims in negligence for failed sterilisation depend not on the performance of the operation[2] but on the degree of warning of failure that was given, and on the consequential question—would the plaintiff have taken contraceptive precautions had he or she been informed of the risk? Essentially, the cases are exercises in 'informed consent' (for which, see page 473).

With a sound technique competently performed, the risk of pregnancy after female sterilisation is very small indeed—but not non-existent. Sterilisation in the male is not so straightforward. When the subjects are tested for the presence of sperm in the ejaculate, it is found that a small number of motile organisms are still present six months after the operation in some 40% of the men treated. Very occasionally, sperm are found later in those who were apparently sterile three months after the operation but, in these instances, the organisms are probably dead. The most serious complication is spontaneous recanalisation of the ducts which may occur in up to 1% of cases

All these considerations must be explained to the patient and to the spouse before consent can be valid. Having done so, the usual rules covering medical negligence apply—if the patient fully understood the risks, if the operation was properly performed and if the procedure was one that was accepted as proper by competent colleagues in the profession,[3] then the mere fact of pregnancy would not be proof of negligence. The proper procedure must, however, include adequate follow-up: this consists of routine examination of the ejaculate[4] and proof by microscopy that the correct tissue was removed.

However, given the fact that negligence has been established, the problem still remains as to what, and under what heads, damages are to be awarded. The solution has traced a chequered pattern through the courts and it suffices, here, to say that the matter has now gone before the House of Lords.[5] The House decided that, while damages were available for the pain and suffering, loss of earnings etc associated with pregnancy, compensation is not available for the birth, albeit unexpected, of a healthy child. Their Lordships left open the question of the birth of a defective infant.

Divorce

Divorce in England and Wales can only be granted on the basis of an irretrievable breakdown of marriage.[6] The position is similar in Scotland, where the grounds for divorce are now consolidated under the general heading of irretrievable breakdown of marriage in the Divorce (Scotland) Act 1976 but a number of specific conditions are taken, either together or individually, to show that this situation exists. One or more of the following must be proved: the fact that the respondent has committed adultery; that the respondent has behaved in such a way that the

2   *Allan v Greater Glasgow Health Board* (1993) 17 BMLR 135, 1998 SLT 580 is an example.
3   The so-called '*Bolam*' test: *Bolam v Friern Hospital Management Committee* [1957] 2 All ER 118.
4   An acceptable regimen would be to require two negative specimens two weeks apart taken two months after the operation followed by a third negative specimen one month later before pronouncing the operation satisfactory.
5   *McFarlane v Tayside Health Board* [1999] 4 All ER 961. This case has been discussed by the author in J K Mason 'Unwanted Pregnancy: A Case of Retroversion?' (2000) 4 ELR 191.
6   Family Law Act 1996, Pt II.

petitioner cannot reasonably be expected to live with the respondent; that the respondent has been in desertion for two years; that the spouses have lived apart for two years and the respondent consents to a divorce; and that the parties have lived apart for five years—in which case, the respondent's consent to divorce is not required.

The English statute insists on, and the Scots legislation encourages, attempted reconciliation; in particular, the continuation of resumption of cohabitation for a limited period—for example, after the discovery of adultery—does not bar a petition and, hence, spouses are not deterred from an attempt to make up.

There is, therefore, surprisingly little forensic medicine associated with divorce. The greater part will involve proof or disproof of adultery and this, in practice, is mainly a matter of paternity. Occasionally, however, the length of pregnancy will be decisive, as may be evidence of sexually transmitted disease that could not have been contracted from the spouse.

Non-accidental injury to married women

Medical evidence must play an important part in the application of the Family Law Act 1996 (Pt IV) when a wife is seeking an injunction against molestation.[7] But what if the doctor notices evidence of physical ill-treatment in a female patient when she has consulted him for other reasons? There is strong evidence that non-accidental injury in married women is a problem comparable in extent with that in children (see Chapter 19).

There is, however, less medical literature on the subject of 'wife-battering', probably because there are essential differences in the aetiology and management of these two types of household violence. The wife who is being ill-treated is adult and capable of taking her complaint to the appropriate authorities. There is no need for the doctor to protect a helpless patient, as applies to babies, and if there is no need there may be no justification for disclosure of confidential information; indeed, there is evidence that many women, whether because of genuine choice or of fear, would themselves resent such an intrusion.[8] The role of the doctor is perhaps limited to counselling not only as to his women patients' course of action but also as to the advisability of the husband being induced to seek medical help; in contrast to fathers who injure their children, many of those who seriously assault their wives are older and suffer from psychiatric disease—in the event of trial, a higher proportion of hospital orders are made than in cases of child abuse. The keeping of accurate records by the doctor, particularly including an assessment of the mental state of the women and of injuries noted in examination but of which no complaint is made, is of equal importance; such evidence might be invaluable in subsequent criminal or civil proceedings.

The concept of the 'battered woman syndrome' has received considerable publicity as a defence available to women who kill their husbands. The defence of provocation involves a 'sudden and temporary loss of self-control' and this is rarely apparent in the circumstances envisaged. It is said, however, that despair,

7   For Scotland, see the Matrimonial Homes (Family Protection) (Scotland) Act 1981.
8   But many wives do seek help, especially from voluntary organisations. See J J Gayford 'Wife battering: a preliminary survey of 100 cases' (1975) i BMJ 194.

anger and fear, rather than anger and loss of self-control, are characteristic of the battered woman syndrome—such a woman would, therefore, react relatively slowly to provocation and the defence would not be wholly denied by the loss of control being associated with what has been described as a 'slow burn'. This was partially accepted in the Court of Appeal in *R v Ahluwalia*,[9] where the 'syndrome' was regarded as relevant to a defence of diminished responsibility—and it may be that the courts will receive a plea of diminished responsibility more sympathetically than they will one of provocation in future similar cases.[10] It is, perhaps, worth noting that the concept of the battered woman syndrome is not welcomed unreservedly by all commentators in that it may make successful defences dependent upon women conforming to a socially restricted image of femininity.[11]

9 [1992] 4 All ER 889.
10 However, the change of emphasis between *R v Thornton* [1992] 1 All ER 306, CA and *R v Thornton (No 2)* [1996] 2 All ER 1023 is to be noted. Here, a woman prepared a knife before stabbing her husband but, by the time of the second appeal, it was agreed that the 'battered woman syndrome' was relevant to consideration in a defence of provocation.
11 See D Nicolson and R Sanghvi 'Battered Women and Provocation: The Implications of *R v Ahluwalia*' [1993] Crim LR 728. For a somewhat cynical approach to 'syndromes' in general, see I Freckleton 'Contemporary Comment: When Plight Makes Right—The Forensic Abuse Syndrome' (1994) 18 Crim LJ 29.

18

Unnatural death of the fetus and the newborn: abortion, child destruction and infanticide or child murder

Few aspects of forensic medicine have changed so far and so rapidly in the last half century as have the legal, medical and social attitudes to the unborn fetus. Induced miscarriage was certainly regarded as one of the more serious offences under the early medico-legal codes and it is specifically proscribed in the Hippocratic oath. Yet, today, the extent to which abortion services are provided is regarded as something of a measure of the community's state of civilisation—and England, with an annual rate of some 12 lawful terminations per 1,000 women aged 14–49, is well up in the premier league.[1] Abortion—or, more correctly, 'procuring the miscarriage of a woman'—is, therefore, no longer an important aspect of forensic pathology. None the less, lawful termination of pregnancy remains an important constituent of medical jurisprudence—murders are committed by opposing sides in the United States[2]— and it is surprising how ill-understood is the relevant law in the United Kingdom. It is mainly from this aspect that the subject will be addressed in this chapter.

The law on abortion, child destruction and infanticide

In England and Wales

The historical background to the present position in relation to both abortion and neonatal killing is most easily described by way of the statutory English, Welsh and Northern Irish law which is contained in the Offences Against the Person Act 1861. This states:

> '58. Every woman, being with child, who with intent to procure her own miscarriage, shall unlawfully administer to herself any poison, or other noxious thing, or shall unlawfully use any instrument whatsoever with like intent, and whosoever, with intent to procure the miscarriage of any woman, whether she be or be not with child, shall

1 The comparable rate for Scotland is about 10 per 1,000 women of child-bearing age.
2 See the Editorial Comment 'This Is a Deadly Game' (1993) 342 Lancet 939.

unlawfully administer to her, or cause to be taken by her, any poison or other noxious thing, or shall unlawfully use any instrument or other means whatsoever with like intent, shall be guilty of an offence.[3]

59.   Whosoever shall unlawfully supply or procure any poison or other noxious thing, or any instrument or thing whatsoever, knowing that the same is intended to be unlawfully used, or employed, with intent to procure the miscarriage of any woman, whether she be or be not with child, shall be guilty of an offence.'

This Act has not been repealed. Abortion remains an offence and subsequent legislation, including the Abortion Act 1967, does little more than define the word 'unlawfully'. There is no mention in the 1861 Act of therapeutic abortion, which was not recognised until the passing of the Infant Life (Preservation) Act 1929.[4]   This enacted (s 1) that child destruction is committed when any person, with intent to destroy the life of a child capable of being born alive, by any wilful act causes a child to die before it has an existence independent of its mother; provided that the prosecution must prove that the act was not done in good faith for the purpose only of preserving the mother's life. For the purposes of the Act, evidence that a woman had at any material time been pregnant for a period of 28 weeks or more shall be prima facie proof that she was at that time pregnant of a child capable of being born alive.[5]

Thus, the Infant Life (Preservation) Act recognised the legal right of a child to a separate existence after the 28th week of intrauterine development and, at the same time, established the unusual crime of child destruction. A child being born naturally cannot be the subject of criminal abortion; on the other hand, a fetus that has had no separate existence—which depends, inter alia, on the neonate having '*completely proceeded* in a living state from the body of its mother'—cannot be murdered. The 1929 Act, in establishing an offence that included killing a child during the process of birth, closed the door on what was, admittedly, more of a permissible defence than a practical likelihood;[6] at the same time, the exemption of 'preserving the mother's life' exonerated the doctor performing a craniotomy for impacted labour— which was by far the most likely form of 'child destruction'.[7]

The relationship between the 1929 Act and therapeutic abortion was, however, both tenuous and uncertain. In referring only to a child 'capable of being born alive', it theoretically had no effect on the existing prohibitions on termination of early pregnancies and these, of course, constituted the great majority of unlawful abortions. Even as regards late termination, the qualification 'for the purposes only of saving the life of the mother' was ambiguous; it was left to case law to establish the limits within which a doctor could legally terminate a pregnancy.[8] A main purpose of the Abortion Act 1967 was to clarify the therapeutic position.

---

3   Amended by the Criminal Law Act 1967, s 12(5).
4   Repeated in Northern Ireland in the Criminal Justice Act (Northern Ireland) 1945, s 25. The 1929 Act does not run to Scotland.
5   The 28-week presumption is retained despite changes in allied legislation: Abortion Act 1967, s 1(1)(a); Still-Birth (Definition) Act 1992, s 1.
6   There is no similar provision in the Criminal Code of Canada, where the case of *R v Sullivan* (1991) 63 CCC (3d) 97 demonstrates the lacuna well.
7   Caesarian section was far less common at the time of the passing of the Act than it is today.
8   The most important being *R v Bourne* [1939] 1 KB 687, the thrust of which was twofold: it effectively extended the therapeutic exemption to early pregnancies and defined 'preserving the mother's life' in terms of 'preserving the physical and mental health of the woman'.   See also *R v Newton and Stungo* [1958] Crim LR 469.

At one time, considerable confusion surrounded the semantics of fetal development. This arose mainly from the use of the phrase 'capable of being born alive' in the 1929 Act and the substitution of this by 'viable' in the Abortion Act 1967, s 5(1). The distinction is of some practical importance, as 'capable of being born alive' merely describes an anatomic-physiologic state; the concept of viability, however, extends this into actually being alive—and even, perhaps, into being alive for a measurable time. Thus, viability results from an amalgam of a physical state and a health care ambience—a fetus may be anatomically capable of being born alive but whether it is viable depends, to a large extent, on the medical support that is available at birth and on the uses of increasingly sophisticated technology. In point of fact, the 'viable fetus' is an American concept based on the three-trimester division of pregnancy established by the Supreme Court in *Roe v Wade*[9]—the state, it was said, had a compelling interest in the survival of the fetus after viability, which was set at somewhere between the 24th and 28th weeks of pregnancy. For obvious reason, the court refused to go further, stating that the diagnosis of viability was essentially one for medical expertise. Thus, viability in this context is a creation of American constitutional law and it has been said that the term has no place in British law.[10] Any difficulties have, however, now been put to rest. First, it was held that a fetus of 18–21 weeks' gestation was incapable of being born alive because it was unable to breathe through its own lungs—with or without the use of the ventilator;[11] the concepts of live birth and viability were, therefore, brought very close together. Later, the court in *Rance v Mid-Downs Health Authority and Storr*[12] put the matter from the other aspect in stating that a child was born alive if, after its birth, it existed as a live child, that is to say was breathing and living through the use of its own lungs alone; the court believed that the word 'viable' was used in the original Abortion Act 1967, s 5(1) as convenient shorthand for 'capable of being born alive'. Finally, s 5(1) has now been substituted[13] and the word 'viable' has disappeared from the statute book. As a corollary, it is important to note that neither case law nor the Infant Life (Preservation) Act defines any age at which the fetus is *not* capable of being born alive. An infant who has proved his or her will to live by breathing after birth has been born alive irrespective of his or her gestational age.

These considerations also have a bearing on the law protecting the infant shortly after birth. The Infanticide Act 1938 provides that the offence of infanticide is committed when a woman by any wilful act or omission causes the death or her child, being under the age of 12 months, but, at the time of the act or omission, the balance of her mind was disturbed by reason of her not having fully recovered from the effect of giving birth to the child or of lactation consequent upon the birth. Thus, the gestational age of the fetus has no relevance to a charge of infanticide per se; all that is required is that the child should have been capable of being killed—that is, it had lived and achieved a separate existence.

When a charge of infanticide is made, it is presumed that the child was born dead unless the prosecution can show proof to the contrary; any doubts that may

---

9 93 S Ct 705 (1973).
10 For discussion, see K McK Norrie 'Abortion in Great Britain: One Act, Two Laws' [1985] Crim LR 475.
11 *C v S* [1988] QB 135.
12 [1991] 1 QB 587.
13 By virtue of the Human Fertilisation and Embryology Act 1990, s 37(4).

exist must be resolved in favour of the mother. The pathological evidence thus assumes major importance and will be discussed later in this chapter. For the present, it is simply emphasised that it may be impossible, even in the presence of only early decomposition, to give positive evidence in respect of a live birth. In such cases, s 60 of the Offences Against the Person Act allows for an alternative charge of concealment of birth. This section makes it an offence for any person to endeavour to conceal the birth of a child by secret disposition of its dead body— that is, disposition in a place where there is no normal access for the public— whether the child died before, at or after its birth; the questions of viability and separate existence are, therefore, immaterial.

The comparative law in Scotland

With one exception, there are no comparable statutes in Scots law, the relevant offences being derived from common law. In general, abortion has been regarded as less of a problem in Scotland than was the case in England and this applies particularly to operations performed by medical practitioners.[14]

In Scotland, as in England, a woman must be shown to have been pregnant before she can be charged with self-inflicted criminal abortion. Moreover, the intention on the part of an outsider to procure an abortion is criminal in both countries—the fact that the attempt is unsuccessful is immaterial; the major difference is that, for a charge in Scotland to be competent, the woman must be pregnant and it is the responsibility of the prosecution to prove that pregnancy. It would be a defence in both England and Scotland to show that the fetus was dead prior to abortion.

There is no Scottish equivalent to the English Infant Life (Preservation) Act. Some very old case law refers to the possibility of destruction of the fetus during birth; it was originally regarded not as homicide but as a serious, albeit unnamed, crime but this view was later disputed.[15] Fortunately, the need for such a charge must be excessively rare.

Nor does the Infanticide Act 1938 apply to Scotland; the comparable crime under Scots law is child murder. None the less, it has long been appreciated that the special conditions surrounding the killing of a neonate by its mother point towards leniency and, in practice, diminished responsibility—which is a product of Scots law—is generally assumed; the crime of child murder is thus reduced to one of culpable homicide. The extenuating conditions can be applied only to the mother in both jurisdictions.

The Concealment of Birth (Scotland) Act 1809 is the only statute relevant to Scotland in the present context and provides that a woman may be convicted if she 'conceals her being with child during the whole period of pregnancy and does not call for and make use of help or assistance at the birth and the child be found dead or be amissing', the presumption being that the child would have been born alive and would have lived unless it had been concealed. This enactment is, in practice, more difficult to apply than is s 60 of the English Offences Against the

14 It is doubtful if Mr Bourne, fn 8 above, would have been prosecuted in Scotland.
15 *HM Advocate v M'Allum* (1858) 3 Irv 187. G Gordon *The Criminal Law of Scotland* (2nd edn, 1978) p 727 prefers the view of Lord Young in *HM Advocate v Scott* (1892) 3 White 240 at 244, to the effect that it makes no difference whether the fetus has or has not completely extruded from the body.

Person Act, principally because the concealment must be total and must be maintained for the whole pregnancy—it must, moreover, be shown that the child was viable not only in the legal but also in the medical sense. A prosecution can, however, succeed in the absence of a body.

The Abortion Act 1967

The precise extent of criminal abortion in the mid-twentieth century is not easy to establish, but it was generally regarded as being so common as to provide the main stimulus to reform of the law on abortion. Even so, the Abortion Act 1967, although widely approved, was controversial at the time and has remained so, despite the fact that the debate in the United Kingdom is relatively muted.[16]

The Act extends to England, Wales and Scotland but not to Northern Ireland.[17] It is remarkable for having remained unchanged for almost a quarter of a century until it was amended by the Human Fertilisation and Embryology Act 1990, section 37. The bones of the Act are still contained in s 1, which now states:

'(1)'. . . a person shall not be guilty of an offence under the law relating to abortion when a pregnancy is terminated by a registered medical practitioner if two medical practitioners are of the opinion, formed in good faith:
   (a) that the pregnancy has not exceeded its twenty-fourth week and that the continuance of the pregnancy would involve risk, greater than if the pregnancy were terminated, of injury to the physical or mental health of the pregnant woman or any existing children of her family; or
   (b) that the termination is necessary to prevent grave permanent injury to the physical or mental health of the pregnant woman; or
   (c) that the continuance of the pregnancy would involve risk to the life of the pregnant woman, greater than if the pregnancy were terminated; or
   (d) that there is substantial risk that if the child were born it would suffer from such physical or mental abnormalities as to be seriously handicapped.
(2) In determining whether the continuance of a pregnancy would involve such risk of injury as is mentioned in paragraph (a) and (b) of subsection (1) of this section, account may be taken of the pregnant woman's actual or reasonably foreseeable environment.'

As has already been stressed, this is not the definitive law on abortion; it is no more than enabling and, indeed, the Act states that 'anything done with intent to procure the miscarriage of a woman is unlawfully done unless authorised by section 1 of the Act'.

The intention of the 1967 Act was to clarify the law in relation to therapeutic abortion and it remains a statute governed by medical considerations. That it was never intended to be a licence for 'abortion on demand' is clear from the number of regulations that must be satisfied to make the operation legal—not least of which is that the operation must be *recommended* by two medical practitioners; moreover, a legal abortion must be carried out in a hospital of the National Health Service or in a place specifically approved for the purpose by the relevant minister.[18]

16 The reunification of Germany, for example, almost foundered on the abortion issue.
17 The situation there can be described loosely as 'post-*Bourne*'.
18 Section 3A, inserted by the 1990 Act, makes special provision for medically induced terminations.

Standardised forms must be used for recommending the abortion and for reporting that an emergency abortion has been performed—in which case, the need for two opinions is waived, as it may be for terminations carried out under s 1(1)(b) and (c). A statutory form notifying the termination of pregnancy must be completed and sent to the relevant Chief Medical Officer within seven days of the event; this contains a number of questions designed to improve the statistical basis of any future legislation.[19]

Nevertheless, the phrasing of the Act is very open and the scope for legalised abortion is considerable—this author has argued that it is extremely difficult for a registered medical practitioner to perform an *unlawful* termination provided the regulations are observed.[20] If nothing else, the risks of termination before the 24th week are almost certainly less than those of a full term pregnancy. Similarly, the legality of termination on the grounds of the fetus' sex appears unlikely at first glance; but it is hard to rebut the argument that the addition of *any* child to the family must have an effect on the existing children of that family, while the addition of a female to the families of some ethnic minorities is certainly likely to affect the mental health of the pregnant woman.[1] Such results probably run contrary to the intentions of the original legislators; yet Parliament and the medical and legal professions have consistently demonstrated their satisfaction with the status quo. Despite this apparent liberality, it is probably true to say that the restrictions contained in the 1967 Act are such that it would be declared unconstitutional in the United States.[2]

It is, in many ways, surprising that such a controversial piece of legislation should have survived unamended for nearly a quarter of a century until a flurry of Parliamentary activity led to some alterations during the passage of the Human Fertilisation and Embryology Act 1990. These changes represented a form of quid pro quo for the contestants. Thus, on the one hand, the fetal age beyond which a termination would not be lawful was reduced from 28 to 24 weeks in respect of those performed for so-called 'social' reasons (s 1(1)(a)). This recognised the paediatricians' increasing ability to maintain and rear the premature infant. On the other hand, no time-bar was imposed on terminations designed to save the life of or to prevent grave damage to the health of the pregnant woman and therapeutic abortion was divorced from the Infant Life (Preservation) Act 1929. Section 5 of the 1967 Act[3] now reads: 'No offence under the Infant Life (Preservation) Act 1929 shall be committed by a registered medical practitioner who terminates a pregnancy in accordance with the provisions of this Act.' This, coupled with the removal of the existing bar of 28 weeks' gestation on terminations because of fetal abnormality, has eliminated at least some of the surgeon's worries when performing a late termination. Previously, delays associated with fetal diagnosis—and especially of chromosomal disease—often placed the surgeon in

19 Abortion Regulations 1991, SI 1991/499; Abortion (Scotland) Regulations 1991, SI 1991/460.
20 For discussion see J K Mason *Medico-Legal Aspects of Reproduction and Parenthood* (2nd edn, 1998) ch 5.
1 In general, it is to be noted that the father has no legal standing in relation to an abortion decision: *Paton v British Pregnancy Advisory Service Trustees* [1979] QB 276; *Paton v United Kingdom* (1980) 3 EHRR 408. For Scotland: *Kelly v Kelly* 1997 SCLR 749.
2 The 'medicalisation' of lawful abortion is a main bone of contention for the women's rights movement. For a very easy commentary, see S McLean *Old Law, New Medicine* (1999) ch 4.
3 Substituted by Human Fertilisation and Embryology Act 1990, s 37(4).

an invidious position;[4] he now faces no criminal charges if he aborts a fetus deemed capable of being born alive, but the problem of the disposal of the living abortus remains.

Terminations after the 20th week are relatively rare and many surgeons who undertake them avoid the dilemma by using deliberately feticidal methods. Others would, however, find this improper[5]—in which case the result may well be an abortus who is breathing or showing other signs of life. Given modern neonatal intensive care, it is difficult to see how a deliberate failure to support such viable entities can, in theory, escape being an offence, including the possibility of manslaughter. On the other hand, the surgeon performing an abortion has effectively contracted to eliminate a fetus and may, therefore, be in an ambiguous position. In the writer's opinion, this should be resolved in favour of the normal neonate but a 'quality of life' decision might be correct in the case of a defective child (see below). Clearly, however, the question of whether or not there was life after abortion may need to be determined—in which case, the pathologist's difficulties will be those discussed at page 266 below but exaggerated by virtue of extreme prematurity. The author feels, however, that a prosecution is very unlikely in the current social climate.

Difficulties also arise at the beginning of gestation which is, itself, ill-defined in United Kingdom law. The Human Fertilisation and Embryology Act 1990 states that a woman is not to be treated as carrying a child until the embryo has become implanted (s 2(3)). This, however, is restricted to being 'for the purposes of this Act'. None the less, since the 1990 Act includes amendments to the Abortion Act 1967 (at s 37), it seems probable that the definition, at least, applies to both pieces of legislation. It is of additional significance that the Attorney-General has said that: 'the phrase "to procure a miscarriage" cannot be construed to include the prevention of implantation';[6] interceptive methods of contraception can, therefore, be excluded from the ambit of the Abortion Act. Rather more difficulty attaches to displanting methods. The Act makes no reference to the duration of pregnancy and it is, therefore, possible that the use of intrauterine devices, which are believed to displace the fertilised ovum, might be illegal.[7] The practice of menstrual extraction, in which the possibility of pregnancy is anticipated by the gynaecologist, is, on the face of things, even more open to question. All such situations deal, in the main, with the theoretical criminality of actions taken by doctors acting from honest clinical motives. Displantation is clearly to be preferred to abortion and it is to be hoped, and expected, that the existing law would be interpreted pragmatically for the benefit of both the profession and the patients.

An example of such reasonable interpretation is provided by the technique of aborting by means of an infusion of prostaglandin rather than by surgery. It has

4   The diagnosis of fetal chromosomal disease involves culturing cells from the fetus or from the chorion—the interface between the fetus and its mother. The practical result is that, in the best circumstances possible, the fetus will be of some 18 weeks' gestation before a diagnosis of, say, Down's syndrome can be made. See, for example, *Gregory v Pembrokeshire Health Authority* [1989] 1 Med LR 81.
5   In 1996, for example, the President of the United States vetoed a Bill of Congress that prohibited so-called 'partial birth abortions'.
6   Parliamentary Debates, Official Report (6th series) col 239, 10 May 1983. In *R v Dhingra* (1991) Daily Telegraph, 25 January, p 5, the judge dismissed the case against a doctor charged under the Offences Against the Person Act 1861, s 58 on the grounds that a woman whose embryo had not implanted could not have been pregnant 'in the true sense of the word'.
7   In *R v Price* [1969] 1 QB 541, CA a doctor was successfully prosecuted under the Offences Against the Person Act 1861, s 58 for so doing but the woman was *known* to be pregnant.

been argued that, in such a situation, it is the nurse who administers the infusion over a period of hours who is performing the abortion, thus contravening the requirements for termination by a registered medical practitioner. It has been resolved that termination of pregnancy is a team effort, the instructions of the doctor being the effective instrument; but it is interesting that this decision was reached by the narrowest of margins with, in sum, a majority of five to four judicial opinions taking the opposite view.[8]

Much of the emotion which surrounds abortion is activated by the health carers' 'Hippocratic conscience'.[9] Surprisingly, however, by far the greatest publicity is given to religious principles—in particular, to those regulated by Roman Catholicism. This author's own inquiries suggest that the Roman Catholic doctrine is not as severe as has been supposed, in that the practice of medicine is a subjective exercise and that the doctor is entitled to follow the dictates of his own conscience.

Be that as it may, many would see feticide for 'social' reasons as lying on a different ethical plane. Despite the arguable claims in favour of women's rights, the moral conflict imposed at this level dictates the need for a 'conscience clause', excusing professionals of a duty to participate in abortions; this is provided in s 4 of the 1967 Act. The dispensation applies only to those directly concerned with the termination. It has been decided at the highest judicial level that s 4 does not apply to secretarial staff[10] but, elsewhere, the situation might not be so clear cut. What, for example, of the hospital porter? And what of the pharmacist in the event that medical abortifacients become 'pharmacy medicines'? No conscientious objection to terminating pregnancy is allowed under the Act when the operation is necessary to save the life of, or to prevent serious permanent injury to, the woman and, irrespective of conscience, any doctor is at risk of civil action should a decision not to terminate be shown in the end to have been professionally wrong.[11] It would obviously be improper for a doctor to attempt to influence his patient on grounds other than those he believes to be in that patient's best interests and, while the Act excuses the medical profession from participating in the treatment authorised, there is no exemption from advising a patient as to the correct medical course—and this will, at the least, dictate that the doctor refers the patient to another who will undertake treatment. Finally, s 4 does not absolve the doctor from treating conditions that have arisen by virtue of an abortion; his duty of care to his patient remains irrespective of his disapproval of the cause of ill health.[12]

---

8 *Royal College of Nursing of the United Kingdom v Department of Health and Social Security* [1981] AC 800.
9 The original 'oath' holds: 'Nor will I give a woman a pessary to procure abortion.' The modern restatement in the Declaration of Geneva (amended 1994) includes: 'I will maintain the utmost respect for life from its beginning.' Full texts of this and other declarations can be found, inter alia, in J K Mason and R A McCall Smith *Law and Medical Ethics* (5th edn, 1999) Appendices A–F.
10 *Janaway v Salford Area Health Authority* [1989] AC 537.
11 In the event of a handicapped neonate being born, an action raised by the mother for wrongful birth would be competent; an action for wrongful life—in which the defective neonate claims the right to have been aborted—is not available in United Kingdom law: *McKay v Essex Area Health Authority* [1982] QB 1166. The problem is, essentially, one of causation—the doctor who fails to recommend a termination under the Abortion Act 1967, s 1(1)(d) has not *caused* the infant's disability.
12 Whereas, in Scotland, a simple statement on oath establishes the doctor's legal position, the burden of proof of conscientious objection in England rests on the person claiming it.

Criminal abortion

Infanticide or child murder, child destruction and criminal abortion are closely related, as all are ultimately referable to an unwanted pregnancy. The pattern and incidence of the basic offence of abortion—and, indirectly, of the other two—has been completely altered by the Abortion Act 1967. There is simply no *need* for unlawful abortion in Great Britain, other than in quite exceptional circumstances—indeed, as we have seen, the only cases which currently come to light involve medical practitioners who either find it convenient to attempt to bypass the Act or who probably do not realise that they may be offending against the law. Fatalities are unlikely in either case and it is improbable that any modern forensic pathologist will see a classic abortion case in Great Britain.

For these reasons, Figure 18.1 has been retained almost solely for historical reasons. In the unlikely event of an abortion-associated death occurring, there is sufficient in the rather large legend for the practitioner to appreciate the problems involved.

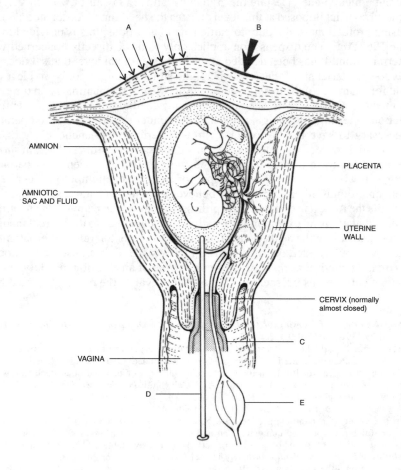

Figure 18.1 Methods available to the criminal abortionist. (A) *The use of abortifacient drugs* include simple purgatives, emmenagogues (the main function of which is to increase menstrual flow) and ecbolics—which promote uterine muscular contraction and which

constitute probably the only group which has a pharmacological effect—prostaglandins are used extensively as a lawful means of termination. It is, however, to be noted that some ecbolics—such as ergot and quinine—have medical as well as abortifacient properties; to be classified as 'noxious substances', they would have to be present in concentrations exceeding accepted therapeutic levels. (B) *Direct violence* may well still occur as a result of a sudden impulse on the part of the male partner. It is, however, more likely to be precipitated in late pregnancy and, if it does not cause the mother's death—which is a very possible outcome—it will more probably result in child destruction. *Criminal instrumentation*: the most common form of criminal abortion involved the use of instruments of some sort. The function of these can be understood by reference to normal pregnancy and delivery. The fetus obtains its nourishment from an interwoven network of blood capillaries on the uterine wall which, at three months, is condensed into the placenta. If this connection is broken the fetus becomes a non-viable foreign body and may be expelled. This mechanism forms the basis of the injection of pastes or of the use of the enema syringe to procure abortion (E). In this connection, it is noteworthy that relatively toxic substances—such as hypertonic saline or urea solutions—are sometimes used in lawful abortions, particularly in late terminations when the possibility of a live abortus arises. Their use significantly increases the risks of late abortion to the pregnant woman but they will be used less often now that child destruction and therapeutic abortion have been dissociated. The fetus is maintained in a fluid medium within the amniotic sac. Drainage of this fluid results in compression of the fetus by the uterine muscle and ultimate expulsion. Any instrument that perforates the amnion may precipitate abortion and there can be few pointed objects—from quill-feather pens to surgical catheters—that have not been employed by criminals for the purpose (D). Dilatation of the cervical canal (C) initiates the normal discharge of a fetus. Artificial dilatation may, in effect, deceive the uterine muscle into believing the time for contraction to have arrived. Certain vegetable substances will absorb water and swell when placed in the cervical canal which is thereby opened. This is the mode of operation of slippery elm bark which was such a favourite of the criminal abortionist because it was likely to leave no trace of interference. Both the lawful and unlawful abortionist may, of course, combine these methods in the surgical operation of cervical dilatation and curettage or suction of the uterine cavity.

Death may follow uterine instrumentation immediately; it may occur fairly soon after the event or it may be delayed. *Immediate death* is the classic 'abortion death' and can arise in two main ways. *Neurogenic inhibition of the heart* can follow any severe abnormal sensory stimulus and has already been discussed in Chapter 1. In the present context it is contact with the inner surface of the cervical canal which precipitates cardiac arrest. *Moderately delayed death*: even if air was not pumped into the circulation, the fluid used, often containing strong soap or toxic antiseptics, could be introduced in the same way. Death from *fluid embolism* might then be fairly rapid but was as likely to be delayed until the effects of tissue necrosis or blood haemolysis had become evident. *Haemorrhage* following laceration of the tissues was relatively common largely due to the laypersons' ignorance of the direction of the vaginal and cervical canals and of the size and position of the pregnant uterus. *Delayed death: sepsis* was once the commonest cause of death after criminal abortion and this was often caused by organisms normally present in the faeces. The most dangerous of these were those causing gas gangrene and tetanus. Many of the complications of criminal abortion are essentially 'shocking' and *renal failure* ensued even if the woman had survived the original crisis. Some deaths were probably associated with *disseminated intravascular coagulation* although the syndrome had scarcely been identified by the time criminal abortion was a problem of the past. Theoretically, all these conditions can follow any surgical procedure but they will be quite exceptional within a modern hospital ambience.

Air embolism

The one exception to this format lies in the condition of air embolism. Certainly, the criminal use of the Higginson's syringe was the most common cause of the condition 50 years ago. It still occurs, however, as a catastrophic complication of several techniques involving insufflation of the pelvis and this remains a suitable point at which to give it mention.

Essentially, the condition of air embolism can be set up whenever there is a combination of the use of gas under pressure in the potential presence of ruptured venules or small veins through which gas bubbles can enter the circulation. The cardiovascular system finds it hard to deal with large gas bubbles; what amounts to an air-lock is established in the heart and death may result. This commonly occurs within about ten minutes of the gas being introduced, although cases have been reported of survival for two hours. The amount of air needed to kill depends on the degree to which the vital organs are embolised—10 ml have been lethal while, in other cases, the injection of 100 ml has been survived.

Nowadays, air embolism may be seen as a result of attempted insufflation of the fallopian tubes for diagnostic or therapeutic purposes; it has also been reported in pregnant women following oral sex-play and as a mishap in the course of lawful suction termination of pregnancy. It could arise as a consequence of laparoscopic investigation and surgery in which carbon dioxide is instilled within the abdominal cavity under pressure. Theoretically, it could occur whenever an intravenous infusion runs out of fluid but this is very unlikely in practice, as the necessary element of pressure is missing. The essential pathological finding which distinguishes death from air embolism from the incidental appearance of air bubbles in the circulation is the 'churning' of air and blood in the right side of the heart into which the veins drain. The circulation of the blood, including that through the coronary system is, thus, halted abruptly.[13] It is to be noted that the production of apparent bubbles in the cerebral circulation is a common artefact induced by removal of the skull at post-mortem dissection; the competent pathologist is, however, aware of this and well able to distinguish such a localised abnormality from the full-blown picture of fatal air embolism.

Potential evidence from the expert witness

Lawful abortion

Death during lawful abortion is extremely uncommon. When it occurs, it is most likely to be due to haemorrhage. As a consequence, the risks of termination of pregnancy increase significantly as gestation progresses beyond the twelfth week.

It is conceivable—although very unlikely in practice—that a pathologist may be called on to establish whether an offence has been committed against the Abortion Act 1967, s 1(1)(a) by reason of the fetus being of more than 24 weeks' gestation. The best assessment[14] is that, by that time, the fetal crown-rump height is 233 mm (range 216–255 mm). The fetus may, however, be mutilated in the

---

13 Air embolism also occurs as a complication of deep sea diving (see Chapter 16) but, here, the mechanism is quite different and the effects are generalised rather than being concentrated on the chambers of the heart.
14 The majority of the measurements in this chapter are taken from W M Krogman *The Human Skeleton in Forensic Medicine* (1962).

process—in which case it may be possible to take the foot length which varies from 42–48.5 mm (with a mean of 45.2 mm) at 24 weeks; it is difficult to measure this accurately and there is considerable overlap—the foot length at 23 weeks, for example, is said to vary from 39–45.5 mm.[15] An alternative would be to consider the presence of centres of ossification of which the most important in the present context are those of the heel—a centre is demonstrable in the calcaneus between the 21st and 25th weeks, while that in the talus can be found between the 24th and 28th weeks. The pathologist's remit may, on the other hand, be to decide whether the fetus lived following extraction; in that case, the methods described under infanticide below should be applied.

Concealment of birth or of pregnancy

Only the mother may be available for expert medical examination in cases involving these unusual charges and proof of recent delivery will depend largely on the clinical findings. The child is likely to have been close to or at full term and manifest enlargement of the uterus may well be found together with evidence of recent stretching of the abdomen—the typical recent red *striae gravidarum*. The uterus remains easily palpable for about ten days after giving birth and the cervix may be flabby and/or torn. A typical bloody discharge, the lochia, persists for some three days to be replaced by a more normal appearing post-partum discharge which lasts for a further week; microscopy of this may prove its nature. Evidence of tearing of the perineum can be of great value—it need not necessarily occur and tears could conceivably be due to causes other than the passage of the fetus; but this is the most likely cause and the extent of laceration may suggest the maturity of the child.

Some time can elapse in cases of concealment—or of infanticide or child murder—before the need for examination becomes apparent. There will, then, be wide variation in the findings, as some women return to normal much faster or slower than the average; it is generally accepted that positive proof of delivery, sufficient to satisfy the court, will be difficult to obtain in the living person after a lapse of eight to ten days. If the body of the infant is discovered, its examination will follow the lines indicated below in the following sections (Child destruction and Infanticide or child murder); it has been noted that there is a rebuttable presumption of a live birth in the Scottish offence of concealment of pregnancy.

Child destruction

The main medical evidence peculiar to this charge concerns the statutory presumptive viability of the child—has it or has it not achieved the 28th week of intrauterine life? The evidence will, again, be based on the general appearance of the fetus and the presence of centres of ossification in various bones.

By the 28th week, the fetus will have developed easily recognisable external sex organs but the testes are not descended into the scrotum; it will have head and body hair together with eyebrows and eyelashes; the skin will be developed and creased; and the nails will almost have reached the ends of the digits. The length from crown to heel is classically 35 cm. This is based on the formula that, after the fourth month, the length of the fetus in centimetres is five times the month of gestation. There will be significant variations about this mean—at seven months

15 Taken from J K Mason *Paediatric Forensic Medicine and Pathology* (1989) Appendix D.

the possible scatter is likely to lie between 33 and 38 cm. The weight at this point is generally between 1.1 and 1.6 kg.

The centres of ossification that appear at or around critical periods include:

24th week:	calcaneus bone of heel;
24th week:	manubrium (upper end) of breast bone;
28th week:	talus bone of heel, first segment of the sternum (breast bone)
32nd week:	last segment of breast bone;
At term:	lower end of femur (thigh bone); cuboid bone of the foot, upper end of tibia (shin bone).

The appearance of these centres is very variable. The table has been simplified and the dates given approximate to the maximum age for, in general, it is the presence of ossification centres that has greatest significance; the negative evidence of their absence is less valuable.

Child destruction is an offence alternative to murder or manslaughter of a child or to procuring a miscarriage unlawfully. As a result, it is very rarely charged on its own and instances are confined to intrauterine death of the fetus following an assault on the mother with intent to harm her fetus;[16] even so, the age of the fetus is important as there is no offence of feticide per se in the United Kingdom.[17]

Infanticide or child murder

The great majority of instances of child murder or infanticide occur during the first 24 hours of the infant's life. The basic pathological problem is, therefore, to distinguish between wilful killing and stillbirth, which has been defined on page 78. It is for the prosecution to prove a live birth and the medical evidence divides logically into two main categories—first, as to whether the child was, in fact, born alive and achieved a separate existence and, secondly, as to indications of an unnatural death.

The pathologist's problem as to 'born alive' stems from the fact that there are two limbs to the diagnosis—to satisfy the legal requirements, the child must not only have 'breathed or shown other signs of life' but it must also have been completely extruded from the mother. Even if there is evidence as to the former, it may be impossible to be certain as to the latter. It may, however, be possible to assert that a live birth was, at least, improbable. The capacity to be born alive depends, as we have seen, on the capacity of the lungs to aerate the body independently of the mother; thus, it is unusual for an immature infant of less than 22 weeks' gestation to be born alive, although the technical skills of the neonatal intensive care unit are continually improving and, at the same time, reducing the theoretical gestational base-line. Monstrous abnormalities of various sorts—in particular anencephaly (lack of a brain)—may or may not be incompatible with life of a sort but the pathologist can generally give a firm opinion; maceration is

16 See *R v Virgo* (1988) 10 Cr App Rep (S) 427, CA, where a man was convicted in such circumstances. Murder cannot be charged because the fetus in utero is not a 'person in being'

17 But if the fetus is born alive and dies of injuries sustained in utero, it can be said to have been killed by dangerous driving: *McCluskey v HM Advocate* 1989 SLT 175. It can also be the subject of a manslaughter charge but not of murder if the intention was confined to injury to the mother: *A-G's Reference (No 3 of 1994)* [1998] AC 245.

certain evidence of this type as it constitutes *aseptic* degeneration of the fetal tissues following death in utero.

Positive evidence of a 'life' may, however, be derived from the post-mortem examination. Major interest then centres on the condition of the lungs which, as described in Chapter 1, are not only without function in utero but are also relatively isolated from the general fetal blood circulation. Fetal lungs are, therefore, virtually solid organs, homogeneous in consistency and colour. The effect of reflex inspiration of air at birth is to expand the lungs, a process which, in turn, initiates the post-natal pulmonary blood circulation; both these processes take time—a matter of minutes—and, until they are fully established, the lung tissue may vary from place to place as to the degree of aeration and of vascularisation. Thus, as the lungs fill the chest cavity, they change in colour from purple to mottled pink and they increase in weight. These general changes can be further demonstrated by the so-called hydrostatic test or by microscopy.

The basis of the hydrostatic test is that an organ containing air will float in water whereas one that does not will sink. Since early aeration will be irregular, the lungs should, theoretically, be tested for aeration one by one and then lobe by lobe—the rationale being that the neonate can be said to have breathed if any parts float. It is customary to decry the hydrostatic test as being both anachronistic and imprecise[18] and, taken to its extreme, it almost certainly is. It appears to the writer, however, to be an adequate practical test which has suffered from being given too great a 'scientific' significance as a single observation; this has resulted in the elaboration of theoretical objections that would be invalid if the post-mortem findings were taken as a composite whole. It is true, for example, that a child could have a separate existence and then develop disease of the lungs of such a type as to make them sink in water; but it is clear that such disease would constitute a natural cause of death and, despite a 'false' result, no harm would be done because the charge of infanticide would rightly fail. The occurrence of a spurious flotation of the lungs is a far more important, and a more practical, objection to the test. This might arise in two ways. First, there is the possibility of artificial mouth-to-mouth respiration having been given. It is said that satisfactory aeration of the fetal lung by this means is difficult to achieve and that, even were it to be effective, the pulmonary circulation would not be started— the appearances of the lungs would, therefore, be different from those of normal breathing. It could, however, be a difficult pathological decision to make. Secondly, there is a very real problem of putrefaction and of pseudo-aeration of the lungs by gas-forming bacteria. Compression of the lung tissue, which fails to remove inspired air but does discharge putrefactive gases, has been recommended to distinguish the two but the manoeuvre is clearly open to inadequate performance and to misinterpretation. It is a matter in the main of common sense and looking at the overall picture—if there is putrefaction of the lungs there will be putrefaction elsewhere. Even so, the near impossibility of diagnosing live birth by way of the pulmonary findings in the presence of even early decomposition is stressed by all authorities and any doubts must be resolved in favour of a failure to breathe. The most objective differentiation is to be made through microscopy; there is little histological similarity between freshly aerated and markedly putrefied lungs but the appearances of aeration *combined with* putrefaction may be very confusing. Some of the microscopic changes that indicate the occurrence of normal breathing

18 For severe criticism, see B Knight *Forensic Pathology* (2nd edn, 1996) p 441.

are subtle, while others depend upon survival for some time; there is no space for their detailed discussion here and the interested reader is referred to the very old, yet still classic, article by Osborn.[19]

Following the definitions of live birth given in *C v S*[20] and *Rance v Mid-Downs Health Authority*,[1] it is doubtful if 'any other signs of a separate existence' are now relevant. Nevertheless, the pathologist will almost certainly be questioned on the subject. The presence of gulped air in the stomach and intestine has been suggested as being valid evidence; anoxic convulsions are not, however, evidence of life and this is the type of sign which could well arise before complete separation from the mother. Presence of food in the stomach or bowel would, of course, be evidence of a separate existence but this would imply long-term survival. The main evidence of this degree of survival is to be found in the umbilical cord, which characteristically shows an inflammatory disposal reaction at the abdominal wall approximately two days after birth. The cord is shed on the fifth or sixth day but the time may be longer or shorter; the umbilical scar is healed in 10–12 days.

There remains the evidence to be drawn as to whether the infant's death was, in fact, due to 'some wilful act or omission'. There are very few limits to the way in which an infant may be murdered—widespread generalised violence, suffocation in its many forms, strangling, including the use of the readily available umbilical cord, drowning and wounding by one method or another are the commonest methods of infanticide. The pathology of all is described elsewhere in this volume and needs no repetition here.

It should, however, be stressed that the differentiation of homicide from accident or from natural disease is exceptionally difficult in the newborn period. Thus, the distinction between death due to natural asphyxia of central origin and that due to the application of a pillow to the face may be impossible, while frightened mothers can and do suffocate their infants accidentally; intracranial haemorrhage due to natural birth trauma may be indistinguishable from that due to deliberate violence; precipitate labour *does* occur and newborn infants *can* slip through the hands to the floor; an infant *may* drown in its own amniotic fluid; the umbilical cord *does* sometimes entangle with the child's neck and distraught mothers may attempt to kill a baby that has never lived. So much depends in each case on the circumstantial evidence and, again, it is the total picture that counts; it would be a brave pathologist who was convinced that he could correctly diagnose every neonatal death on his unsupported post-mortem findings alone.[2]

Nothing has been said about infanticide by omission, and it is the experience of most authorities that deliberate killing of babies by abandonment alone is surprisingly rare. A large proportion of embarrassing dead newborn infants are, however, hidden and this is irrespective of stillbirth or of whether death was due to natural or unnatural causes. Discovery is often delayed and in many instances changes due to putrefaction or animal scavengers may be so severe that the pathologist can do no more than state that there is no way of proving a separate existence. The possible procedures then include a charge of concealment of birth or, far more often, the issue of a certificate of stillbirth.

19 G R Osborn 'Pathology of the Lung in Stillbirth and Neonatal Death' in C K Simpson (ed) *Modern Trends in Forensic Medicine* (1953).
20 [1988] QB 135.
 1 [1991] 1 QB 587.
 2 In practice, custodial sentences for women found guilty of infanticide are very uncommon. For further discussion of the ambience of infanticide, see J K Mason *Medico-legal Aspects of Reproduction and Parenthood* (2nd edn, 1998) p 382 et seq.

19

Injury and death in infancy and childhood

Although only a small proportion of deaths in infants and children are of criminal origin, many of them are obscure and may give rise to suspicion. Lawyers and doctors may find the pathological, sociological and criminological aspects more complex than appears at first sight.

Natural death in childhood

Natural death in the first two or three days of life is especially important, as it is in this phase that child murder is most probable. The proportion of 'neonatal deaths'[1] that arise in the first 24 hours of life is high, varying between 30% and 40%, largely according to the medical skills available; a further 15% occur between 24 and 48 hours after delivery. Thus, approximately half of all such deaths take place within the first two days of life. There is a very close association with prematurity. Over 50% of all stillbirths and neonatal deaths occur in premature babies and the smaller the infant, the less are its chances of survival. Thus, the mortality rate for infants of 26 weeks' gestation is said to be in the region of 44% in the best possible hands; this rises to 100% at 22 weeks and, indeed, the indications are that a biological barrier to survival exists up to 23–25 weeks' gestation. Current survival rates are unlikely to improve using existing techniques and expertise.[2]

Lack of oxygen resulting from damage to the placenta or cord is a common cause of stillbirth but the signs of hypoxia (see Chapter 13) are found in only some 10% of neonatal deaths due to natural causes. Indeed, an autopsy indication of oxygen starvation in a mature infant should give pause for thought. However, deaths due to birth trauma make up what is an important group from the medico-legal aspect because they may be difficult to distinguish from homicidal injury. They are rare in well-conducted obstetric practice and probably account for less than 5% of deaths that follow live birth. Prematurity plays its part here too—the brain of a small baby is particularly susceptible to injury—but, obviously, the unusually large infant is also at risk. Although subdural haemorrhage is rare in

---

1   The 'neonatal' period is defined as the first 28 days of extrauterine life.
2   N Rutter 'The Extremely Preterm Infant' (1995) 102 Brit J Obstet Gynaecol 682.

fetal fatalities taken as a whole (it has a general incidence of about 4%), it is an almost invariable finding in death due to birth injury; since this lesion also results from homicidal injury to the infant's skull, its forensic significance needs no emphasis. In the end result, the true interpretation of a fetal injury discovered in this period may depend upon the combined evidence of the obstetrician, the pathologist and the police authority. It is, perhaps, ironic that the main medico-legal importance relates not so much to the death of an infant during delivery as to the *survival* of one who is, thereby, brain damaged. The law reports are full of negligence actions brought against obstetricians for this reason.[3] It is important to appreciate that the mere fact that an infant is born brain-damaged does not prove that the damage was due to avoidable trauma or oxygen starvation during birth. Many such cases may well result from intra-uterine complications which have no basis in negligence;[4] the problems are, however, too specialised for discussion in a book of this nature.

After the immediate postnatal period, the majority of infant deaths are the result either of infection or of congenital abnormalities. The former are being rapidly eliminated as a result of improved antenatal and postnatal care; major interest currently concentrates on the transmission of the human immunodeficiency virus from mother to child, either across the placenta or through breast-milk.[5] Congenital defects that may result in sudden death of the neonate are confined in practice to the cardiovascular and central nervous systems and to biochemical abnormalities that are not apparent on ordinary post-mortem dissection.

Congenital disease

Congenital disease of all sorts may be due to no more than chance; the more specific diseases, however, can be associated with chromosomal disorders, with genetic abnormalities or with environmental factors. Attitudes and understanding of this group of diseases are changing almost daily as the complexities of the human genome—or the fundamental human genetic constitution—are unravelled. Most readers will now have a good idea of the salient facts but, before considering the actual conditions involved, it will still be appropriate to outline the principles involved as the results of genetic or chromosomal aberrations provoke a fair proportion of medically based family litigation.

Elementary genetics

The normal human nucleus, which defines the 'personality' of the cell, contains 46 chromosomes arranged in two sets of 23 pairs. The sex cells, ova or spermatozoa, are unique in containing only a single series of 23 chromosomes, but this series is

---

3   Of which the type-specific instance is *Whitehouse v Jordan* [1981] 1 All ER 267.
4   Some 23% of infants born between 22 and 25 weeks' gestation will demonstrate severe developmental or neurological deficits at the age of 30 months: N S Wood, N Marlow, K Costeloe et al 'Neurologic and Developmental Disability after Extremely Premature Birth' (2000) 343 New Engl J Med 378.
5   See, for example, European Collaborative Study 'Mother to Child Transmission of HIV Infection' (1988) 2 Lancet 1039. Congenital infection is said to occur in 30% of children born to infected mothers.

formed from a random choice between the constituents of two paired chromosomes present in each parent.

Chromosomes consist of large numbers of genes. These are formed from deoxyribonucleic acid (DNA) and function as templates from which further identical genes can be formed at will through the medium of ribonucleic acid (RNA) which acts as a 'messenger' or carrier of a carbon copy. The original genetic pattern of the fertilised ovum is thereby maintained as the fetus and free-living body are developed.

Save in abnormal circumstances, each paired chromosome will contain one of a pair of genes that refer to the same genetic characteristic; each gene is derived from either the father or the mother but both cannot come from a single parent. These paired genes are known as *alleles*. The allelic genes may be the same, in which case the individual is said to be *homozygous* for that particular factor, or they may be different, resulting in the *heterozygous* state. In the simplest heterozygous state, one of the pair of genes will express itself—or demonstrate its presence—and is therefore said to be *dominant*; the other member of the pair is known as *recessive*—it is still present and available for transmission to the offspring but is overshadowed or obscured by its dominant partner. This can be illustrated in simple fashion by hair colour for which characteristic the 'black hair' gene is dominant over the 'red hair' gene. Figure 19.1 shows that, if a man (or woman) homozygous for black hair mates with a woman (or man) homozygous for red hair, all the offspring will be heterozygotes but all will be black-haired because the gene for red is recessive. But if two such heterozygotes mate, one of four offspring will be red-haired and three will be black-haired; two of the latter will, however, be 'carriers' of a recessive gene for red hair.

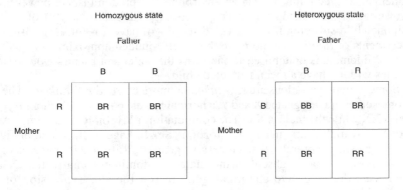

Figure 19.1 Homozygous and heterozygous matings. Either of the genes present in one parent may be paired with either of the genes present in the other; see text for explanation.

A moment's thought will, however, show that the position has been oversimplified, since only a few people in whom it is not a racial characteristic have jet-black hair. In other words, dominance, save in some well-defined all-or-nothing situations, is relative; the capacity of a dominant gene to express itself is described as its degree of *penetration*—a gene of weak penetration may express itself only rarely when all the circumstances are in its favour—and the circumstances will include the status of other genes which may exert an influence on its function.

The concept of the genetic environment is important. It is customary to speak of *monogenetic* disease, in which a disease can be easily attributed to a single gene,[6] and to contrast this with *environmental* disease in which any genetic influence is non-existent or minimal. In fact, the situation is in the nature of a continuum in which genetic and environmental components are always interacting—in other words, almost all genetic disease is of *multifactorial* type. As a consequence, while we may know that a deleterious gene is present, we may well not know what form of disease it will cause nor, indeed, if it will express itself at all. This is one justification for genetic counselling and of all that it implies; if a very weakly penetrating harmful gene expresses itself once in a family, we need very careful analysis as to whether the conditions that encouraged its expression are likely to recur or whether possession of that gene is of no consequence to the bearer.

None the less, the principle of monogenetic, or of predominantly genetic disease, remains of major importance in genetic counselling and, at the same time provides a reason for prohibiting certain degrees of consanguineous marriage. Save in unusual circumstances, it is scarcely possible for a truly disadvantageous gene to be dominant and for the strain to survive;[7] 'in-breeding' must, however, increase the possibility of recessive genes meeting as alleles—the gene which is innocuous in the heterozygous state is then free to express itself with increasing frequency in a dangerous homozygous configuration.

It will also be appreciated that the pattern of genetic counselling changes according to the importance of the genetic component—or the *heritability*—of congenital disease. In the illustration shown in Figure 19.1, we can say that one in four children of the marriage is likely to have red hair; we can, in short, make a mathematical prediction. Given an environmental predominance, however, the best we can say, for example, is that experience tells us that some 10% of families with one child suffering from a given disease will have a recurrence. But such assessments of *liability* are no more than well-founded approximations and the parents' dilemma is epitomised if one turns the statement round—90% of such families will *not* have a second affected child.

Some genetic variations are *sex-linked* or, more correctly, *X-linked*.[8] The sex chromosomes are designated X and Y; a normal female possesses the homozygous alleles XX while the male is XY. The combination YY is biologically impossible since Y is available only in a spermatozoon. Sex linkage is illustrated in Figure 19.2 on the simple premise that a recessive gene is positioned in that area of the X chromosome that is absent in the male. A dominant 'unaffected' X arm suppresses the recessive abnormal gene in the female; expression of the abnormality can only occur in the male while the female remains a 'carrier—the only way for a female to express an X-linked gene is for her to possess two abnormal X chromosomes, a possibility that is unlikely in the absence of 'in-breeding'.

6   Cystic fibrosis is the commonest example in Caucasian populations.
7   Though it can be done. The dominant gene for Huntington's disease, for example, persists because the disease does not manifest itself until after the subject has reached procreative age.
8   Haemophilia and Duchenne muscular dystrophy are prominent examples.

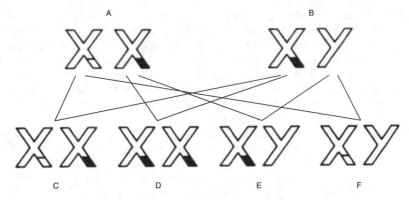

Figure 19.2 Sex linkage. In the illustration, the normal gene absent from the Y chromosome is designated in black, while the abnormal variant is white. A is a female carrier of the abnormal gene which is suppressed by the normal; B is a normal male. Their possible progeny are as follows: C, a normal 'carrier' female similar to her mother; D, a normal female—the disease has been eliminated from that strain; E, a normal male; F, a diseased male—there is no normal X-linked gene available to suppress the abnormal.

Certain severe abnormalities are the direct result of an abnormal number of chromosomes being present—Down's syndrome is, perhaps, the classic example. The numerical abnormality is always an *addition* or *trisomy*—the *deletion* of a chromosome, leading to *monosomy*, is, save in very rare cases, incompatible with fetal survival. It will be seen that, in the majority of cases, chromosomal disease is a matter of chance which can be predicted only in vague terms. Currently, the most important factor determining chromosomal abnormality is maternal age; Down's syndrome is some 15 times more common in the children of mothers aged 40 years (1 in 100 births) than it is in those aged 20. It is, however, to be remembered that chromosomal disease due to translocation—that is when part of one chromosome becomes attached to another—is transmitted to future generations in much the same way as is genetic disease and is independent of maternal age.[9]

Manifestations of congenital disease

Congenital abnormalities of the cardiovascular system are mainly associated with failure of the heart to establish its four chambers with normal relationships—if, for example, the interventricular septum (see page 6) is inadequately developed, one is left with the classic 'hole in the heart' baby. Alternatively, the distinction between systemic and pulmonary circulations may not be achieved or the intrauterine cardiac anatomy (see page 7) may persist into extrauterine life. Many such abnormalities are now detectable in utero using ultrasonography. In general, their occurrence is random with a very low heritability value. However, severe cardiac abnormality is present in some 15–20% of cases of Down's syndrome and is even more frequent in the less common forms of chromosomal trisomy.

9   A very instructive case is to be found in *Gregory v Pembrokeshire Health Authority* [1989] 1 Med LR 8. In practice, the chances of a child being affected are 1:3 rather than 1:4, as the fetuses rendered monosomous will die in utero.

The main physical abnormalities of the central nervous system with medico-legal significance include anencephaly—that is, absence or partial absence of the brain—which often results in stillbirth. Otherwise, there may be obstruction to the normal flow of cerebrospinal fluid that results in hydrocephalus ('water on the brain'), or the protective skeletal covering of the spinal cord may develop inadequately which leads to herniation of the spinal cord or of its surrounding membranes—so-called 'spina bifida'. Again, such abnormalities, which are collectively known as neural tube defects, are now readily detectable before birth; failure to do so has been the basis of several actions for 'wrongful birth'.[10] Only half the cases of congenital mental retardation can be associated with genetic factors;[11] at least one third of these are associated with chromosomal abnormalities but the extent of retardation in, say, Down's syndrome is very variable.

Biochemical defects may be concerned with the metabolism of carbohydrates, of proteins or of fats; when they occur in the neonate they are known as 'inborn errors of metabolism'. Some of these—for example, phenylketonuria—may cause severe and irreparable brain damage; many can be contained by dietary modification—early neonatal diagnosis is, therefore, essential if brain damage is to be avoided.

Environmental factors may interfere with the development of the fetus by reason of a specific insult, the end result depending greatly upon the actual time of the adverse stimulus. Basically, the more primitive the tissue at the time of attack, the more profound will be the effect; hence, infection in the mother—particularly by the rubella (or German measles) virus—or by drugs that interfere with the proper development of the fetus—of which thalidomide is the classic example—will have maximal effect in the first three months of pregnancy. By contrast, the effect of environmental factors that act upon the developed fetus, as opposed to the developing embryo, will increase *pari passu* with growth; in such conditions, of which incompatibility to the Rhesus blood group (see Chapter 31) is a good example, premature birth may be a positive advantage.

These general observations indicate that major medico-legal interest centres on the relationship between congenital disease and the application of the Abortion Act 1967, s 1(1)(b) (see Chapter 18). What, in effect, are the chances of accurately predicting—and preventing—the birth of a seriously handicapped child?

Prenatal diagnosis of congenital defects

The available predictive methods are divisible into so-called non-invasive techniques and those that involve penetration of the fetal environment—that is, the amniotic sac.

Of the non-invasive methods, the use of X-rays to examine the fetus is certainly contraindicated and the technique has now been overtaken by ultrasonic scanning.[12] Estimation of the levels of α-fetoprotein in the serum of the mother

10 In which the mother sues for negligent failure to offer her the option of medical termination of pregnancy. See *Rance v Mid-Downs Health Authority and Storr* [1991] 1 QB 587. Neural tube defects can be markedly reduced by the use of folic acid supplements in pregnancy: N J Wald and C Bower 'Folic Acid and the Prevention of Neural Tube Defects' (1995) 310 BMJ 1019.

11 The Fragile-X syndrome, which is part genetic and part chromosomal in origin, is the commonest cause. As the name implies, it is also x-linked.

12 Whether or not routine ultrasonography is justified is not proved beyond doubt. There are also problems as to consent—eg does the woman who submits to routine examination, say, for estimation of fetal maturity, understand the implications if an abnormality is discovered?

may demonstrate severe defects of the fetal central nervous system before 20 weeks' pregnancy and is effective in some 80–90% of cases. A positive test is, however, probably best regarded as an indication of the need for amniocentesis (see below). For reasons which are less clear, a low level of maternal α-fetoprotein is associated with Down's syndrome in the fetus[13] and there are several other maternal markers of this condition that can be applied.[14] More recently, it has been claimed that ultrasonography of the fetal neck can identify 80% of cases of Down's syndrome at 10–14 weeks' gestation.[15]

The best known invasive technique—amniocentesis— involves the withdrawal of amniotic fluid from the fetal sac (see Figure 18.1, page 262 above) and is more definitive. The fluid obtained can be used for:

- Direct diagnosis, by biochemical analyses, of open lesions of the fetal central nervous system—in particular, anencephaly and spina bifida.
- Culture of cells from the amniotic fluid to detect chromosomal abnormalities— which can be identified after 10–20 days in tissue culture—or to demonstrate inborn errors of metabolism which may entail culture for six weeks before adequate enzyme assays can be made.

The technique has its difficulties. First, there is a 5–10% failure rate in obtaining fluid in the early stage of pregnancy and this may necessitate repeated investigation; elective abortion, if proven to be advisable, may, then, have to be performed rather later in pregnancy than is desirable. Secondly, every amniocentesis carries with it the risk of miscarriage, which follows the procedure in about 0.5% of cases. Thirdly, and perhaps of greatest medico-legal importance, neither positive nor negative accuracy can be guaranteed; although about 95% of the diagnoses of central nervous system lesions and of chromosome abnormalities are correct in skilled hands, enzymatic testing has not yet achieved such accuracy.[16]

The technique of chorionic villus sampling, which involves the removal and study of early placental cells within the first trimester of pregnancy, has been widely used in attempt to overcome these problems. It cannot be used for the diagnosis of neural tube defects; moreover, the technique results in more doubtful chromosomal analyses and in a larger number of miscarriages than does amniocentesis. There is, in addition, a fear that early sampling of the placental tissues may result in limb abnormalities in the fetus.[17] Amniocentesis and chorionic villus sampling are procedures that demand from the diagnostic subject a full

13 H S Cuckle, N J Wald and R H Lindenbaum 'Maternal Serum Alpha-fetoprotein Measurements: A Screening Test for Down's Syndrome' (1984) 1 Lancet 926.
14 A standard 'triple test' is used but this is steadily being developed; the most modern techniques employ four tests: N J Wald, J W Densem, L George et al 'Prenatal Screening for Down's Syndrome using inhibin-A as a Serum Marker' (1996) 16 Prenatal Diagnosis 143. This is said to give a 70% detection rate with a 5% false positive rate. An action for not providing such a test was mooted but does not seem to have materialised: A Ballantyne 'Mother Sues over Lack of Down's Test' *The Sunday Times*, 23 August 1992, p C5.
15 R J Snijders, P Noble, N Sebire et al 'UK Multicentre Project on Assessment of Risk of Trisomy 21 by Maternal Age and Fetal Nuchal-translucency Thickness at 10–14 Weeks of Gestation' (1998) 352 Lancet 343.
16 A combination of the modern techniques of chorionic villus sampling and of recombinant DNA methods has significantly altered the picture.
17 For review, see L C Stranc, J A Evans and J L Hamerton 'Chorionic Villus Sampling and Amniocentesis for Prenatal Diagnosis' (1997) 349 Lancet 711.

understanding not only of all its hazards but also of the implications of the tests. Consent of a special nature is needed—not least as regards what is to be done in the event of a positive result.

The medico-legal consequences of an error in diagnosis include the possibilities of an action for damages on the part of the woman for failure to advise a termination of pregnancy—the so-called 'wrongful birth' action—and by the neonate on the grounds that he or she has been condemned to a life of diminished quality—the 'wrongful life' action. The normal 'rules' of the negligence action will apply (see Chapter 30) and the latter will not succeed in the United Kingdom on the grounds of causation; the laboratory—and a high proportion of such cases involve laboratory mishaps—or radiologist may have missed the diagnosis but they did not *cause* the fetal abnormality;[18] moreover, courts all over the world have found policy difficulties in being seen to prefer death by abortion to life—albeit a diminished life. It is to be noted that the neonate who has been *negligently injured* while in utero has a right of action so long as he or she survives.[19] By contrast, the 'wrongful birth' action is likely to succeed provided the woman can convince the court that she would have agreed to termination had she been given the opportunity;[20] the only common problem may be the quantum and distribution of the damages awarded.[1]

Sudden death in infancy

Sudden natural death in infancy still poses a baffling problem to forensic pathologists, despite the fact that such deaths have declined by some 70% in the last decade.[2] Medical and sociological attitudes are subject to swings of mood which are accentuated by changes in definition which, in turn, depend very much on the current theory as to causation. Some 1:1,000 live-born infants will die suddenly and unexpectedly in their sleep; it is, therefore, customary to speak of these as 'cot deaths' or, in America, as 'crib deaths'. This, however, refers only to the common locus of death and, since this is not invariably the case, it has been the practice for many years to attribute such deaths to the sudden infant death syndrome (SIDS). Briefly, the condition presents as an apparently healthy child being put to bed by unsuspecting parents and being found dead either at the next feed or at normal waking time. The process may be extremely rapid and silent.

Cases may occur between the ages of two weeks and two years—the main incidence is at three to four months. They are reported all over the world but have a seasonal association, the majority of deaths being in the colder months. There is a rather indefinite association with the lower socio-economic groups which

---

18 *McKay v Essex Area Health Authority* [1982] QB 1166, CA. There is a long line of US cases which reach the same conclusion.

19 Congenital Disabilities (Civil Liability) Act 1976; the neonate must survive for 48 hours to be eligible and actions by the neonate against its mother are not available in the present context. The right has always existed in Scotland by way of the common law and an action has probably always been available in England: *Burton v Islington Health Authority; de Martell v Merton and Sutton Health Authority* [1992] 3 All ER 833.

20 *Gregory v Pembrokeshire Health Authority* [1989] 1 Med LR 81.

1 *Salih v Enfield Health Authority* [1991] 3 All ER 400.

2 T Dwyer and A-L Ponsonby 'Sudden Infant Death Syndrome: After the "Back to Sleep" Campaign' (1996) 313 BMJ 180.

may masquerade as an ethnic variation;[3] no type of family is, however, immune—the children of doctors are often stricken. Trends in the incidence of cot deaths are notoriously difficult to assess, as much depends on definitions and on the availability of diagnostic resources—including the use of autopsy as a diagnostic tool; the preferences of doctors in stating the cause of death will also affect the mortality statistics profoundly.[4] Thus, while there does seem to be a significant fall in the number of cases in the United Kingdom, there is less evidence to that effect in the United States and the incidence seems to be rising in France.[5] The condition still presents a major health problem. It also has great social importance. The tragedy in losing an infant child needs no emphasis; added to this, the death, being unexplained and of uncertain cause, attracts a medico-legal inquiry by definition.

SIDS has been defined as the sudden unexpected death of an infant for which no cause can be discovered. The search for a 'cause' of the condition is, therefore, something of a contradiction in terms and, certainly, no satisfactory answer has been reached. Many explanations—ranging from trace-metal deficiency to allergy to cows' milk and including, most recently, exposure to toxic antimonial compounds[6]—have been proposed but no theory can account for *all* cases. The best that can be done is to identify risk factors which predispose to apnoea in sleeping infants. Of these, the New Zealand researchers, among others, have identified socio-economic disadvantage, youth of mothers, lack of breast feeding, prone sleeping position of the child, maternal smoking and bed sharing[7] as being the most significant which, together, may account for the underlying cause of some 80% of cot deaths. Most observers, however, are now content to regard prone sleeping as the major hazard.

There are three definable groups of SIDS. In one group, the death is wholly inexplicable. In the second, which is the largest, some minor abnormality—often in the form of a mild upper respiratory tract problem—can be recalled in retrospect. In the third and smallest group, a manifest illness, unsuspected in life, is detected at post-mortem dissection—but, while such deaths may be 'cot deaths', they should not, according to definition, be regarded as SIDS. Such distinctions are,

---

3   See, for example, E A Mitchell, A W Stewart, R Scragg et al 'Ethnic Differences in Mortality from Sudden Infant Death Syndrome in New Zealand' (1993) 306 BMJ 13, where the high incidence among Maori families was found attributable to risk factors other than ethnicity. Similar factors probably account for the fact that 'cot deaths' in Israel are far more common in Arab families than among the Jewish community.

4   As a result, something of a reaction to the concept of SIDS has developed. See J L Emery 'Is Sudden Infant Death Syndrome a Diagnosis?' (1989) 299 BMJ 1240, in which it is asked if the entity is not a convenient diagnostic dustbin.

5   A useful collection of trends is collected under the heading 'Cot Deaths' (1995) 310 BMJ 7.

6   P J Fleming, M Cooke, S M Chantler and J Golding 'Fire Retardants, Biocides, Plasticisers, and Sudden Infant Death' (1994) 309 BMJ 1594. This suggestion has, in fact, been virtually eliminated: D W Warnock, H T Delves, C K Campell et al 'Toxic Gas Generation from Plastic Mattresses and Sudden Infant Death Syndrome' (1995) 346 Lancet 1516.

7   R Scragg, E A Mitchell, B J Taylor et al 'Bed Sharing, Smoking, and Alcohol in the Sudden Infant Death Syndrome' (1993) 306 BMJ 1312. The importance of bed sharing is an interesting reversal to the problems of 'overlaying' (see p 180). The authors' further studies, however, suggest that bed sharing is a major risk factor only when associated with maternal smoking. For a succinct overview of modern concepts and a review of the literature, see T Dwyer and A-L Ponsonby 'Sudden Infant Death Syndrome: After the "Back to Sleep" Campaign' (1996) 313 BMJ 180.

however, unhelpful, as the effect on the parents—who may have intense feelings of guilt on their own part—will be similar irrespective of the pathological findings.

Sympathetic counselling is, therefore, called for and the medico-legal investigation must be designed so as to cause the minimum additional distress. At the same time, it has to be said that such an investigation, including post-mortem dissection, is needed in every case to exclude the possibility of unlawful killing. The 'cot death story' is widely known and it has been authoritatively estimated that some 10% of cot deaths occurring in an English city a decade ago were, in fact, filicides.[8] The difficulty is to see how such an estimate can be made with accuracy as the autopsy findings in a true SIDS death are, to all intents, indistinguishable from those of suffocation (see page 179). The post-mortem dissection may disclose evidence of criminal activity in the form, for example, of specific external injuries and it is designed to do so. But such findings will be the exception; it would be a brave pathologist who would claim to be able to identify even a majority of filicides in the face of a resolute history of cot death—and it would be even more difficult to prove that they were criminal beyond reasonable doubt.[9] A further complication is that 'confessions' by women to infanticide or child murder subsequent to disposal of a case as a cot death are by no means uncommon. The author's opinion is that the majority of such 'confessions' result from severe psychological stress brought on by feelings of guilt; in any event, since an exhumation is extremely unlikely to provide any substantive evidence, it may well be pragmatically best to regard them as such.

None the less, one cannot ignore the authoritative warnings that are being raised as the known incidence of fatal or near-fatal child abuse rises.[10] Despite the increased distress it would cause the great majority of parents in this position, it might, perhaps, be best to admit to our uncertainty and adopt the habit of stating 'cause of death unascertained' when that is a true reflection of the findings. But to do so would involve a major change of medico-legal policy.

Accidental death in childhood

Many forms of accidental death that are likely to occur in childhood are discussed in specific terms under the various headings in this book. Childhood deaths do, however, form a special group—first, because there is a volume of legislation aimed at protection of the very young and, as a consequence, an offence may have been committed despite the undisputed fact that death was accidental, while, secondly, the most common defence against a charge of infanticide, child murder or homicide of a young person is to suggest that the fatal injury resulted from an accident—the pathological distinction is of major importance and may be very difficult to make.

Many accidental deaths in this age group are asphyxial in nature and, of these, death from burning is comparatively common—some 100 children die from this

---

8 J L Emery 'Infanticide, Filicide, and Cot Death' (1985) 60 Arch Dis Childh 505. Similar claims have been made more recently: R Meadow 'Unnatural Sudden Infant Death' (1999) 80 Arch Dis Childh 7.

9 For a good example of the subjectiveness involved, see 'In the matter of an inquest into the death of Adam Bithell, deceased' (1986) 150 JP 273.

10 Eg M A Green 'Time to Put "Cot Death" to Bed?' (1999) 319 BMJ 697.

cause in England and Wales each year.[11] Infants and children may be left unattended and be killed as a fire engulfs a whole house or hotel; this is the commonest form of death by burning. Non-fatal thermal injury is more common when children accidentally pour boiling liquids from the stove on to themselves as a result of curiosity or they are exposed to an unguarded fire. Very severe injuries can result if the clothes are then accidentally lit—but this source of injury and death has been greatly reduced by regulations.[12] Moreover, it is an offence for any person of the age of 16 or over having charge of a person under the age of 12 (or 7 in Scotland), without taking reasonable precautions, to allow the child to be burned or scalded by reason of being in a room containing an open-fire grate or any heating appliance insufficiently protected to guard against the risk of the child being injured.[13]

The same Acts[14] also refer to the relationship of acute alcoholism and suffocation by overlaying in bed, a charge of neglect being possible if a child under three years old has been overlaid by a person aged 16 years or more who was under the influence of drink. Asphyxial deaths in sleeping accommodation—be it crib, pram, cot or parents' bed—pose special problems. They may, as discussed before, be natural and they may be accidental. It has, however, to be reiterated that accidental asphyxia in infancy must be accepted as a cause of death with caution. Just as in distinguishing a cot death from child murder, it may be difficult, if not impossible, from the pathological findings alone, to distinguish a baby that has been accidentally trapped face down on its pillow from one that has been forced; a visit to the scene and discovery of ancillary evidence may be essential to the correct diagnosis. Similar considerations surround the occasional case in which, for example, an infant is strangled by its restraining harness; such deaths do certainly occur but, again, the correct diagnosis depends very much on the circumstantial evidence.

Accidental drowning in children may, of course, occur amongst the older age group while at play or among toddlers who fall into unprotected garden pools or swimming pools; the latter is scarcely a hazard in the United Kingdom but has been a very potent cause of childhood deaths in, for example, Australia where the incidence has been markedly reduced by the use of isolation fencing.[15] Drowning in infancy happens not uncommonly in the bath; death, when accidental, is often due to neurogenic inhibition of the heart—the baby slips backwards and water contacts the nasopharynx and larynx; as in adults, the finding of the conventional signs of drowning after death in the bath should arouse suspicion. A surprising number of infant drownings occur in buckets—the child slips head-first into to a large container and has no means of egress.[16]

---

11 See D Cohen 'Accidental Injury in Childhood' in J K Mason (ed) *The Pathology of Trauma* (2nd edn, 1993) ch 12.
12 Nightwear (Safety) Regulations 1985, SI 1985/2043, as amended by Nightwear (Safety) (Amendment) Regulations 1987, SI 1987/286.
13 Children and Young Persons Act 1933, s 1; Children and Young Persons (Scotland) Act 1937, s 22. Should death or serious injury result, the penalty on summary conviction is a fine not exceeding £50!
14 Section 1(2)(b) of the 1933 English Act and s 12(2)(b) of the Scottish Act.
15 Interestingly, there is considerable debate in Australia as to whether pool fencing should be enforced by statute: V F Carey 'Childhood Drownings: Who is Responsible?' (1993) 307 BMJ 1086.
16 M I Jumbelic and M Chambliss 'Accidental Toddler Drowning in 5-gallon Buckets' (1990) 263 J Amer Med Ass 1952. See also J C Giertsen 'Drowning' in J K Mason and B N Purdue (eds) *The Pathology of Trauma* (3rd edn, 2000) ch 16.

Asphyxia of central nervous system origin usually results from drug overdosage and is a tragically common cause of accidental death in younger children. The subject is discussed in greater detail in Chapter 21. Deaths in older children due to solvent abuse are also still common in the larger cities.[17]

Infant deaths due to road-traffic accidents are relatively rare, due mainly, one suspects, to the improbability of drivers being drunk when transporting the baby. In older infancy and early childhood, automobile tragedies occur through inadvertent opening of car doors; child safety locks provide problems of their own, particularly in relation to escape from a post-crash fire. The importance of adequate harness restraint for children in cars has been discussed in Chapter 10; death due to cervical spinal fracture used to be common in children subjected to quite minor deceleration trauma while standing unrestrained in vehicles. The frequency of pedestrian deaths in childhood needs no emphasis. In one major study, 76% of fatal head injuries in children (median age 10) were sustained in road-traffic accidents; 69% of the victims were pedestrians.[18] Deaths of this type are doubly distressing, in that they have emotional effects not only on the bereaved parents but also on the driver who, especially where this age group is concerned, may well have been blameless.[19] Children may fall down the stairs or out of windows; again, the distinction between accident and homicide must depend very largely on the circumstantial evidence.

Children at play present a special problem. The provision of playgrounds is now expected and the apparatus is often used by children older than those for whom it was intended. Moreover, swings and roundabouts tend to be operated by the older children to an extent beyond the capacity of toddlers. Head injury and limb fractures are not uncommon results and, reverting to Sharples' study,[20] 53% of fatal accidents occurred while the child was at play; interestingly, the great majority of these were due to falls, which accounted for 12% of all the deaths.

The isolated head injury presents a difficult diagnostic problem in infant deaths. Such injuries are often explained as 'the baby slipped off my shoulder while I tried to turn on the light', or 'I fell down the stairs with the baby in my arms'. There is no doubt that such accidents do occur and it may be impossible purely through the pathological findings to distinguish the resultant injuries from those caused by deliberate dropping of the baby from comparable positions. False explanations of this type are, however, used to cloak deliberate injury of a different type—homicidal head injuries in infancy are often caused by direct manual violence or by swinging the child by the feet against a wall or other solid object. Certain features may help to distinguish these injuries in the post-mortem dissection. First, there is the degree of injury that may be greatly in excess of that likely from the given explanation. Secondly, the position and external appearances

17 C H Ashton 'Solvent Abuse' (1990) 300 BMJ 135. Deprivation is a common associate: A Esmail, B Warburton, J M Bland et al 'Regional Variations in Deaths from Volatile Solvent Abuse in Great Britain' (1997) 92 Addiction 1765.

18 P M Sharples, A Storey, A Aynsley-Green and J A Eyre 'Causes of Fatal Childhood Accidents Involving Head Injury in Northern Region, 1979-86' (1990) 301 BMJ 1193.

19 In Sharples' study, ((1990) 301 BMJ 1193, fn 18 above), it was concluded that the child's unsafe behaviour was the primary cause of the accident in 89% of pedestrian deaths.

20 Fn 18 above. See also older the Australian experience in J Nixon, J Pearn and I Wilkey 'Death during Play: A Study of Playground and Recreation Deaths in Children' (1981) 283 BMJ 410.

of the injury may give rise to suspicion. Thus, a blow from the hand may leave no external mark and the resulting deep bruising and fracture may be markedly localised to one side of the head, whereas injuries due to a fall which is uncomplicated by bruising of the shoulder or arm are more likely to be vertical in presentation. The most important cause for suspicion is the unexpected finding of a head injury in a death purported to be natural—the great majority of genuine accidental injuries will be reported immediately to the doctor.

Child abuse

Despite the manifest improvements in social welfare and the widespread availability of services such as counselling, child abuse persists in all communities, including those of the western world. Until relatively recently, it has been customary to equate child abuse with physical abuse or deliberate injury of children.[1] It is, however, now apparent that abuse can take other, and sometimes more subtle, forms so as to include:

* physical abuse;
* sexual abuse;
* child neglect;
* emotional abuse;
* child poisoning;
* Münchhausen syndrome by proxy.

Some of these conditions are dealt with elsewhere in this book. Here, it is intended to concentrate mainly on those aspects which demonstrate visible physical signs and, especially, those which may lead to death.

Physical abuse or non-accidental injury in childhood

From approximately 1945, a syndrome describing head injury and multiple limb fractures in children[2] was regarded as a clinical entity; only in the mid-1950s was it realised that these children were suffering from repeated injury inflicted by those responsible for their care—generally including one or both parents. This condition—'repetitive non-accidental injury in childhood'—is commonly known as the 'battered baby' syndrome, an emotional term which was chosen deliberately by Kempe, to whom must go the major credit for bringing the subject to public notice.[3]

Children often come to autopsy as a result of such treatment, but death of the child is seldom anticipated in the circumstances under consideration. The main bulk of sufferers present as clinical and sociological problems; one of the most

---

1 For a useful overview, see B Knight 'The History of Child Abuse' (1986) 30 Forens Sci Internat 135.
2 For the historically minded, the original paper is J Caffey 'Multiple fractures in the long bones of infants suffering from chronic subdural hematoma' (1946) 56 Amer J Roentgenol 163.
3 The original paper is by C H Kempe et al 'The Battered Child Syndrome' (1962) 181 J Amer Med Ass 17. For a lawyer's appraisal of 'syndromes' in general, see I Freckelton 'When Plight Makes Right—The Forensic Abuse Syndrome' (1994) 18 Crim LJ 29.

disturbing features is that violence breeds violence—a high proportion of those who deliberately injure their children were themselves the objects of similar assault. Estimates vary as to the number of children who will die each year as a result of being 'battered' in Great Britain. It has been put as high as between 450 and 750, but a more realistic figure, supported by the NSPCC, is in the region of 100 per annum.[4] These derive from a total of some 5,000 affected; 20% of these will be seriously injured. These figures are based on rather old statistics and comparable more modern estimates are hard to find—largely because of changing and extended definitions. A significant finding was, however, reported in 1987, when the incidence of *severe* injury was found to be falling while that of relatively minor nature was increasing markedly.[5] The probable explanation is that the *reporting* of rather than the *incidence* of injuries was increasing, and this is very much an area in which it is difficult to compare like with like over time because fashions in definition and reaction fluctuate. While there is no intention to underestimate the importance of the condition, it is only right to point out that, on occasion, the pendulum may swing too far and injuries that are truly accidental are reported as being non-accidental; in one study, 2.6% of referrals for physical abuse were found to have been wrongly diagnosed.[6]

While it is not to be supposed that conditions are similar in the United Kingdom and the United States, more recent figures from the latter country indicate that demonstrable serious harm actually increased from 2.3 to 8.5 cases per 1,000 children between 1986 and 1993. At the same time, the incidence of fatal injury remained steady at 2 per 100,000 children and that of moderate injury was also little changed (13.9 rising to 14.7 cases per 1,000 children in 1993). Some suggestion that increased awareness and/or reporting was operating arises from the figures for 'endangered' children, which rose from 4 to 15.4 per 1,000 children in the same period.[7]

The clinicosocial expression of the condition is difficult to summarise but, in general, the following may be found:

- The family is often inadequate, maladjusted, immature and under social stress.
- The child is usually aged less than four years and over half the cases, both fatal and non-fatal, are reported in the first two years of life.
- There is often a delay in, or failure of, reporting the injuries to the medical practitioner and a false explanation of their cause is then given.
- The commonest injuries are bruises and fractures, the latter being predominantly of the chest cage (especially the back), long bones and skull. Burns and bite marks are sometimes seen and severe injury to the abdominal viscera may occasionally be present. Injuries to the inside of the lips or the

4   The higher figure was given in 'A guide to management of non-accidental injury in children' prepared by a Working Party in the Department of Child Health, University of Newcastle-upon-Tyne (1973) iv BMJ 657. The *Report of the Committee on Child Health Services* (S D M Court (Chairman) (Cmnd 6684, 1976)), quoted, without comment, figures from the British Paediatric Association indicating an annual mortality of 350–400. A far lower estimate was given in A D M Jackson 'Wednesday's Children' (1982) 75 J Roy Soc Med 83.
5   J Jenkins and O P Gray 'Changing Incidence of Non-accidental Injury to Children in South Glamorgan' (1987) 294 BMJ 1658.
6   D M Wheeler and C J Hobbs 'Mistakes in Diagnosing Non-accidental Injury: 10 Years' Experience' (1988) 296 BMJ 1233.
7   D Sharp 'Preliminary Results of Latest US Child Abuse Survey Released' (1996) 348 Lancet 606.

gums and dislocation of the teeth are almost diagnostic. Bizarre variations include injuries due to immersion. The child nearly always shows evidence of emotional and, sometimes, physical deprivation.
* The most important diagnostic feature is that the injuries have been caused at different times.

Examination of the living should include, whenever possible, photography and radiography—these provide invaluable evidence of a permanent nature. Expert radiological support is also essential in eliminating diseases of bone which may predispose to accidental fracture—such as osteogenesis imperfecta and copper deficiency—and in distinguishing conditions which mimic healing fractures—such as scurvy or, although now improbable, congenital syphilis; radionuclide imaging may also be employed with advantage.[8] A re-examination of a child suspected of being 'battered' some 24–48 hours after suspicions have been aroused is often helpful—bruises, in particular, may become more obvious and new ones may have appeared.

These classic clinical signs will be mirrored in fatal cases at post-mortem dissection, which must include a full radiological study as a routine—the plates are invaluable not only as evidence of injury and its dating but also in assessing the role of bone disease as a causative or contributory factor. The examination should also include a microscopic study of the wounds in an attempt to establish their various ages. Death is often due to some terminal excessive injury resulting in cerebral or abdominal haemorrhage. The former is almost always in the form of sub-dural haemorrhage and results not so much from direct violence as from shaking the child—the relatively large size of the head renders the very young child especially susceptible;[9] the latter is commonly due to direct violence and involves either the liver and/or the bowel where tethered and mobile segments meet—as at the duodeno-jejunal junction.

Considerable advances have been made in the care of children at risk, responsibility for the safety of whom rests with the Director of Social Services of the relevant local authority. The social services, the NSPCC or the police may apply to the court to have a child placed in care.[10] The police have strictly constrained emergency powers to keep a child in a safe place for up to 72 hours if they believe that the child might otherwise suffer significant harm[11] and the court may, on application by an officer of the NSPCC or other designated person, make a care or a supervision order which may last, at first instance, for eight weeks;[12] this is subject to satisfaction that the child is suffering, or is likely to suffer, significant harm and that the harm results either from inadequate parental care or from the child being beyond parental control.[13] As a preliminary or as an alternative

---

8 See K T Evans and G M Roberts 'Radiological Aspects of Child Abuse' in J K Mason (ed) *Paediatric Forensic Medicine and Pathology* (1989) ch 19, for thorough discussion.
9 For an outstanding review, see J K Brown and R A Minns 'Non-accidental Head Injury, with Particular Reference to Whiplash Shaking Injury and Medicolegal Aspects' (1993) 35 Develop Med Child Neurol 849; H Carty and J Ratcliffe 'The Shaken Infant Syndrome' (1995) 310 BMJ 344.
10 The court may be the Family Proceedings Court, the County Court or the High Court (Children Act 1989, s 92(7)). See Family Proceedings Courts (Children Act 1989) Rules 1991, SI 1991/1395; Children (Allocation of Proceedings) Order 1991, SI 1991/1677.
11 Children Act 1989, s 46.
12 Children Act 1989, s 31.
13 Children Act 1989, s 31(2).

to this, the court may make a child assessment order, the conditions for which are likely to cause less conflict with the parents.[14] The whole system is designed for the benefit of the child and the child's interests must be paramount in respect of any decisions taken;[15] the court must arrange for the child to be represented by a guardian ad litem or a solicitor unless satisfied that it is an unnecessary safeguard of the child's interests.[16] Appeal against the decision of the Family Proceedings Court is to the High Court. The evidence given by the person seeking a care or supervision order is confidential and the informant's name need not be divulged to the parents; moreover, the local authority are not liable in damages for its actions in child care cases.[17] It is to be noted that the common law right to apply for wardship of a child is not removed by the 1989 Act and the High Court retains its inherent jurisdiction—albeit with considerable ring-fencing (1989 Act, s 100). The High Court can also issue a specific issue order for the purpose of determining a specific question that has arisen in respect of any aspect of parental responsibility.[18]

The care situation in Scotland is regulated by the Children (Scotland) Act 1995, under which the protection of children at risk is vested primarily in the Reporter to the Children's Panel. The conditions under which a child may be considered to be in need of compulsory measures of supervision are detailed in s 52(1), where it will be seen that they are more detailed and more specific than is the case in England. Each local government area has an established Children's Panel made up of members of the community approved by the Scottish Ministers (Sch 1). Cases are heard at a Children's Hearing (s 39(3)) and appeal, by child or parent, is to the sheriff or to the Court of Session on a point of law. Emergency procedures very similar to those in England are available. Under both jurisdictions, the reporting in the newspapers or elsewhere of proceedings involving children is forbidden.

Non-accidental childhood injury raises questions of medical confidentiality. Doctors, possibly alerted by the health visitor, are likely to see the injured baby first and the medical profession cannot abnegate its obligations for eliminating a condition that, in morbidity alone, is a serious problem for society. Since the doctor's responsibility is to the patient, who is, in this case, the child, there can be no ethical contraindication to reporting the case[19] but such reports should be

---

14 Children Act 1989, s 43. It is to be noted that the application of the traditional wardship jurisdiction is now strictly limited by the Children Act 1989, s 100: *Re T (a minor) (care: termination of contact)* [1994] Fam 49. Placing children in care, coupled with refusal of further parental contact, does not conflict with the parents' human rights: *Re F (minors) (care proceedings: contact)* [2000] 2 FCR 481.

15 And this will include such factors as the effect of having a 'father' on the child's self-esteem: *Re C and V (minors) (prenatal responsibility order)* [1998] 1 FLR 392.

16 Children Act 1989, s 41. The guardian ad litem would also be a suitable co-ordinator to collate the reports of expert witnesses: In *Re C (Children Act: expert evidence)* [1995] 1 FLR 204.

17 *D v National Society for the Prevention of Cruelty to Children* [1978] AC 171; *X v Bedfordshire County Council* [1995] 2 AC 633. The European Commission of Human Rights considered an application for review of the latter case to be admissible but no further reports are available: *TP and KM v United Kingdom* (Application 28945/95).

18 Children Act 1989, s 8. For example, *Camden London Borough Council v R (a minor) (blood transfusion)* [1993] 2 FLR 757.

19 Indeed, the General Medical Council regards the reporting of cases to the appropriate authority as being close to a requirement: *Guidance to Doctors: Confidentiality* (1995) para 11.

made in the first instance to the Department of Social Services (or the children's department of the Area Health Services)—who have a clear 'right to know'—rather than to the police, whose right to know is secondary to the establishment of criminal activity. The practical alternative is to arrange for admission to a paediatric hospital with the express purpose of protecting the patient; the wide consultation that is regarded as important in the management of the children is best arranged from such a unit. Primary among such procedures will be the calling of a case conference. Doctors may fear that their attendance at such conferences involves a breach of medical confidentiality; none the less, such a breach is justified in the patient's best interests and it could be that a doctor who jeopardised the management of his child patient by refusal to participate could be held to be negligent.[20]

There are other practical problems in relation to repetitive non-accidental childhood injury which lie in the sphere of criminology. The predisposing conditions must be dealt with correctly and, in fatal cases, the pathological examination has its role to play in fully defining the nature and the sequence of the injuries discovered. This may affect the outcome of any criminal trial. A murderous attack on a child can seldom be excused on medical grounds; by contrast, the establishment of a true 'battered baby syndrome', which is widely accepted as the outcome of a psychosocial disorder, may properly result in conviction for culpable homicide or manslaughter rather than murder and be followed by equally enlightened sentencing. However, some disillusionment is becoming evident among paediatricians. Certainly, there would seem to be two essentially different groups involved. On the one hand, there are those unstable parents who, in a perpetual state of exasperated inability to cope with family life, resort to violence as the only apparent escape from such pressures; these persons may well be treated as social invalids. On the other hand, parents who subject their children to deliberate torture by seating them on electric fires, burning them with cigarettes, biting and the like cannot deserve public sympathy. The pathologist makes a major contribution to criminology in distinguishing between these two types of inflictors of injury.

Deliberate injury to children is a social evil which cannot be solved by unilateral action—be it on the part of the medical profession, the health visitors, the social workers or the police. It is a problem that emphasises particularly well the interdependence of forensic and community services in the protection of the individual.[1] Emotion is, however, an uneasy motivator and it is well to remember the alternative view which is that the existence of 'at-risk registers' and the like may serve to frighten parents who have no cause for guilt; children who are genuinely accidentally injured may, as a result, be deprived of necessary treatment. The placing of children on an 'at risk' register is a serious matter, which is subject to judicial review, albeit rarely.[2] Finding the correct balance of views may be less easy than appears at first sight.

---

20 A Harris 'General Practitioners and Child Protection Case Conferences' (1991) 302 BMJ 1354.
1 See the Department of Health and Social Security *Working Together* (1988).
2 *R v Norfolk County Council, ex p M* [1989] QB 619. The court will maintain a strict attitude as to what constitutes parental abuse and the line between correction and abuse may, at times, seem unclear: *R v East Sussex County Council, ex p R* [1991] 2 FLR 358.

Sexual abuse

While physical abuse of children was, perhaps, a major disclosure of the mid-twentieth century, sexual abuse has only come to the fore in its later decades; there is little doubt that the greater part of any increase in reported abuse can be attributed to the sexual component. It is best discussed in Chapter 20. Here, it need only be said that the difficulties associated with suspicion, diagnosis and disposal that have been described in relation to physical abuse are magnified in the ambience of sexual abuse where the physical signs are very much more open to interpretation. Individual examiners also have differing approaches to their work. The clinical paediatrician, sponsored by the social services, is happy to see his 'patient' being offered satisfactory therapy; moreover, the burden of proof of abuse for the purposes of the Children Act 1989 is on the civil standard of a balance of probabilities.[3] The police surgeon, by contrast, knows that his evidence is likely to be tested beyond reasonable doubt in the criminal court. Conceptual conflicts are bound to occur but will be minimised if joint examinations are carried out[4]—a practice which also limits the *number* of examinations and which is, therefore, greatly to the benefit of the child concerned.

A relatively recent report has looked at the subject from the angle of prosecution of those accused.[5] Just under 40% of males accused of sexual abuse were taken to court and 86% of these were convicted; interestingly, none of nine women accused were prosecuted. The results probably reflect a 'prosecution policy' rather than a true estimate of the extent of the problem. The whole subject has now come to be clouded by what is termed the 'recovered memory' or, significantly, 'false memory' syndrome, as a result of which, it is claimed, adults can retrieve memories of unpleasant incidents—especially involving sexual abuse—that occurred in childhood. Clearly, it is possible to instil false memories by repeated interviewing and the distinction from a true repression of memory may be difficult to make.[6] The subject is considered in Chapter 27.

Child neglect

Neglect is probably that form of abuse which is most likely to lead to death. The results are often horrific and cases, when discovered, tend to generate a great deal of public concern.[7] The subject has, however, been discussed in Chapter 14. Neglect inevitably involves an element of *emotional abuse*. Physical signs when the latter is operating alone are, however, of a collateral significance only. The distinction between relatively normal family stresses and emotional abuse may be difficult and, in general, there must be evidence of harm or, at least, a likelihood

---

3   In *Re G (a minor) (child abuse: standard of proof)* [1987] 1 WLR 1461.
4   As recommended in Lady Justice Butler-Sloss (Chair) *Report of the Inquiry into Child Abuse in Cleveland, 1987* (1988). It is noted that the courts believe that the recommendations in this report should be followed in all cases: In *Re E (a minor)* (1991) 1 FLR 420.
5   C S Lazaro, A M Steele and L J Donaldson 'Outcome of Criminal Investigation into Allegations of Sexual Abuse' (1996) 75 Arch Dis Childh 149.
6   For a recent overview, see S Brandon 'Recovered Memories: Some Aspects of the Controversy' (1999) 67 Med-Leg J 25. The majority of actions under this umbrella would be time-barred in the United Kingdom: *Stubbings v Webb* [1993] AC 498, HL.
7   See, for example, *Report of the Committee of Inquiry into the Care and Supervision Provided in relation to Maria Colwell* (1974).

of harm before a child can be put on the child protection register.[8] The subject is essentially one for the specialist paediatric psychiatrist.[9]

Münchhausen's syndrome by proxy

This unusual condition, first described in 1977,[10] is also of primary interest to psychiatrists but, because of its effects, it is equally important to physicians and surgeons. The condition, which consists essentially of the fabrication of illness in a child by its mother or other carer, throws up a number of anomalies. Ought it to be regarded as a maternal illness that should be managed by doctors or as, primarily, a matter of child abuse that should lie in the province of the local authority? It is said that the underlying motivation is the mother's concern for supposed illness in her child which will go unattended by the doctors unless they can be convinced by symptoms; others, however, contend that the mother is seeking attention for herself, as was described by Meadow in his prototype case. It is also to be noted that, in so far as the child may be 'dosed' or injured so as to manifest physical signs, he or she is put in double jeopardy as the physicians—or surgeons—make increasing efforts to diagnose and treat what is a fictitious disease.

It is possible that the so-called single syndrome is, in fact, including two—or more—different conditions. The one may be medically orientated as described above; alternatively, there may be a distinct group of women who are engaged in deliberate infanticide or murder—it is significant that the majority of modern literature on the subject is concerned with intentional smothering.[11] Indeed, major interest now centres on the morality of covert video surveillance as an aid to diagnosis.[12] But, if there are two conditions, where does one place inappropriate medication—is this part of the 'medical' syndrome or is it, in fact, *child abuse by poisoning*? Such distinctions are, perhaps, not of major practical significance because, on any interpretation, the infants concerned are at grave risk; Münchhausen's syndrome by proxy is a condition of which every paediatric physician and surgeon should be aware.

8 Moreover, emotional abuse per se must be persistent or severe: *R v Hampshire County Council, ex p H* [1999] 2 FLR 359.
9 A good general review is to be found in A Gath 'The Emotional Abuse of Children' in J K Mason (ed) *Paediatric Forensic Medicine and Pathology* (1989).
10 R Meadow 'Münchausen Syndrome by Proxy: The Hinterland of Child Abuse' (1977) ii Lancet 343.
11 See D Brahams 'Video Surveillance and Child Abuse' (1993) 342 Lancet 944; Editorial Comment 'Spying on Mothers' (1994) Lancet 1373.
12 See D M Foreman and C Farsides 'Ethical Use of Covert Videoing Techniques in Detecting Münchausen Syndrome by Proxy' (1993) 307 BMJ 611 and reply by D P Southall and M P Samuels at 613. At the time of writing, video recording is the subject of a government inquiry.

20

Sexual offences

Expert medical evidence will be called in relation to a number of criminal offences associated with sexual activity, among which the following will be discussed in some detail:

* rape;
* inflicting clandestine injury on a woman;
* indecent assault;
* lewd, indecent or libidinous practices;
* indecency with children;
* homosexual offences;
* incest.

In addition, this is an appropriate place in which to consider sexual abuse of children in a general context.

The law

The majority of sexual offences are defined in England and Wales by the Sexual Offences Acts 1956 to 1993. There is a principally psychiatric medico-legal interest in the Indecency with Children Act 1960 (and with indecent exposure—dealt with by the Vagrancy Act 1824, s 4).

In Scotland, the more serious sexual offences are dealt with at common law. Otherwise, sex law is, to a large extent, consolidated in the Criminal Law (Consolidation) (Scotland) Act 1995 and the Crime and Disorder Act 1998.

Consent and age in sexual offences

Rape is defined in England and Wales by statute.[1] A man commits rape if he has sexual intercourse with a person (whether vaginal or anal) who at the time of the

1   Sexual Offences Act 1956, s 1, as amended by the Criminal Justice and Public Order Act 1994, s 142.

intercourse does not consent to it and, at the time, he knows that the person does not consent to the intercourse or he is reckless as to whether that person consents to it.[2] This definition derives from the Heilbron Committee,[3] which was established largely as a result of the decision that, when a man accused of rape honestly believed the woman to have consented, the reasonableness of the accused's mistake was irrelevant as a matter of law.[4] The 1994 Act does, however, represent a further major change in the law in that it admits of 'male rape' and of rape *per anum*. It thus follows a trend in sex law which has been pioneered in several Commonwealth jurisdictions. The offence of rape has, for example, been abandoned in Canada and in New South Wales in favour of a concept of aggravated assault.[5] In Victoria, the definition of rape now includes non-consensual penetration of the penis into the vagina, mouth or anus of any person, male or female, or the introduction of any other part of the body or of an inanimate object into the vagina or anus—including a surgically constructed vagina.[6] The law in England and Wales is now aligned save that it excludes non-consensual oral penetration and also the use of instruments—which can, of course, nevertheless be prosecuted as indecent assaults.[7]

In Scotland, rape is a crime at common law defined as 'the carnal knowledge of a female by a male person obtained by overcoming her will'.[8] It follows that, throughout the United Kingdom, so long as there is no consent, the age of the victim is immaterial to a charge of rape; age, however, becomes important in the event of apparent consent by a young person.

Irrespective of consent, intercourse with a girl under the age of 16 is unlawful. To have intercourse with a girl below the age of 13 years is a very serious, and distinct, offence and there is no defence on the basis of mistaking her age.[9] In Scotland, the common law age for constructive rape is 12 years; it might be possible to raise the defence of error as to age in the event of such a charge being laid.

The age of the victim between 13 and 16 years is significant under both jurisdictions. In England, having or attempting to have intercourse with a girl

---

2 A man also commits rape if he induces a married woman to have sexual intercourse with him by impersonating her husband (s 1(3)). Note that the presumption that a boy below the age of 14 is incapable of sexual intercourse has now been repealed: Sexual Offences Act 1993. There never was such a presumption in Scotland.

3 *Report of the Advisory Group on the Law of Rape* (Cmnd 6352, 1975).

4 *Morgan v DPP* [1976] AC 182, HL—an extraordinary case involving connivance by the woman's husband. An equally surprising case was reported shortly afterwards *(R v Cogan, R v Leak* [1976] QB 217, CA). For Scotland, see *Meek v H M Advocate* 1982 SCCR 613 and *Jamieson v HM Advocate* 1994 SCCR 181.

5 Canadian Criminal Code, ss 246.1–246.3; Crimes Act 1900 (NSW), as amended by the Crimes (Amendment) Act 1989 (NSW) and the Criminal Legislation (Amendment) Act 1992 (NSW).

6 Crimes Act 1958 (Vic), as amended by the Crimes (Sexual Offences) Act 1991 (Vic). South Australia has similar legislation.

7 Although the Act does not specifically say so, it is apparent that, for the purposes of the criminal law, the definition of sexual intercourse is extended from penetration of the vulva to include penetration of the anus. It is probable that it is also rape to penetrate the 'vagina' of a surgically converted male-to-female transsexual: M Hicks and G Branston 'Transsexual Rape—A Loophole Closed?' [1997] Crim LR 565 quoting Hooper J in *R v Matthews (John)* (1996) unreported.

8 Hume *Commentaries* I, 301. The Criminal Justice and Public Order Act 1994 does not extend to Scotland and, at the time of writing, there seems to be a serious dichotomy in the sex law of the United Kingdom.

9 Sexual Offences Act 1956, s 5; Criminal Law (Consolidation) (Scotland) Act 1995, s 5(1).

above the age of 13 and under 16 years constitutes the offence of having or attempting to have unlawful sexual intercourse, rather than rape. Section 5(3) of the 1995 Act defines a similar offence in Scotland.[10] It is a defence under both codes for a man under the age of 24, who has not been previously charged with a like offence, to prove he had reasonable cause to believe that the girl was aged 16 or over.[11]

Age notwithstanding, consent to sexual intercourse is considered impossible in the case of a mental defective as defined by the Sexual Offences Act 1956, s 7 or the Mental Health (Scotland) Act 1984, s 106(6). The situation is similar to that of a normal girl below the age of 16. It is a defence for the accused to prove that he did not know and had no reason to suspect that a girl was a defective and any consent given, although invalid in law, would certainly mitigate the offence.[12]

Age and consent are relevant also in the offence of indecent assault—an offence that falls short of rape, generally because of absence of penetration, although this may not necessarily be the reason.[13] Under the 1956 Act it is an offence in England and Wales to commit an indecent assault on a man or woman. Children under 16 cannot give legal consent and, therefore, indecent assault on them must always be an offence; s 14(2) provides specific statutory support for this generalisation. The potential defence of error as to age by a young man is not available against a charge of indecent assault, unless it should arise in association with 'marriage'.

An actual assault is necessary to establish a charge of indecent assault and, to cover those cases in which no assault was alleged, the Indecency with Children Act 1960 was applied to England and Wales; under the Act, it is an offence for a person to commit an act of gross indecency with or towards a child under the age of 14. In Scotland, these cases are loosely referred to as 'lewd and libidinous practices', which are offences at common law when associated with children below the age of puberty (12 years in relation to girls).[14] Between the ages of 12 and 16, the offence is defined in the Criminal Law (Consolidation) (Scotland) Act 1995, s 6; consent is no defence nor is error as to age.

Age is important in relation to homosexual offences. The Sexual Offences Act 1967, s 1 and the Criminal Justice (Scotland) Act 1980, s 80 are now amended so that an adult is defined, for the purposes of the Act, as any person more than 18 years of age.[15] Age is also significant as regards sentencing where the importance

---

10 Note that the offence is that of 'having sexual intercourse with a girl'. It is quite incorrect to speak of the 'age of consent to sexual intercourse'. See *Gillick v West Norfolk and Wisbech Area Health Authority* [1985] 3 All ER 402 at 431, per Lord Brandon.

11 In the event of a man 'marrying' a girl below the age of 16 it is a defence throughout Great Britain, irrespective of the man's age or of the number of convictions, that he believed her to be his wife and had reasonable cause for that belief (Marriage Act 1949; Marriage (Scotland) Act 1977; Sexual Offences Act 1956, s 6(2); Criminal Law (Consolidation) (Scotland) Act 1995, s 5(5)). A similar exception is made in connection with a charge of indecent assault.

12 The meaning of 'mental defective' in s 7 of the 1956 Act, as amended by the Mental Health Act 1959, s 127, was further modified by the Mental Health (Amendment) Act 1982, s 65(1) and Sch 3, Pt I, para 29.

13 See *HM Advocate v Logan* 1936 JC 100.

14 *Boyle v Ritchie* 1999 SCCR 278—what action constitutes an offence depends entirely on the circumstances.

15 Criminal Justice and Public Order Act 1994, s 145. The age limit is similar in Northern Ireland (Homosexual Offences (Northern Ireland) Order 1982, art 3, as amended by s 145(3) of the 1994 Act—the result of the European Court of Human Rights decision in *Dudgeon v United Kingdom* (1981) 4 EHRR 149).

of the age differential is acknowledged; the youth of the victim is important—buggery of a person below the age of 16 is punishable by life imprisonment.

Medical evidence in alleged rape of a woman

The medical evidence to be obtained in a case of alleged rape will clearly differ according to whether the victim is a man or a woman. The former is conveniently discussed under the heading of homosexual offences. This section will be limited to the evidence surrounding female rape which can be directed to answering the questions implied in the wording of the definitions—was there sexual intercourse, was there lack of consent and, if so, what was done by the man to overcome the woman's will? The evidence may be derived from a medical examination both of the victim and of the accused.

One source of confusion as to definition has now been removed. Until relatively recently, it has been assumed that a man cannot be charged with the rape of his wife unless, for example, the parties were separated either legally or by agreement.[16] The archaic nature of such a presumption and its consequent dubiety were widely appreciated and the courts in both England and Scotland finally disposed of the concept at much the same time.[17] Clearly, however, this should be a matter for statute rather than case law and the word 'unlawful', which was assumed to mean extra-marital, has now been removed from the definition of sexual intercourse as applied to rape.[18] There is thus no reason why medical evidence should not be required in cases of alleged husband/wife rape although, as will be seen below, it is likely to be even more difficult to obtain and to interpret than it is in the case of stranger rape.

Examination of the genitalia

Limiting discussion, here, to sexual intercourse *per vaginam*, the medical examiner may well have little difficulty in saying positively that sexual intercourse has taken place when a previously virginal hymen has been recently penetrated, particularly if this has been accompanied by some force. The external genitalia are often bruised or swollen and obvious lacerations of the hymen, together with bleeding, may well be present, the main problem being to differentiate the latter from menstrual efflux. Difficulties arise when such typical signs are lacking as may well be the case in the non-virginal state. The absence of lacerations does not necessarily exclude penetration even when previous intercourse can be discounted; the hymen may be naturally lax and sufficiently patent to admit a penis or it may have been rendered so by the use of tampons or by masturbation. The certain sign of penetration is the finding of spermatozoa in the deeper portion

16 There was a long line of cases both in England and in Scotland which steadily eroded the concept of marital immunity. See, for example, *R v Steele* [1977] Crim LR 297, CA; *HM Advocate v Paxton* 1984 JC 105.
17 *R v R* [1991] 4 All ER 481, HL; *Stallard v HM Advocate* 1989 SCCR 248. *R v R* was confirmed in the European Court of Human Rights: *S W v United Kingdom, C R v United Kingdom* [1996] 1 FLR 434, (1996) 21 EHRR 363.
18 Criminal Justice and Public Order Act 1994, s 142, amending Sexual Offences Act 1956, s 1. Rape being undefined by statute in Scotland, the matter is settled in *Stallard v HM Advocate* 1989 SCLR 248.

of the vagina. It has been stated that recognisable spermatozoa can be found three days or more after intercourse and that morphologically perfect specimens with tails are present up to 16 hours after deposition during intramarital intercourse.[19] In the author's experience, such survival is the exception rather than the rule; while being abundant at two hours, perfect forms are rare at 12 hours, the usual finding at that time being of 'scanty bodies indistinguishable from degenerating spermatozoal heads'. In any event, the taking of adequate swabs from within the vagina is an essential step in the examination of the suspected victim, certainly within 24 hours of the alleged offence. It is the positive finding that is of evidential value; a failure to identify spermatozoa is of less consequence as, in law, emission is not essential to sexual intercourse.

The difficulties facing the medical examiner have not yet been exhausted. Full penetration is not required to constitute rape, sexual intercourse being held to mean 'a degree of penetration of the vulva by the penis'; quite clearly, the doctor cannot, and should not be expected to, provide positive evidence on this point on the basis of a simple physical examination. Again, however, a search for spermatozoa may be of very great value; superficial swabs should be taken from the area between the labia in addition to those taken deeply, as a positive finding in them would, save in exceptional circumstances, be very good evidence of intercourse within the legal definition.[20]

The examination of the suspect for evidence of sexual intercourse is generally unrewarding. The glans is very seldom found to be injured beyond what might be anticipated after legal sexual intercourse. Attempts to identify the woman's secretor substance on the male penis—somewhat after the fashion in the examination of bite marks (see Chapter 28)—would theoretically be useful, particularly in cases involving multiple potential assailants, but have proved disappointing in the author's experience. Others have suggested a search for cells from the vaginal epithelium, which have fairly individual staining properties, but the time during which they will be recognisable must be limited.

The use of force or fear

Lack of consent is the basic ingredient of rape in England and Wales. The concept of lack of consent has been broadening so that it can now include what might be described as resigned acquiescence.[1] It follows that evidence of the use of force is not essential to a successful prosecution but it still represents very strong corroboration of lack of consent; it is, perhaps, now mainly of relevance in relation to the definition of and proof of rape in Scotland.

---

19 From the now rather dated work of A David and A Wilson 'The Persistence of Seminal Constituents in the Human vagina' (1974) 3 Forensic Sci 45. A H Heger 'Sexual Violence' in J K Mason and B N Purdue (eds) *The Pathology of Trauma* (3rd edn, 2000) ch 12, quotes anything from 100–25% retrieval of vaginal sperm during the first 24 hours. The present author believes that survival of sperm is far shorter in the hostile environment of rape than it is in consensual conditions. The time can be very much longer in the dead body.
20 An interesting defence on the grounds that refusal of consent to sexual intercourse only *after* penetration did not substantiate a charge of rape has been rejected by the Privy Council: *Kaitamaki v R* [1985] AC 147. Confirmed in an unreported UK case, see F Gibb '"No" Means No at any Point' *The Times*, 26 February 1993, p 3.
1 *R v Olugboja* [1982] QB 320.

The ultimate evidence of force is the death of the victim.[2] A careful pathological assessment of the mode of dying is then essential both to the prosecution and to the defence. However, the remainder of this section will be confined to rape that is uncomplicated to this extent.

It used to be said that the victim's resistance must be 'to the utmost', but this absolute term must be interpreted in a relative fashion; the important feature is unwillingness to take part *throughout* the act. The medical examiner is often in great difficulty here, it being a frequent finding that there is little tangible evidence of force or resistance either in the victim or in the assailant; this may be due to a gross disparity in size and power between victim and rapist, which will be exaggerated if several men have been involved. The alleged assailant must certainly be examined carefully for evidence of scratching, bite marks and the like, Even if these are discovered—and they are infrequent—they must not be *assumed* to be associated with the offence; a note must be made of their probable duration. The examining doctor must also be wary of an almost inescapable element of subjectivity—in the circumstances, it is all too easy to attribute significance to injuries that are, in fact, no more than the result of normal activities.

Many potential injuries in the victim are prevented by the interposition of clothing, and examination of the clothes is an essential part of the complete medical inspection. All doctors will be aware of the possibility of artefacts induced by the accuser herself but real difficulty occurs surprisingly seldom. An association with blood or seminal stains is evidence of genuineness but it is particularly important to examine with care the precise relationship between stains and tears, as these may demonstrate anomalies as to timing; the scientific investigation of clothing is a matter for the laboratory but the doctor must be allowed to make his own assessment at the time of examination.

Overcoming the victim's will

Injury to the accused may also be minimal because she is afraid to resist. Her reaction may be modified by fear, say, of reprisals against a third party, and there can be little or no medical evidence to be drawn on this score—other than a dubious inference from the lack of injury. There is some difference between the English and Scots law on this point. In the former jurisdiction, a charge of rape would still stand under this type of duress. Scots law would, however, require threats of immediate harm rather than of future action; the Criminal Law (Consolidation) (Scotland) Act 1995, s 7(2) prescribes a specific offence of procuring or attempting to procure by threats a woman to have unlawful sexual intercourse. Medical evidence might, however, be sought in the event that the will of the female is said to have been overcome by drugs—of which alcohol used to be, and may still be, the commonest.[3] In practice, the medical examiner would be unlikely to be able to do more than take the necessary samples for laboratory analyses. The law is, again, of interest and importance. It is an offence under the Sexual Offences Act 1956, s 4, 'to administer any drug, matter or thing to a woman

2   In England, the Homicide Act 1957, s 1 abolished the concept of 'constructive malice' whereby the victim's death as part of the process of rape would have amounted to murder. In Scotland, death during rape would be murder only if the cause of death was unrelated to the act of rape (see G H Gordon *The Criminal Law of Scotland* (1978) p 745).
3   The use of drugs such as Rohypnol is now becoming a real problem.

with intent to stupefy or overpower so as thereby to enable any person to have unlawful sexual intercourse with her'; there is a similar provision in the Criminal Law (Consolidation) (Scotland) Act 1995, s 7(2)(c). It is accepted under common law in Scotland that rape itself can be committed by drugging a woman so that she becomes incapable of resisting the accused—drugging, in that it constitutes a means of overcoming the will of the victim is, in effect, a loose form of force. Only alcohol can have any real relevance and the main points are, first, that the woman must be plied with drink *in order* to overcome her resistance—the process of merely 'softening up' by excessive social drinking would be insufficient to substantiate a charge of rape[4]—and, second, that the woman must be deprived of the ability to consent or refuse consent to intercourse.

It is not rape in Scotland to have intercourse with a woman who is insensible through alcoholism or her own making or who is asleep[5]—if such a thing be possible. The reason given is that since the helplessly intoxicated woman is incapable of consenting or refusing consent, there can be no rape because rape involves intercourse against the woman's will.[6] Such cases provide examples of the Scottish offence of inflicting clandestine injury to a woman; they would constitute rape in England due to the absence of positive consent, the alternative of indecent assault being precluded by the act of intercourse. Medical evidence would certainly be called but since there was, by definition, no resistance and previous virginity would be unlikely, the evidence would probably be limited in practice to the demonstration of spermatozoa in the vagina; calculations of the likely alcohol value at the time of the offence might also be needed and the assessment of the primary or synergistic effect of drugs would depend upon adequate analyses.

Intercourse by fraud

Examples of rape by fraud include impersonation of the woman's husband, an offence defined as rape in both the Sexual Offences Act 1956, s 1(3) and in the Criminal Law (Consolidation) (Scotland) Act 1995, s 7(3).[7] Obtaining intercourse by pretending to be giving medical treatment has been regarded as rape in England[8] but might be regarded as only fraud in Scotland. Again, the medical evidence would be likely to be limited to demonstration of emission in such cases.

Scientific evidence of a medical nature in rape

During the medical examination, the doctor will seek and retain certain specimens for laboratory study and analyses; these may be of non-human or of human biological nature.

The former need not be dealt with here as they will lie in the province of the forensic science laboratory—obvious examples would be the retention of any loose fibres, grass or seeds about the person or clothing which might provide rebutting or corroborative evidence of circumstantial detail.

---

4   *HM Advocate v Logan* 1936 JC 100.
5   *HM Advocate v Sweenie* (1858) 3 Irv 109.
6   *HM Advocate v Grainger and Rae* 1932 JC 40.
7   But the word 'husband' is to be interpreted according to the standards of today: *R v Elbekkay* [1995] Crim LR 163.
8   *R v Flattery* [1877] 2 QBD 410.

Although the biological specimens will also probably be examined in a science laboratory, the interpretation of results may well fall to the medical witness. Those that may most often be of value include:

1. *Seminal stains from the clothing of both suspect and complainant.* Direct positive observation under the microscope is certainly the most acceptable proof that a stain is of seminal origin. Spermatozoa are very stable on fabric from which they can be recovered in recognisable form for up to six months after emission; admixture with other body fluids may, however, result in their early disappearance.

   The great majority of individual seminal stain analysis is now a matter of DNA profiling (for which, see below). However, for historical and, very occasionally, for current practical reasons, it is to be noted that such stains can be examined using traditional serological techniques. These depend on the so-called 'secretor state' of the donor. Water-soluble blood-group antigens can be found in the body fluids of approximately three-quarters of the population. Secretion of blood groups is limited to A, B and H substances and the chances of failure to distinguish between two individuals on the basis of seminal 'grouping' are of the order of 45% of secretors; the medico-legal usefulness of such testing is, therefore, virtually confined to exclusion or to the role of no more than an adjunct to other evidence of identification of the man responsible. It is clear that, for any value to be obtained, blood and saliva specimens must also be obtained from the suspect—the former to establish the blood group status and the latter to identify secreted substances. (See also page 435.)

   It is self-evident that stains may be mixed—the tights of a rape victim, for example, may be contaminated both with vaginal and with seminal fluids and may, therefore, give the reactions of both. Only in very exceptional circumstances would it be possible to distinguish between them using standard techniques.[9] This is an area where the use of single probe DNA analysis has influenced forensic evidence profoundly.

2. *Blood stains.* Blood stains can be grouped relatively easily on the ABO system and they may well be fresh enough to allow the demonstration of additional group antigens, 'serum groups' and specific enzyme systems. The blood group systems are considered in a little more detail in Chapter 31. For the present it need only be stressed that serological methods can never identify the donor of a stain specifically. They may provide corroboration of other evidence and, more significantly, they can be used to exclude a suspect. However, sufficient nuclear material may be available to allow for positive identification by way of DNA analysis.

3. *Pubic hair combings from both victim and accused.* The presence of foreign hair will at least show proximity. Hair known to be from the two principles— ie obtained by plucking—must also be available for comparison and, since it contains nuclear material, will be available for DNA testing.

4. *Nail scrapings.* To be examined for blood or tissue from the other party.

5. Any potential *bite marks* should be examined for the presence of saliva, as described in Chapter 28. The use of similar preparations from the glans penis has been discussed above.

---

9   For an exemplary case, see *Preece v HM Advocate* [1981] Crim LR 783.

DNA profiling

The technique of DNA profiling is a matter for the forensic science laboratory and will not be discussed in detail (see page 30 for a broad outline). It is, however, in the criminal field that the process has gained most notoriety and in which it is probably finds its greatest use. The test is, to an extent, the victim of its own success.[10] As with any new test, the problems are twofold—first, that of methodology and, secondly, that of interpretation. As to the first, human error can never be eradicated but laboratory standards can be assured to some extent, for example, by accreditation.[11] It is the second, or statistical, basis of the test which has caused greatest problems—particularly in the US courts[12]—and which is especially associated with the absence of databases for ethnic minorities.[13]

It could be that the initial enthusiasm for DNA profiling—and its enormous potential for positive identification of the origin of nuclear material—has resulted in something of a backlash;[14] it is reasonably easy to throw doubt on claims for a match probability, or chance that an unrelated individual will match the defendant's DNA profile, of the order of one in several hundred million. Many would agree with the American geneticist who is reported as saying: 'I don't care—even if it's 1 in 10,000 that's more than enough'[15]—but that is not the way of the adversarial system of criminal justice; the danger is that the right answers are being given to the wrong question and that, in this particular circumstance, the expert is usurping the function of the jury.[16] The issue has been before the English Court of Appeal; while not doubting the validity and value of DNA testing in general, the court considered that the problems of statistical interpretation as related to ethnic minorities had not been sufficiently explored in the evidence and ordered a retrial.[17] DNA profiling is now very reliable in expert hands; challenges are likely to become fewer and fewer.

The introduction of new techniques such as the use of the polymerase chain reaction (PCR) allows for the amplification of the DNA presentation and, as a result, the successful examination of samples which would have, previously, been inadequate; PCR may also be efficient when the test material is old or degraded. It is this capacity that allows for the reopening of cases which had been inadequately

10 Eg J Sufian 'Forensic Use of DNA Tests' (1991) 303 BMJ 4. For a relatively new and cautionary analysis, see M Redmayne 'Doubts and Burdens: DNA Evidence, Probability and the Courts' [1995] Crim LR 464.
11 Possibly through the National Measurement Accreditation Service. See Lord Runciman (Chairman) *Report of the Royal Commission on Criminal Justice* (1993). Semi-official bodies set up to ensure the quality of the DNA service include the European DNA Profiling group (EDNAP) and the European Network of Forensic Science Institutes has a standing DNA Working Group.
12 Eg *People v Castro* 545 NYS 2d 985 (1989).
13 In the unreported Australian case of *R v Tran*, the defence succeeded largely because there was no evidence as to the statistical match probabilities in the Vietnamese—see N McLeod 'English DNA Evidence Held Inadmissible' [1991] Crim LR 583.
14 See P Alldridge 'Recognising Novel Scientific Techniques: DNA as a Test Case' [1992] Crim LR 687.
15 R Rhein 'US Courts Challenge Evidence from DNA Fingerprinting' (1992) 305 BMJ 973.
16 D J Balding and P Donnelly 'The Prosecutor's Fallacy and DNA Evidence' [1994] Crim LR 711. Much the same view was taken by J Cohen and I Stewart 'Beyond All Reasonable DNA' (1995) 345 Lancet 1586.
17 *R v Gordon (Michael)* [1995] 1 Cr App R 290. But it is understood the accused subsequently tendered a plea of 'guilty'.

examined previously. It is to be noted that the police are now engaged in compiling a National DNA Database which facilitates not only matches of suspects to a crime but also matches from one crime scene to another. Statute law has been amended to allow for this (see page 298 below).

Consent to the provision of specimens

The nature of consent on the part of the person being examined is important (see also Chapter 30). An examination without consent is a potential assault and of at least doubtful evidential value. In cases of rape, there is little difficulty as to the victim because she—or he—will generally appreciate that an examination is an essential adjunct to the accusation; even so, it is well that the doctor should specifically warn her or him of the intimate nature of the examination as this may, albeit surprisingly, not be understood, particularly when the prime complainants are the victim's parents. It is also important to emphasise that there is no confidentiality as regards the findings. The problem is more complex in the case of the accused, to whom the advantage of examination may be dubious. There is no doubt that consent must be sought and that this must be after telling the accused person the object of the examination and that the results of the examination will be reported—whatever they may be. The action to be taken in the event of refusal to be examined is not entirely clear. It is probable that, provided the subject was under arrest and that the examination was expressly for the purpose of confirming or disproving the subject's involvement in a recordable offence,[18] authority for an examination could be given in England and Wales by a police officer of the rank of superintendent or above. In Scotland, the correct procedure would be to obtain a sheriff's warrant. In either case, it is suggested that reasonable force might be used[19] but the statute only gives such authority to a police officer and the examiner would still do well to remember that he might have to justify his action. A satisfactory examination of a resisting subject would be difficult to undertake and, in the face of determined opposition, the doctor might do well to abandon the effort, having warned the subject that inferences might be drawn from his refusal to co-operate.

The *taking of samples* is fully governed by the Police and Criminal Evidence Act 1984, ss 61–65,[20] in which bodily samples are divided into intimate and non-intimate. The taking of the former[1] is subject to both authorisation by a police officer of at least the rank of superintendent *and* the consent of the examinee when he is in police detention—and, in certain circumstances, when he is not detained (s 62). No intimate sample may be taken in the absence of written consent but the court or jury may draw such inferences from the refusal as appear proper when determining the person's guilt (s 62(10)). Non-intimate samples can be taken without written consent if the subject is in police detention or custody—and if he is not and either a specimen has not been taken or one that has been

---

18 A recordable offence is, roughly, one that is punishable by imprisonment.
19 Police and Criminal Evidence Act 1984, s 117; Criminal Procedure (Scotland) Act 1995, s 19B, as amended by the Crime and Punishment (Scotland) Act 1997, s 48(2).
20 As amended by Criminal Justice Act 1988 and Criminal Justice and Public Order Act 1994.
1 An intimate sample means a sample of blood, semen or other tissue fluid, urine, or pubic hair, a dental impression or a swab taken from a person's body orifice other than the mouth (1984 Act, s 65, as amended by 1994 Act, s 58).

taken has proved inadequate—and the procedure is authorised by a police officer of at least the rank of superintendent who has reasonable grounds for suspecting that the subject may be involved in a recordable offence. Non-intimate samples involve samples of hair other than pubic hair, samples from a nail or from under a nail, swabs taken from any part of the body, including the mouth but not any other body orifice, saliva and a footprint or a similar impression of any part of a person's body other than a part of the hand. Hair roots contain blood or tissue fluid in addition to nucleated cells; however, s 63A(2) of the 1984 Act now states that head hair can be plucked and constitutes a non-intimate sample.

In Scotland, the taking of samples is governed by the Criminal Procedure (Scotland) Act 1995, s 18.[2] A constable can take, or require the person to provide, such relevant personal data—defined as fingerprints, palm prints and other prints and impressions of an external part of the body—as he thinks appropriate to take from or require of him in view of the nature of the case (s 18). Given the authority of an officer no lower than the rank of inspector, he may take specimens of hair, other than pubic, by cutting, combing or plucking, of nails or nail scrapings and of blood or other body fluid or material by swabbing or rubbing an external part of the body; a mouth swab may also be taken (s 18(6)). There are interesting differences from the English statute. First, consent is not mentioned and the authority of a comparatively junior officer is all that is required for taking what would be, in English terms, non-intimate samples; somewhat surprisingly, the constable needs neither consent nor authority to take fingerprints (cf Police and Criminal Evidence Act 1984, s 61). Secondly, the list is specific and relatively short. There is no statutory authority for obtaining what would be regarded as intimate samples in England. However, the common law power to obtain a sheriff's warrant is preserved (s 18(8)(c)) and this would have to be invoked were the subject to refuse consent for a medical practitioner to take any samples other than those listed.

Though there are statutory provisions for the destruction of samples that have been taken if the person concerned has been cleared of the offence,[3] the law has now been amended to enable the police to retain records in certain circumstances— for example, where the offence is one in which another person has been convicted (1984 Act, s 64(3A)) or where it might involve destruction of a sample lawfully held in relation to another person (1995 Act, s 18(4)). The majority of recent amendments, which cannot, for want of space, be detailed here, are associated with developments such as electronic 'live-scan' fingerprinting and the establishment of databases.

Charges against practitioners

Charges of rape, of attempted rape or, more commonly, of indecent assault are not infrequently made against doctors and dentists in the course of their practice. The more serious charges commonly result from delusions, possibly wishful, arising under anaesthesia; dentists are, therefore, particularly at risk when they

---

2   As amended by Crime and Punishment (Scotland) Act 1997, ss 47(1), 62(2), Sch 3 and Crime and Disorder Act 1998, s 119, Sch 8, para 117.
3   Police and Criminal Evidence Act 1984, s 64(1), (2) and (3); Criminal Procedure (Scotland) Act 1995, s 18(3).

operate and anaesthetise single-handed, while the practice of 'horizontal dentistry' is psychologically predisposing to sexual fantasy on the part of the patient. The general medical examination would go far to exclude the possibility of rape but, in the event of deliberate premeditated fabrication, the 'patient' would be likely to inflict damage on her clothing and person. An interesting situation could arise in the event of the charges being substantially true. It would clearly be rape to give a woman an anaesthetic *in order* to have intercourse; on the other hand, Gordon[4] suggests that it is not rape to have sexual intercourse having drugged a woman for a lawful purpose such as to give an anaesthetic for an operation—*Grainger and Rae*[5] would presumably apply.

The doctor is particularly open to charges of indecent assault—some of which arise from a genuine misunderstanding of the nature of an intended examination. It was once a truism that a male doctor should not allow himself to be isolated with a female patient; such are the present staffing conditions, however, that the counsel of chaperoning at all times cannot always be followed. It would, however, be foolhardy for a male doctor to examine the genitalia or the breasts in the absence of a female witness. Even then, it is strongly advised that *specific and informed* consent should be obtained before undertaking such an intimate examination.

Medical evidence in attempted rape or indecent assault

The examination of a victim of assault with attempt to commit rape would follow the lines of investigation of any case of assault. Medical evidence would be called to assess the severity of the assault and this might derive from an examination of both parties.

Indecent assault, which is not a specific offence in Scotland, may be perpetrated homosexually or heterosexually by either sex. It must be overtly sexual, with an element of immodesty, and may be accompanied by violence ranging from severe to mere touching—indeed, the assault need only be psychic if physical contact is threatened; medical evidence becomes of decreasing value as the element of assault diminishes. It is to be noted that, even before the marital exemption from a charge of rape was withdrawn, there was no such exemption for a husband who indecently assaulted his wife.[6]

Possibly the least traumatic sexual offences are the commission of indecency with or of lewd or libidinous practices against children for which no physical contact is required. It may well be that the medical examination that is often required in such cases does more psychological harm to the very young people who are involved than does the occurrence itself; the offence is limited to practices against children under the age of 14 in England and Wales and against girls under 16 and boys under 14 years in Scotland, the only alternative in the case of offended adults being a charge of what is loosely known as 'indecent exposure'.

4   G H Gordon *The Criminal Law of Scotland* (1978) p 886.
5   *HM Advocate v Grainger and Rae* 1932 JC 40.
6   *R v Kowalski* (1988) 9 Cr App R (S) 375.

Incest

Incestuous relationships differ in England and Scotland. In England the Sexual Offences Act 1956 makes it an offence for a man to have intercourse with his mother, sister, daughter, granddaughter or half-sister; there may, of course, be alternative charges, of both general and specific type, if the female is aged below 16 years.[7] Similar relationships with the sexes reversed are also forbidden but a girl must be over 16 years old to be guilty of incest. The law in Scotland is contained in the Criminal Law (Consolidation) (Scotland) Act 1995, ss 1–4. The prohibitions by way of consanguinity are still wider than those in England and include intercourse with a grandmother, aunt, niece, great-grandmother and great-granddaughter. Incest cannot now be committed by those related only by affinity and the absurdity of incest being impossible between bastard relatives is removed. The Scots incest and marriage laws are brought into conformity in that incest may be committed with an adoptive mother or daughter and a separate offence of having intercourse with a stepchild under the age of 21, who has cohabited with the stepparent when aged below 18 years, is included. More significantly and farsightedly, a person aged over 16 years who is in a position of trust or authority over a child and who has sexual intercourse with that child when aged less than 16 years commits an offence which is punishable by imprisonment up to and including for life. The element of an abuse of trust, which is so essential to the concept of incest, is thus given due notice.

The conditions for proof of incest are the same as those for rape—there must be penetration but, in respect of incest, this must be vulval. Medical and medico-scientific evidence in incest is largely confined to establishing the fact of intercourse in the female and either not excluding or excluding the suspect male. Cases seldom come to light immediately and it may well be that pregnancy provides the evidence of intercourse. In addition, the relationships might have to be tested as described in Chapter 17. Both parties are equally guilty of the offence but, in practice, the female is very rarely prosecuted. Deviate intercourse cannot be incest.

Homosexual offences

Homosexual relationships between consenting women do not constitute an offence unless one of them is under 16 years of age and is, therefore, unable to consent to an indecent assault.

In England, sodomy is a form of buggery and consists of connection per anum with any other person; the term is slightly more restrictive in Scotland and refers to unnatural carnal connection between men.

Buggery is an offence in England under the Sexual Offences Act 1956, s 12, but the Sexual Offences Act 1956, s 1A,[8] provides that it is not so when performed in private by consenting parties who have both attained the age of 18.[9] Homosexual

---

7   Eg incitement to incest—Criminal Law Act 1977, s 54.
8   Inserted by the Criminal Justice and Public Order Act 1994, s 143. Note that, as a result, anal intercourse with a consenting adult woman in private is no longer an offence. The same rules apply in Northern Ireland.
9   This will shortly be 16 in both jurisdictions—the necessary legislation has had a chequered career through Parliament.

acts between merchant seamen and between members of the armed forces are now no longer criminal.[10] Sodomy in Scotland is a separate common law crime. The Criminal Law (Consolidation) (Scotland) Act 1995, s 13 allows for private homosexual practices between consenting adults as in England.

Effectively, therefore, medical evidence in cases of consenting homosexual practice will be limited to the examination of young men—the prosecution may prove that an act between adults was not conducted in private but the value of and need for medical evidence in such cases must be limited. Proof of penetration of the anus is needed to establish unnatural carnal connection but proof of emission is not required. The examining doctor may be in great difficulty in the event of incomplete penetration but, in practice, serious resistance by the passive partner is unlikely to occur—full distension of the anus is probable. The signs likely to be discovered depend, therefore, on the habituation of the passive partner. In the case of a first occurrence, tenderness, oedema and, perhaps, bruising or laceration will be present around the anus. The orifice of the habitual passive sodomist by contrast becomes dilated and smooth, the sphincter is lax and, of greatest importance, loses its elasticity; the surrounding skin may become horny and may also show scars from earlier lacerations. The presence of traces of lubricant may provide suggestive evidence and the finding of spermatozoa on swabs prepared either from within the canal or from the anal mucosa will prove the act almost beyond dispute. But it must be admitted that, in many cases, there will be insufficient evidence for the doctor to reach a firm conclusion that unnatural intercourse has occurred. The pathologist examining a dead man may have difficulty in distinguishing true sodomy from the effects of post-mortem change; cases are often seen, particularly in young persons, where an apparently grossly patulous anus can only be ascribed to a post-mortem phenomenon.

The examination of the active partner is unlikely to provide much firm evidence. Certainly, the glans may be damaged—but this is not proof of anal connection; remnants of faeces or lubricant may be present beneath the foreskin in the unlikely event of a suspect not having washed himself before examination. In practice, convictions are more likely to follow on a charge of gross indecency than on a charge of sodomy.

Intercourse with animals

The English offence of buggery includes bestiality, which can be committed by either a man or a woman with an animal.[11] Bestiality consists of intercourse per vaginam although, in view of the recent revision of the definition of rape, it may well be that it can also be committed per anum. It is a common law crime in

---

10 Criminal Justice and Public Order Act 1994, s 146. However, the authority to discharge or dismiss on the grounds of homosexual conduct is retained in both the armed forces and the merchant navy (s 146(4)). This was held not to be irrational: *R v Secretary of State for Defence, ex p Smith* [1996] QB 517, CA, nor was it thought to offend against the European Council Directive as to Equal Treatment (76/207/EEC (OJ 1976 L39/40)): *R v Secretary of State for Defence, ex p Perkins (No 2)* [1999] 1 FLR 491. It does, however, contravene the European Convention on Human Rights, art 8: *Lustig-Prean and Beckett v United Kingdom, Smith and Grady v United Kingdom* (1999) 29 EHRR 548.
11 Sexual Offences Act 1956, s 12.

Scotland for a man to have 'unnatural carnal connection' with an animal;[12] it is doubtful if a woman could be so charged.

The offence is committed when there is penetration; emission is not essential. Veterinary evidence would be important if a small animal was used but the only medical evidence likely to be led in most cases would relate either to the presence of human sperm in an animal or to demonstrating an animal origin of sperm in a human orifice. Spermatozoa differ in size and shape according to species, some cells are, however, very similar to the human and the origin of stains and material on diagnostic swabs would probably be most easily demonstrable by serological methods or DNA profiling. Most acts of bestiality are conducted in privacy and there can, therefore, be little forensic medical experience of the offence; but the emphasis on bestiality in 'hard' pornography suggests that the subject may exert a surprising fascination.

Sexual abuse of children in general

It will be seen that there is very little scope for sexual activity with children that is not proscribed either by statute or by common law; the doctor is, therefore, most likely to become involved through the police and the principles of examination and interpretation discussed above will apply.[13] Alternatively, however, sexual abuse of children may be seen as a social problem and the primary investigation is, then, in the hands of the social services department. The problem then is whether the child should be taken into care—something which can be done with relative ease and for which the evidence need only be based on the standard of probability;[14] indeed, such may be the repercussions of a 'missed' case, that little more than suspicion often suffices.[15] As a consequence, the examining doctor is left with problems of interpretation which must be based on minimal or controversial evidence.[16]

Such cases are commonly dealt with without publicity but, increasingly, allegations of ritual or other group abuse are made which illustrate the difficulties vividly. Such an instance arose in Cleveland in 1987 when over 200 children were placed in care on the grounds of parental sexual abuse.[17] Many of these disposals were made on the basis of what was called the 'sign' of reflex anal

---

12 Hume *Commentaries* I, 469.
13 For a very good analysis of the somewhat pragmatic approach to, and results of, criminal investigation, see C San Lazaro, A M Steele and L J Donaldson 'Outcome of Criminal Investigation into Allegations of Sexual Abuse' (1996) 75 Arch Dis Childh 149.
14 Children Act 1989, s 31(2)(a); Children (Scotland) Act 1995, s 52(2). In *Re G (a minor) (child abuse: standard of proof)* [1987] 1 WLR 1461 it was suggested that the probability should be stronger when a parent was accused of abuse than when some other person was involved; but see *Re B (minors) (care proceedings: practice)* [1999] 1 WLR 238 when more than one child is involved. For Scotland, see *Reporter to Central Region Children's Panel v F*, Inner House (1990) Scotsman, 7 November.
15 Children have no right of action against a local authority for mistakes either way in this connection: *X (minors) v Bedfordshire County Council* [1995] 2 AC 633.
16 It is well to remember that sexual abuse of children is not confined to abuse of females, although that is by far the more common form. See R Wilkins (1990) 'Women who Sexually Abuse Children' (1990) 300 BMJ 1153.
17 There have been others—notably in Manchester in 1990 (see in *Re A (minors) (child abuse: guidelines)* [1991] 1 WLR 1026, CA) and the Orkney Islands in 1991, both of which resulted in severe judicial criticisms of the systems used.

relaxation and dilatation whereby gentle traction on the buttocks resulted in relaxation of the anal sphincter—a reaction attributed to previous sexual penetration of the anus. The diagnostic value and the interpretation of this sign were strongly disputed and it is not proposed here to take sides in the argument. The important lesson to be learnt is that no one physical sign can, at the present time, be regarded as being uniquely diagnostic of child abuse.[18] Equally important are the attitude of mind to the diagnosis and the avoidance of subjectivity—there is a wide difference between awareness of the existence of sexual abuse of children and a determination to demonstrate its presence. The importance of dual examinations to the well-being of the child has been stressed in Chapter 19; a further advantage is that excessive motivation on either side is likely to be curbed in a co-operative atmosphere. It is only by reducing the level of anxiety to obtain positive results that satisfactory solutions will be found to what are, almost always, very real dilemmas.

18 Department of Health and Social Security *Diagnosis of Child Sexual Abuse: Guidance for Doctors* (1988) para 12.20.

21

Poisons and poisoning

Poisoning can be seen from the medico-legal viewpoint as being of two main types—that which affects large sections of the community and that which involves individuals only. Environmental and industrial poisoning provide the main components of the former category; the number of deaths and the extent of disability directly attributable to poisoning of the community reaches serious levels in most industrialised countries and their limitation is often a matter of legislation. Individual intoxication may be accidental, iatrogenic, suicidal or homicidal. While the last has certainly the greatest forensic significance, it is now rare compared with some decades ago; far more individuals die from accidents or suicide.

Environmental poisoning

Environmental poisoning results either from the effects of emissions into the atmosphere or from the presence of specific substances or elements in the surroundings as a whole. The main contributors to the former are smoke-producing fires or furnaces and motor car exhausts.

The major source of atmospheric pollution used to be domestic coal fires, the products of which, when reacting with a simple fog in windless conditions, produced the classic London 'pea-souper'. If a fog precipitated in an already polluted atmosphere is not dispersed, there is a massive build-up of smoke particles and of the gas sulphur dioxide. Mortality and morbidity are related closely to the combined concentration of these substances, the majority of deaths occurring in those already suffering from disease of the lungs or heart. The most effective way of controlling this type of poisoning is through the limitation of smoke—it is doubtful if sulphur dioxide, which is the main atmospheric contaminant due to furnaces, is harmful by itself.[1] The conditions responsible for this source of community ill-health have now been either eliminated or drastically reduced by empowering the local authority to declare the whole or part of their district a smoke control area—the Secretary of State can impose the use of such powers

---

1   Even so, the sulphur content of oil fuels for furnaces is strictly controlled: Clean Air Act 1993, s 31; Sulphur Content of Liquid Fuels (England and Wales) Regulations 2000, SI 2000/1460.

should he be confronted by what he sees as a reluctant authority.[2] As a result, domestic pollution is virtually a thing of the past and the 'pea-souper' has disappeared along with it. Concurrently, there has been a reduction in the associated cardiopulmonary disease which can, therefore, be counted among those medical conditions that are controllable by legislation.[3]

The production of smoke from non-domestic furnaces is now governed by the Clean Air Act 1993, which prohibits the emission of 'dark smoke' (Pt I) and lays the ground for controlling the emission of smoke, grit, dust and fumes—effectively, every new furnace installed must be, so far as is practicable, smokeless; approval of all non-domestic furnaces is the function of the local authority (Pt II). This two-pronged attack on smoke emission is responsible for one of the greatest improvements in living standards to have been achieved in the course of the last century.

The effects of motor car exhausts stem from several factors. Depending on the efficiency of the engine, the exhaust gases contain between 2% and 10% carbon monoxide and this is reflected in the carboxyhaemoglobin levels in persons such as policemen on traffic duty. Although the levels reached—of the order of 5–6%—will not cause deterioration in function, the condition is of minor medico-legal importance in that it has been claimed that it is the carbon monoxide derived from smoking—and, therefore, also from other environmental sources— that is, to some extent, responsible for the development of coronary heart disease;[4] it is thought, however, that this view would get little support today. Other important forms of carbon monoxide poisoning are discussed later in this section but, in the present context, the main significance of the gas when derived from motor car exhausts lies in its potential as a cause of vehicular accidents, especially in a synergistic role; this has been discussed in Chapter 10.

The hydrocarbons liberated in exhaust gases due to incomplete combustion of the fuel are more important from the environmental aspect. The interaction of sunlight and exhaust vapour produces an atmosphere that is irritating to the nose and eyes—the characteristic 'smog' of the Western USA. Unlike the British fog, 'smog' has little permanent effect on human beings but has been reported as being damaging to crops.

Many motor car exhaust gases also contain lead, which forms a link with the second aspect of environmental pollution—that is, pollution by specific elements. Apart from radioactive pollution (discussed in Chapter 26), the outstandingly significant substance in this class is lead. Lead poisoning is, in the main, a matter of industrial medicine but outbreaks of subclinical poisoning occur at an environmental level, particularly in areas close to lead works. Lead present in the soil, as well as that present in the air, then constitutes a significant part of the

2   Clean Air Act 1993, ss 18–20. In Scotland, this power rests with the Scottish Environment Protection Agency (s 19, as amended by Environment Act 1995).
3   The prescription of processes, irrespective of the medium which may be contaminated, the appointment of inspectors and the authorisation of types of fireplace are governed by the Pollution Prevention and Control Act 1999 (Environmental Protection (Prescribed Processes and Substances) Regulations 1991, SI 1991/472 as amended). For the powers of local authorities in respect of smoke from private dwellings, see Clean Air Act 1993, ss 24, 25. See also the Smoke Control Areas (Exempted Fireplaces) Order, SI 1999/1515, for Scotland SI 1999/58.
4   See, for example, N Wald et al 'Association between atherosclerotic disease and carboxyhaemoglobin levels in tobacco smokers' (1973) i BMJ 761.

health hazard and children, who are more susceptible to the metal, are at greatest risk.[5] The contribution of motor cars to this risk is not clear. Certainly there is more lead in the atmosphere of urban streets than there is in country areas but absorption into the body is not proportionately increased; nevertheless, all industrial countries are legislating to reduce the amount of lead in motor car fuels.[6]

The list of environmental contaminants is, however, growing as manufacturing methods and the materials used diversify. Planners' problems are increased by the uncertainty of and the measurement of any health hazards posed by emissions. Statistical proof of a causative relationship between an agent and a disease is generally based on a 95% confidence limit—that is to say, the relationship is proved when the likelihood of a chance association only is 5% or less. This, however, is a far more stringent test than is required in the civil courts, where no more than a 51% likelihood of a causative association is required for a successful action in negligence.[7] Furthermore, developers must now submit environmental impact assessments for every project and these must include the 'possible' impact of the development on humans[8]—and a possible impact is an even lower standard of proof than is a 51% probability. The planner is thus not only faced with establishing a standard to which he or she must work but, having done so, must also accept that it is a standard which is likely to vary with the severity of the possibly associated disease; moreover, the risks must be balanced against the benefits of the intended development.

There have been several examples of the difficulties involved over recent years. Perhaps the best known is the alleged association between a polluted environment surrounding nuclear power stations and childhood cancers; after an extremely long hearing, the court concluded that the plaintiffs had failed to prove their case.[9] A rather similar allegation—that of an association between the electromagnetic fields emanating from electric power lines and malignant disease of childhood—has yet to come to the British courts; once again, the difficulty of proving causation of personal injury by way of epidemiological evidence is exemplified.[10] Mention should also be made of the environmental effects of modern warfare. Large numbers of diseases have been attributed to the use of Agent Orange and its contained dioxin which, although legitimately used in agriculture, was sprayed without precautions in the Vietnam war; once more, epidemiological studies are inconclusive. More recently, we have the 'Gulf War

---

5 A lead level of 40–50 mg/100 ml blood in a child is regarded as requiring investigation, whereas the level at which an industrial worker is considered in danger of developing lead poisoning is 80 mg/100 ml.

6 Clean Air Act 1993, s 30. The lead content of petrol used in the United Kingdom must now be reduced to 0.15 g/l in leaded fuel or 0.013 g/l in unleaded fuel (Motor Fuel (Composition and Content) Regulations 1999, SI 1999/3107).

7 The calculations are further complicated by introducing the concept of relative risk. Thus, the 51% standard of proof equates with a relative risk of 2—that is, exposure to the agent has at least doubled the risk of contracting the disease. See R Meeran 'Scientific and Legal Standards of Proof in Environmental Injury Cases' (1992) 339 Lancet 671.

8 E C Council Directive on the Assessment of the Effect of Certain Public and Private Projects on the Environment 85/337 (OJ L175, 5.7.85), implemented by Town and Country Planning (Environmental Impact Assessment) (England and Wales) Regulations 1999, SI 1999/293.

9 *Reay v British Nuclear Fuels plc* [1994] 5 Med LR 1. It is suggested that the cause is likely to have been a common unidentified infection triggered by population mixing.

10 D A Savitz 'Power Lines and Cancer Risk' (1991) 265 J Amer Med Ass 1458.

Syndrome', in which not only are the symptoms indefinite but, also, the suspected atmospheric pollutant, or other causative agent, remains unidentified; thus far, no scientific panel has validated any claims attributed to the syndrome.[11] Finally, it is to be remembered that, although environmental poisoning is overwhelmingly due to atmospheric pollution, the importance of marine and waterway pollution is being increasingly noted—no doubt, for example, far more will be heard of the suggestion that congenital limb deformities are causally related to maternal bathing in our polluted coastal waters.[12]

Industrial poisoning

Industrial poisons may be absorbed through the skin, they may be ingested or they may be inhaled; inhalation is by far the most important source, not only on physiological grounds but also because it is largely outwith the control of the individual. Much of the preventive legislation is, therefore, concentrated on the maintenance of a pure atmosphere in the workspace.

Industrial poisons are given threshold limit values (TLV), which are expressed as the airborne concentration of the given substance to which it is believed that nearly all workers may be repeatedly exposed without ill effects. Such values, which are expressed either in weight per cubic metre or in parts per million, are to some extent artificial and are well compared with the 30 mph speed limits on roads—not all accidents will be prevented by such a limit but it is an arbitrary standard below which it is impractical to go; in industry, the TLV is the level thought likely to be injurious if exceeded.

Dust or fumes of a potentially dangerous character are now subsumed under the general category of substances that are hazardous to health. An employer must ensure that exposure of his employees to such substances is either prevented or, when this is not reasonably practicable, it is adequately controlled.[13] When there is exposure to a substance for which a maximum exposure has been specified,[14] then, so far as the inhalation of the substance is concerned, the employer's efforts will be regarded as adequate only if the level is, again, reduced so far as is reasonably practicable and, *in any case*, is reduced to below the maximum exposure limits defined in the regulations. It is interesting that, a few exceptions aside, the measures taken should not be limited to the provision of personal protective clothing—the Act calls for active rather than passive measures. All practicable measures—not just some—must be taken when stipulated and practicality refers only to the technical possibilities according to current knowledge[15]—cost, for example, does not enter into the equation. Active elimination by extraction is incomparably the best means of preventing industrial poisoning and it must be used—ideally sited as close to the source as possible—when the conditions make

11 F M Murphy 'Gulf War Syndrome' (1999) 318 BMJ 274. It is pointed out that ill-defined 'syndromes' arise after most military conflicts. See K C Hyams, F S Wignall and R Roswell 'War Syndromes and their Evaluation' (1996) 125 Ann Intern Med 398.
12 A James 'Marine Pollution and Limb Reduction Defects' (1994) 343 Lancet 990. For legislation as to water pollution in general, see Water Resources Act 1991, Pt III, as amended.
13 Control of Substances Hazardous to Health Regulations 1999, SI 1999/437.
14 SI 1999/437, Sch 1.
15 *Brooks v J and P Coates (UK) Ltd* [1984] ICR 158.

it practicable. It scarcely needs emphasis that the extraction cannot be haphazard and care must be taken to ensure that contamination of the local community is kept to a minimum.

In addition, health surveillance must be provided for employees exposed to substances listed in the 1994 regulations, Sch 5. These substances include vinyl chloride monomer, nitro or amino derivatives of phenol and benzene, benzene (including benzol), carbon disulphide, carbon tetrachloride and trichlorethylene.[16]

The early identification of cases of poisoning forms one check on the lack of efficiency[17] of a factory's preventive methods. It is for this reason that a number of conditions (listed in Appendix N) are scheduled as diseases that are notifiable to the Health and Safety Executive.[18] These diseases must be distinguished from those prescribed under the Social Security Contributions and Benefits Act 1992 (see page 214); although nearly all notifiable diseases are also prescribed, the method and purpose of reporting are different. Many of the notifiable conditions are specific; others—for example, 'blood dyscrasia'—are usefully non-specific in that they open possibilities for clinical notification of dangerous conditions before they are specifically defined by regulations.

Poisoning in industry is a vast subject which is constantly changing in emphasis and growing in extent—a matter which is, for example, recognised in the Notification of New Substances Regulations.[19] The subject will, therefore, be dealt with only in general terms, attention being drawn to the main categories of hazard.

First, there is poisoning by heavy metals of which, as has been seen, lead is the outstanding example; industrial processes involving lead are subject to the Control of Lead at Work Regulations 1998.[20] Although ingestion is also considered hazardous, industrial intoxication by lead is almost entirely a matter of inhalation. This is also a matter of great interest to public, as opposed to employees', health—hence the importance attached to the control of emissions from factories processing toxic substances.[1] Emission of noxious or offensive substances imposes a duty on the persons having control of the premises to use the best practical means for preventing the emission of such substances and for rendering them harmless or inoffensive.

The main danger of lead lies in its cumulative effect; the vast majority of industrial cases are examples of chronic intoxication—colic, joint pains, anaemia, muscle paralyses and generalised brain dysfunction (encephalopathy) may result and are probably due to the fact that lead is basically a poison to enzymes. Other metallic poisons that are dangerous mainly by way of inspiration include beryllium and cadmium, which are intensely harmful to the lungs, and manganese and mercury, chronic poisoning from both of which causes extensive abnormality of the central nervous system—the latter metal, in particular, giving origin to the term 'mad as a hatter'. The effects of chronic metallic poisoning may be delayed for many years; much responsibility rests on the medical profession when establishing a cause-and-effect relationship.

---

16 SI 1999/437, reg 11(1) and (2).
17 Efficiency is positively identified by monitoring or measuring the atmosphere at regular intervals.
18 Reporting of Injuries, Diseases and Dangerous Occurrences Regulations 1995, SI 1995/3163.
19 SI 1993/3050, amended by Ionising Radiation Regulations 1999, SI 1999/3232.
20 SI 1998/543.
 1 See Health and Safety (Emissions into the Atmosphere) Regulations 1983, SI 1983/943. Schedule 2 lists a large number of emissions described as noxious or offensive substances (see Appendix O).

The second major group of industrial poisons consists of the hydrocarbons, of both aromatic and of aliphatic type. Again, intoxication is generally by inhalation but absorption through the skin plays a significant part in many cases.

Poisonous aromatic hydrocarbons include benzene itself, which in its chronic form causes an anaemia of very specific type; nitrobenzene, which may be acutely fatal if splashed on the skin; nitroglycerine, again absorbed rapidly through the skin and capable of causing a fatal fall in blood pressure; and trinitrotoluene, which was responsible for a large number of industrial deaths in both World Wars, the outstanding features being cyanosis, anaemia and, occasionally, toxic jaundice—jaundice, or yellowness, being a visible indication of liver failure. Aliphatic hydrocarbons may be dangerous industrial chemicals when halogenated—that is, combined with chlorine or bromine. The simplest of these compounds—methyl chloride and methyl bromide, which can be used as refrigerants or, in the case of the latter, as a fire extinguisher—are acutely poisonous to the brain. Otherwise, the common characteristic of this group of poisons is their action on the liver and, to a lesser extent, the kidney. Halogenated hydrocarbons are used principally as cleaning agents or industrial solvents. Most have a narcotic action and the least toxic can be used as anaesthetics. Carbon tetrachloride, tetrachlorethane and, especially, dichlorethane are severely damaging to the liver and are the main sources of industrial toxic jaundice. Tetrachlorethane was a serious cause of illness in early aircraft workers, when it was used to tighten the fabric of aeroplanes. The variations in toxicity of the halogenated hydrocarbons offer wide opportunities for substitution and, as a result, the extent of the industrial hazard is diminishing.

Finally, attention is drawn to the potential association of cancer with some industrial processes. Many of these conditions are of historic interest—for example, the 'mule spinner's cancer' induced by chronic friction between the skin and clothing impregnated with mineral oil. Others, for example, malignant disease of the liver associated with vinyl chloride, have appeared only relatively recently—carcinogenesis is, however, being increasingly appreciated as being work related. For an association with occupation to be clear, a cancer must, generally, be of a fairly rare type; it is possible that some common tumours are related to specific substances—the association of carcinoma of the lung with asbestosis and smoking is an example (see page 219)—but, for the purposes of the Social Security Contributions and Benefits Act, it may be difficult to show that they 'do not constitute a risk to the whole population'. Examples of unusual cancers that are prescribed include carcinoma of the nasal membrane in workers exposed to nickel fumes (disease No C.22) or to wood dust (disease No D.6); although it can arise independently, mesothelioma (disease No D.3) is sufficiently rare to be firmly attributable to asbestosis. Disease No C.23, cancer of the bladder, is interesting, as the most common industrial association of this tumour is with workers in aniline factories; the condition is, in fact, due to the presence as an impurity of the prescribed substance naphthylamine. Vinyl chloride monomer is associated with angiosarcoma of the liver.

Agricultural poisons

Agricultural poisoning merits isolation from other industrial hazards because, apart from potential effects on the workers, there may well be secondary ecological effects; the community as a whole may also be at risk if a toxic substance is distributed widely in the environment or is incorporated in foodstuffs. Excluding manifest abuses such as using defoliation as a weapon of war, toxic agricultural chemicals of the insecticide, the fungicide or the herbicide groups may be poisonous to man when used legitimately;[2] the art of their production and use lies in limiting their toxicity to the species it is intended to destroy.

Control of the problems of non-specificity lies with the Advisory Committee on Pesticides.[3] The committee must be provided with full details of a proposed pesticide—including its justification for use, its toxic properties and its potential residual effects in foodstuffs; particular importance is placed on possible harm to the human users and consumers of treated crops, to livestock and to wildlife. Products so notified are given trials clearance—usually for a limited period—which may involve destruction of all treated material until the remaining safety measures have been taken. Following trials, there is usually a period of limited clearance, during which regulated sales may be permitted; if this is passed satisfactorily, a provisional commercial clearance is granted which allows the product to be marketed commercially for a defined period. If the exhaustive inquiries demanded during these phases have indicated that the product is safe to use[4] and is free from serious ecological ill-effects, a full commercial clearance may be given subject to recommendations as to labelling, as to the method of treatment of and the choice of crops and as to the protection of man, livestock and wildlife. The committee keeps any chemical under review and may vary the regulations in the light of any fresh evidence that accrues during normal use.

In addition to this monitoring system, several statutory controls are imposed. Those chemicals that are seriously toxic to the user are specified under the Chemical (Hazard Information and Packaging for Supply) Regulations 1994;[5] a main danger of most agricultural toxins is that, in addition to inhalation, entry to the body through the skin is a common method of poisoning. Contact in the agricultural environment is inevitable; regulations are, therefore, very much concerned with the provision of protective clothing.[6] Other chemicals, which constitute a hazard if improperly used, are listed in the Farm and Garden Chemicals Regulations 1971;[7] a main purpose of the regulations is to ensure that toxic chemicals are adequately labelled and carry appropriate warnings.[8] Less specifically, certain chemicals that may be used as pesticides are subject to

2   All such agents, including rodenticides, are known collectively as pesticides. Rodenticides will not be discussed at this point.
3   Food and Environment Protection Act 1985, s 16 (SI 1985/1390).
4   Note that a chemical may be poisonous but, when used in a specific way taking normal precautions, it may not necessarily be hazardous—paraquat is a prime example of such a substance (see below).
5   SI 1994/3247, which included the dinitrophenol compounds; endrin; the organophosphorus compounds; fluoroacetic acid compounds; organomercury sprays; arsenic; the organotin compounds; nicotine; and sulphuric acid.
6   SI 1999/437, reg 7.
7   SI 1971/729.
8   See also Chemicals (Hazard Information and Packaging for Supply) Regulations 1994, SI 1994/3247, as amended.

the Poisons Rules[9] made under the Poisons Act 1972; the Act is described in greater detail in Chapter 22.[10]

In assessing the poisonous properties of an agricultural chemical, due note must be taken of the advantages offered. Some of the organochlorines are theoretically if not actually poisonous;[11] but the benefits to mankind resulting from the widespread reduction of insect-borne diseases, including malaria and sleeping-sickness, greatly outweigh any such considerations. Similarly, paraquat (see below) has revolutionised the agricultural economy of many developing countries; an occasional suicide in such areas must be accepted as a price to pay for the community benefit. Certain insecticides or herbicides will, however, be specifically mentioned in view of their medico-legal interest on other than industrial grounds.

The most important group among the insecticides is that of the organophosphorus compounds, which can enter the body through the inspired air, the skin or even the eye. They owe their profound effect to altering the normal mode of action of the nerves on the muscle masses and to antagonising the effects of the sympathetic nervous system. The most common preparation, parathion, has been used homicidally; because the action of the organophosphates is essentially physiological, the detection of such cases presents a formidable forensic challenge.

Nicotine is a common fungicide which is a powerful poison when concentrated;[12] it enters the body through either the lungs or the skin. The effect of the latter will increase as the body-size decreases—the author has been concerned with two deaths in small children that could only be attributed to contamination with a commercial nicotine spray.

The herbicide that has caused most public and medical concern is paraquat. This remarkable substance is immediately destroyed on contact with the ground—used normally it is, therefore, remarkably safe and highly efficient. Unfortunately, it became a frequent medium for suicide in farming communities; accidental poisoning was also common and there have been at least three convictions for murder by its use in the United Kingdom. Death from paraquat poisoning is singularly unpleasant.[13] Its major action is on the lungs and consists, essentially, of acute oxygen poisoning; the treatment of a patient who is, nevertheless, dying of oxygen *lack* presents a major therapeutic dilemma.

One other slightly bizarre medico-legal aspect of chemical agriculture deserves mention—crop spraying has the highest mortality of any type of aviation. This is related almost solely to the difficult flying conditions; actual poisoning of pilots by their chemical cargo is extremely rare, though minor effects, such as those of the organophosphates on the eyes, could be very dangerous in this situation.

---

9 SI 1982/218, as amended.

10 Several statutes deal with the preservation of the ecology in general or in respect of specific species of wildlife. The most important consolidating Act is the Wildlife and Countryside Act 1981, Pt I.

11 In fact, the Research Committee on Toxic Chemicals reported in 1970 that no evidence had been produced of risks to man resulting from the use of DDT or dieldrin when these were applied properly nor when occurring as residues in a normal diet. Other members of the group—eg Aldrin—might be more hazardous.

12 Nicotine is free from restriction when sold in an aerosol containing not more than 0.2% nicotine (Poisons Rules 1982, Sch 4).

13 Paraquat is restricted as to sale save in its weak, pellet form (Poisons Rules 1982, Sch 4).

Iatrogenic and suicidal poisoning

These forms of poisoning are interlinked and can be discussed under one heading.

Large numbers of new medicinal compounds, which are of increasing complexity both as to their multiplicity of content and as to the effects of the individual drugs contained, appear regularly on the market; doctors are under constant pressure to try new remedies; and, in the conditions of an overworked practice, there is a positive economy of surgery time to be gained by prescribing drugs in such quantity as will serve the patient for a considerable period. Accidental poisoning can occur, therefore, in the normal process of medical practice and, in essence, mishaps can be put down to one of four sources of error:

1. overprescribing the quantity of a single drug;
2. the cumulative effects of drugs;
3. adverse reactions on bodily systems other than that being treated;
4. drug interactions with one another or with articles of diet.

The statutory defence against the majority of these mishaps is provided by the Medicines Act 1968, which is described in Chapter 22. The Act, inter alia, authorises the establishment of a Medicines Commission.[14] The commission, which consists of a chairman and not fewer than eight members, advises the licensing authorities and, to this end, appoints committees which are charged with overseeing the safety, quality or efficiency of medicines and with promoting the collection and investigation of information relating to adverse reactions to drugs on which such advice will be based.[15] The most relevant committee in the present context is that on the Safety of Medicines.[16] This committee meets monthly to review the position of drugs on trial and has a subcommittee to consider notifications of adverse drug reactions that have been made by practitioners. When satisfied that a hazard may exist, the committee, on its own authority, dispatches warning notices drawing the attention of practitioners to areas of danger.[17] All manufacturers of drugs are now required to circulate data sheets in association with advertisements sent direct to practitioners;[18] these data sheets must give all reasonable information as to dosage, effect, contraindications, adverse reactions and the like. The information is consolidated annually by the Association of the British Pharmaceutical Industry as a Data Sheet Compendium which is issued free to doctors. There is, therefore, now ample opportunity for doctors to appreciate the hazards of drug therapy and failure to heed the many warnings given is likely to be construed by the courts as negligence.

It is unusual for a drug to act on only one system—for example, a high proportion of those usually prescribed for disorders of the central nervous system

14 The Medicines Commission and Committees Regulations 1970, SI 1970/746.
15 Medicines Act 1968, s 4(2) and (3).
16 Medicines (Committee on Safety of Medicines) Order 1970, SI 1970/1257.
17 A classic example was the warning issued in 1988 against long-term treatment with benzodiazipines. A massive class action related to benzodiazipine addiction was ultimately struck out due to its minimal chances of success: *AB v John Wyeth & Brother Ltd (No 3)* [1997] 8 Med LR 57, CA. See H Ashton 'Risks of Dependence on Benzodiazepine Drugs: A Major Problem of Long Term Treatment' (1989) 298 BMJ 103 for the background.
18 Medicines Act 1968, s 96. See also Medicines (Advertising) Regulations 1994, SI 1994/1932, as amended.

also have a profound effect on the heart and blood vessels; the danger here is that the prescribing doctor may fail to make himself aware of the patient's total condition. Occasionally, drugs may have serious side effects in humans that did not show up in preliminary animal testing. Unexpected cumulative effects may arise if the patient's capacity for metabolism or excretion of a drug is reduced by disease, for example, of the liver or kidney that has passed unnoticed. Drug interactions are extremely common—they may be complementary or antagonistic, the effects may be dangerous or, on occasion, may be desirable; in many instances, a known effect can be counterbalanced by modifications of the dose. Occasionally, a catastrophe may occur because of unawareness on the part of the practitioner, but the most common cause of adverse interactions results from the use by patients of drugs remaining from a previous prescription—repeated self-medication may be dangerous if the patient is by then receiving another drug for another complaint.

This introduces the problem of overprescribing, which may be unintentional as, for example, when a doctor prescribes two preparations each of which contain an element of the same drug. But the far greater problem lies in semi-elective overprescribing forced by pressures of work; a not uncommon pattern is of a large primary issue followed by repeated prescriptions without adequate confirmation of the patient's need. This, being the practice of probably a majority of doctors, can scarcely be regarded as professional negligence but, as a direct result, there are few households in which an excess of potentially dangerous medicines is not to be found; while some persons would take their own lives no matter how carefully their prescriptions were regulated, there is little doubt that a degree of responsibility for many deaths due to suicidal or accidental poisoning must be laid on the pressures of National Health Service practice.

The pattern of suicidal poisoning varies over the years. Ingestion of toxic substances has, however, always been the commonest form of suicide and, in some areas, as many such victims are admitted to intensive care units as are derived from road-traffic accidents. A further virtually invariable finding is that, whereas, in general, men commit suicide more often than do women, the ratio is reversed and females predominate in suicides by ingestion. As regards the men, those who are single and, particularly, widowers seem to be at risk; the divorced and separated of both sexes are also especially prone to this form of suicide, which seems to have aroused less public concern as a cause of death than it merits

Variations in the drugs most commonly used depend upon several factors. Availability is prominent among these and legislation has a strong affect in this context. Thus, the very marked reduction in the number of suicides due to barbiturate poisoning must be attributed, at least in part, to their inclusion as Class B controlled drugs in 1984;[19] the strenuous efforts made by the medical profession itself to outlaw barbiturates from treatment schedules will also have contributed significantly. It is reasonable to suppose that depressives, who are at greatest risk of suicide, will use the materials close to hand; the pattern will thus depend to an extent on the popularity of the various drugs available for the treatment of depression—and the tricyclic anti-depressants feature prominently in most series of suicides studied and reported. The 'tranquillisers' as a heterogeneous group also account for a large number of suicides—again, these drugs must always be obtained on prescription and many diazapines are now

19 Misuse of Drugs Act 1971 (Modification) Order 1984, SI 1984/859, as amended.

classified as Class C controlled drugs.[20] The tendency for some tranquillisers to cause depression is well known and it may well be that death in such overdose cases may be due to some other factor. The majority of modern anxiolytics are, in fact, remarkably innocuous when taken in excess alone and the additional factor which alters this property is often found to be alcohol. The cause and effect relationship of alcohol to death from ingestion of drugs is complex and is discussed further in Chapter 24. It does, however, often complicate the problem of death certification in these cases.

A major difficulty in establishing the cause of death in drug poisoning lies in the great variation in post-mortem tissue levels that have been reported in fatal cases; this is discussed more fully in Chapter 25. Certainly, there are obvious features that may make one person more susceptible to a drug than another—the route of absorption and the presentation of the drug (ie how it is dissolved or otherwise compounded) may be of significance; an unwell patient is likely to be less tolerant of a given poison than is one who is fully fit—a fact that emphasises the importance of a full autopsy to assess the real significance of drugs in the mode of death; by and large, children and old persons are more susceptible to poisons than are those in other age groups. But, very often, these features will not, in themselves, explain apparently anomalous findings and both the pathologist and the toxicologist are dependent largely on the circumstantial evidence; certainly, attempts to estimate the dose taken that are based on a single post-mortem tissue analysis are liable to very wide error. And it must always be remembered that drugs discovered *within* the intestinal tract are, strictly speaking, *external* to the tissues; the discovery of large numbers of tablets within the stomach does not necessarily mean that they are the cause of death.

Other common suicidal poisonings are associated with substances that are available on general sale, the most important group being the analgesics taken for headaches, etc. Despite the efficiency of modern treatment, there are still an appreciable number of deaths due to aspirin; and, although paracetamol has had a vogue as a suicidal agent, the discovery of a specific antidote has relegated its 'success' to those cases which remain undiscovered for some time. The occurrence of sudden 'waves' of poisoning by specific drugs leads to the suspicion that it is publicity which determines trends in suicide although, in fact, this subjective impression is hard to substantiate. The author has been surprised at the number of deaths due to lysol or similar corrosive poisons that still occur—these seem to be confined to the elderly. Other suicidal poisonings are rare and their individual nature often indicates severe mental derangement; many cases of suicidal paraquat poisoning exhibit this feature. There is also a small group of suicidal poisonings which are linked to occupation—often by way of an exception being made in restrictive legislation for professional purposes; thus, for example, suicides due to cyanide ingestion are virtually confined to photographers and laboratory workers.

There remains carbon monoxide poisoning which, 25 years ago, was as common a method of suicide as was barbiturate poisoning. It was always rare in the USA, where domestic gas supplies were almost universally of natural origin; the introduction of natural gas into British homes has, in the same way, greatly reduced the incidence of carbon monoxide suicides. Such cases as now occur are

20 Misuse of Drugs Act 1971 (Modification) Order 1985, SI 1985/1995, with amendments.

nearly all associated with motor car exhaust fumes. Generally, some method of increasing the certainty of success—eg by passing a tube from the exhaust to the interior of the car—is used. In the absence of such apparatus, the distinction between suicide and accident may be very difficult to make; in fact, poisoning by exhaust fumes from motor cars is probably more often accidental than suicidal.

Accidental poisoning

Accidental poisoning is of considerable medico-legal significance; first, because of its frequency and, secondly, because of the not uncommon difficulty met in distinguishing it from suicide or homicide. It is best discussed in two phases—as related to children and as related to adults.

Children are most often poisoned by reason of genuine mistake. Perhaps the most dangerous factor lies in the similarity between some medicinal tablets and some widely advertised brands of sweets. Alternatively, poisonous berries growing naturally may be mistaken for fruits seen more commonly in the greengrocer's shop. Children may also be victims of their natural inquisitiveness—there is a strong urge to discover what is so pleasant about the 'sweets' kept beside the parents' beds. The prevention of accidental poisoning in children is a matter, first, of adequate security of containers,[1] medicine cupboards, cleaning closets, garden sheds and the like, coupled with adequate surveillance when in an unusual environment—as, for example, on picnic outings.[2] The determination and agility of children is well known; locks are essential wherever potentially poisonous substances are stored. The distinction between accidental poisoning of children and Münchhausen's syndrome by proxy has been discussed at page 287.

Accidental poisoning in adults is, again, of dual origin. First, there are incidents involving errors of perception—the dose of a drug is misread due to age or ill health, medicines are poured out in the dark or when half-asleep; such errors are potentiated by the effects of alcohol. It may be very difficult to distinguish genuine error from a deliberate act. Secondly, there is involuntary error—the taking of poison in the belief that it is an innocuous substance. As in the case of children, this may occur in nature or in the home. Examples in the former situation include the eating of the poisonous fungus *Amanita* in mistake for the edible mushroom *Agaricus* or the use of aconite root instead of horse-radish. Poisoning due to involuntary error in the home is almost always a matter of improper labelling—the frequency with which intensely poisonous substances are stored in open areas in beer or lemonade bottles while these still retain their original labels is astounding. Rarely, the possibility of deliberate substitution has to be considered.

Carbon monoxide is a common agent of accidental poisoning which may, on occasion, give rise to unusual findings at the scene of death. The subject has been discussed in detail in Chapter 13. The diagnosis often depends upon awareness

1   For aspirin and paracetamol, see Medicines (Child Safety) Regulations 1975, SI 1975/2000, as amended.
2   The number of child *deaths* among cases of poisoning is surprisingly small, possibly due to the fact that children are closely observed at home. See S M Cordner and J Ozanne-Smith 'Injury and Death in the Home' in J K Mason and B N Purdue (eds) *The Pathology of Trauma* (3rd edn, 2000) ch 21.

of the possibility—it is surprising how many people fail to appreciate that death from carbon monoxide poisoning can occur in the kitchen even when natural gas is in use; curious mistakes, such as attributing death to food poisoning rather than to carbon monoxide, have resulted from inadequate post-mortem examination.

Homicidal poisoning

The pattern of homicidal poisoning has also changed over the years. Not only have the types of poison used altered, but the condition as a whole appears to have become very uncommon. This must be due largely to steadily more useful legislation. The facilities of the National Health Service (see below) must have a considerable effect while, amongst other factors, the direction of social change is such as to reduce the overall need for the disposal of wives or husbands; when a poisoning occurs it is often found to have unusual background features such as a motivation on eugenic or other humanitarian grounds.[3]

Poisoning is a crime at common law in Scotland. The English Offences Against the Person Act 1861 is more precise and deals with endangering life or with causing grievous bodily harm by poisoning (s 23) and even goes so far as to specify an intention to annoy (s 24). No distinction is made under either jurisdiction between a drug and a poison; both may be noxious things but, as regards the former, the dose given is relevant to the definition, as is its mode of presentation—that is, for example, whether or not the substance is in the form of a reputable pharmaceutical preparation. There is no attempt to specify a noxious substance; it is the intention of the individual user that is of paramount importance.

Very occasionally, homicidal poisoning may be associated with medical treatment, when the injurious substance may be introduced by injection. In the vast majority of cases, however, such poisons are administered by mouth and the victim must suffer to some extent from symptoms of gastroenteritis; the great majority of poisons used with intent to murder will cause vomiting with or without diarrhoea. This is particularly true of the well-known irritant metallic poisons, of which arsenic is the most infamous, and of phosphorus.[4] Nevertheless, natural food poisoning (see below) or diarrhoea and vomiting due to virus disease or to psychiatric causes are far more common than is homicidal poisoning. The practitioner may well be excused for failing to diagnose such a case at first glance[5] but when his suspicions are aroused he is faced with an ethical dilemma. He must

3   There is no automatic recognition of 'mercy killing' in the United Kingdom, although the majority of offenders will be charged with manslaughter rather than murder. This is a statutory reduction in the case of a survivor from a suicide pact in England and Wales: Homicide Act 1957, s 4.
4   Many of the poisons used in the famous cases of the past were incorporated in rodenticides—thallium is, perhaps, the most modern example and its supply is now strictly controlled. No rat poison may now contain strychnine, the use of which is authorised only for the killing of moles or foxes; the use of monofluoroacetic acid in rat control is mainly restricted to use in ships or sewers (Poisons Rules 1982, Sch 12). Yellow phosphorous and red squill cannot be used for the destruction of any mammalian animal: Animals (Cruel Poisons) Act 1962; see Animals (Cruel Poisons) Regulations 1963, SI 1963/1278. Rat poisons are now largely compounded of biological substances but acquired resistance may dictate a return to chemical control.
5   The same might be said about the dermatologist because chronic poisoning may manifest itself in unusual skin conditions.

have the interests of his patient as his main concern; yet to take action that might be interpreted publicly as implying suspicion of foul play could result in serious charges in the event that it was ill-founded.

The doctor in this position should continue to treat his patient but should take extra precautions against the time when his evidence may be needed in court. Thus, particularly careful notes ought to be made of statements, of relevant times and of specific points that are considered unusual. The normal specimens of vomit and faeces should be taken and labelled accurately; there would seem to be no reason why a toxicological analysis should not be arranged in parallel with bacteriological examinations provided confidentiality is assured and the test can be justified as being in the best interests of the patient. Ideally, specimens of food might be obtained and sent for similar analysis but this could be extremely difficult to achieve if a homicidal attempt were really being made. The ultimate test is to remove the patient to hospital and, in practice, this is what will usually happen in the conditions of a National Health Service. By the time a practitioner is sufficiently concerned to suspect poisoning, he will have been already anxious to obtain improved conditions for his patient on purely medical grounds; this will be particularly so if he finds, as may well happen, that he has been called in late to the case. The homicidal process is thus effectively aborted – although it is remarkable in how many suspicious cases it is found that a relative is still bringing food into the ward.

If deliberate poisoning is proved to the satisfaction of both the practitioner and the hospital consultant, then it would be right for a confidential report to be made to a senior police officer; few doctors would, however, like to do so without the support of their defence or protection society. In the event of a death that arouses suspicion, the doctor's duty is clear and unequivocal—the case must be reported to the fiscal or to the coroner; this applies also to deaths due to natural poisoning.

Natural poisoning

Food poisoning

Food poisoning as a cause of accidental death has been already mentioned, as has its importance in the differential diagnosis of homicidal poisoning. This is probably its main forensic significance, although actions for tort or delict might well be brought against suppliers, restaurants and the like when damage is suffered; criminal charges could be brought in the event of transgression of the statutory law.[6]

Acute poisoning may result from the ingestion of either living virulent bacteria or of toxins or toxic principles which, in turn, can derive from bacteria or may be normal components of the foodstuffs. An important distinction is that bacteria, unless present in the form of resistant spores, are killed by heat; toxins, however, may be thermostable, particularly when they are mixed with or are part of the food.

---

6   The greater part of food safety legislation is to be found in the Food Safety Act 1990 (as amended by the Food Standards Act 1999), the Food and Environment Protection Act 1985 and in the remnants of the Food Act 1984—backed by massive secondary legislation. For an interesting analysis of the powers of the local authorities, see *R v Secretary of State for Health, ex p Eastside Cheese Co* [2000] EHLR 52, CA.

Strictly speaking, bacterial food poisoning will include any disease transmitted through food or water or by a food handler—for example, typhoid fever, cholera, dysentery of either bacterial or of amoebic (protozoal) type or poisoning by pathogenic forms of *E. Coli*.[7] However, while a few other bacteria may cause very similar symptoms, the term is confined by popular usage to infection by organisms of the *Salmonella* group, virulent *Staphylococci* or *Clostridium welchii*—an organism that also causes gas gangrene. *Salmonellae* are essentially parasites of animals and may pre-exist in the foodstuff or be introduced by contamination; the food shows no evidence of putrefaction and symptoms may be due to the presence of preformed toxin or to proliferation of the bacteria in the human host. *Staphylococci*, on the other hand, are nearly always introduced from a human carrier during the processing of food such as ice-cream or bakery products. In either case, the symptoms of abdominal pain, vomiting and diarrhoea may closely simulate those of acute metallic poisoning. *Cl. welchii* typically contaminates raw meat, poultry or stews; outbreaks of food poisoning in institutions are often due to this organism.

Although it is very rare, botulism is the classic food poisoning due to the presence of preformed bacterial toxin. The organism (*Cl. botulinum*) lives in soil and can, therefore, be transmitted in vegetables; it grows only in the absence of oxygen and will flourish in canned or bottled foodstuffs. Home bottling of vegetables is probably the least uncommon source of the condition but meat products are also implicated. The disease is generally of great severity and is often fatal; it causes paralysis of the central nervous system and the usual symptoms of food poisoning are absent. Cases are very rare in the United Kingdom.

Poisoning by reason of the nature of the food may result from ingestion of both vegetable and animal matter. The fungi, which are most likely to be eaten in error, are the best known of the very many vegetables that have poisonous properties. Fungi of the genus *Amanita*, eaten in mistake for the common mushroom *Agaricus*, contain toxins that may cause severe gastrointestinal upset with accompanying surgical shock or, through the action of the alkaloid muscarine, may interfere with the nervous stimulation of the muscles. The toxic principles of some fungi are hallucinogenic and are at the root of a modern social problem. The most dangerous fungus, *A. phalloides*, is toxic even having been cooked. On the other hand, many fungi apart from the common field mushroom are palatable and non-toxic.

Animal foods that are toxic in the absence of bacterial contamination mostly derive from fish.[8] The poisonous principle is neurotoxic and is concentrated maximally in the gonads and the liver at spawning time. Alternatively, fish such as tuna and mackerel may be secondarily poisonous due to inadequate storage conditions; so-called scombroid poisoning is a well-recognised entity due to bacterial contamination which produces an allergic form of disease – death is uncommon. Poisonous fungi and poisonous fish are used both homicidally and suicidally in primitive societies—the usual responsible substance, tetrodotoxin, is one of the most powerful natural toxins known.

7   The majority of strains of *E. Coli* are non-pathogenic when in the bowel. Further controls have been introduced in both England and Scotland as a result of a serious outbreak: Food Safety (General Food Hygiene) (Butchers' Shops) Amendment Regulations 2000, SI 2000/930. For Scotland, SI 2000/93.

8   The dangers of most shellfish and molluscs stem not only from their primary toxicity at certain times of the year but also from their lifestyle as scavengers and their frequent contamination with disease-producing organisms. It is interesting that many religious taboos—especially those of Judaism—are founded on good public health principles.

Poisons naturally injected

Many animal species inject venom either as a defence mechanism or as a means of immobilising their prey. Of these, snakes are by far the most important both medically and in the forensic context.

There are two main families of venomous snake—the *Viperidae*, all of which are poisonous, and the *Colubridae*, many of which are non-poisonous but which include the very dangerous cobras and kraits. Venom is injected reflexly through the fangs when the snake strikes or bites. All venoms contain a mixture of toxic principles but, in general, the colubride venom is neurotoxic and kills rapidly due to paralysis while that of the viperidae acts on the blood and kills slowly by destroying the red cells and altering the clotting mechanisms. Tragedies have occurred in mistaking the staggering gait and slurred speech of the victim of cobra bite for drunkenness.

Snake venoms are not of equal potency, nor is each injection equally efficient; but the concentration of the dose depends upon the body weight and it follows that snake bite, or any other venomous injection, is more dangerous in the case of children than in adults. The prognosis is also greatly influenced by the availability of efficient treatment.

The treatment of snake bite is both general and specific. It is the latter, in the form of antivenin therapy, which causes most medico-legal concern. Horses can be immunised against snake venom and thus provide antisera for the treatment of humans. The most specific antisera will be the most efficacious but their use depends upon accurate identification of the specific snake; in practice, therefore, the doctor is often forced to use a less efficient, 'wide-spectrum' antivenin. At the same time, there is always a risk of severe reaction by the patient to the 'horse' components of the injection (see page 94). There may well be a therapeutic dilemma. Little doubt would be raised in areas in which poisonous snakes abounded—provided that the patient was seen within eight hours of being bitten, antivenin would be given without hesitation. At the other extreme, the only poisonous snake that exists in Great Britain, *V. berus*, injects a venom that is only slightly toxic—its bite may well be less dangerous than is the use of the available antivenin. The decision could be a hard one in the case of a small child; if antiserum was given, test dosing followed by very careful administration and desensitisation (eg by the use of adrenalin) would be mandatory. It is believed that snake bite kills some 40,000 persons annually throughout the world, the most dangerous areas being Asia, Central America and Australia. Most Asian practitioners would probably agree, however, that a number of otherwise violent deaths are incorrectly attributed to snake bite.

The sting of the scorpion, which does not live outside the subtropics, is perhaps the second most common serious envenomation on a world-wide basis; at the very least, the sting is intensely painful, while the venom of certain species is as dangerous as is that of some snakes. All spider bites are potentially poisonous but dangerous poisoning is far less common than is generally supposed. The most serious bite is that of the species *Latrodectus*—the 'black widow'—which tends to lurk under rustic latrine seats. Antivenins are available both for scorpion sting and for spider bite and, again, the seriousness of the prognosis is inversely proportional to the body weight of the person attacked.

Few insect stings are completely free from danger, particularly if they are multiple. The sheer pain may induce a vagal type of shock, whereas unduly sensitive persons may die from an antigen/antibody reaction. It is also to be noted, not only in the present context but also as a generalisation in forensic medicine, that the *conditions* under which an incident occurs may have a profound effect on the outcome. A bee sting may well be innocuous when sitting in a deck-chair; it could be fatal if sustained while driving a car at high speed.

22

The law relating to drugs and poisons

The law relating to environmental and industrial poisoning is a wide subject very largely beyond the control of the individual. The purpose of this chapter is to outline only the statutory control of poisons and drugs that are dispensed through the pharmaceutical and medical professions.

Thus limited, there are three groups of enactments of major importance. The Poisons Act 1972 is concerned entirely with non-medicinal poisons and, in the main, regulates the storage of poisons and their sale and supply to the public and to the health professions. The Medicines Acts 1968 and 1971 are, as their names indicate, related to medicinal drugs; they cover many administrative aspects of the advertisement and sale of medicines and essentially regulate the standards of pharmaceutical practice. The Misuse of Drugs Act 1971 deals with only a limited list of drugs; nevertheless, it is that part of drug legislation that is most closely associated with forensic medicine, being both directly and indirectly related to criminality.

Sale of non-medicinal poisons to the public

The Poisons Act 1972 provides for:

- the registration of sellers of poisons;
- the categorisation of poisons in relation to how they may be sold or supplied;
- the drawing up of Poisons Rules and their review.

The last two provisions are amongst the functions of the Poisons Board, which advises the Secretaries of State on both aspects.[1]

The Poisons List[2] is divided into two parts. Part I poisons may be sold only by pharmacists from registered premises; Part II poisons may be sold only by

1 The Poisons Board consists of five members appointed by the interested government departments, the Government Chemist, five persons approved by the Pharmaceutical Society of Great Britain, four members appointed by echelons of the medical profession, one by the Royal Institute of Chemistry and any additional members thought necessary.
2 Poisons List Order 1982, SI 1982/217, as amended.

pharmacists or, from specified premises, by persons who are approved by the local authority as listed sellers of Part II poisons. The Poisons Board has authority to recommend the precise listing of poisons but, in general, Part II poisons are those to which it is reasonable for the public to have adequate access—they thus include those substances which, although poisonous if misused, are in everyday household use.

The sale, supply and storage of listed poisons are controlled by the Poisons Rules,[3] in which the word 'poison' means a non-medicinal poison. Much of the meat of the rules is to be found in the Schedules. Poisons that are listed in Schedule 1 are restricted in that the retail purchaser must either be known to the seller or must provide a certificate signed either by a householder known to the pharmacist or by a police officer in charge of a station; full details of the sale must be entered in a book kept for the purpose, and the purchaser must sign the entry.[4] Since the 1972 Act deals only with non-medicinal substances, there is no reason why doctors and other health carers should not be subject to the same controls; when a Schedule 1 poison also has a medicinal role, it is subject to the provisions of the Medicines Act 1968 (see below) when prescribed for that purpose. Schedule 1 poisons held in a shop or similar premises must be stored in a cupboard or drawer reserved solely for the storage of poisons or in a part of the premises to which the public have no access; strict precautions must be taken to avoid contamination of food.[5] Schedule 4, by contrast, contains a number of exemptions from the Act and from the rules; these include, first, general exemptions related to articles and preparations in common use which may contain poisonous substances and, secondly, many special exemptions related both to the use of and the concentration of poisons in the listed substances.

Schedule 5 regulates the sale by listed sellers of Part II poisons of certain poisons used mainly in agriculture and horticulture; Part A itemises the forms in which they are exempted from control, while Part B lists those poisons which may be sold only to persons engaged in the trades or businesses of horticulture, agriculture or forestry for the purposes of such trade or business—thus, the public distribution of many potent pesticides that are dangerous to humans is specifically controlled. The remaining Schedules are concerned, in the main, with the control of rodenticides—in particular, strychnine—and are of very specific application. Even so, the various Poisons Acts have undoubtedly been largely responsible for the decline in homicidal poisoning by non-medicinal substances that has been so evident over the past 50 years.

The Medicines Act 1968

This massive Act is concerned, in the main, with the regulation of the manufacture and supply of medicinal products, which are defined (s 130) as any substances (not being instruments, apparatus or appliances) that are manufactured, sold, supplied, imported or exported for use by being administered to human beings or

3   Poisons Rules 1982, SI 1982/218, as amended. The labelling of poisons is now controlled by the Chemicals (Hazard Information and Packaging for Supply) Regulations 1994, SI 1994/2247, as amended.
4   Poisons Act 1972, s 3(2).
5   Poisons Rules 1982, r 21.

animals for a medicinal purpose or that are ingredients of a substance or article used for medicinal purposes. A 'medicinal purpose' implies treatment or prevention of disease, diagnosis, contraception, induction of anaesthesia or interference with a normal physiological function in either a negative or positive fashion.

Part II of the Act introduces licences and certificates relating to the sale, wholesale and manufacture of medicinal products with general exceptions from the restrictive regulations for doctors, dentists, veterinary practitioners and pharmacists; clinical trials on patients and medicinal tests on animals are also controlled (ss 31 and 32). Part III deals with the sale of medicinal products. Part IV defines pharmacists and pharmacies and their registration. Part V deals with the labelling, packaging and identification of medicinal products and Part VI lays down criteria on the important subject of advertising—particular attention is paid to the problems of false or misleading advertisements and representations.[6]

While the Act defines a number of offences, all of which may come within the ambit of the lawyer, very few of these involve directly the doctor or the dentist—indeed, they are specifically excluded from the majority of the provisions; a detailed discussion is, therefore, beyond the scope of a text on forensic medicine. We must, however, consider the special points concerning the supply of medicines to the general public.

The basic provision in this respect lies in s 51 of the Act, which introduces the category of General Sale List Medicines.[7] These drugs are of generally innocuous type and a few are listed as being saleable in automatic vending machines. Medicinal products used in eye drops or ointments or those intended for injection may not be on general sale (SI 1984/769, Sch 3). A medicine may be sold or supplied only from a registered pharmacy unless it is categorised as a general sale list medicine.

Section 58 of the Act defines the category of 'Prescription Only Medicines'.[8] As the name implies, such drugs can be sold or supplied by retail only in accordance with a prescription given by a doctor or dentist as appropriate.[9] The general classes of such drugs include all products containing one or more of the substances listed in Sch 1 to the 1997 Order, medicinal products containing any drug specified in Sch 2 to the Misuse of Drugs Act 1971[10] and medicinal products that are for parenteral administration, irrespective of whether or not they contain a prescription-only drug.[11]

6 Medicines Act 1968, s 93; Medicines (Advertising) Regulations 1994, SI 1994/1932, as amended by Medicines for Human Use (Marketing Authorisation etc) Regulations 1994, SI 1994/3144 and SIs 1996/1552 and 1999/267. The meaning of false or misleading was addressed in *R v Roussel Laboratories Ltd; R v Good* (1988) 88 Cr App Rep 140, CA.
7 Specified in Medicines (Products other than Veterinary Drugs) (General Sale List) Order 1984, SI 1984/769, as amended.
8 Prescription Only Medicines (Human Use) Order 1997, SI 1997/1830, as amended.
9 Registered nurses, midwives and health visitors are able to prescribe certain 'prescription-only' medicines: Medicinal Products: Prescription by Nurses etc Act 1992. The rest of the chapter should be read with this in mind.
10 There are exceptions to this whereby certain drugs—eg codeine, morphine and medicinal opium—are excluded when present below a specified strength.
11 The effect of the Act is that no one can administer a parenteral injection (other than to himself) unless he is an appropriate practitioner or is acting under the instructions of one. Insulins are no longer excluded from the category of prescription-only drugs: Prescription Only Medicines (Human Use) Amendment Order 1998, SI 1998/108, reg 2. Certain other drugs can be administered parenterally by anyone in an emergency, SI 1997/1830, reg 7.

There remains a group of drugs that are covered by neither of the above sections. These are known as 'Pharmacy Medicines', which are not on general sale and can be offered for retail sale only through a retail pharmacy business.

There are very stringent rules governing the labelling of medicinal products and, in particular, pharmacy and prescription-only medicines must be clearly labelled 'P' and 'POM' as appropriate.[12] All medicinal products must be labelled 'Keep Out of the Reach of Children'. A record must be kept of every sale or supply of a prescription-only medicine unless the medicine was prescribed through the National Health Service and this includes medicine dispensed in an emergency (see below); records and prescriptions must be preserved for two years.

Article 15 of the 1997 Order details the requirements for a valid prescription of a prescription-only medicine. These can be summarised so that it:

'1. Shall be written in indelible ink.
2. Shall contain the following particulars:
    (a) The address and usual signature of the practitioner giving it;
    (b) the date on which it was signed by the practitioner giving it;
    (c) such particulars as indicate whether the practitioner giving it is a doctor, a dentist, a veterinary surgeon, a veterinary practitioner or a nurse practitioner.
    (d) where the practitioner is a doctor or a dentist or a nurse practitioner, the name, address and the age (if under 12 years) of the person for whose treatment it is given; and
    (e) where the practitioner is a veterinary surgeon or a veterinary practitioner the name and address of the person to whom the prescription-only medicine is to be delivered for the treatment of animals.
3. Except where it is a repeat prescription, shall not be dispensed for the first time later than 6 months after the date referred to in 2 (b) above.
4. Where it is a repeat prescription, shall not be dispensed other than in accordance with the direction contained therein.
5. Where the prescription is not a repeat prescription but contains a direction that the prescription be repeated without specifying the number of times it may be dispensed, shall not be dispensed on more than two occasions unless it is an oral contraceptive when it may be dispensed up to 6 times in the 6 months following the date of prescription.'[13]

If a doctor is unable to provide a prescription, the pharmacist may supply the medicine under art 8, subject to the doctor undertaking to rectify the position within 72 hours; no repeats are allowed and the medicine must contain no substances subject to full control under the Misuse of Drugs Regulations 1985, Schs 1, 2 and 3.[14] In extreme emergency, the pharmacist may also supply at the request of the patient so long as he is satisfied that an emergency exists and that the patient had previously been prescribed the medicine requested. The total supply must not be sufficient for more than five days' treatment and the medicine must not contain any controlled drug (Misuse of Drugs Regulations, Schs 1, 2 and 3) other than a barbiturate for the treatment of epilepsy.

---

12 Medicines (Labelling) Regulations 1976, SI 1976/1726, reg 14B and C; Medicines for Human Use (Marketing Authorisations etc) Regulations 1994, SI 1994/3144.
13 Note that, irrespective of the drug prescribed, the doctor is liable to the patient in negligence if the poor quality of his handwriting results in damage due to the supply of the wrong drug: *Prendergast v Sam and Dee Ltd* [1989] 1 Med LR 36.
14 SI 1985/2066.

Otherwise, Part I of the 1968 Act—its administration—is apposite in that it establishes the Medicines Commission which, in turn, has the power to recommend to the minister the setting up of committees with particular responsibility for the safety and efficacy of medicinal drugs. These functions have been discussed already.

Drug abuse

The Misuse of Drugs Act 1971 is now the consolidated legislation dealing with drugs of addiction and others that are thought to constitute a social problem. The major regulations flowing from the Act are the Misuse of Drugs Regulations 1985,[15] the Misuse of Drugs (Safe Custody) Regulations 1973[16] and the Misuse of Drugs (Supply to Addicts) Regulations 1997.[17]

The 1971 Act does four things of major importance to the doctor:

1. It establishes an Advisory Council on the Misuse of Drugs.
2. It classifies certain drugs as Controlled Drugs.
3. It takes steps to regulate doctors who are deemed unsuitable to prescribe or administer controlled drugs (ss 12 and 13).
4. It empowers the Advisory Council to advise on the establishment of centres for treatment, rehabilitation and after-care of persons affected by the misuse of drugs.

The Act is, therefore, more than simply repressive in type and represents a great advance in social legislation over the statutes it repealed.

The Advisory Council, as presently constituted, consists of not fewer than 20 persons with wide and recent experience in the specialities of medicine, dentistry, veterinary medicine, pharmacy, pharmaceutical manufacturing, chemistry and social work involving the misuse of drugs. The remit of the council has the very great advantage of flexibility. It must monitor the national situation in regard to drug abuse and can advise on measures to be taken in the light of changing circumstances. Drugs can, therefore, be controlled rapidly; alternatively, drugs that seem at any time to have ceased to be a problem can be released from restriction. Equally important functions of the Advisory Council include the promotion of co-operation between all the social services involved in the eradication of drug abuse and the education of the public—and especially the younger public—as to the dangers of the misuse of drugs.

Historically, dangerous drugs have been equated with narcotic drugs. The pharmaceutical industry has, however, made such advances in the production of drugs that have powerful effects outwith their intended therapeutic roles that drug abuse has escaped from its previous confines. Stimulants, hallucinogens and the like may be just as dangerous or antisocial as are the narcotics, particularly when they are used as mixtures. This is the trend that s 2 of the Act is designed to combat. Under this section and its resultant regulations,[18] certain drugs are listed

---

15 SI 1985/2066, as amended.
16 SI 1973/798, as amended.
17 SI 1997/1001.
18 Misuse of Drugs Regulations 1985, SI 1985/2066, Schs 1–3 as amended.

as 'controlled'. Controlled drugs are classified into classes A, B and C, the classes being determined by the punishment specified for the offences of their production, supply and possession. The penalties are greatest in the case of Class A and least in the case of Class C drugs[19] and, in all cases, are more severe in relation to production and supply than as to possession. It is a logical consequence that, in practice, the most harmful drugs are placed in Class A. A distinction is made, however, in the case of drugs that are both harmful and have negligible therapeutic application; these drugs are listed in Sch 1 to the 1985 regulations. Whereas many professional persons—including doctors, dentists, etc—may legally possess controlled drugs for the purpose of carrying on their profession, a special licence is needed for the possession of those in Sch 1.[20]

The lawful supply of controlled drugs is carefully regulated. A prescription given by a doctor must be in ink or otherwise indelible and, unless it contains phenobarbitone only, must be written in the prescriber's own hand; it must be signed and dated by him and must state the name and address of the person to be treated and of the prescriber unless it is written on a National Health Service prescription form; and the dose of the controlled drug must be written both in words and in figures. Repeat prescriptions are not permitted and, should it be the intention to dispense the prescription by instalments, the total amount of controlled drug to be given in each instalment and the intervals to be observed must be stated. The pharmacist must either know the signature of the prescriber or must have no reason to doubt its genuineness.[1] These restrictions are intended to detect or discourage forgery and to prevent the stockpiling of controlled drugs by individuals.

The 1985 regulations maintain the requirements for recording the supply and administration of controlled drugs. Unless the drugs are supplied to a patient on prescription, an entry must be made in a bound register of receipt and supply of all drugs in Classes A and B and of all those in Sch 1 to the regulations (regs 19 and 20). A doctor must keep such a register and must produce this for inspection on request when so directed in writing by the Secretary of State. Controlled drugs must be kept in a locked safe, cabinet or room or in a locked container that can only be opened by the person legally in possession[2] but Sch 1 to the 1973 regulations lists relaxations in respect of many Class B and Class C drugs. A locked car would not be considered a locked receptacle for the purposes of the regulations,[3] but a locked glove compartment in a locked car would probably qualify.

The Misuse of Drugs Act includes statutory controls over the rights of doctors to prescribe and possess drugs. Under s 12, the Secretary of State may direct that a doctor who has been convicted of an offence under the Act[4] shall be prohibited from possessing or prescribing controlled drugs; such a direction is operative once it has been served on the practitioner to whom it applies but can be cancelled or suspended at any time.

---

19 Rather surprisingly, the only difference between Class A and Class B drugs relates to the punishment for possession of a controlled drug (Sch 4 to the 1971 Act).
20 This is not stated positively but would appear to be so by a process of deductive reasoning—it is certainly the policy adopted by inspectors appointed under s 23 of the Act.
1 SI 1985/2066, regs 15 and 16.
2 Misuse of Drugs (Safe Custody) Regulations 1973, SI 1973/798, as amended, reg 3.
3 *Rao v Wyles* [1949] 2 All ER 685.
4 Or certain offences in connection with the Customs and Excise Management Act 1979.

Sections 13 and 14 are of more practical concern to the lawyer. Under the former, the Secretary of State may prohibit a practitioner from possessing or prescribing controlled drugs either if the doctor prescribes controlled drugs to an addict[5] or if he contravenes reg 3, which states that heroin, cocaine and dipipanone can only be prescribed under licence unless it be for treatment of organic disease or injury. The Secretary of State may also impose a prohibition if he believes that the practitioner has been prescribing controlled drugs in an irresponsible fashion. It is to be noted that these regulations put a curb on the doctor's clinical freedom.

Section 14 describes the procedure to be followed in all these circumstances. In the first instance, the case is referred to a tribunal,[6] which may find that there is no reason for a direction of prohibition to be made; in that case, the practitioner is so informed. Should the tribunal find against the practitioner, a recommendation is made to the Secretary of State, indicating those controlled drugs that he should be forbidden to possess or prescribe. The proceedings before the tribunal are private, unless a public hearing is requested by the respondent, and the parties may be legally represented. Representations against the findings of a tribunal are referred to an Advisory Body which consists of a Queen's Counsel as chairman, a medical (or dental or veterinary) practitioner in government employ, and a further member appointed by the respondent's profession; legal representation is again allowed. The Advisory Body may recommend a direction of prohibition either accepting or modifying the advice of the tribunal, it may refer the case back to the tribunal or another tribunal, or it may advise that no further proceedings be taken.

A further disciplinary power exists when there appears to be considerable urgency over the need to suspend a practitioner's right to supply controlled drugs (1971 Act, s 15). In these circumstances, the Secretary of State refers the case to a professional panel which consists of three members of the respondent's profession appointed by the Secretary of State. In the event that the panel advises the need, the Secretary of State may issue a direction of temporary prohibition for a period of six weeks but must, at the same time, refer the case to a tribunal. The temporary prohibition may be extended, subject to the agreement of the tribunal, for periods of 28 days.

This control of a doctor's or dentist's practice by statute is a departure from the established regulation of professional conduct by the General Medical or Dental Councils (see Chapter 29); the seriousness of this step is reflected in the intricacy of the procedure. Nevertheless, it is noteworthy that, with the exception of the legal chairmen, the respondent's case is still tried entirely by his peers. It is clear, however, that a decision by the tribunal need not necessarily be the same as that taken by the General Medical Council; the former is concerned with the misuse of controlled drugs and the latter with the ethical standards of the medical profession.[7]

---

5 Misuse of Drugs Act 1971, s 10(h); Misuse of Drugs (Supply to Addicts) Regulations 1997, SI 1997/1001. The 14 drugs to which the regulations currently refer are listed in the Schedule to the regulations.

6 Misuse of Drugs Act 1971, Sch 3; Misuse of Drugs Tribunal (England and Wales) Rules 1974, SI 1974/85. The tribunal consists of a lawyer of at least seven years' standing as chairman and four members from the medical (or dental or veterinary as appropriate) profession.

7 *Desrath Rai v General Medical Council* (1984) i Lancet 1420, PC.

23

Drug addiction

Malcolm Bruce

Change is slow for some topics within this book. For example, a stab wound 20 years ago is still a stab wound today. Drug use in society, however, is changing rapidly along a number of parameters—including the length of use, the type of drug, the dose, the adulterants, the environment, the frequency and route of use, the combination of drugs and society's major areas of concern. The current drug laws[1] reflect this dichotomy between history and changing attitudes and practice. At the time of writing, two reports have been published which attempt to inform and to raise the debate above polarised 'sound-bite' positions:[2]

> 'In the long run, society will only be at ease with its drug control policies if they are based on a rational assessment of the risks associated with different psychoactive substances and an objective appraisal of the consequences of previous policy changes, rather than on moral postures, the mistaken assumptions of the past and the accidents of history'.[3]

It is less than 200 years since the United Kingdom defended its right to an open free market in trading opium in the 'opium wars' with China. There was no legislation related to drugs in the United Kingdom prior to the Pharmacy Act 1868, which restricted sale of opium to pharmacists only. It was only during the First World War that, due to concern about the fighting ability of the soldiers, cocaine and opium were restricted to supply by prescription only under the Defence of the Realm Act 1914. Subsequently, the Dangerous Drugs Act 1920 added morphine and heroin to the list. Committees have reported to government in 1926,[4] 1961 and 1965.[5] The resulting legislation, the Dangerous Drugs Act 1967,

---

1   Mainly the Misuse of Drugs Act 1971.
2   Report of the Independent Inquiry into the Misuse of Drugs Act 1971 *Drugs and the Law* (2000); Report of the Joint Working Party between the Royal College of Psychiatrists and the Royal College of Physicians on Drug Misuse and Public Policy in the UK *Drugs, Dilemmas and Choices* (2000).
3   Joint Working Party Report, fn 2 above.
4   Ministry of Health, Report of the Departmental Committee on Morphine and Heroin Addiction (1926) (also known as the Rolleston Committee Report).
5   The Second Report of the Interdepartmental Committee (1965) (also known as the Brain Committee Report).

limited the prescribing of drugs to 'addicts' and created the UK 'addicts index' by way of mandatory notification which was stopped in May 1997. The Misuse of Drugs Act 1971 set up the Advisory Council on the Misuse of Drugs (ACMD) as a standing committee. It also introduced the subdivision of controlled drugs into 'Classes' A, B and C, a unique differentiation within Europe. The rationale for the Class system is not defined within the Act, but it is widely accepted that the drugs that cause the most harm should be seen as Class A, and that those that cause less harm need to be distinguished from the more dangerous drugs and placed in a lesser Class of B or C.

International agreements on drug control, in which the United Kingdom has been a major participant, have to be considered when looking to the future of domestic law. The Police Foundation Report[6] unearthed a general belief that these obligations rule out the possibility of changes to our law. However:

> 'although they rule out the legalization of any prohibited drug other than for medical, scientific or limited industrial purposes, the conventions allow more room for manoeuvre than is generally understood. It is in the area of drug use, possession and related acts that the scope left by the international conventions for different approaches is widest. We have found that it is not well understood that, for such offences, there is express provision for imposing measures such as treatment, education, rehabilitation or social reintegration; These measures may be imposed either in addition to or, more importantly, as an alternative to conviction or punishment.'

Aetiology of drug use and misuse

The aetiogical factors vary, depending on what stage of drug use one is examining. Factors that determine the initiation of drug use differ from those that influence the continuation of drug use, the move into dependent use and the causes of relapse.

Initiation of drug use

Mankind has used psycho-active drugs at all stages of history:

> 'Most men and women lead lives at worst, so painful, at the best, so monotonous, poor and limited, that the urge to escape, the longing to transcend themselves only for a few moments, is always and has been one of the principal appetites of the human soul.'[7]

It is estimated that 95% of the population take drugs that are active on the brain, in the form of caffeine, tobacco, alcohol or illicit drugs. As the majority of the population is law abiding, most do not take illegal drugs. However, in any one year, at least 3% of the adult population of Great Britain—some 1.4 million people—will do so.[8] Most of these take cannabis, and most use it only occasionally. Population averages can, however, be misleading when applied to young adults and school children. A longitudinal study of knowledge and experience of young

6   *Drugs and the Law*, fn 2 above.
7   A Huxley *The Doors of Perception* (1940).
8   Institute for the Study of Drug Dependence *National Audit of Drug Misuse in Britain, 1997* (1998).

people regarding drug misuse has been monitored every five years since 1969 in one English town. The proportion of people who knew someone taking drugs increased in this period from 15% to 65% and the proportion who had been offered drugs increased from 5% to 45%. The major change occurred primarily between 1989 and 1994. Stimulants were more commonly mentioned than were opiates.[9] Cross-sectional studies in the United Kingdom have shown that at least 40% of pupils aged 15 to 16 had used illicit drugs at some time, mainly cannabis. Geographical variations also occur—levels of drug use are, for example, higher in Scotland than in England. A typical cross-sectional study in Scotland, which involved all local council areas and 189 different schools with just under 10,000 pupils aged between 11 and 17 participating, found that the use of cannabis was reported most commonly in at least 40% of the group of 14 to 15 year olds and then, in descending order, pain killers, solvents, amphetamine, magic mushrooms, LSD, tranquillisers, ecstasy, cocaine and heroin—only 1.2% had tried heroin. Fourteen per cent of the group used drugs once a week or more, with a further 15% using it once a month and 10% once a year.[10]

Whether an individual will take a particular drug depends on its availability, cost, legal status, the alleged effects and risks of so doing and, in some cases, the form of the drug. Why one person will choose to use a drug alongside another who chooses not to, given the same situation, is more complex. Personality traits, such as rebelliousness and curiosity, are thought to contribute to drug experimentation, as is a wish to express independence or hostility. The search for peer group approval may also contribute. Individuals are also influenced by families and by society and, here, role models and group pressure may cause some individuals to take drugs when others would not. In some instances, initiation to drug use is iatrogenic—for example, in the treatment of severe pain. It is in the initiation of drug use that the moral judgmental model is strongest. An assumption of freedom of choice lies behind all 'just say no' campaigns.

Continued use

A steady increase in the numbers of casual drug users continues, especially in the case of those who use cannabis.[11] Another feature of casual drug use in the last decade has been the very substantial increase in the numbers of young people using a wide combination of drugs, particularly stimulants, in leisure settings. While the factors involved in the initiation of use may have a varied influence on subsequent drug behaviour, additional factors come into play when people continue to take drugs. An individual drug must give positive effects and minimal negative effects if its use is to be maintained. These positive effects provide the beginning of the development of 'positive outcome expectancy' which, with continued reinforcement, will later develop into craving. The onset of classical conditioning and conditioned responses become more apparent with use and the pharmacology of the drug then determines much of what users then choose to do. At the individual level, continued use is associated with general non-conformity. Our understanding

9 J Wright and L Pearl 'Knowledge and Experience of Young People Regarding Drug Misuse, 1969–1994' (1995) 310 BMJ 20.
10 Fast Forward Positive Lifestyle Ltd *Scottish Schools Drug Survey, 1996* (1996).
11 Institute for the Study of Drug Dependence (ISDD) *National audit of drug misuse in Britain 1998* (1999).

of the genetic contribution to individual differences in sensitivity to drugs and their influence on behaviour are not fully developed, but will play its part in the future analysis of the aetiology of the movement from experimental to recreational use and, then, to dependence. Individual distress or unrecognised psychiatric illness can lead some in search of self-medication and the short-term alleviation of symptoms to continued use.

Dependent use

The trend over the past 20 years of a substantial and steady increase in problem drug use in the United Kingdom is clear; it is now estimated that there are up to 200,000 problem drug users, of whom the majority are heroin users, often injectors.[12] The largest increase over the last five years has been among those under 21. There is a high correlation with social deprivation and urban residence. Once the dependence syndrome has developed, tolerance and withdrawal symptoms are frequent features of the condition and the quality and severity of withdrawal is primarily determined by the substance of use. Avoidance of withdrawal then becomes a major factor in continued drug use. At the individual level, personality traits in people dependent on drugs, particularly heroin addicts, certainly differ from those of normal controls. There is an increased incidence of low self-esteem, submissiveness, dependence on others and a craving for approval; lack of self-confidence, a learnt helplessness, low expectations for the future and a tendency to give up easily are also found in excess. However, prospective studies have failed to disclose whether this is a cause or an effect of the dependence syndrome. Much is said about individual denial of problems related to drug use, or at least a lack of awareness. Alternatively, dependent drug users may choose to persist because the benefits of giving up are not outweighed by the advantages of continued use. A further theory underlying persistent drug use in dependent users is that they have not developed mechanisms for coping with problems that present themselves and that the use of drugs is their main management strategy. As mentioned above, classical conditioning and learning theory play an increasing role the longer the drug is used.

For most of those involved, drug misuse is a chosen, relatively controlled lifestyle following a period of either experimental or 'recreational' use which has been adopted in full knowledge of the range of risks involved, including breaking the law. This chapter will not consider the criminal aspects and is confined to consideration of the mental and behavioural disorders associated with psychoactive substance use.

Disorders associated with drug misuse

Drug misuse may result in a wide variety of disorders, which differ in severity from harmful use and uncomplicated intoxication to obvious psychotic disorders and dementia. The system of classification used in the diagnosis of these various conditions lies in ICD-10.[13] Initial subdivision is by substance type and the

---

12 ISDD, fn 11 above.
13 World Health Organisation 'The ICD-10 Classification of Mental and Behavioural Disorders: Clinical Descriptions and Diagnostic Guidelines' *International Statistical Classification of Diseases and Related Health Problems* (10th edn, 1992).

substance causes the 'mental and behavioural disorders' attributed to it. The substance involved is indicated by two digits after the letter F, as indicated below:

F10.   alcohol;
F11.   opioids;
F12.   cannabinoids;
F13.   sedatives or hypnotics;
F14.   cocaine;
F15.   other stimulants, including caffeine;
F16.   hallucinogens;
F17.   tobacco;
F18.   volatile solvents;
F19.   multiple drug use and use of other psychoactive substances.

The identification of the psychoactive substance used may be made on the basis of self-reported data, objective analysis of specimens of urine, blood, etc, or other evidence—including the presence of drug samples in the patient's possession, clinical signs and symptoms or reports from informed third parties. It is always advisable to seek corroboration from more than one source of evidence relating to substance use. Objective analyses provide the most compelling evidence of present or recent use, although these data have limitations with regard to past use and current levels of use. Hair analysis and plasma levels are currently being developed and may prove more useful in the future.[14] Many drug users take more than one type of drug, but the diagnosis of the disorder is classified according to the most important single substance (or class of substances) used. The F19 code is used only in cases in which the patterns of psychoactive substance taking are chaotic and indiscriminate.

Further subdivision into the clinical conditions is by the fourth and fifth characters (as listed below). Not all four-character codes are applicable to all substances, and specialist texts should be referred to for further clarification.[15]

F1x.0 Acute intoxication

This is a transient condition following drug use that results in disturbances in the level of consciousness, cognition, perception, affect or behaviour or other psychophysiological functions and responses. This diagnosis is only used in cases where more persistent substance-related problems are absent. Acute intoxication is usually closely related to dose levels but a small dose of a substance may produce a disproportionately severe intoxicating effect in some individuals with underlying organic conditions (eg renal or hepatic insufficiency). Disinhibition due to social context—eg behavioural disinhibition at parties or carnivals—should also be taken into account. The intensity of intoxication lessens with time and the effects eventually disappear in the absence of further use of the substance. Symptoms of intoxication need not always reflect the primary actions

---

14 J Strang, J Black, A Marsh and B Smith 'Hair Analysis for Drugs: Technological Breakthrough or Ethical Quagmire?' (1993) 88 Addiction 163. For comments, see (1994) 89 Addiction 295.
15 J H Lowinson, P Ruiz and R B Millman (eds) *Substance Abuse: A Comprehensive Textbook* (1997).

of the substance; benzodiazepines, for instance, may have apparently stimulant effects on behaviour at low dose levels, lead to agitation and aggression with increasing dose levels and produce clear sedation at higher levels. The effects of substances such as cannabis and hallucinogens may be particularly unpredictable. Recovery is complete following uncomplicated intoxication. The following fifth-character codes may be used to indicate whether the acute intoxication was associated with any immediate complications:

.00 Uncomplicated.
An example for opiate intoxication symptom cluster would include:
* relief of pain (mental state of detachment);
* euphoria;
* poor concentration, extending to sleep with increasing dose;
* depression of respiration, extending to cessation and death with increasing dose;
* suppression of the cough reflex, extending to absence of reflex and aspiration and death with increasing dose;
* depression of gastrointestinal tract;
* central nervous effect, inducing nausea and vomiting;
* 'pin-point' pupils (miosis).
.01 With trauma or other bodily injury.
.02 With other medical complications.
.03 With delirium.
04 With perceptual distortions.
.05 With coma.
.06 With convulsions.
.07 Pathological intoxication. This currently applies only to alcohol, but there is little good scientific reason why that should be so. It is described as a sudden onset of aggression and often violent behaviour, which is not typical of the individual when sober, very soon after drinking amounts of alcohol that would not produce intoxication in most people.

F1x.1 Harmful use

Here the pattern of use is causing damage to health. The damage may be physical—as in cases of acquired HIV from the self-administration of shared injected equipment—or mental—eg episodes of depressive disorder secondary to consumption of stimulants. A harmful pattern of use is usually observed by others. Adverse social consequences, such as marital arguments or arrest, are not, in themselves, evidence of harmful use from a health perspective. The fact that a pattern of use or use of a particular substance is disapproved of by another person or by the ambient culture is not seen as being clinically relevant.

F1x.2 Dependence syndrome

This syndrome is a cluster of physiological, behavioural, and cognitive phenomena, in which the use of a substance becomes the main focus of the user's lifestyle. A definite diagnosis of dependence is usually made only if three or more of the following have been present together at some time during the previous year:

- a strong *desire* or sense of compulsion to take the substance—this is an essential characteristic;
- *difficulties in controlling* the substance-taking behaviour in terms of its onset, termination or level of use;
- a physiological *withdrawal* state (see F1x.3 and F1x.4 below) when substance use has ceased or been reduced, or used to relieve or avoid withdrawal symptoms;
- evidence of *tolerance*, such that increased doses are required in order to achieve the effects originally produced by lower doses;
- progressive *neglect* of alternative pleasures or interests because of psychoactive substance use; increasing amount of time needed to obtain or take the substance or to recover from its effects;
- *persistence* with use of the substance despite clear evidence of overtly harmful consequences, such as depressive mood states consequent upon periods of heavy substance use or drug-related impairment of cognitive functioning.

The fifth character code further specifies the dependence syndrome:

.20 Currently abstinent.
.21 Currently abstinent, but in a protected environment (eg in a rehabilitation unit or prison drug-free hall).
.22 Currently on a clinically supervised maintenance or replacement regime (eg with methadone, nicotine gum or nicotine patch).
.23 Currently abstinent but receiving treatment with aversive or blocking drugs (eg naltrexone or disulfiram).
.24 Currently using the substance (ie active dependence).
.25 Continuous use.
.26 Episodic use.

F1x.3 Withdrawal state

This consists of a cluster of symptoms arising on absolute or relative withdrawal of a substance after repeated, and usually prolonged and/or high-dose, use. The onset and course of the withdrawal are time-limited and are related to the type of substance and the dose being used. Physical and psychological symptoms—eg sweating, tremor, anxiety, depression and sleep disorders—vary according to the substance being used. Typically, the patient is likely to report that withdrawal symptoms are relieved by further substance use. Rarely, withdrawal symptoms can be induced by conditioned/learned stimuli in the absence of immediately preceding substance use. In such cases a diagnosis of withdrawal state is made only if it is warranted in terms of severity. The fifth character code further specifies the withdrawal state as follows:

.30 Uncomplicated.
    An example for opiate withdrawal symptom cluster is:
    - sweating;
    - running eyes and nose;
    - yawning;
    - feeling hot and cold;
    - anorexia and abdominal cramps;

- nausea, vomiting and diarrhoea;
- tremor;
- insomnia and restlessness;
- generalised aches and pains;
- rapid heart beat and high blood pressure;
- gooseflesh;
- dilated pupils;
- increased bowel movements and sounds.

.31　With convulsions.

F1x.4　Withdrawal state with delirium

This diagnosis is at present only found in association with alcohol-induced *delirium tremens.* It may be that other sedative drugs, such as the benzodiazepines, also cause these states and should be coded here.

F1x.5　Psychotic disorder

This diagnosis is not straightforward. Some drugs induce distortions of perception or hallucinatory experiences as their primary effects—eg lysergiside (LSD). In this case intoxication is a more appropriate diagnosis. A typical psychotic disorder occurs during or within 48 hours after drug use. Late-onset psychotic disorders (with onset more than two weeks after substance use) may occur but should be coded as Flx.75. Psychoactive substance-induced psychotic disorders may present with varying patterns of symptoms. The cluster of phenomena that occur are characterised by vivid hallucinations (typically auditory but often in more than one sensory modality), misidentifications, delusions and/or ideas of reference (often of a paranoid or persecutory nature), psychomotor disturbances (excitement or stupor) and an abnormal affect, which may range from intense fear to ecstasy. Thinking is usually clear but some degree of clouding of consciousness, though not severe confusion, may be present. The disorder typically resolves at least partially within one month and fully within six months.

Particular care must also be taken to avoid a mistaken diagnosis of a more serious condition (eg schizophrenia) when a diagnosis of psychoactive substance-induced psychosis is appropriate. Many psychoactive substance-induced psychotic states are of short duration provided that no further amounts of the drug are taken. False diagnosis in such cases may have distressing and costly implications for the patient and for the health services. Dual diagnosis also makes management of these cases difficult in that the substance use can aggravate or precipitate the other mental health condition—these typically being: schizophrenia, mood disorder, paranoid or schizoid personality disorder.

Flx.6　Amnesic syndrome

This syndrome is associated with chronic prominent impairment of recent memory; sometimes, remote memory is impaired, while immediate recall is preserved. Disturbances of time sense and ordering of events are usually evident, as are difficulties in learning new material. Confabulation may be marked but is not invariably present. Other cognitive functions are usually relatively well preserved and amnesic defects are out of proportion to other disturbances.

The primary requirements for this diagnosis are:

- memory impairment, as shown in impairment of recent memory (learning of new material); disturbances of time sense (rearrangements of chronological sequence, telescoping of repeated events into one, etc);
- absence of defect in immediate recall, of impairment of consciousness and of generalised cognitive impairment;
- a history or objective evidence of chronic (and particularly high-dose) use of alcohol or drugs.

Personality changes, often in the nature of apathy and loss of initiative, and a tendency towards self-neglect may also be present but should not be regarded as necessary conditions. Although confabulation may be marked, it is not always present.

F1x.7 Residual and late-onset psychotic disorder

In this category, a psychoactive substance-induced change of cognition, affect, personality or behaviour persists beyond the period during which a direct psychoactive substance-related effect might reasonably be assumed to be operating. The disorder should be carefully distinguished from withdrawal-related conditions (see F1x.3 and F1x.4 above) remembering that, in certain conditions and for certain substances, withdrawal state phenomena may be present for a period of many days or weeks after discontinuation of the substance. The clinical differentiation from pre-existing mental disorder may be difficult. Mental states—for example, a phobic anxiety, a depressive disorder—or schizophrenia may have been masked by substance use and may reappear as the effects related to the psychoactive substance fade.

This diagnostic group may be further subdivided by using the fifth character code:

.70 Flashbacks—which may be distinguished from psychotic disorders partly by their episodic nature, frequently of very short duration (seconds or minutes), and by their duplication (sometimes exact) of previous drug-related experiences.
.71 Personality or behaviour disorder.
.72 Residual affective disorder.
.73 Dementia.
.74 Other persisting cognitive impairment.
.75 Late-onset psychotic disorder.

A natural history and drug career perspective

Clinical management must be considered in the context of the natural history of drug misuse. An awareness of the different stages through which drug misusers pass can help in the understanding of the clinical responses. For example, the needs of a 16-year-old intermittent oral stimulant user, newly involved in drug misuse, are very different when compared with an individual who has been injecting heroin for over 20 years.

The natural history of most regular drug users is typified by general reductions in consumption and increased cessation rates with age. There are many social pressures dissuading adults from ongoing drug use and to do so results in marginalisation of those who persist in the practice. Thus, many older drug misusers are motivated to accept treatment. Most young people who take drugs stop as part of the process of growing up. However, rates of cessation among dependent opiate users are significantly lower than are those for users of other drugs.

The stages of change model applied to drug misuse

The stages of change model described by Prochaska and DiClemente,[16] linked to the technique of motivational interviewing, has important practical applications for assessment and treatment. Motivation is considered to be a precondition for effective treatment and this model assists the clinician to encourage motivation in a more effective way.

The model recognises that established drug misusers often only actively engage in change, or treatment for change, when they have passed through various key stages:

- *Pre-contemplation*: A stage where drug misusers are not aware that they have a problem, and therefore do not seriously think about change. It is others who recognize that there are problems and that change is required. This stage may last for years but treatment can encourage the move to the stage of contemplation, eg using specific forms of motivational interviewing and providing basic harm-reduction advice, eg clean needles.
- *Contemplation*: A stage where individuals begin to weigh up the pros and cons of their drug misuse; they feel somewhat ambivalent about their behaviour. The subject considers that there may be a problem and that change might be necessary. Contemplators also need encouragement to make a decision and enter the action phase of treatment.
- *Decision*: A hypothetical stage where the balance of change is influenced and a point is reached where the misuser makes a decision to do something, or possibly nothing, about his or her behaviour.
- *Action*: The process or stage of doing something—eg undertaking detoxification, regular clinic attendance etc. The person chooses a strategy for change and pursues it, taking steps to put the decision into effect. This is traditionally where 'motivation' for treatment would begin. Maintaining the positive effect of treatment involves structured and active follow-up to build on changes already made. This may take months or years.
- *Maintenance*: During this stage the task is to maintain the gains that have been made in order to avoid a return to undesired previous patterns of behaviour. Failure to consolidate progress may result in a relapse.
- *Relapse*: At a point of relapse, the individual would return to previous patterns of behaviour either at the pre-contemplative or the contemplative stage. However, relapse in itself would not be considered a treatment failure but a positive learning experience, potentially increasing the successful outcome next time round. Relapse is seen as the norm in treatment response.

16 J O Prochaska and C C DiClemente 'Towards a Comprehensive Model of Change' in W R Miller and N Heather (eds) *Treating Addictive Behaviours: Processes of Change* (1986).

It follows that clinical interventions must be tailored for particular stages and needs in a drug misuser's life. For example, there is no strong clinical indication to offer a package of detoxification to a drug misuser at the stage of pre-contemplation. However, there is a clinical responsibility to encourage the client to begin to contemplate his problem and to provide advice in relation to harm reduction.

Goals of treatment

The use of this heading may seem obscure because the overall goal of treatment is cure. However, cure has been associated with abstinence and has become an expectation of society—including the medical profession. An attempt to achieve the sole goal of abstinence in drug users with a dependence syndrome has led to a sense of therapeutic nihilism and, to avoid this in the future, it is important to elaborate on the goals of treatment. Most of the clinical conditions outlined above are self-limiting and require no more than supportive management. A few residual states exist where the management is no longer directed at drug use but towards helping people live with their changed state. Difficulty arises when people continue to use drugs, or are dependent on drugs, and require help in moving away from a lack of awareness of the problems that their drug use is causing. The hierarchy of goals and harm reduction for intravenous drug users with an active dependence syndrome is as follows:

* reduction of the sharing of injecting equipment;
* reduction in injecting;
* reduction in street drug use;
* stabilisation on substitute prescribing;
* management of features associated with the dependence syndrome;
* reduction in substitute prescribing;
* maintenance of abstinence from psycho-active drugs.

Health professionals are primarily focused on health issues. However, it has to be accepted that, as HIV infection becomes less of a driving force for establishing and maintaining services for drug users, drug-related crime and its prevention will become a relatively more important source of motivation in cost benefit terms. The costs sustained by victims of drug-related crimes committed by dependent heroin users alone is estimated as between £58m and £864m annually.[17] The cost to the criminal justice system of dealing with drug users is similarly substantial, being around £500m per year.[18] Similar papers by the political parties also support this view.[19] So far, the rehabilitation of dependent drug users by the criminal justice system is less positive than is that done through the health system. Diversion from the criminal justice system into health care may become more

17 The figures relate to 1994.
18 M Hough 'Drug Misuse and the Criminal Justice System: A Review of the Literature' (1996) Home Office Drug Prevention Initiative Paper, 1996/15.
19 J Straw *Breaking the Vicious Cycle: Labour's Proposals to Tackling Drug-related Crime* (1996).

important in the next decade. This view is supported by the development of the new Drug Treatment and Testing Order.[20] This order requires a consenting offender to undergo treatment for their drug problem with regular testing to monitor compliance. The order will often be given in association with an existing community sentence, though in some instances it may stand alone. Since 1 October 1998, the Home Office has been piloting the order in parts of England (Croydon, Gloucestershire and Merseyside) to examine its effectiveness; a parallel pilot in Scotland is also ongoing. The intention is to implement the strategy nationally after the pilots have run for 18 months.

The criminal justice system

Police custody

Many drug misusers come into conflict with the law and are taken into police custody; in that setting, they may be seen by a police surgeon (forensic medical examiner) who has particular experience in assessing detainees for appropriate treatment.[1] In those police stations where an arrest referral scheme operates, forensic medical examiners who suspect a detainee of drug misuse may wish to recommend that an arrested person is seen by an arrest referral worker for specialist assessment and advice. Particular problems may arise at the time of interview from intoxication, withdrawal states or treatment requirements if the detainee is dependent on drugs.

The Probation Service

At least a third of individuals who are under the supervision of the Probation Service are drug misusers. In Scotland, responsibility for work with offenders in the community lies with the criminal justice arm of local authorities' social work departments. The fact that an offender misuses drugs will be relevant to certain key probation functions:

- pre-sentence reporting and preparation of an outline supervision plan where a community sentence is proposed;
- providing information to help courts make bail decisions;
- supervision of community sentences, including those with treatment as a condition of probation; sentence planning and supervision of prisoners and ex-prisoners after release;
- referral to drug misuse treatment and advice agencies;
- referral to medical services within prison and in the community.

The Prison Service

The Prison Service has been making progress in introducing a range of treatment services for drug misusing offenders in prison since it introduced its strategy for

---

20 Established under the Crime and Disorder Act 1998, s 61.
 1 Guidelines for management are available: *Substance Misuse in Detainees in Police Custody: Guidelines for Clinical Management* (1994).

England and Wales—*Drug Misuse in Prison*;[2] these now closely reflect those in the community. The Scottish Prison Service published its policy on Drug Misuse in Prison in 2000.[3]

It is recognised that prison is a unique operating environment with specific security requirements within which drug services have to be delivered safely and clinically responsibly. However, many of the principles of good practice still apply in this context. Wherever possible, effective treatment that had been established before imprisonment should be continued in the prison. Young offenders need special consideration in the light of the increased suicidal risk in young prisoners with a history of alcohol and drug misuse.

Prisoners should be warned of the risk of drug overdose on leaving prison, due to possible loss of tolerance. It is to be hoped that links with community services can promote continuity of care both for reception into prison and for release into the community.

Drugs and driving

Driving licence requirements

The Driver and Vehicle Licensing Agency (DVLA) has recently distributed a new edition of their *At a Glance Guide,* which sets out the medical standards that are required for the holding of licences.[4] This document outlines the new regulation on persistent misuse of drugs.

Holders of a driving licence are required to inform the DVLA of ' . . . any disability likely to affect safe driving'.[5] The DVLA regards drug use as a disability in this context, whether or not it amounts to dependency. Additionally, the use of prescribed medication to treat drug/substance misuse constitutes a relevant disability. The responsibility for notification lies with the holder, not the prescribing doctor or drug service.

A drugs-related patient seeking a Group 1 driving licence will be required to undergo a short independent medical examination which will include a urine screen for drugs. If there are only methadone metabolites in the urine, a licence will usually be issued for one year at a time, until three years have elapsed since the cessation of treatment. The issue of a licence is subject to the person being on a supervised methadone withdrawal course and that the application is supported by a favourable report from a consultant. The patient will have to undergo a further medical examination on re-application; this will again include a urine screen for drugs. Patients will be called back for further annual medical examinations until three years after the methadone treatment has finished.

The DVLA will not issue or renew a Group 2 (HGV/PSV) licence to anyone receiving methadone treatment. Patients with a Group 2 licence who inform the DVLA that they are receiving methadone on prescription will have their licence withdrawn for a minimum of three years.

2 A revised Prison Service Strategy was published in 1998.
3 Scottish Prison Service *SPS Action on Drugs, Partnership and Co-ordination: Revised Guidelines on the Management of Drug Misuse in Scotland's prisons* (2000).
4 Driver and Vehicle Licensing Authority *At a Glance Guide to Medical Aspects of Fitness to Drive* (1998).
5 Road Traffic Act 1988, s 92, as amended by Road Traffic Act 1991, s 18.

The DVLA will withdraw a licence for one year if a urine screen carried out as part of a DVLA medical examination indicates persistent misuse of cannabis. They will withdraw a licence for a minimum of one year if the urine shows positive for any other drug, but this may be for up to three years in cases of persistent misuse. There will be another medical examination on re-application and every year for the first three years after the licence has been returned.

Driving under the influence of drugs

It is an offence to drive or to be in charge of a vehicle if 'unfit to drive through drink or drugs'.[6] It is to be noted that the mere fact that a person has taken a drug does not mean that he or she is unfit to drive—each occurrence is an individual case to be decided by the court on its own facts. Whether or not practitioners should breach confidence and inform the DVLA without their patient's consent if they are concerned about their patient's ability to drive—or if the patient is driving a passenger or heavy goods vehicle—is a complex but real ethical issue. The matter is discussed in greater detail in Chapter 30.

The assessment and management of clinical conditions

Every doctor is now likely to see patients who misuse drugs: the intensivist in the Accident and Emergency Department concerned with acute intoxication; the general practitioner confronted with concerns around the harmful use of various substances in the home; the obstetrician faced with a pregnant patient whose drug use has been disclosed because of concerns about the child; the police surgeon in the cells with a patient who is psychotic due to a drug-induced state; the house officer in the general ward face-to-face with a patient undergoing withdrawal from drugs; the psychiatrist having to differentiate drug induced psychopathology from other causes; or the specialist in the drug service trying to help a patient with a dependence syndrome who has already failed to give up the substance by himself. In any case, a low index of suspicion of drug misuse is required before assessment; early detection is preferable to the later management of the dependence syndrome. Assessment is based on standard clinical skills of history examination and investigation, with emphasis given to:

* drug use and previous treatment;
* areas of conflict: relationships, jobs, debt, the law;
* support structure;
* mental state;
* objective signs of withdrawal;
* needle marks;
* urinary toxicology;
* co-morbid, physical and mental conditions, eg HIV infection.

Distinct principles of management can be applied within each clinical condition induced by drug use:

6   Road Traffic Act 1988, s 4.

Acute intoxication may involve the medical or surgical management of injury incurred secondary to the intoxication. It may also require observation of any head injuries. Life support may be required in the event of coma and in some instances, eg opiates, antagonists may be available and given to reverse drug effects.

Harmful use. Education is required as to the dangers of drug use and the options about how to change that behaviour must be explained. Some patients may not see their drug use as a problem and the process of motivational interviewing can be used to effect change towards awareness and a wish to move away from harmful drug use.

Dependence syndrome. Once this is developed, management will depend on the patient, the drug in use and the patient's environment:

* If the patient is continuing to use, the aims of management should be as those outlined above for harmful use.
* If abstinent and in the community, the focus should be on the prevention of relapse.
* The patient may be abstinent but in a protected environment. These may be divided into four groups: rehabilitation houses; religious units; community crisis rehabilitation units; and residential 12-step programmes.
* The patient may be abstinent but receiving treatment with antagonist drugs (eg opiate addicts receiving naltrexone).
* The final category consists of those patients who are in a clinically supervised maintenance or replacement regime (controlled dependence).

It is this final category, and its subsequent management, that continues to attract the most interest. This is partly due to the size of the group—which is probably the largest and growing—and to the fact that substitute prescribing involves perpetuating the addiction with a safer substitute, some of which finds its way onto the illegal drug market. Because of this, the Department of Health has published guidelines to support clinical management.[7] These set out the minimum responsibilities of the prescribing doctor and include advice as to the decision to prescribe and, most particularly and in greatest detail, the circumstances in which the prescription of substitute drugs should be considered and monitored.

The guidelines emphasise that substitute medication, such as methadone, should not be prescribed in isolation—a multidisciplinary approach to drug treatment, including regular discussion with other members of the team, is essential. In particular, the prescribing doctor should liaise regularly with the dispensing pharmacist about the specific patient and the prescribing regime and no more than one week's drugs should be dispensed at one time, except in exceptional circumstances. None the less, prescribing is the particular responsibility of the doctor signing the prescription. The responsibility cannot be delegated.

Withdrawal state, with our without delirium. Withdrawal states may be managed by symptomatic supportive measures or, more commonly, by the use of substitute

---

7   Department of Health *Drug Misuse and Dependence – Guidelines on Clinical Management* (1999). The interested lawyer should consult the original, which clearly expresses the extent of the problem.

medication followed by a graduated, more humane withdrawal over a period of time. The types of withdrawal and the drugs that maybe used are discussed below.

Drug induced *psychotic disorder* requires similar management to that of any other psychotic disorder. It typically resolves at least partially within one month and fully within six months and is unlikely to recur so long as the patient remains drug-free.

The management of *residual and late onset psychotic disorders* is symptomatic.

The prevention of relapse

There has been limited outcome research to support the various models designed to maintain freedom from drug dependence in addictions other than that to alcohol. However, an understanding of the nature of relapse is fundamental to developing effective interventions for long-term management of substance misuse which needs to be seen as a *chronic relapsing disorder*. Progress in the field is hampered by uncertainty in the definition of relapse itself. The continuing development and harmonisation of accepted standards of outcome measures makes it likely that the results of future studies of individual groups can be generalised beyond the setting of the particular research. Thus, the analysis of studies into alcoholic relapse undertaken by Miller et al[8] could be extrapolated to other substances. In addition to pre-treatment characteristics, they identified five theoretical areas predisposing to relapse:

* negative life events;
* cognitive appraisal, including self-efficacy, expectancy and motivation for change;
* client coping resources;
* craving experiences;
* effective/mood status.

From this, key themes to treatment have been developed which depend on a supportive regime that is largely devoted to helping the patient understand the nature and predisposing causes of relapse.

Specific drugs and treatment options

Opiates

Acute intoxication with opiates can result in respiratory depression and sometimes death. This is not an uncommon event. A recent Australian study of heroin users indicated that two-thirds had had a drug overdose and a third within the past year.[9] Part of the reason for this may be that the purity of heroin can vary such

8   W Miller, V Westerberg, R Harris and J Tonigan 'What Predicts Relapse? Prospective Testing of Antecedent Models' (1996) 91 Addiction Supp: S155.
9   S Darke, J Ross and W Hall 'Overdose among Heroin Users in Sydney, Australia: I. Prevalence and Correlates of Non-fatal Overdose' (1995) 91 Addiction 405.

that, when injecting, the exact dose being taken is unpredictable. Alternatively, taking a dose of drug that brings the user near to the edge of death may form part of the euphoric effect. Methadone overdose is an increasing presentation of opiate intoxication. The reasons for this are complex, but there is no doubt that methadone now provides a more common route into opiate dependence than does heroin. Methadone overdose can be difficult to control and follows an unpredictable course in non-tolerant patients, who are at risk of sudden death. Clinical management is along general guidelines. The opiate antagonist, naloxone, may be used to reverse respiratory depression but, as it is short acting and the overdose may be of a long acting drug such as methadone, repeated infusion may be required. Concern as to the mortality of accidental opiate overdose has made some advocate the 'take-home' of naloxone by opiate addicts.

Patients with an opiate dependence syndrome traditionally constitute the bulk of specialist drug services' work. Their management depends on their current drug use and is, in general, based on the strategies that have been discussed already. There has been some promising work using naltrexone[10] as a condition of treatment for people who repeatedly offend in order to finance their drug habit. A select group of patients may elect to go into drug-free rehabilitation programmes, but there is often a high drop-out rate if patients do so while still using opiates. The majority of patients with opiate drug dependence syndrome tend to be managed, at least at some point, in a maintenance programme. Repeated reviews of the literature have confirmed that this treatment retains people in treatment, reduces illicit drug use, reduces criminal activity, and lowers the risk of seroconversion for HIV, hepatitis B and hepatitis C; it also improves re-socialisation.[11] It needs to be remembered, however, that methadone itself is not the treatment, and has to be given in conjunction with a full package of care. Doses of methadone in the United Kingdom were primarily aimed at the minimum dose to avoid withdrawal symptoms, but a higher dose is usually needed if the goal is the reduction of illicit drug use. A typical dose may be in the region of 60 mgs methadone mixture, 1 mg/1 ml per day. Doses of 40 mgs and above have been associated with death in naïve drug users. An additional variable between the United Kingdom and other countries is that more 'take-home' medication is prescribed in the former; the majority of medication in the United States and Australia is provided on a daily dispensing basis—often with supervised consumption at the point of collection.[12]

The withdrawal syndrome has been outlined in the example given above under F1x.30. The severity and length of withdrawal depends on the drug of abuse, shorter acting drugs tending to have more severe withdrawal symptoms over shorter periods as compared with those of longer acting drugs, which are more protracted but less severe. Some describe withdrawal as a 'flu-like illness' but others demonstrably have a severe reaction. This may in part be due to expectation but is also affected by the levels of tolerance and dependence on the

10 Naltrexone is a new opiate antagonist which can be administered orally and the effect of which lasts for 24 hours.
11 M Farrell, J Ward, R Mattick et al 'Methadone Maintenance Treatment in Opiate Dependence: A Review' (1994) 309 BMJ 997; G Bertschy 'Methadone Maintenance Treatment: An Update' (1995) 245 Europ Arch Psychiat Clin Neurosci 114.
12 J Strang, J Sheridan and N Barber 'Prescribing Injectable and Oral Methadone to Opiate Addicts: Results from the 1995 National Postal Survey of Community Pharmacies in England and Wales' (1996) 313 BMJ 270.

drug. The withdrawal is managed by substitution of the opiate, usually with methadone, and a gradual reduction is then carried over a period of time. The shortest period advocated is 24 hours but treatment then needs to be carried out in an Intensive Care Unit and involves naltrexone induced withdrawal accompanied by heavy sedation.[13] More typical withdrawal periods are of 10 to 21 days as in-patients or of longer maintenance in abstinence programmes as out-patients. Further symptomatic treatment can be provided by the use of α_2-adrenergic agonists but these drugs have no effect on the insomnia, craving and muscle aches associated with withdrawal. The medical management of opiate withdrawal is not complicated other than when using the very short procedures—the difficulty lies in achieving continued abstinence.

Stimulants

Intoxication with stimulants appears less common, possibly because the pleasurable effect is lost at high doses; it becomes, instead, associated with paranoia and psychosis and may end up with convulsions. Treatment is along general symptomatic lines. Patients with a stimulant dependence syndrome usually abuse amphetamines but are increasingly turning to cocaine and, in some areas, crack cocaine. As, with any other substance, harm reduction advice is essential if the patient is continuing to use a stimulant. However, treatment options are limited, in that therapy is exclusively abstinence-orientated with the majority of models involving residential settings.[14] The main focus, therefore, is on relapse prevention. Various drugs have been suggested as being useful in the stimulant dependence syndrome but their use as part of a standard therapy is not justified by research. Similarly, there are no randomised controlled trials that support the use of maintenance prescribing or maintenance to abstinence prescribing for the syndrome, although some prescribing along these lines does occur in the United Kingdom. Stimulant withdrawal has been suggested by some to be a tri-phasic state, with 'crash', 'withdrawal' and 'extinction' phases. The crash typically occurs within 30 minutes and may last up to 40 hours. The withdrawal phase tends to peak at two to four days and various depressive symptoms, including hypersomnia, fatigue, anhedonia, sadness, suicidal ideation and general malaise, last for several weeks after that. There is no specific symptomatic treatment and the majority of stimulant users end their dependence without resorting to medical support.

Sedatives and hypnotics

Illicit use of drugs in this group is now almost exclusively confined to the benzodiazepines although, historically, barbiturates have been important. The management of benzodiazepine acute intoxication is along general principles although the benzodiazepine antagonist flumazenil may be used to reverse the onset of respiratory depression and coma. This class of drugs is commonly used in conjunction with others, particularly stimulants and alcohol. Their harmful use is extensive and results in increased risk behaviour amongst intravenous drug users, an increased association with accidents, aggression, deterioration in

13 J J Legarda and M Gossop 'A 24-h Inpatient Detoxification Treatment for Heroin Addicts: A Preliminary Investigation' (1994) 35 Drug Alcohol Depend 91.
14 M A Schuckit 'The Treatment of Stimulant Dependence' (1994) 89 Addiction 1559.

performance and amnesic effects which can be used medically to good purpose as pre-medication for surgery. Iatrogenic initiation of the benzodiazepine habit and subsequent dependence remains a concern; this is despite the recommendations from the Committee on Safety of Medicines to limit treatment to short courses only.[15] Medical negligence may be claimed in these cases and long-term use requires careful supervision.[16] Numerically speaking, iatrogenic benzodiazepine drug dependence is a greater problem that that due to high dose illicit use, which usually occurs in the context of poly-drug use. The latter group pose a significant clinical challenge but have been studied the least. The clinical management of the former has been reviewed and guidelines have been issued.[17] The best outcome in this group is associated with younger patients, who have fewer withdrawal symptoms and demonstrate less personality disturbance six months after withdrawal; the ideal management of the high-dose, illicit use dependence syndrome may, however, be different. The withdrawal state has features which are clinically similar to and sometimes indistinguishable from anxiety states. Additional features include hypersensitivity in all the senses, de-realisation and de-personalisation. Late presentations of withdrawal include psychotic states and convulsions. The management of withdrawal involves substitute prescribing of a long-acting benzodiazepine (eg diazepam) combined with gradual controlled withdrawal over a period of months. Rapid in-patient detoxification may be unsafe.[18]

Hallucinogens

A large variety of hallucinogens may be used and can produce clinical conditions. These include psilocybin and mescaline (primarily found in fungi), lysergic acid diethylamide (LSD) and 3, 4-Methylene dioxy methamphetamine (MDMA) and many other compounds with a botanical origin. The main drugs used which have clinical importance are LSD and MDMA. Hallucinogenic intoxication usually presents only when there is a 'bad trip', which depends primarily on the mental set and the environment of the user. An unrelaxed atmosphere, pressures of time, arguments and major resentments are important in the latter context; solitary experimentation in an over-stimulated environment can also precipitate bad experiences, which usually wear off before medical intervention is sought. Treatment, when given, should be directed to preventing the patient from physically harming themselves or others. The somatic (dizziness, paraesthesia, weakness and tremor), perceptual (altered reality) and psychic (labile mood, dreams, altered time sense and de-personalisation) changes may be so severe as to require neuroleptic medication. Some of the adverse reactions that occur are not due to LSD itself but to contaminants such as phencyclodine (PCP). There appears to be no significant dependence syndrome or withdrawal state for the hallucinogenic groups and there is no evidence of any neuro-toxic effects due to LSD; this, however, is not so in the case of MDMA.

15 Committee on Safety of Medicines *Benzodiazepine Dependence and Withdrawal Symptoms* (1988) Current Problems 21.
16 C Hallstrom 'Benzodiazepines and Medical Negligence' (1990) Hospital Update 569.
17 Substance Abuse Committee of the Mental Health Foundation *Guidelines for the Prevention and Treatment of Benzodiazepine Dependence* (1992).
18 M Robertson and J Bell 'Are Rapid Inpatient Benzodiazepine Detoxifications Unsafe?' (1993) 158 Med J Austral 578.

Acute intoxication with MDMA can produce a condition similar to the serotinergic syndrome and the neuroleptic malignant syndrome—which consists of hyperthermia, muscle rigidity and impaired consciousness. The harmful use of MDMA results from tolerance, as a consequence of which users may increase the dose to get the original effect achieved. Subjects may take large doses which result in neurotoxicity.

Cannabis

As with hallucinogens, the pre-morbid state and setting are influential in determining the reactions to acute ingestion of cannabis. Acute intoxication can result in disturbances of perception and, in severe cases, psychotic states in a dose-response manner.[19] A dependence syndrome undoubtedly occurs in a small minority of cannabis users; but treatment tends to be geared towards reduced consumption and abstinence. Withdrawal symptoms have also been reported in high-dose, chronic users. Little evidence of adverse long-term consequences for chronic users has been found.[20] That being said, marijuana smoke contains the same carcinogens as does tobacco smoke, usually in somewhat higher concentration; long-term physical health, therefore, may well be at risk. Cannabis has recently been made available on prescription in two American States. This is limited to symptomatic treatment in conditions such as cancer, AIDS, anorexia, chronic pain, spasticity, coma, arthritis and migraine. However, the Federal Government of the United States is concerned about this development.

Solvents

Acute intoxication by solvents can result in coma and death and, in addition, there are quite specific problems of sudden death that are usually related to cardiac arrhythmias or neurogenic inhibition resulting in cardiac arrest. There seems to be no place for harm reduction in solvent misuse and the sole goal is one of abstinence. There is limited evidence that a dependence syndrome with specific withdrawal symptoms occurs. Residual states due to long-term use can arise as protracted use leads to multiple organ damage. The main foci for solvent management are prevention, early detection and abstinence.[1]

The law and tackling drug misuse

Drug misuse cannot be eradicated. The aim of the law should be to control and limit the demand for and the supply of illicit drugs in order to minimise the serious individual and social harms caused by their use. It also needs to be accepted that the law is only part of the public response to the problem; prevention, education and health are as important and no one element is capable of dealing with the issue alone. The deterrent effect of the law per se has been very limited. Despite large increases in the number and quantity of seizures of all drugs, there is no strong evidence that they have become harder to obtain or more expensive.

---

19 H Thomas 'Psychiatric Symptoms in Cannabis Users' (1993) 163 Brit J Psychiat 141.
20 Institute of Medicine *Marijuana and Health* (1982).
 1 Advisory Council on the Misuse of Drugs *Volatile Substance Abuse* (1995).

Nor has there been any decrease in purity. At the same time, the range of available synthetic drugs has grown. All the evidence suggests that the law plays no more than a minor part in deterring demand. It is of prime importance, therefore, that the law should accurately reflect relative harm in terms of current knowledge and experience. Only then can it support a public health agenda of education and prevention.

The recent report of the Independent Inquiry into the Misuse of Drugs Act 1971[2] concludes that:

> 'one of the most dangerous messages of all is the message that all drugs are equally dangerous. When young people know from their own experience that part of the message is either exaggerated or untrue, there is a serious risk that they will discount all of the rest. Recent evidence indicates that there is a pressing need to refocus education and attention on the pre-eminent harm of heroin and cocaine.'

At present, possession offences dominate the operation of the law in the fight against drug abuse. They constitute around 90% of the total of offences against the Misuse of Drugs Act 1971 and they take up a very large amount of the time and resources of the criminal justice system. Offences associated with the possession of cannabis constitute by far the largest category of all drug related offences—78,000 out of a total of 113,000 in 1997. Cannabis is not a harmless drug. But by any of the main criteria of harm—mortality, morbidity, toxicity, addictiveness and relationship with crime—it is less harmful to the individual and society than any of the other major illicit drugs, or than alcohol and tobacco.

The Independent Inquiry into the Misuse of Drugs Act 1971 took the view that:

> 'if the sanctions for cannabis possession and cultivation, both in the law and its enforcement, were to be substantially reduced, there would be a risk that more people would use it. But the international evidence does not suggest that this is inevitable or even likely. Given the current widespread availability and use of cannabis, we judge that more would be gained in terms of credibility, respect for the law and the police, and accurate education messages than would be lost in potential damage to public and individual health. It would promote the targeting of enforcement on those drugs and activities which cause the greatest harm.'

2   *Drugs and the Law* (2000).

24

Medico-legal aspects of alcohol

The main social significance of alcohol rests on its being a drug of dependence. It has been estimated that there are some 90,000 alcoholics in Great Britain and, for some time, alcohol has been regarded as the drug that is most widely used in the country;[1] this probably holds true today despite the recent rise in the use of the more flamboyant recreational substances. Clearly, the more alcohol that is drunk, the more alcohol related problems will arise and the more will alcohol related illness express itself. Alcohol is intimately associated with crime, suicide and accident. There can be no doubt that it merits a section to itself in a work on forensic medicine.

Alcohol is a cortical depressant. Since it is the highest and the most recently evolved brain functions that are first affected by depressants, the immediate effect of a dose of alcohol is to inhibit those cerebral functions that are associated with orderly community behaviour and with finer critical judgments; an illusion of cerebral stimulation is thus established with few physical ill-effects other than those of cerebrospinal dehydration. Chronic alcoholism, however, almost inevitably leads to physical and social degeneration, inability to retain employment, disruption of the family and the like, followed by generalised cerebral deterioration. Dependence is often of extreme degree and the high cost of alcoholic drinks has two major effects—first, increasingly cheap and, concurrently, toxic forms of alcohol are consumed and, secondly, there is often a lapse into petty criminality designed to obtain and conserve supplies. The criminal alcoholic who develops has to be distinguished from the intoxicated criminal—that is, the person with criminal inclinations which are potentiated by consumption of alcohol.

This chapter will not deal with alcoholism as a disease. The present concern is, in the main, to consider the association of acute alcoholism with injury and sudden death and to outline the resulting legal consequences.

Physiology of consumption of alcohol

Alcohol is absorbed from the stomach but more especially from the upper intestine—absorption and transfer to the blood stream is likely to be more rapid

1 Royal College of Psychiatrists *Alcohol: Our Favourite Drug* (1986).

than normal, and its effects more obvious, if the stomach empties unduly fast, as in persons who have had by-pass surgical operations. At the same time, alcohol retained in the stomach is degraded by the gastric enzyme alcohol-dehydrogenase and this accounts for the commonly observed 'sobering' effect of a full stomach which delays emptying. The patient who has had his or her stomach removed is, therefore, in double jeopardy because any empirical data as to the absorption and peak distribution of a dose of alcohol will be based on the normal emptying of the normal stomach—these going hand in hand with normal destruction in the stomach of a proportion of the alcohol ingested.[2] Once absorbed, the alcohol is dissolved in the body water and is distributed according to the water content of the tissues—thus the blood, in which there is much solid material, contains less alcohol, volume for volume, than does, say, the cerebrospinal fluid. The amount of alcohol circulating in the body—and, hence, affecting the brain—is expressed in the United Kingdom in terms of milligrams of alcohol per 100 millilitres of the fluid under examination; this has, traditionally, been blood on the grounds that it is blood that is in direct contact with the brain.[3]

The greater part of the ingested alcohol that is absorbed is destroyed by the liver through the action of the hepatic alcohol-dehydrogenase. Approximately 10% is excreted in the urine, sweat and breath. The combined effect of destruction and elimination is to reduce the blood alcohol by an amount that is variously estimated but which can, for practical purposes, be regarded as equivalent to 15 mg/100 ml blood/hour. This, however, can only be regarded as a most likely figure; in practice, the metabolic rates for individuals can vary within relatively uncertain limits. From the lawyer's point of view, it is convenient to accept these as lying between 10 and 25 mg alcohol/100 ml blood/hour—these being the limits which were not disputed in the leading case in the House of Lords.[4]

Since alcohol diffuses uniformly in the body water, it will be present in the urine which is formed in the kidneys. But, as urine contains very little solid materials, there will be more alcohol per 100 ml of urine than per 100 ml of blood and, in order to compare the two fluids, a ratio of 1.3:1.0 is usually accepted. This, however, assumes that the urine and blood are in equilibrium, and this cannot be so in practice because urine is isolated and stored in the bladder. The nearest one can get to equivalence of blood and urine is to empty the bladder and test the smallest amount that can next be voided naturally—a matter of some 20 minutes' excretion by the kidneys. Of greater importance in relation to current practice is the fact that the breath also contains water which is derived from the alveolar air that has been in immediate contact with the blood in the capillaries; theoretically, a constant breath/blood ratio should be achieved and this is accepted as approximately 1:2,300. While it is true that a breath sample contains an inconstant amount of tidal air which has not been in contact with the blood, this can be compensated for in the method of testing. Nevertheless, so many variables are involved that direct conversions between blood, urine and breath are too inaccurate to be accepted with certainty.[5]

2   J Caballeria, M Frezza, R Hernández-Munoz et al 'Gastric Origin of the First-Pass Metabolism of Ethanol in Humans: Effect of Gastrectomy' (1989) 97 Gastroenterology 1205.
3   In all the EU countries, the expression is in grams per litre ('Promille'); the result is that the bald number quoted in the United Kingdom is 100 times that quoted for a similar concentration on the Continent.
4   *Gumbley v Cunningham* [1989] AC 281.
5   I have discussed this in J K Mason 'Conversion on the Road to Auchtermuchty' 1996 SLT 33.

Test results should be given in terms either of blood, urine or breath alcohol and this is the practice that is accepted—and imposed—by the courts.[6]

The amount of alcohol present in the tissue fluids at any time is determined by many more factors than the simple measure of the quantity ingested. It depends on the method of dosing, on the amount destroyed in the stomach before absorption, on the rate of absorption, on the available water for distribution—which is reflected in the body weight and stature and, hence, on the sex—and on the capacity of the liver to metabolise the dose. All these variables are commonly operating in the context of normal social drinking where the intake, itself, is likely to be sporadic both as to timing and quantity. Consequently, the chances of converting a supposed intake to prospective blood or breath values with scientific accuracy is remote. The literature on the subject is vast and many tables, nomograms and the like have been produced[7] in an effort to provide ready conversion figures but none overcomes the problems inherent in an individualised biological process; unfortunately, many lawyers find this difficult to appreciate. The present writer is content to use the original tables prepared by the British Medical Association,[8] which give very adequate results in practice,[9] despite their antiquity and the criticism to which they have been subjected. At the same time, their limitations should be emphasised. The major need to undertake such conversions lies in the road-traffic legislation, where particular emphasis rests on the defences available to alleged contraventions.

Motor vehicle accidents and alcohol

There is abundant evidence that alcohol is a potent source of automobile accidents. The results of four old but well-controlled surveys are summarised in Table 24.1; although the figures differ in degree, the association of accidents with rising alcohol concentrations is clearly reproducible. Some interest attaches to the consistent finding that very small amounts of alcohol actually reduce the accident rate. It is submitted that this does not represent a beneficial effect of alcohol but, rather, demonstrates that persons who know they may be at risk are at particular pains not to be discovered.

The current relevant United Kingdom (excluding Northern Ireland) legislation is contained in the Road Traffic Act 1988, as amended by the Road Traffic Act 1991. At this point, discussion will exclude causing death by driving and will be limited to those offences solely concerned with the ingestion of drugs or alcohol

---

6   *Lockhart v Deighan* 1985 SCCR 204.
7   See, for example, L A King 'Nomograms for Relating Blood and Urine Alcohol Concentrations with Quantity of Alcohol Consumed' (1983) 23 J Forens Sci Soc 213.
8   *Relation of Alcohol to Road Accidents* (1960). See *R v Somers* [1963] 3 All ER 808.
9   The tables do not, however, allow sufficiently for the relatively slow absorption and, hence, increased gastric destruction of the alcohol contained in large quantities of beer— and this has to be taken into account. The majority of nomograms and the like do this by using a different 'Widmark factor' according to whether beer or spirits have been drunk. But, since the Widmark factor refers to the ratio between the water content of the whole body and the water content of the blood, and was designed to account for this, there seems very little scientific basis for so doing. It is more logical to build in a 'gastric destruction' factor which can, of course, only be empirical.

Table 24.1 Alcohol and traffic accidents

Approximate band of alcohol concentration (mg/100 ml)	Ratio of accident/non-accident drivers			
	I	*II*	*III*	*IV*
0—50	0.7	0.8	0.3	0.9
50—100	3.3	1.3	2.4	1.5
100—150	8.7	2.1	10.2	4.0
Over 150	33.1	8.1	41.8	18.0

The figures have been modified from the following reports: *I* R L Holcomb (1938) Journal of the American Medical Association, **111**, 1076. *II* G W H Lucas, et al (1955) in Proceedings of the 2nd International Conference on Alcohol and Road Traffic, Toronto, p 139. *III* M Vamosi (1961) *Traffic Safety and Research Review* 4.8. *IV* F Borkenstein, et al (1964) *The Role of the Drinking Driver in Traffic Accidents*, Indiana University Department of Police Administration.

and its effect on fitness to drive.[10] Within that limitation, there are two basic offences. Section 4(1) prescribes the offence of driving or attempting to drive a motor vehicle on a road or other public place while unfit to drive through the action of drink or drugs; s 4(2) relates to being in charge of a car in a similar condition. Section 5(1) prescribes an offence if a person (a) drives or attempts to drive a motor vehicle on a road or other public place or (b) is in charge of a motor vehicle on a road or other public place after consuming so much alcohol that the proportion of it in his breath, blood or urine exceeds the prescribed limit. Section 11(2) defines the prescribed limits as 35 µg alcohol per 100 ml breath, 80 mg alcohol per 100 ml blood and 107 mg alcohol per 100 ml urine.

Charges under s 4 are now rare and are largely confined to cases where there is a possibility of driving or being in charge while under the influence of drugs—there is, however, no reason why the police should not prosecute under s 4 when they have a 'negative' breath analysis for alcohol. In such a case, a medical examination must be undertaken and the results of this are certainly open to the court as matters of fact; police surgeons do have, as a point of policy, a standardised form of examination and reporting which eliminates much argument. None the less, proof that a driver's ability to drive is impaired by way of drugs is often difficult.[11] A specimen of blood or urine can be taken, but only on the advice of a medical practitioner that the driver's condition may be due to drugging; even then, the mere finding of a drug is not proof of cause and effect. Ultimately perhaps the most important function of the clinical examination from the medico-legal aspect is not so much the detection of drugging as the exclusion of other causes of abnormal behaviour. Head injury or disorders of carbohydrate metabolism spring immediately to mind but other, less urgent, considerations apply— slurring of speech, for example, may be due to neurological disorder and it is important to the accused that this be recognised.

The basic practical effect of the legislation is to use the breath test as the definitive test to establish charges under s 5(1)(a). The preliminary procedure is

10 Section 3A, inserted by the Road Traffic Act 1991, s 3, combines the two by defining the offences of causing death by careless driving while, at the time of driving, either being unfit to drive through drink or drugs or having a proportion of alcohol in the breath, blood or urine that exceeds the prescribed limit.
11 It is a defence to s 4(2) that the person was not intending to drive the car while still unfit to drive. But, since this depends on a clinical examination at the time, it is virtually impossible to pursue.

laid down precisely in s 6 but, in general, a constable can require any person driving or attempting to drive a motor vehicle who is suspected of having, or having had, alcohol in the body or has committed a traffic offence while the vehicle was in motion, or any person who was driving and was involved in an accident, to provide a specimen for a breath test; the specimen can be taken at the site of the incident, nearby or in a police station and failure to provide a specimen constitutes an offence. If the breath test is positive or if the subject refuses a test, the constable can arrest him without warrant; the police in England and Wales can also enter a place by force in order to obtain a specimen when there is reasonable suspicion that injury has been sustained by another person.[12] Other than when the accused is in hospital, the definitive investigation must be undertaken at a police station, where he will be asked to provide two specimens of breath (s 7(1)(a)) for testing in an 'approved device'; the lower of the two readings is then recorded as the accused's breath alcohol concentration. Again, refusal to provide a specimen constitutes an offence tantamount to having alcohol in the specimen above the prescribed limit (s 7(6)); the police are, however, required to inform the accused of the consequences of refusal (s 7(7)).[13] A specimen of blood or urine may be taken at the police station if the accused cannot provide a specimen of breath for medical reasons,[14] or if no reliable breathalyser is available, or if he is suspected of being under the influence of a drug—this last requirement is subject to the provisions noted above. The choice of blood or urine rests with the constable.[15] A blood specimen must be taken by a registered medical practitioner and only with the consent of the accused. A specimen of urine must be taken within one hour of the requirement being made and after providing a previous specimen which is discarded. Specimens of blood or urine required in hospital can only be obtained on the authority of the medical practitioner in charge of the case, who may object if the undertaking of the test or the warning given would be prejudicial to the care of the patient (s 9(2)).

It is apparent that the use of definitive breath testing deprives the accused of a right to a test by his own analyst; this is covered by allowing him the option that his blood or urine be used for analysis if the lower breath result is no higher than 50 μg alcohol/100 ml breath (s 8(2))—and the police constable must inform him of that right.[16] The choice between blood and urine is, again, at the discretion of the constable but the driver should be advised of this when being informed of his right; he should also be told that his only right to object to a sample of blood being taken would be for medical reasons to be determined by the medical practitioner called to obtain the sample.[17] A further concession exists in Scotland, where it has been stated that, as a matter of public policy, a prosecution will not be mounted if the breath specimen gives a value of more than 35 but less than 40 μg alcohol per 100 ml.[18] In

12 Section 6(6). Section 6(7) excludes Scotland from this power—but this is simply because the power was always there (see *Cairns v Keane* 1983 SCCR 277).
13 *Murray v DPP* [1993] RTR 209—and this is irrespective of whether prejudice is caused to the motorist.
14 Which can include intoxication per se: *Young v DPP* [1992] RTR 328.
15 *DPP v Warren* [1993] AC 319, HL—the previous belief that the driver's preference should be ascertained was held to be bad law.
16 *Anderton v Lythgoe* [1985] 1 WLR 222. Moreover, no pressure must be applied to dissuade an accused from exercising the right: *Green v Lockhart* 1985 SCCR 257; *Rush v DPP* [1994] RTR 268.
17 *DPP v Warren* [1993] AC 319 per Lord Bridge. For analysis, see *DPP v Jackson (Failure to Provide Specimen)* [1999] 1 AC 406.

the event of such a result, the police cannot cajole the accused into providing a blood or urine specimen under the terms of s 8(2);[19] this is of some importance as the effective *de minimis* rule applies to the breath specimen only.[20]

The use of a motor car is almost essential for the discharge of many professions and the obligatory disqualification for driving consequent upon conviction for driving or attempting to drive with a tissue alcohol concentration in excess of the prescribed limit can be draconian in its effects. It is not surprising, therefore, that a mass of case law has been built up on the basis of all conceivable methods of outwitting the statute. Conversely, the courts have become increasingly anxious to apply the law rigidly and a number of surprising—and often contradictory— decisions have been taken. Thus, inter alia, the police have been allowed to regard the approved apparatus as reliable even though the first reading was 87 µg and the second 58 µg alcohol/100 ml breath;[1] a person may be convicted of refusing to provide a specimen even though he was not the driver;[2] most importantly, the fact that a person has been wrongfully arrested does not render the specimen inadmissible in evidence.[3] In fact, the definition of a specimen now specifically includes cases where the specimen was not provided in connection with the alleged offence.[4] In so far as this is arguably inconsistent with Road Traffic Offenders Act 1988, s 15(4)— which holds that a specimen of blood is to be disregarded unless it was taken from the accused with his consent by a medical practitioner[5]—it is difficult to see quite what it means. The probability is that it does no more than pre-empt defences based on no more than procedural errors. A far more disturbing possibility is that the alcohol content of a specimen of blood taken, for example, for clinical and diagnostic purposes could be seized upon by the prosecution; it is very unlikely, however, that Parliament could have intended such a meaning.

One further aspect—that of what constitutes reasonable excuse to provide a specimen—merits comment. The recent increase in cases of asthma and the adult respiratory distress syndrome make this a real possibility—certainly, the roadside test, at least, demands reasonably adequate lung function.[6] Other genuine conditions, aside from injury in the accident, must be rare.[7] The middle-aged man with prostatic hypertrophy may be at a serious disadvantage if asked to provide a specimen of urine[8] but such requests are now very rare. The situation as regards blood, which involves an invasive technique for its provision, is rather different.

18　'Drinking and Driving' (1983) 28 JLSS 405.
19　*Benton v Cardle* 1987 SCCR 738.
20　*Lockhart v Deighan* 1985 SCCR 204. It may be that the rule was introduced to safeguard against a margin of error in the device used at the time: see 'New Breath Test Device' (1999) 44 JLSS (8) 15. The prosecution cannot evade the concession by 'back calculating' to the time of the incident: *Hain v Ruxton* 1999 SCCR 243. For discussion, see J K Mason 'Back-calculation and the Crown Agents' Letters' (2000) 5 SLPQ 25.
1　*Carson v Orr* 1992 SCCR 260.
2　*Bunyard v Hayes* [1985] RTR 348; *R v Ashford and Tenterden Magistrates Court, ex p Wood* [1988] RTR 178.
3　There are many cases in point, the leading authority being *R v Fox* [1986] AC 281.
4　Road Traffic Offenders Act 1988, s 15(2), introduced by the Road Traffic Act 1991, Sch 4, para 87.
5　Arguably inconsistent in that consent is valid only if the subject is sufficiently informed to be able to make a reasoned choice (see 'informed consent', p 473).
6　But there must be a direct relationship between the excuse and the failure: *DPP v Furby* [2000] RTR 181.
7　'Shock' or 'stress' following the incident may or may not be an excuse: *DPP v Ambrose (Jean-Marie)* [1992] RTR 285 (disallowed); *DPP v Pearman* [1992] RTR 407 (allowed).
8　And it can occur: *DPP v Winstanley* [1993] RTR 222.

One can imagine certain conditions—for example, a severe skin disease or a horror of injections—that might constitute good reason for not wishing to undergo a needle prick.[9] Yet, even here, the criteria for reasonable excuse are very strict: 'no excuse can be adjudged reasonable unless the person from whom the specimen was required was physically or mentally unable to provide it or the provision of the specimen would entail a substantial risk to his health.'[10] Virtually the only concession made is that, once a specimen has been provided, it is perfectly proper for the accused to refuse to give a second one; neither the police nor the police surgeon can retrieve a technical error made by them.[11] Recently, however, the possibility of challenging the accuracy of the test device has been revived.[12]

Effectively, however, the accused motorist is, nowadays, confined to statutory defences—and these are limited. A defence to charges under s 5(1)(a) lies in Road Traffic Offenders Act 1988, s 15(3), which has it that the assumption that the proportion of alcohol in the accused's breath, blood or urine at the time of the alleged offence was not less than that discovered in the specimen shall not be made if the accused can show that he drank alcohol between the alleged offence and the provision of the specimen and that, if he had not done so, the proportion of alcohol in his breath, blood or urine would not have exceeded the prescribed limit.[13] The first condition is a matter of credibility; the latter is one for deduction by an expert witness. In effect, this entails establishing the gross 'value' of the post-incident drinking using whatever tables or other method the expert prefers, adjusting this for metabolic loss between ingestion and analysis and arriving at a net post-incident value. The 'scientific' limb of the defence (s 15(3)(b)) is established if the final figure derived by subtracting the net post-incident value from the observed value is less than the prescribed limit. It is clear that, whatever method is used, a number of assumptions, as discussed above (see page 351), must be made and these must be freely admitted. The inevitable inaccuracies, both as to fact and as to calculations are recognised, at least in Scotland, in that the court can proceed on the basis of reasonable approximations.[14] The onus of proof lies on the defence, the standard being that of the balance of probabilities.

A second statutory defence, this time against charges under Road Traffic Act 1988, ss 4(2) and 5(1)(b), is provided by Road Traffic Act 1988, ss 4(3) and 5(2). These hold that it is a defence for the accused to prove that, at the time he is alleged to have committed the offence, the circumstances were such that there was no likelihood of his driving the vehicle while he was still unfit to drive or while the proportion of alcohol in his breath, blood or urine remained likely to exceed the prescribed limit. We have already noted that, in most cases, the former involves a clinical opinion which is almost impossible to provide. As to the latter, although the Act does not say so, it is reasonable to assume that expert evidence

---

9 But, to be accepted, it would have to amount to a medically recognisable phobia: *Johnson v West Yorkshire Metropolitan Police* [1986] RTR 167. See also *DPP v Jackson* [1999] 1 AC 406.
10 *R v Lennard* [1973] RTR 252.
11 In *Beck v Watson* [1980] RTR 90 the specimen was dropped; the analysis of a second specimen was considered invalid.
12 *DPP v Spurrier* [2000] RTR 60. It is, however, difficult to see how this defence can be upheld in the face of a positive roadside test.
13 The defence can also be used against charges brought under the Road Traffic Act 1988, ss 3A, 4 and 5(1)(b) if a test result is being used as evidence.
14 *Hassan v Scott* 1989 SCCR 49.

as to the accused's metabolism of alcohol will be required.[15] Theoretically, knowing the accused's intake and the time between ingestion and breath analysis, one could calculate his actual metabolic rate and, hence, the time at which his tissue alcohol levels would reach the prescribed limits. In practice, most persons so charged have only the haziest recollection of their intake and the exercise is self-defeating. In this writer's view, it is far better to adopt the parameters that were not disputed in *Gumbley v Cunningham*[16] (see above, page 350) and, thus, present the court with a bracket involving the fastest, slowest and most probable times it would have taken for the accused to be legally fit to drive.

There remains the plea of special reasons why the person guilty of driving with excess tissue alcohol levels should not be disqualified from driving. In the present context, which is only one particular aspect of 'special reasons', this involves proof that the accused was given alcohol unknowingly and that, had he not been, his tissue alcohol levels would not have exceeded the prescribed limit. There is considerable evidence of the courts' antipathy to this plea and, as a result, the law in the area is confused. The general tenor is to be found in *Adams v Bradley*,[17] in which it was held that a mere mistake as to the quality of drink being taken is no excuse to offer against disqualification; there must be an element of intervention by a third party 'or a misleading of the motorist by a third party . . . by reason of someone having misled him or given him false information'.[18] Once again, the successful plea depends on two limbs—the fact that the drink was 'laced' must be proved and, following this, that the amount of alcohol ingested involuntarily was sufficient to account for, at least, the difference between the observed value and the prescribed limit. Expert evidence is required for the latter unless the situation would be obvious to the non-expert.[19] The 'scientific' process is simply one of evaluating the value of the 'lacing' drinks and subtracting these from the observed value; the estimation of the net 'lacing value' is, however, complicated by the fact that some acknowledged alcohol is almost always also present. Even if all the necessary evidence is proved, disqualification may still follow on the grounds that the prudent person should have realised that his or her intellectual capacity was impaired beyond normal expectation.

A word should be said as to some other, non-procedural, defences that are sometimes raised. Prominent among these is the ingestion of petrol while syphoning. Petrol vapour will affect the devices used in both England and Scotland but experimental data indicate that the effect of any 'mouth' petrol will be eliminated in some 15–20 minutes, during which time the suspect will almost certainly have been under police surveillance; the same applies to alcohol-containing salves applied to the lips. Throat or mouth sprays containing alcohol will also be eliminated within the period of police observation—as will mouth alcohol remaining from a previous drink.[20] The author has been unable to demonstrate that exposure to alcohol containing vapour, say, while at work will affect the tissue alcohol concentrations significantly[1] and this has been confirmed

---

15 *DPP v Frost* [1989] RTR 11, relying on *Pugsley v Hunter* [1973] 2 All ER 10.
16 [1989] AC 281.
17 [1975] RTR 233. For a contrary result, see *Alexander v Latter* [1972] RTR 441.
18 Per Lord Widgery [1975] RTR 233 at 236.
19 *Pugsley v Hunter* [1973] 2 All ER 10.
20 As a result, the police are instructed to wait until 20 minutes after the last drink before testing.
 1 J K Mason and D J Blackmore 'Experimental Inhalation of Ethanol Vapour' (1972) 12 Med Sci Law 205.

as regards industrial solvents within the usual parameters of testing.[2] The most common medical 'defence' raised is that of the excretion of acetone in the breath of diabetics; both the English and Scottish approved devices are designed to compensate for this other than, possibly, for a concentration of acetone which would arise only in a state of diabetic coma. Current interest, however, rests on the possible apparent elevation of tissue alcohol levels in those who drink while under treatment with H_2-receptor antagonists—which are used widely in the treatment of dyspepsia and gastric ulceration.[3] This makes sense in that the agents are likely also to inhibit the action of gastric alcohol-dehydrogenase and, thus, to increase the amount of alcohol available for absorption. The evidence is not all one-sided but it is sufficient to induce the Danish authorities to include a compulsory labelled warning of a possible increase in blood alcohol concentration after drinking when such a drug is taken at the same time.[4]

Aside from any connotations with the Road Traffic Act, the determination of alcohol levels in all persons killed or injured accidentally is of further practical importance on at least two counts. First, virtually all personal accident insurance policies carry an exclusion clause for injuries sustained 'whilst under the influence of intoxicating liquor' and this applies in a temporal sense, no causal relationship being required.[5] Secondly, a realisation that the driver is drunk amounts to contributory negligence by a passenger who accepts a lift from him;[6] the blood alcohol concentration must go a long way to establishing the likelihood of such an appreciation. It is to be noted, however, that the defence of *volenti non fit injuria*—ie that the plaintiff consented to the conditions—is not now available to the driver who is negligent in respect of his duty of care to his passengers through drink; an element of moral turpitude may, by contrast, prohibit such a passenger from obtaining damages.[7]

A person who, while riding a cycle on a road or other public place, is unfit to ride through drink or drugs commits an offence (Road Traffic Act 1988, s 30). There is no offence of riding a cycle with a tissue alcohol above the prescribed limit and there is no power to demand a specimen of breath, blood or urine in these circumstances.

Studies of pedestrians killed in road-traffic accidents indicate a very similar pattern of alcohol association to that shown by drivers. *All* persons killed in traffic accidents should be examined post-mortem for evidence of alcoholic intoxication; the knowledge that a killed pedestrian was drunk to the state of muscular inco-ordination should be available to the defence of a driver.

2   R C Denney 'Solvent Inhalation and "Apparent" Alcohol Studies on the Lion Intoximeter 3000' (1990) 30 J Forens Sci Soc 357.
3   See, for example, C DiPadova, R Roine, M Frezza et al 'Effects of Ranitidine on Blood Alcohol Levels after Ethanol Ingestion' (1992) 267 J Amer Med Ass 83. By contrast, there is no evidence that the so-called proton pump inhibitors, which are used for the same purpose, have a similar effect: R Roine, R Hernández-Munoz, E Baraona et al 'Effect of Omeprazole on Gastric First-Pass Metabolism of Ethanol' (1992) 37 Digest Dis Sci 891.
4   M Andersen and J S Schou 'Are H_2 Receptor Antagonists Safe over the Counter Drugs?' (1994) 309 BMJ 493.
5   *Louden v British Merchants Insurance Co Ltd* [1961] 1 All ER 705, per Lawton J. 'Influence' was here defined as 'a disturbance of the quiet, calm and intelligent exercise of the faculties' but it is understood that most insurance companies would pragmatically accept a blood alcohol level in excess of 80 mg/100 ml as evidence of intoxication.
6   *Owens v Brimmell* [1976] 3 All ER 765.
7   Road Traffic Act 1988, s 149. See *Pitts v Hunt* [1991] 1 QB 24.

The expert witness will also be asked what was the likely practical effect of a given tissue concentration of alcohol. Again, the answer is this can only be given in wide terms. Much depends on the conditions for drinking, the availability of food, etc; there is also no doubt that habituation to alcohol occurs—the reason for this not being entirely clear—and the same blood concentration will have a lesser effect on the regular drinker than on the novice. However, the following table of blood alcohol concentrations represents an acceptable average assessment:

10—100 mg/100 ml: Loss of self-control, an increase in self-confidence, talkativeness and alterations in judgment.

100—200 mg/100 ml: Distinct loss of skill, slurring of speech and commencing loss of co-ordination.

200—300 mg/100 ml: Loss of equilibrium, decrease in pain sense, marked disturbances in vision.

300—400 mg/100 ml: Increasing dissociation, stupor and probably coma.

400+ mg/100 ml: Coma (with its attendant hazards such as hypothermia) and possible death.

These are, however, subjective criteria. Objective measurements show that even low concentrations—of the order of 50 mg/100 ml—cause a lengthening of the reaction time in response to a complex situation and a decrease in visual function. If one adds to this the impulsive psychological effects, there is good reason to suppose that the most dangerous person on the roads with respect to alcoholism is the man who is only moderately intoxicated; while he is not able to react in an emergency in the normal way, he is, at the same time, unable to appreciate the deterioration in his performance.

Such subtle changes are not disclosed by normal clinical tests—probably only those with a blood level of more than 150 mg alcohol/100 ml are detected as being unfit to drive by this means. This is, perhaps, the main reason why virtually all countries with a drink/driving policy have adopted the imposition of statutory tissue limits—and the limits in the United Kingdom are higher than in most.

Aircraft accidents and alcohol

A momentary digression to aircraft accidents is excusable since they illustrate an important point in relation to alcoholism.

It is not generally appreciated that, just as in the case of cars, a proportion of light-aircraft accidents are alcohol associated—and it hardly needs emphasis that any effects of alcohol are likely to have more serious repercussions in the air than on the roads. The figures shown in Table 24.2 are old but, nevertheless, illustrate an interesting feature. The fact that 13% showed alcohol concentrations that would be significant in any circumstances is, in itself, interesting. However, the authors of the study noted that since the Federal Aviation Authority had introduced a regulation forbidding private flying within eight hours of alcoholic intake, the proportion of fatal accidents associated with a *very high* blood alcohol had, in fact, risen.[8] Only one conclusion is possible. There is one cadre of drinkers who

8   L C Ryan and S R Mohler 'Intoxicating Liquor and the General Aviation Pilot in 1971' (1972) 43 Aerospace Med 1024.

are amenable to reason and regulation—that is, the social drinkers; at the other end of the scale lie the hardened alcoholics who are indifferent to moral pressures or punitive measures. The same thing probably occurs in motorists and it is difficult not to infer that, if there are two classes of offender, there should, on general criminological grounds, be two types of penalty.[9]

It is an offence to fly anywhere any aircraft registered in the United Kingdom or any other aircraft within the United Kingdom, when acting as a member of the crew, while under the influence of drink or drugs so as to impair the capacity of the crew member so act.[10] Surprisingly, there is no authority to test the biological fluids of living pilots for alcohol content comparable with that which exists for drivers of automobiles and trains.[11] In the absence of statutory provisions as to aviation, there is no reason why the defence of volenti (see above) should not be available to a drunken pilot in respect of his willing passengers.[12]

In fact, attitudes to aviation and drinking are changing and most modern studies indicate that it is far less of a problem than was once supposed. A more recent British analysis, for example, found only seven out of 485 fatalities studied to be associated with ingestion of alcohol.[13] Aircraft accident fatalities are, however, likely to be severely injured, thus allowing for a serious possibility of the spurious post-mortem bacterial production of alcohol; up to 50% of positive findings may be so attributed, including results exceeding 100 mg alcohol/100 ml blood[14] (see page 365).

Table 24.2 Intoxicating liquor and the general aviation pilot in 1971

Fatal accidents studies for ethanol		256
Number positive (more than 15 mg/100 ml)		52 (20%)
15–49 mg/100 ml	= 25%	
50–99 mg/100 ml	= 12%	
100–149 mg/100 ml	= 21%	
150 mg/100 ml +	= 42%	

The proportion of 'Ethanol Positives' has remained stable since 1968 and the proportion of accidents with ethanol 50 mg/100 ml or more is fairly stable. However, the proportion of accidents with ethanol 150 mg/100 ml or more is higher since the introduction in 1970 of an eight-hour abstinence period before flying.

9   As the Blennerhassett Committee *Report of the Departmental Committee on Drinking and Driving* (1976) acknowledged. The suggestion was not, however, taken into legislation where the possibility is covered by the courts' discretion to extend the period of disqualification and to order retesting and by the 'totting-up' procedure (Road Traffic Act 1988, s 35, as amended by the Road Traffic Act 1991, Sch 4).
10 Air Navigation (No 2) Order 1995, SI 1995/1970, art 57(2).
11 In the United States, Federal Aviation Regulations prohibit operating an aircraft with a blood alcohol level of more than 40 mg/100 ml. Even so, 7.9 % of pilots involved in fatal general aviation accidents between 1989 and 1993 were 'above the limit': D V Canfield et al quoted by S A Cullen and H C Drysdale 'Aviation Accidents' in J K Mason and B N Purdue (eds) *The Pathology of Trauma* (3rd edn, 2000) ch 19.
12 *Morris v Murray* [1991] 2 QB 6.
13 I R Hill 'Toxicological Findings in Fatal Aircraft Accidents in the United Kingdom' (1986) 7 Amer J Forens Med Pathol 322.
14 See J J Kuhlman, B Levine, M L Smith and J R Hordinsky 'Toxicological Findings in Federal Aviation Administration General Aviation Accidents' (1991) 36 J Forens Sci 1121. In Hill's series (1986 7 Amer J Forens Med Pathol 322), 172 fatalities had raised blood alcohol levels; all but seven were discarded as being artefactual.

Alcohol and the railways

A significant number of railway accidents occur and, very often, these are of an unusual nature with an obscure cause. It has always been a disciplinary offence for railway workers to be drunk on duty but the matter is now codified in the Transport and Works Act 1992. Section 27(1) and (2) cover alcohol related offences by railway or tramway drivers, guards, and signalmen or those in a maintenance capacity (including those in a supervisory capacity). The offences may be, either, consuming alcohol so that the ability to perform one's task is impaired or working with a breath, blood or urine alcohol concentration in excess of the prescribed limits—which are the same as for car drivers. The statute provides a suspicious constable with rather wider powers to request a sample for analysis than is the case for car drivers, as there is no requirement that the subject be driving or in charge of the train or tram—the fact that he or she is at work is sufficient provided the constable has reasonable grounds to suspect that drink has been taken. Moreover, if a dangerous incident occurs, it is the tissue alcohol at the time of the incident that is significant—and this clearly allows for back calculation by the prosecution. The 'responsible operator' or the employer can also be liable for the alcoholic status of the employee. Otherwise, the regulations for obtaining, analysing and reporting the tissue samples follow those laid down in the Road Traffic Act 1988 very closely. Section 34 of the 1992 Act specifies a defence for railway staff against charges under s 27(2) similar to that which is available to motorists under Road Traffic Offenders Act 1988, s 15.

Accidental death of other types associated with alcohol

Consumption of sufficient alcohol to remove the constraints of normal care is very often associated with accidental firearm injuries.[15] Theoretically, the level of blood alcohol might be expected to be of diagnostic significance in this connection. Reported results are, however, equivocal, in that a high proportion of suicidal gunshot wounds are alcohol associated; moreover, there is no reason why a drunken argument should not end in a shooting. The finding of alcohol in a victim of a gunshot incident is but one piece of evidence to be assessed in conjunction with the findings discussed in Chapter 9.

Other accidental deaths associated with alcohol are directly related to the more severe physiological effects. At a level of about 200 mg alcohol/100 ml blood, a loss of equilibrium will be superimposed on inhibition of the critical faculties. Falls from heights, particularly out of windows, are likely to be precipitated and it may be extremely difficult to establish the total innocence of the death in conditions of group alcoholism; very little force will be required to overbalance an intoxicated person and any minor marks sustained in a mêlée might be obscured by, and would certainly be difficult to differentiate from, the effects of terminal impact. Similarly, drowning is associated with alcohol, particularly in docks or canals beside which the less uninhibited would be wary of walking and where the high sides make escape from the water very difficult. However, this writer has been impressed by the high incidence of artefactually

15 Before issuing a firearms certificate, the Chief Constable must be assured that the applicant is not of intemperate habits (see Chapter 9).

raised blood alcohol levels in cases of drowning and this possibility should be excluded before a firm association is accepted in individual cases.

Stupor is likely at higher blood levels and this is a very common underlying cause of death from burning, a cigarette dropped from the hand setting light to the bedclothes; many such deaths are due to the synergistic effects of alcohol and carbon monoxide poisoning. Other forms of carbon monoxide/alcohol deaths include the situation in which the subject 'passes out' in front of a carboniferous source of heat which burns with decreasing efficiency. Overlaying of small children while in alcoholic stupor is fortunately uncommon now that adequate housing is more widely available; it is an offence both in England and Wales and in Scotland for a responsible person to be drunk while in bed with a small child (see page 180). At comatose levels, hypothermia constitutes a major hazard, the physiological protection provided against the cold by constriction of the peripheral blood vessels being countered by the pharmacological action of alcohol; the person who lies down in a field on a cold night on the way home after a drinking bout is at great risk. At even higher levels of intoxication, accidental death may be due to no more than the action of the alcohol itself; this may well be the tragic ending to the 'dare' or race to drink an entire bottle of spirits which, if done rapidly, can elevate the blood alcohol level to an order of 600 mg/100 ml.[16] The problem of asphyxia due to inhalation of aspirated stomach contents has been discussed in Chapter 13; while many experts are sceptical, the author believes massive inhalation of vomit to be a genuine cause of death that is particularly associated with intoxication by drugs or alcohol.

Suicidal alcoholism

Deliberate suicide through the use of spirits that are ordinarily consumed must be extremely rare, though it has been reported. There are, however, two other aspects that are relevant. First, suicide may well be effected by the consumption of toxic alcohols, of which ethylene glycol, available mainly as antifreeze, is the most probable. Secondly, ethanol is most commonly associated with suicide when both alcohol and drugs have been taken together. An additive effect undoubtedly occurs—indeed, the action of very many drugs, especially the cerebral depressants, is enhanced by alcohol—and some apparent suicides may be accidents that are due to sheer ignorance of the possible consequences. Others have suggested that these deaths are accidental in that the subject, who is accustomed to taking a hypnotic as a routine, fails, in a state of alcoholic confusion, to distinguish the number of capsules he or she is taking; this seems unlikely. Many such deaths are undoubtedly suicidal but, even then, it is doubtful whether the alcohol component is taken with deliberate self-destructive intent; it is more probable that a state of alcoholic depression contributes to the suicidal frame of mind. These distinctions have become of less importance since the passing of the Suicide Act 1961; in addition, a coroner's verdict of self-killing is now virtually unknown in the absence of confirmatory circumstantial evidence.

16 The cause of death provided may be significant in relation to insurance policies. Death due to alcoholic poisoning would not be classed as an 'accident' but asphyxia due to inhalation of vomit might well be so categorised: *Dhak v Insurance Company of North America (UK) Ltd* [1996] 2 All ER 609.

One form of alcoholic suicide, which probably occurs more often than is recognised, is the deliberate contrivance of a vehicular crash while under the influence of alcohol. In one case that the author has investigated, a man with flying experience and of unstable personality had a series of altercations with his family and, on being left alone, went to an airfield where he borrowed a light aircraft; he crashed after 60 minutes' flying which was observed to be of progressively more dangerous character. A broken half-bottle of spirits was discovered in the wreckage and the post-mortem blood alcohol level was 313 mg/100 ml. Similar cases have been reported by others both in aircraft and in motor vehicles. The function of the alcohol in these tragedies is probably of two types. Either it is consumed in the certainty that it will ultimately precipitate an accident—a type of subconscious guilt transference; or the alcohol consumed merely serves, deliberately or otherwise, to inhibit a normally dominant moral rejection of self-destruction.

Alcohol and serious assaults

The most obvious association of alcohol with serious assaults is the typical 'pub brawl', so liable to end in a fatal stabbing. In English law, drunkenness in itself is no excuse to a criminal charge. However, if the crime charged is one that requires proof of a specific intent (eg murder or wounding with intent to do grievous bodily harm), then, but only then, evidence of drunkenness may be admitted as evidence of lack of that specific intent.[17] Acceptance of such evidence reduces the guilt of murder to that of manslaughter. The legal rules concerning drunkenness are based on policy rather than on logic. In Scotland, a charge of murder cannot be reduced to one of culpable homicide on the basis of self-induced intoxication— the recklessness in getting drunk to that extent compensates for any debatable question of intent.[18] The distinction rests on the fact that, whereas intent is all-important in England, 'wicked recklessness' constitutes an alternative basis for murder in Scotland.[19]

In essence, voluntary intoxication is not a defence to any crime for which recklessness is enough to constitute the necessary mens rea in either England or Scotland—rape being a example.[20] There are, however, some subtle distinctions as to the relationship between alcohol and rape in England and Wales and in Scotland and these are discussed in Chapter 20.

Similarly, acute alcoholic intoxication—as opposed to the potential disease of chronic alcoholism—cannot substantiate a plea of diminished responsibility by reason of mental abnormality in a case of homicide.[1] However, the mere fact of drinking is insufficient to set up the necessary conditions for establishing the major statutory form of adult homicide—that is, causing death by dangerous

---

17 *DPP v Beard* [1920] AC 479; *DPP v Majewski* [1977] AC 443; *R v Garlick* (1980) 72 Cr App Rep 291, where it was held that the correct question to be put to the jury was whether the drunken man formed the intent rather than whether he was capable of forming the intent.

18 *Brennan v H M Advocate* 1977 JC 38, in which the court overruled previous decisions suggesting that the decision in *DPP v Beard* [1920] AC 479 conformed with Scots law.

19 J H A Macdonald *The Criminal Law of Scotland* (1867) p 140.

20 *R v Fotheringham* [1988] Crim LR 846.

 1 *R v Tandy* [1989] 1 All ER 267.

driving; before using such evidence, the jury must be convinced that enough alcohol had been drunk as to affect the driver adversely.[2] As a counter to this, the Road Traffic Act 1991, s 3 introduced[3] the offence of carelessly causing death while driving, either, when unfit to drive through drink or drugs or having consumed so much alcohol that the proportion of it in the breath, blood or urine at the time exceeded the prescribed limit. This section contains some innovations. First, it refers to the tissue alcohol level *at the time of driving,* whereas the significant time under s 5(1) is thought to be that of the breathanalysis. Secondly, it renders a suspect liable to provide a specimen at any time up to 18 hours after the incident. There is, therefore, clear evidence that 'back-calculation' of the alcohol level is anticipated; it has yet to be decided whether this extension is specific to s 3A or whether it can also be applied to s 5(1).[4]

As discussed elsewhere (see Chapter 13), there is an association between death due to neurogenic inhibition of the heart and a state of alcoholism in the victim and, generally, the intoxication is of moderate degree only. There is little doubt that the finding of a level of, say, 150–200 mg alcohol/100 ml blood in a fatality resulting from an assault—particularly one involving the neck—could be taken as supporting a claim by the assailant that the death was unexpected.

Excessive alcoholic intake is positively associated with wife battering. In criminal proceedings, the general principles derived from *Tandy*'s case would almost certainly apply and alcoholic intoxication would have to be recognisable as insanity if it was to be used as a successful special defence. The insanity could be either temporary or permanent by reason of alcoholic brain disease; otherwise, any mental or pathological condition short of insanity is relevant only to the question of mitigating circumstances and sentence. The same thinking would apply both in England and in Scotland. In civil law, not even true alcoholism would provide a defence for a husband accused of behaviour such that his wife could not reasonably be expected to live with him.

Alcohols other than ethanol

Alcoholic addiction is not confined to ethanol intended especially for human consumption; unusual preparations containing alcohol—such as cheap eau-de-Cologne—are often used, while hand lotions and rubbing alcohols can be ingested; the alcohol involved is isopropyl alcohol, which is more toxic than is ethanol.

The main alcohols other than ethanol that are of medico-legal significance are methanol (methyl alcohol) and ethylene glycol. The latter requires only a brief mention—it is the basic ingredient of many antifreezes and produces much the same effects as does ethanol but in far more exaggerated form. There is severe involvement of the central nervous system and death in coma is to be expected when more than 100 ml is drunk. Severe damage to the kidneys may persist in the event of survival from the immediate effects.

Methyl alcohol is absorbed in the same way as is ethyl alcohol but it is metabolised far more slowly by the liver. As a result, a cumulative effect is added

2   *R v Woodward (Terence)* [1995] 3 All ER 79.
3   By inserting Road Traffic Act 1988, s 3A.
4   For discussion, see JK Mason 'Back-calculation and the Crown Agents' Letter' (2000) 5 SLPQ 25.

to its inherent toxicity. Methanol is used in industry and is a constituent of some antifreezes but it is more generally available as 'methylated spirits' or 'surgical spirit'. Industrial methylated spirits, consisting of ethanol with 5% methanol added, is widely used in medicine and can be obtained from pharmacists on a written order by medical practitioners, laboratories and the like; not more than 1 pint can be dispensed to a patient at any one time and the container must be marked 'for external use only'. The ordinary household equivalent is known as mineralised methylated spirits, which is 9% methanol in ethanol with added disgustants and colouring matter.

A blood level of 80 mg methanol/100 ml is dangerous, the toxic action being twofold—the body is rendered severely acidotic and there is depression of the central nervous system. Methanol almost specifically affects the eyes and, even if a generally toxic dose is survived, visual impairment of permanent or temporary nature, or even complete blindness, may persist. Very occasionally, methanol poisoning is caused by the use of lotions containing the substance but, in general, it results from either involuntary of voluntary ingestion. Involuntary ingestion is associated with drinking ordinary commercial spirits that have been deliberately or accidentally contaminated. Voluntary 'meths' drinking—often in association with a cheap source of palatable ethanol—is a resort of many impoverished alcoholics; there is no doubt that some habituation to methanol, similar to that seen in ethanol drinkers, must occur. The sale of methylated and surgical spirit has been simplified in Scotland but sale to a person known to be under the age of 14 is still prohibited.[5]

Alcohol and disease

Alcoholism is associated with disease both directly and indirectly.

Direct association is represented by disease of the mind—alcoholic dementia— and by conditions that are primarily centred on the gastrointestinal system.

Alcoholic dementia—of which the most prominent examples are Korsakov's psychosis and delirium tremens—is of little direct medico-legal importance other than as to testamentary capacity. It is sufficient only to emphasise that crime committed while suffering from such conditions is clearly committed within the legal concept of insanity. The question of whether chronic alcoholism or the alcohol dependence syndrome—associated with a scarcely resistable compulsion to drink—constitutes a disease of the mind in legal terms is vexed; much would depend on whether the brain was impaired or, short of this, whether the condition was sufficiently advanced to render the drinking involuntary.[6] In addition to causing mental disturbance, alcohol also has a direct toxic effect on the peripheral nerves (alcoholic peripheral neuropathy).

Alcohol-associated gastrointestinal disease may be of relatively minor character, such as the so-called alcoholic gastritis, which is a degenerative process in the stomach lining rather than a true inflammation. This condition may lead to malabsorption of essential foodstuffs; an unsatisfactory diet may compound a

5   Methylated Spirits (Sale by Retail) (Scotland) Act 1937, as amended by Deregulation (Methylated Spirits Sale by Retail) (Scotland) Order 1998, SI 1998/1602.
6   The expert witnesses in *R v Tandy* [1989] 1 All ER 267 were divided as to whether the condition was or was not a disease.

deficiency of protein and of vitamins. Coincidentally, there is degeneration of the liver of fatty type with, ultimately, fibrous destruction of the liver tissue; the condition of alcoholic cirrhosis is established and this may well be fatal—and be a cause of *sudden* death.

Indirect association of disease with alcohol is of little medico-legal significance. Most examples stem from the inhibition of higher critical faculties and consequent social and physical degeneration.

There is a distinction in the medico-legal disposition of alcohol-associated deaths in England and Wales on the one hand and in Scotland on the other. In the former, the mere mention of alcohol in the death certificate—eg liver failure due to chronic alcoholism—would dictate reference to the case to the coroner by the registrar.[7] There is no such obligation on the procurator fiscal in Scotland unless the death was sudden and unexpected—as, for instance, an accidental death associated with acute alcoholism.

Alcohol and the doctor

Alcoholism and drug misuse provide major reasons for disciplinary action against doctors and dentists by the General Medical and Dental Councils.

The subject is discussed in greater detail in Chapter 29. Any court conviction of a medical or dental practitioner will be reported to their respective disciplinary bodies. Proven motoring offences are reportable and convictions relating to alcoholism will certainly result in warning letters if not more serious reaction. Less commonly, but certainly more seriously, professional negligence or improper behaviour towards patients resulting from alcoholism virtually 'speaks for itself' and will inevitably result in a complaint to the GMC or GDC. In the extreme case, alcohol may be the factor that precipitates a prosecution for manslaughter through criminal negligence—though it is hard to think when such a case last occurred. A doctor, above all persons, should be able to appreciate the likely effect of alcohol on his clinical judgment and expertise; the courts might well be exemplarily harsh in the event of such a case arising. In general, it is to be hoped that the intervention of the Health Committee of the GMC (see page 445) would pre-empt any action in the criminal courts.

Particular problems of post-mortem blood alcohol analyses

Many reviews involving post-mortem determinations of ethanol draw attention to the occurrence of certain artefacts. Although the literature is confused, there is fairly widespread evidence that some bacteria and yeasts can produce alcohol as part of their normal metabolism and that, prominent among these, are bacteria responsible for post-mortem putrefaction.[8] Vehicular, and especially aircraft, accidents produce severe open injuries in which micro-organisms can flourish.

---

7 But the coroner cannot attribute death to chronic alcoholism specifically (Coroners Rules 1984, Sch 4, notes to Form 22, SI 1984/552).
8 An exhaustive review of the complex subject is to be found in J E L Corry 'Possible Sources of Ethanol Ante- and Post-mortem: Its Relationship to the Biochemistry and Microbiology of Decomposition' (1978) 44 J Appl Bacteriol 1.

Post-mortem enzymatic activity may also convert sugar to alcohol. There is, therefore, a potential for falsely raised blood alcohol values to be obtained using post-mortem specimens, and this applies particularly to those derived from accident cases; the possibility of artefact has to be taken into consideration when responsibility for the accident is being considered.

Experience has shown that a sample of urine or vitreous humour of the eye—or, preferably, both—taken post-mortem may be a more reliable qualitative index of ante-mortem intoxication than is blood, but there is no doubt that the courts are more accustomed to blood values; the main function of the urine or vitreous analysis is to check the validity of the blood result. It has been recommended that, if a post-mortem blood analysis is to be interpreted with certainty, blood specimens should be obtained from three different sites in the body and that these should be tested by two gas chromatographic techniques; but it is doubtful whether many laboratories would abide by such counsels of perfection and even less certain that coroners would accept the expense involved. These considerations apply only to putrefying blood specimens; in vivo specimens taken from motorists are placed immediately in bactericidal containers and are very unlikely to show artefacts due to contamination.

As something of a coda to this discussion, mention should be made of the possibility of endogenous production of alcohol during life—the so-called 'autobrewery syndrome'. Theoretically, bacteria which produce alcohol during putrefaction should be able to do the same thing in the bowel; the alcohol so formed could then pass into the bloodstream. One would imagine that the liver would then be able to deal effectively with the small amounts involved and, indeed, no workers have ever claimed a natural production equivalent of more than about 3 mg/100 ml blood. Even that, however, could be important to the driver with a blood level of 81 mg alcohol/100 ml blood or its equivalent in breath value. In the author's opinion, the matter is still undecided—there may be the occasional case where conditions combine to produce demonstrable levels of endogenous alcohol in the blood. Nevertheless, current opinion tends to decry the possibility.[9]

---

9   J A Gatt and P Matthewman 'Autobrewing: Fact or Fantasy?' (2000) 40 Science Justice 211.

25

Forensic toxicology

J S Oliver

The role of the forensic toxicologist lies in the detection, identification and measurement of poisons in human biological materials. This differs from that of the clinical toxicologist, who recognises poisoning from the symptoms and specialises in the care and maintenance of the poisoned patient. Both require knowledge of the physiological action of the poison, the latter for the care of the patient and the former to assist either the police surgeon or the pathologist with the interpretation of the results.

The training of the forensic toxicologist is primarily in the field of analytical chemistry. The instruments available to the analytical chemist are used to detect, identify and measure poisons that are mostly present in trace amounts with respect to the biological material submitted for analysis. In addition, training must take cognisance of the biochemistry and pharmacology of poisons, elementary human physiology and pathology. This aspect is particularly important when interpreting laboratory results.

Poison

The term 'poison', through popular usage, indicates a substance which, when ingested in small amounts, destroys life or impairs health. This definition indicates to the lay person a limited range of substances that, by and large, have gained the reputation of being poisons through past use. Such popular or historical poisons include arsenic, cyanide and strychnine.

A better definition of a poison is a substance which, when taken by any route, has a deleterious action on the body. This definition sets no boundaries on the types of substance involved, the quantities ingested or the route of entry to the body. Far from limiting his field of interest, it dictates that the toxicologist's ability as an analyst must be comprehensive, since practically all substances are poisons when taken into the body in sufficient amounts. There are, for example, many reports of water poisoning resulting from the excessive intake of water.

In practice, the type and range of poisons encountered are determined largely by the availability of the necessary materials. The poisons available in the United Kingdom are mostly illicit drugs, medicinal drugs, alcohol, household and garden chemicals. Chemicals such as solvents have to be added to the list in an industrial environment; industrial pesticides and herbicides would be included in an agricultural area.[1]

Samples and information

Samples for analysis can be provided from either the living or the dead. In the case of the living, specimens are generally blood and urine. Hair and nail clippings can be used to determine chronic exposure, particularly when metallic poisons are suspected. More recently, however, techniques have been developed to use these specimens to detect past usage of drugs in order to prove compliance with prescribed medication or abstinence from drug abuse over a period of months. Post-mortem samples will, in addition, normally include portions of liver, kidney, lung and brain and the contents of stomach and intestine. If an injection site has been found, it should be submitted together with the underlying fat and muscle. Blood samples should be clearly labelled as to the site of origin and should be taken from the periphery of the body so as to minimise the effect of post mortem redistribution of drugs. This can occur by diffusion from the gastro-intestinal tract or from organs such as the liver which may contain elevated concentrations of the drugs. The blood and urine specimens should be divided into two clean containers. One set should be preserved with sodium fluoride in the case of blood and phenyl mercuric nitrate for urine; the other set should be free of preservatives. The preservative is used to prevent the formation of ethyl alcohol should the specimens be contaminated with yeast or bacteria from the atmosphere. The tissue samples should be packaged in clean, sealed and properly labelled polythene bags; hair and nail samples for trace element analysis should also be packaged in clean polythene bags. For drug analysis, about a pencil thickness of hair should be plucked from the vertex of the scalp, wrapped into a bundle using tissue paper (cigarette paper) with a clear indication of the 'root' end. This bundle should be placed into a clean glass jar and clearly labelled. Each centimetre of hair represents approximately one month's growth. An entire lung, tied off at the main bronchus, should be submitted if a volatile solvent is suspected as a possible poison. An aliquot of the trapped air can be taken quickly in the laboratory for analysis and the lung can then be returned to the pathologist for histological investigation. All specimens should be kept cool and transported to the laboratory as quickly as possible. Frozen specimens are not usually required; thawing can cause unnecessary delays.

The information required by the laboratory for record and interpretation comprises name, age, sex, significant post-mortem findings, observed behaviour prior to death and, in the living patient, a report of the symptoms observed by the doctor. In addition, efforts should be made by the reporting officer to ascertain the previous relevant medical history. When death has occurred, medicine containers that are available should be labelled and submitted with the biological specimens, even if they are empty.[2] Drug paraphernalia should also be submitted.

1   It is always useful to know the employment of the subject under investigation (or of his friends or neighbours) because the materials used at work often find their way into the home environment.
2   Note that this often involves a refuse-sack half filled with a lifetime's accumulation of medicines etc.

Since this will usually involve syringes, the investigator should take care to avoid needle-stick injuries whilst handling and must ensure that subsequent unpackaging does not cause injury at the receiving laboratory. Drinking vessels found at the locus, again even if they appear to be empty, can reveal rapidly the nature of a contained toxin when analysed using sensitive laboratory procedures. The remnants of any household chemicals that have been involved must be submitted with the specimens. The information yielded and the subsequent time saved in the laboratory are well worth the effort.

Since the results of the toxicologist's work may be presented in court, meticulous records must be kept of the handling of the specimens from delivery to the laboratory to the subsequent uplift by the police. This chain of evidence must be maintained for as long as the specimens are in the control of the laboratory.

Analysis of specimens

The analysis of a biological specimen for a poison has four steps—the drug must be isolated from the biological matrix, detected, identified and the quantity present measured. The first problem is to isolate a poison that may or may not be present in minute amounts in the sample. An extraction procedure that recovers most of the poison, contaminated with as little co-extractable biological material as possible, is required. The analytical steps are designed to make the poison as insoluble as possible in the biological material and as amenable as possible to the extraction procedure. In the case of volatile solvents, such as alcohol and solvents, simply warming aliquots of material in a closed vial causes sufficient solvent to escape into the vapour above the sample for the analysis to be made. The addition of acid to a blood sample will cause any cyanide present to form volatile hydrogen cyanide and, in a closed system, this vapour can be trapped in dilute alkali prior to further analysis.

Most analysis is carried out for drug substances. This is the area where terminology causes greatest confusion for the non-scientist. The toxicologist is primarily interested in that property of the drug that can be used in its isolation. As a result, drugs are classified as acids, neutrals, bases, amphoterics (which behave as acid or base) or water soluble (such as quaternary ammonium compounds). The pathologist, for example, may request an analysis for drugs, with a particular interest in analgesics. Such a classification is based on the pharmacological action of the drug. Equally, the request could have been to concentrate on one or more of narcotics, hypnotics, anticonvulsants, antidepressants, tranquillisers, etc. Each group can contain chemically related drugs but also may contain others that are totally unrelated. For example, both chlorpromazine and meprobamate are tranquillisers but, chemically, the former is a basic and the latter a neutral drug.

The steps taken in the isolation of the drug are determined by its chemical classification and by a knowledge as to whether it becomes linked to protein in the body or is changed biochemically to a water-soluble conjugate. A protein-bound drug can be released prior to extraction by breaking down the protein either by enzyme digestion, warming with acid or by precipitating the protein. Water-soluble conjugates require hydrolysis with a suitable enzyme to release the conjugating group. Thereafter, the chemistry of the drug is the determining guideline. An acidic drug will be less soluble and more amenable to solvent extraction in an acid solution. Similar principles apply to a basic drug in an alkaline solution. Neutral drugs can be extracted directly into a solvent. Amphoteric drugs can be rendered less soluble in the aqueous medium by careful adjustment of the pH of the solution[3] to the correct narrow range in which the drug changes from being an acid to an alkali. Quaternary ammonium compounds can be extracted after conjugation with 'ion-pair' reagents. These chemicals bind highly water-soluble drugs into complexes that are more soluble in the extraction solvent. After extraction, the 'ion-pair' complex can easily be broken to allow for further analysis. Solvent extraction has been replaced by solid phase extraction in the modern laboratory. The solid phases have similar characteristics to the packing materials used in high-pressure liquid chromatography columns; consequently, they can be selected to optimise the drug recoveries. As outlined above, the drugs are rendered less soluble in the biological matrix to increase their affinity for the extraction phase. In general, only small volumes of biological sample are required; the risk of loss of sample through emulsion formation is removed. Drug recoveries are generally high and reproducible and the procedure can be automated.

This guide is by no means comprehensive. It outlines the initial steps necessary to produce an extract of the biological materials that can then be concentrated and used for further analysis. The extracts produced may be impure and contain co-extractable biological materials, such as lipids, from which the drug must be separated. Extraction processes may change one drug to another or may destroy it completely. Alternatively, materials (artefacts) similar to drugs may be fabricated. It is the forensic toxicologist's job to be aware of this and to proceed accordingly.

Analytical techniques

Chromatography

A poison can be separated from the crude extract for the purposes of detection, identification and measurement by using various forms of chromatography.

The non-scientist can best understand the technique of chromatography by relation to a familiar occurrence—for example, the use of a proprietary dry-cleaning solvent or paraffin to remove a dye stain from a piece of cloth. The technique used is to dab the stain with a tissue soaked in the solvent. Some of the stain transfers to the tissue; some spreads outwards from the stain into the material following the spread of the solvent into the cloth; the solvent, as it spreads through the cloth, has tried to take the dye with it, thus causing it to move over the material. In a laboratory, the cloth can be replaced by a sheet of blotting paper about 10 x 10 cm in size. Making a single dot 1 cm from one edge can reproduce the dye stain. The solvent can be applied by dipping that edge into a trough of solvent while keeping the dye spot above the surface. Capillary action will cause the solvent to flow up the paper. As it passes the dye spot, it tries to carry it along while the binding of the dye to the paper tends to hold it back. The rate at which the dye moves over the paper relative to the solvent is determined by its solubility in the solvent and the strength of the binding between the dye and the paper. Thus, by the time the solvent has reached the other edge of the paper, the dye will have moved a distance determined by its speed of movement.

---

3   See p 28 for the definition of pH.

A different dye will have a different binding strength and a different solubility in the solvent and will, therefore, move at a different rate. As a result, it moves a different distance in the time taken for the solvent to reach the top of the paper. This means that a mixture of the two dyes would separate if the experiment were repeated in that way.

Since the rate of movement of one of the dyes, say A, would be the same if run alone or in a mixture with dye B, it would be a simple matter to identify dye A in the mixture. This could be achieved by dotting the mixture on to the paper and dotting a known sample of dye A on an imaginary line through the spot and parallel with the edge that will dip into the solvent, the origin line. The mixture will separate into two spots, one of which will be directly opposite the spot formed by dye A which has been run as a reference. This identifies one of spots as dye A.

Expand this problem to the situation where the unknown dye may be one of several hundred. Some other criterion is then required, since it will not be practical to spot each dye for reference purposes. This is achieved by making use of what is called the R_f value; this is found by dividing the distance travelled by the spot by the distance travelled by the solvent. Its value is governed by the relative affinity or binding strength of each dye to the paper for a given solvent system.

This system of chromatography can be used to identify dyes by initially chromatographing all the dyes likely to be encountered and tabulating their R_f values. The unknown can then be chromatographed and its R_f value calculated. The dyes with similar values should be listed. The use of a different solvent system will identify another group of dyes with the same R_f values. Comparison of the groups will reveal one dye common to both groups, thus identifying the unknown. Using this dye as a reference, a third system should be chosen with different solvent characteristics to confirm the identity.

This identification procedure using paper chromatography for dyes is identical with that used for drugs except that, whereas dyes can be seen, drugs have to be revealed by spraying or by dipping the chromatogram into a colour-forming reagent. The drug is thus revealed as a coloured spot against a uniform background. The colour formed by the drug may itself, provide an additional aid to identification.[4]

The identification procedure as outlined shows the limitation of this and all other forms of chromatography—they are constrained as means of identification by the availability and comprehensiveness of reference tables.

The technique of paper chromatography was superseded by thin-layer chromatography, in which glass plates coated with a thin layer of absorbent material are used instead of paper. The major advantages are that separation can be achieved over a movement of 10–15 cm in approximately 30 minutes as opposed to several hours when using paper chromatography. Also, corrosive colour-forming reagents can be used directly on the layer.

Although it was possible to achieve reproducible layers and conditions, the technique was used primarily as a screening method to indicate the presence or absence of a drug. It could then be used to confirm the identity of a drug by chromatographing the extract together with a reference of the suspected drug. The procedure could also be used as a purification step prior to the use of other analytical techniques.

---

4   This is the basis of many of the so-called 'spot tests'.

The technique has been superseded in the modern laboratory by instrumental based chromatographic techniques including gas chromatography, high pressure/ performance liquid chromatography, capillary electrophoresis etc.

Gas chromatography

A schematic diagram of the apparatus for gas chromatography is shown in Figure 25.1. The apparatus is complex but its function can be understood by direct analogy to paper chromatography. The paper is replaced by a glass or stainless steel tube packed with a fine granular powder. In gas-solid chromatography, the powder alone is selected for the separation; in gas-liquid chromatography, the powder is coated with a selected wax or grease. The column is mounted in an oven since separations are achieved in the vapour phase. A carrier gas, usually nitrogen or helium, replaces the liquid solvent of paper chromatography.

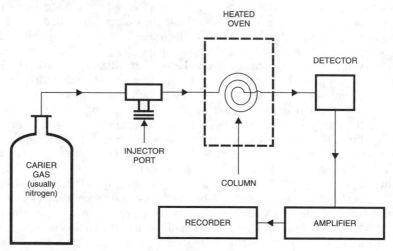

Figure 25.1 Schematic diagram of gas chromatography equipment.

The sample is injected at the start of the column where it is vaporised. The carrier gas sweeps it through the column, where the packing material retards its progress. As a result, components of samples are retarded to greater or lesser extents and are thereby separated; they emerge from the column at various times after injection, these being determined by their speed of progress through the column. This retention time is the characteristic that will ultimately identify the unknown.

As a component emerges from the column, it passes through a detector, which causes an electrical signal to be generated; this signal is amplified and displayed on a strip chart recorder. A typical chromatogram is shown in Figure 25.2. The peaks have been formed by the change in detector signal made as each component emerges. The interval from the time of injection to the appearance of the top of the peak is called the retention time of the component. When this is divided by the retention time of a co-chromatographed reference compound, the resultant relative retention time for the system chosen will be constant and will correct for any minor variations in columns and conditions between laboratories. Comprehensive tables of relative retention times for drugs sought under standard conditions have been compiled and are consulted for the initial identification of a drug.

The amount of component that passes through the detector determines the size of area of the peak and this measurement of area can be calibrated to measure the quantity of drug in the extract. Gas chromatography is most commonly used in the laboratory for the detection and measurement of alcohol in blood samples. Other instruments with different columns and detectors are set to measure drugs, solvents, gases and pesticides. The technique is specific in that it will separate a drug from its metabolites and measure each individually but it is constrained by the availability and scope of reference tables of retention data.

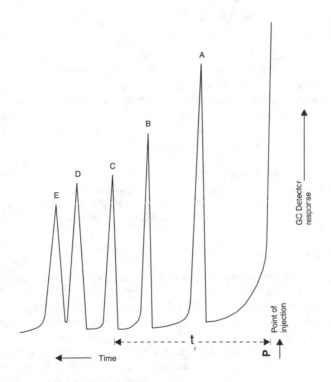

Figure 25.2 Gas chromatogram showing resolution of components of a mixture of substances A–E. t_r = Retention time of substance C.

High-performance liquid chromatography

This technique produces tracings similar to those resulting from gas chromatography. Instead of a carrier gas, a solvent is pumped at high pressure through a short column of tightly packed absorbent material. The extract may be injected directly into the column, although it is better to flush the extract into it using a valve with a sample loop. As before, the passage of the components through the column results in separation. The components are 'seen' by the detector as they emerge and the resultant signal is amplified and recorded. Comparing retention times allows identification of a component; quantitations are achieved using a measurement of the detector response.

The main advantage of this procedure over gas chromatography lies in its ability to separate components that are not volatile. Sample preparation can be minimal and may involve no more than the precipitation of proteins. Also, the separated components can be collected for further analyses since the technique is non-destructive. A possible disadvantage of the procedure is that assays tend to be for small groups of structurally related drugs rather than for the large groups that are possible by the use of gas chromatography for chemically related drugs. Otherwise, the technique has replaced and improved many of the analyses formerly carried out by gas chromatography.

Mass spectrometry

The mass spectrometer is the most powerful analytical tool available in the forensic science laboratory and can be used on its own or coupled to either a gas chromatograph or a high pressure liquid chromatograph. The instrument functions by bombarding the unknown drugs with a stream of electrons that cause the drug to break down reproducibly into charged fragments. Separating and measuring the mass to charge ratio of these fragments results in a cracking pattern for the drug. This is its mass spectrum and is unique for the drug in question. It can be used to identify the drug by comparison with a library of drug spectra. If no matches are found, a skilled spectroscopist can still identify the chemical formula of each fragment and slowly piece together possible structures for the unknown. Comparative spectra can be prepared by obtaining or synthesising indicated reference materials and, hence, an identification can be made.

Ultraviolet spectrometry

Just as the eye can differentiate between coloured dyes in daylight, the ultraviolet spectrometer can record the 'colour' of the drugs in the ultraviolet region of the spectrum. A rainbow displays the various components, or wavelengths, of visible light and the colour of a dye is formed by the molecules absorbing some of these components. The ultraviolet spectrometer sequentially shines different wavelengths of ultraviolet light through a solution of the drug and measures the amount of light absorbed. This measurement is compared with the amount of incident light and is recorded on a scale of absorbance plotted against wavelength.

This plot is an instrumental look at the 'colour' of the drug in the ultraviolet region. It can be used to indicate the identity of a drug by referring to a table of wavelengths at which absorbance is maximal. It is a useful, non-destructive analytical aid. The presence and possible identity of a drug can be indicated when the crude extract is dissolved in acid, alkali or ethanol. The quantity of drug present may be estimated by measuring the absorption but the identification is not absolute since drugs of similar molecular structure can produce identical spectra. Also, the metabolites of drugs will probably have spectra identical with the parent drug. For this reason, the measurement of drug levels should only be related to the total drug present and be used as a guide for further analysis to determine the amount of individual components.

Immunoassays

Radio-immunoassays and enzyme-multiplied immunoassays are techniques that make use of the body's immune response to foreign proteins. Antibodies can be obtained from a host animal that has been injected with a foreign protein to which the drug of interest has been linked. The antibody will recognise and bind itself to the drug molecule in a solution and this binding has been used as the basis of both techniques.

The techniques are sensitive, they require small sample volumes and they are relatively rapid. Unfortunately, they are not totally specific. An antibody raised to recognise morphine will cross-react to a greater or lesser extent with the other opiate drugs. An antibody raised to diazepam will cross-react with other benzodiazepines. As a result, these assays, although useful and highly acceptable in the clinical laboratory, have to be treated with caution for evidential purposes. Without preliminary separations, they are best used in the laboratory as presumptive tests for the presence or absence of a group of drugs.

The interpretation of results

Analytical techniques for detecting and measuring drugs are similar from laboratory to laboratory but are not always identical. The choice of techniques to solve a particular problem is largely a matter for the personal skill and preference of the analyst. Safeguards must be incorporated to ensure that the chosen procedures will have sufficient sensitivity to detect significant amounts of a drug or its metabolite, that the identification is beyond doubt and that the measurement techniques employed yield a true estimate of the quantity of drug present.

All measurements have errors. For example, the measurement of alcohol in blood by gas chromatography in the hands of a careful analyst is known to be accurate within 2% of the true value. However, bearing in mind the range of conditions of tissue and blood, from fresh to badly decomposed, that form the work-piece for the analyst, results are more realistically regarded as lying within 10% of the true value. The procedures used should be tested against standards dissolved in whole blood or tissue slurries as appropriate.

The interpretation of the drug level found should be done in consultation with the clinical or pathological findings. The level of the drug should be checked initially against known therapeutic levels and, if available, levels that have been measured in cases of fatal and non-fatal poisonings. A similar procedure must be adopted if a metabolite has been measured, since some metabolites are more active pharmacologically than is the parent drug. This approach will solve the majority of cases encountered and will generally explain the clinician's or the pathologist's findings when the known pharmacological effects have been considered.

Approximately 40% of all poisoning cases involving drugs also involve alcohol and this combination is, perhaps, one of the most difficult to interpret. When sufficient cases of poisoning by a particular drug have been encountered both with and without alcohol, a statistical analysis of the drug levels should reveal the influence of alcohol on the toxicity of the particular drug. The effect will probably be additive.

A satisfactory explanation of death is not always possible in cases in which several drugs have been detected at low to therapeutic levels. However, careful sifting of the information available in the medical literature may reveal a recorded adverse reaction when two of the drugs have been used together. Observed symptoms should be considered against those recorded.

The relationship of blood alcohol levels to alcohol consumed is the most frequent calculation required of the toxicologist in court. Such requests vary in complexity from the estimation of the quantity of beer or spirits that could account for a particular blood alcohol level to the calculation of the contribution of post-accident consumption of alcohol to the subsequent blood alcohol reading.

As a result of laboratory experiments in which volunteers of known weight consumed known amounts of alcohol, it is possible to predict a blood alcohol level from a known consumption. However, it must be remembered that variations in the order of plus or minus 20% in the maximum readings are usual after the consumption of the same amount of alcohol by volunteers of the same weight. The consumption of some foodstuffs prior to an experiment can slow the rate of alcohol absorption into the blood stream and consequently reduce the predicted maximum level.

Where alcohol consumption has taken place over a period of time, the effect of metabolism must be taken into account. Alcohol is removed from the body at a constant rate for the individual. This rate averages 15 mg per 100ml of blood (6.5 µg per 100 ml breath) per hour but experimentally, it has been shown to vary within the range of 9–27 mg alcohol per 100 ml blood (3.9–11.8 µg alcohol per 100ml breath) per hour. Consequently, a blood alcohol level resulting from the consumption of a known amount of alcohol will lie within a wide range of possible values.

So far as drugs are concerned, it is scarcely possible to do better than to make an educated guess at the relationship between drug levels and consumption. This is because of great variations from person to person. The situation is even more difficult when trying to relate drug levels to effect. A person undergoing long-term amitriptyline therapy may be living normally and driving with blood levels that would be in the fatal region if attained by way of a single dose. The toxicologist must be extremely circumspect when giving evidence on such matters.

Within the United Kingdom, and particularly over the past 20 years, the workload of the forensic toxicologist has changed dramatically from the investigation of the involvement of prescription drugs in fatalities to reflect the growing problem of drug abuse. Driving under the influence of drugs rarely involves individuals who are taking prescription medicines. The majority of cases relate either to drugs of abuse or to abused prescription medicines obtained illegally or to combinations of both.[5] The investigation of fatalities generally includes an analysis for drugs of abuse. In recent years, this usually results in the detection of the use of heroin and a benzodiazepine drug such as temazepam until 1997 and, since then, diazepam. Other drugs are found subject to availability (methadone), fashion (Ecstasy and cocaine) or price (dihydrocodeine). Since there can be a large overlap in drug levels measured in regular users and in fatalities, the interpretation of the analytical findings must take into account the history of abuse to obtain an indication of possible tolerance, or, as in the case of recently released prisoners, a loss of tolerance. Intravenous injection of

5   A Seymour and J S Oliver 'The Role of Drugs and Alcohol in Impaired Drivers and Fatally Injured Drivers in the Strathclyde Region of Scotland, 1995–1998' (1999) 103 Forensic Sci Internat 89.

benzodiazepine drugs can result in severe respiratory depression that is rarely seen from oral administration.

Analysis time

Popular television series often give the impression that an analysis for poisons can be almost instantaneous. Unfortunately, this is not true. If adequate specimens and information have been provided and adequate trained staff and equipment are available, results for most routine toxicology cases should be available, on average, within two working days. This can be, and often is, short-circuited to provide interim verbal reports within a few hours when the need arises and where the indicated poison falls within a group of readily analysable substances. The written report must be prepared only when the full toxicological investigation has been completed.

While the above statements are true for perhaps 99% of cases, unavoidable delays occur when an obscure poison or a complete unknown is encountered. It is impossible to predict an analysis time in such cases—their solution may take from a few hours to several weeks. Occasionally, the poison may remain undetected despite the best efforts of the analyst using the best available equipment.

26

Radiology in forensic medicine[1]

Radiological techniques have many applications in forensic science. Amongst these may be included the examination of fingerprints and of documents. There is, however, no intention to discuss the purely scientific field in this section which deals only with forensic medicine. The forensic *use* of medical radiology falls into two functional categories—those investigations concerned with identification and those directed to diagnosis. Forensic *interest* in radiological techniques is, however, increasing as their range and invasive character develops. Severe injury and even death may follow the use of some modern investigations; inevitably, the law will be involved when problems of medical negligence arise and, equally inevitably, such mishaps fall within the medico-legal ambit.

Radiology and identification

As described in Chapter 3, methods used for the identification of dead bodies may be, first, of a deductive nature. These are designed to indicate the type of person who should be sought in the missing-persons files; this approach is dictated when there is no clue as to identity. But once there is reason to suppose a personal identification, this is proved largely by means of comparative methods. Radiological assistance is valuable in the former circumstances but has a very special place in the latter; only a few of those benefiting from a National Health Service have not been X-rayed at some time during their lives. However, current United Kingdom regulations require the retention of X-rays for five years only and there is no provision for microfilming.

Deductive identification methods

The age of a cadaver at death is particularly well estimated radiologically. In infancy and early childhood, the presence of centres of ossification can be demonstrated with accuracy and ease; the union of these centres can be observed in childhood and adolescence up to approximately 25 years of age; in later life,

1   This section has been kindly reviewed by Dr A J A Wightman.

degenerative changes may give some indication of maturity, but this is only over a wide range—the chief value of X-rays of adult fatalities is to distinguish between two or three bodies who are known as a group but are of unknown individual identity. The main ossification details are given in Appendices G and H. Radiology of the teeth as an aid to assessment of age is discussed in Chapter 28.

The sex of a mutilated or charred body can also be established with some certainty and without the need for extensive cleaning processes if suitable bones are available for X-ray. The pelvis is by far the most useful bone in this respect (see page 49).

Comparative identification

Provided X-rays taken in life are available, any similar radiograph taken after death can be used for comparison. Identification can be based on similarities either in normal or in abnormal structures; the value of the latter in positive identification is proportional to the rarity of the abnormality.

Of the normal structures routinely used for comparison, the skull sinuses—the frontal sinus in particular—are the most satisfactory; the number of variations in shape and size that are potentially available is so diverse as to make a radiographic outline almost unique to the individual; the problem is mainly one of reconciling the view in the cadaver with that obtained in life. If an adequate front view is not available, the general outline of the skull, including the shape of the pituitary fossa, may provide almost equally good evidence.

One particular form of comparison of the normal that should be mentioned is the process whereby a post-mortem X-ray is superimposed on a photograph of the living person. The technical difficulties associated with obtaining a precisely similar scale and orientation are formidable but can be largely overcome by modern electronic methods such as simultaneous video-recording; even without this, the method has been used with success in several classic cases of investigation of homicide.[2] It has been suggested that the main value of this type of investigation lies in *excluding* identification—and this important use is common to all comparative methods of identification.

Abnormalities that may be of value are so numerous that only a few illustrations can be given. Congenital abnormalities such as absence of bones, displacement or malformation may be so rare as to be virtually diagnostic of identity. Others, such as fusion of the ribs, are not uncommon and should only be regarded as confirmatory of other circumstantial evidence. Pre-existing disease—in the form of changes in bone density, arthritic deformities and the like—may provide unequivocal evidence of identity of dead persons from whom films taken in life are available for comparison. Such opportunities are not confined to bone; unusual calcification—of tuberculous origin in the lungs or lymph nodes or due to degenerative changes in the uterus and many other organs—may show a pattern as individual as is that of a fingerprint. The presence of healing fractures in sites known to have been broken in life would obviously provide strong confirmatory evidence of identification but, even more useful, is the presence of surgical prostheses or of supportive implants such as plates, pins or orthopaedic screws— not only can the X-rays be compared but the appliance can be removed from the

2   Of which probably the best known is *R v Ruxton*, Manchester Assizes, March 1936.

cadaver and superimposed. Surgical implants are of very great use in identification after mass disasters; if, for example, one man is known to have a bone plated, it is simplicity itself to screen that bone radiologically in all unidentified bodies.

The importance of dental identification in both the single unknown body and in the mass has already been stressed. Radiography very greatly enhances the contribution of the odontologist. The mere presence of a single or double restoration in one or two commonly filled teeth would be insufficient to prove a positive identification as opposed to an exclusion of identification. The precise shape of the fillings is, however, likely to be unique and it would not be impossible to make a reasonably certain identification from a comparison of post- and ante-mortem radiographs of a single filling. Dental radiography may also show up significant root shapes, socket outlines or abnormalities of tooth eruption, development or decay; it is the policy in the Scandinavian countries, among others, to record the dentition of their commercial aircrew radiographically as a routine.

Another useful adjunct provided by radiology in identification in the mass lies in the occasional localisation of significant possessions that have been embedded in charred tissues; generally, this represents no more than a 'fringe benefit' of radiographic examination for other purposes—such as a search for injuries due to explosives—but it is, none the less, often of great value.

Diagnostic radiology

Diagnostic radiological techniques are of value both in accidental and in criminal deaths.

Accidental deaths

Forensic pathology has a great part to play in satisfying current interest in accidents as a cause of death since all such fatalities are investigated through the medico-legal system. It is doubtful whether a busy forensic pathologist can be expected to demonstrate individually all fractures present after a fatal accident, despite the fact that some of these may be of research significance; routine X-ray coverage of accident cases simplifies the whole procedure. Moreover, some fractures—notably those of the spine—are difficult to demonstrate satisfactorily by post-mortem dissection. The prevention of spinal fracture in vehicular accidents is one of the main objectives of the bio-engineers; in some unusual circumstances—such as escape by ejection from high-speed aircraft—it is, perhaps, the main limiting factor to added safety. Ideally, the complete autopsy in vehicular accidental death should include adequate radiography of, at least, the spine. X-rays may be of great assistance in distinguishing ante- from post-mortem fracture, an observation that may have profound significance in the reconstruction both of accidental and of homicidal deaths. It is to be noted that X-ray diagnosis is not confined to the study of bones; very useful information in relation to soft-tissue changes can also be obtained.

There is, of course, nothing to prevent the pathologist carrying out his own radio-opaque injection techniques and, occasionally, these may be of major advantage. A specific example is that of traumatic subarachnoid haemorrhage (see page 158) in which the critical lesion in one of the intracranial arteries may not only be difficult to demonstrate by dissection but may also be unwittingly simulated artefactually during the process. Injection of the arteries and X-ray examination prior to dissection may provide irrebuttable—and permanent—proof of rupture. But, as already mentioned, such investigations demand considerable foresight from the pathologist.

Homicidal death

The most obvious use of X-rays in potentially homicidal death lies in the demonstration within the body of bullets and other missiles (see Chapter 9). The technical difference between searching for a single bullet in a cadaver with and without the assistance of radiographic localisation needs no emphasis; moreover, even if the missile is recovered, fragments of bullets or of bomb casings or contents can easily be missed in an unaided dissection; much important information, including, say, the track of the missile, might thereby be lost to the ballistics expert. The importance, both to the reconstruction of events and to the subsequent investigation, of localisation of shot from smooth-bore weapons has been discussed in Chapter 9. Any radiographs that have been taken for the purpose of investigation can be retained as permanent records and, if necessary, used as exhibits or productions at trial.

Hijacking of aircraft is a particular modern use of firearms. The diagnosis of sabotage has been discussed at page 130; the possibility of demonstrating hijacking as a cause of a fatal accident would depend, to a large extent, on the finding of bullets in the crew members, a task that would be physically impossible to discharge with assurance in the absence of X-ray facilities. Overall, the importance of radiography in the investigation of shootings or explosions can scarcely be over-stressed.

Other forms of homicide are also well illustrated by way of X-rays. Particularly noteworthy is the radiography of the larynx in cases of strangulation; fractures of the thyroid cartilage or hyoid bone are generally well shown, particularly in the aged, in whom the cartilages are often calcified.

Perhaps, however, radiography and radiology reach their apogee in the examination of suspicious infant deaths. X-ray examination in the non-accidental injury syndrome (discussed in detail in Chapter 19) does more than merely demonstrate the presence of fractures. Its particular value is to prove the infliction of injury at various times—evidence that is essential to the concept of 'battering'. The X-ray picture can demonstrate the difference between healing and fresh fractures clearly and can often differentiate different periods of repair in the former. Attention has also been drawn to the possibility of indicating parental inattention to fractures sustained. Fractures unite by the elaboration of primitive bone known as 'callus'. The deposition of callus is particularly marked when the fracture has not been properly treated by immobilisation. Additionally, the radiologist may be able to demonstrate that a fracture has been caused in an unusual way—as, for example, by severe twisting. Such evidence strongly negates a defence, say, of an accidental fall.

The demonstration of active bone replacement is made more sensitive by using the more modern technique of radionuclide imaging, which depends on the uptake of injected radioisotope-labelled phosphate by bone which is being actively formed.[3] Positive findings are not, however, confined to trauma and it may be necessary to combine the investigation with routine radiography to make a certain diagnosis.

---

3   J R Sty and R J Starshak 'The Role of Bone Scintigraphy in the Evaluation of the Suspected Abused Child' (1983) 146 Radiology 369.

All such evidence is, primarily, designed to prove that physical abuse has occurred. Equity demands, however, that possible alternative causes of multiple fractures are pursued and X-ray evidence is well-nigh essential to this end. The main condition to be excluded is osteogenesis imperfecta, which is, in the majority of cases, a genetically inherited disease associated with abnormally brittle bones; the clinical and radiological differentiation from abuse is, generally, not difficult. There are also a number of conditions which, because of the periosteal reaction they cause, closely resemble one possible end-stage of repetitive injury to the bones. Some of these—such as scurvy and congenital syphilis—are of little more than historical interest. A more topical, and controversial, condition is that of copper deficiency[4]—including the associated enzymatic deficiency disease known as the kinky hair syndrome. While many of these conditions are rare, the lawyer must be aware of them as they will undoubtedly be raised as possibilities in any trial involving serious child abuse.[5]

X-ray examination of the living

Industrial diseases

The importance of X-rays in the assessment of dust diseases is discussed in Chapter 15. The diagnosis and assessment of disability due to coal miners' pneumoconiosis, which are based on the distribution and size of pulmonary nodules, are virtually in the hands of the radiologist.

Angiography

Angiography or arteriography—the study of the arteries by means of X-rays—is performed by injecting radio-opaque material into a blood vessel and observing its subsequent movement and distribution. There are several applications of the technique that are of major medico-legal importance.

First, angiography of the cerebral vessels may be used as a test of brain death. It can be taken that the situation is incompatible with function or revival if serial observations of the brain show the intracranial circulation to have been absent for 15 minutes; the permanence of the films provides lasting evidence of the fact of death and this method of establishing death is increasingly used in Continental Europe in relation to transplantation (see Chapter 12).

Secondly, angiography of the coronary arteries is now an accepted technique for establishing the in vivo state of the coronary vessels and, hence, assessing either treatment options or, more importantly in the present context, the risk of sudden death or disablement in the future. Thus, the technique might be applied to the diagnosis of asymptomatic disease of the coronary arteries in persons in whom sudden collapse poses a particular risk to public safety—the most obvious example is the commercial pilot. Although there have been no case decisions at the time of writing, there is the possibility that failure to diagnose arterial inadequacy prior to an accident attributed to such disease might result in a

---

4   S Chapman 'Child Abuse or Copper Deficiency? A Radiological Review' (1987) 294 BMJ 1370.
5   An excellent overview is to be found in K T Evans and G M Roberts 'Radiological Aspects of Child Abuse' in J K Mason (ed) *Paediatric Forensic Medicine and Pathology* (1989) ch 19.

successful negligence suit; and the diagnosis of coronary artery disease—as opposed to frank disease of the heart muscle which is its consequence—cannot be made with certainty using current standard electrocardiographic techniques. Recourse to more specialised tests is sometimes indicated. The relatively simple exercise electrocardiographic technique, however, gives non-specific results and, although the expertise is, now, very considerable, coronary angiography still has its limitations. First, while the examination may show the presence of the disease, there is no certainty that the disease will prove fatal—in one series of observations, only 60% of persons with 80% narrowing of all three main vessels and, presumably, symptoms at the time of examination, had died from coronary heart disease six years after the test; the six-year mortality for persons with obstruction of only one artery was 20%. It follows that the test might unnecessarily prevent a competent person being properly employed; the risk would have to be balanced against the many other factors involved.[6] Secondly, despite the advances of recent years, the test is not without danger and has some mortality in its own right; the risk of an adult dying in experienced hands is less than 0.05%[7] but this might still be sufficient to make it unacceptable as a screening test—even were such an application feasible on logistical grounds. It follows that it would be unreasonable to suggest its use for this purpose on a routine basis. In the opinion of this writer, coronary angiography has presently little or no place in the *selection* of persons in high-risk occupations unless these are exceptionally specialised—for example, astronauts.

Finally, angiographic contrast methods are widely employed in the diagnosis and management of many conditions attributable to arterial disease, including spasm which may, in turn, be exacerbated by the contrast medium; it should also be remembered that some persons are sensitive to the medium used. It follows that all such techniques carry an inherent morbidity; the main medico-legal importance of this in present-day medicine is that the patient should be made aware of such risks and should be able give a valid consent to them.[8] This, however, is a matter of negligence which is discussed briefly below.

Radiology and negligence

Failure to make an X-ray examination in a case of head injury or in any other situation in which fracture might reasonably be anticipated—and the consequent failure to diagnose the lesion—might, in the conditions of modern hospital practice, be difficult to justify no matter how full the clinical examination may have been. The later development of disability for this reason would almost certainly result in an action for negligence; some cases might be indefensible. The same could well be so were the presence of a foreign body to remain undiagnosed. The presumption of negligence is, however, by no means certain. Lord Denning MR is reported as stating:

---

6   It might, for example, be difficult to find an experienced airline pilot without some degree of coronary narrowing; the results of reducing the overall experience of airline pilots might well be worse than the risks involved in well-organised 'double-crewing' by older men.

7   G A H Miller 'Cardiac Catheterization' in D J Weatherall et al (eds) *Oxford Textbook of Medicine* (2nd edn, 1990) p 13.52.

8   J O M C Craig 'Consent in Diagnostic Radiology' (1988) 39 Clin Radiol 1.

'In some of the earlier cases the doctor had been criticised for not having taken X-rays with the result that they had sometimes been taken unnecessarily. This case showed that the courts did not always find that there had been negligence because a patient had not had an X-ray; it depended upon the circumstances of each case.'[9]

We will see below that the increasing number of radiographic examinations makes a significant contribution to the total dose of radiation delivered to the population; moreover, should it be that a significant number of examinations are unnecessary, this could be a drain on financial resources which a health system of any sort could well do without.

The former problem has been re-addressed by the Royal College of Radiologists and the National Radiological Protection Board[10] and is referred to again below. The latter has been considered more recently[11] and it has been estimated that the National Health Service wastes some £20m on inappropriate X-ray examinations. Guidelines for the appropriate use of radiography prepared by the Royal College of Radiologists are now generally followed in the United Kingdom.[12] It is not, of course, suggested that all, or even a significant number of, unnecessary examinations are made in the casualty department—but the figures indicate not only that there is always room for considering the implications before ordering an X-ray but also that the pressures on junior medical staff to do so are very considerable. Not every failure in what may well be a brand of 'defensive medicine' will be blameworthy—but the circumstances will be all-important.[13]

Mention has been made above of failure to warn patients of the risks associated with invasive radiological techniques—such a failure may well result in a claim in negligence should an undisclosed but foreseeable hazard materialise. This is simply one aspect of the application of the doctrine of informed consent (see page 473) but a surprising number of such actions are related to radiology. The *locus classicus* is *Moyes v Lothian Health Board*,[14] which not only demonstrates well the issues involved but also shows how difficult it is for an action in consent-based negligence to succeed.

Magnetic resonance imaging

Partly due to the anxiety to reduce the dose of ionising radiation delivered to the patient and to the public, and partly due to the inevitable march of science, new methods of imaging are being produced and used increasingly.[15] Among these is that of magnetic resonance imaging which, essentially, involves exposing the

9 In *Braisher v Harefield and Northwood Hospital Group Management Committee* (13 July 1966, unreported), CA. This case was quoted by H Jellie (1966) ii Lancet 235.
10 National Radiation Protection Board *Patient Dose Reduction in Diagnostic Radiology* (1990).
11 Audit Commission *Improving Your Image: How to Manage Radiology Services More Effectively* (1995).
12 Royal College of Radiologists *Making the Best Use of a Department of Clinical Radiology. Guidelines for Doctors* (4th edn, 1998).
13 A salutary news item concerns a doctor who diagnosed a child as being asthmatic and refused requests for an X-ray. Two years later a 1½ inch screw was removed from her bronchus; agreed damages of £10,000 were paid: *The Scotsman*, 8 May 1991, p 2.
14 [1990] 1 Med LR 463; 1990 SLT 444.
15 The newer techniques are, however, often expensive and slow. They may well remain no more than supplementary to X-rays which are cheap and quick to perform.

whole body to an intense magnetic field[16] and detecting the response of the atomic nuclei—in particular, those of the hydrogen contained in body water—which act as minute magnets themselves. Differential response results in computerised tissue images of sectional type. No pathological changes in the tissue have been demonstrated using this technique but the absorption of energy can lead to local heating; a possible future source of damage lies in the production, and improper use, of machines of increasing power. Those working in the field are limited to strict exposures as to time and peak T values—this being a precautionary measure rather than one of need; pregnant women in the first trimester are excluded from examination for the same reason.[17] The main danger of MRI is, however, that any magnetisable objects in the body—or in the bodies of those around—may be affected, but this is something of which all operators will be aware.[18]

The hazards of radiation

The dose of X-rays given to an individual during a single diagnostic procedure is well controlled and the possibility of damage in the form of, say, skin burning is limited to the very large doses which are given as treatment. Nevertheless, radiation used outside the field of clinical medicine may affect the genetic structures or the blood-forming tissues and represents a hazard which is growing in importance along with a national environmental conscience. Radiation injury of all types falls within the ambit of forensic medicine and has potential, and perhaps current, medico-legal significance.

Electromagnetic radiation (see Table 26.1) is of two types—*non-ionising* and *ionising*—the precise type and effect of the radiation depending upon the frequency of the electromagnetic waves. Non-ionising radiation is not without danger.[19] In the industrial field, long exposure to microwaves may result in cataract (or opacity of the lens of the eye), while laser workers may develop burns of the retina; such cases are rare but may increase as the devices become increasingly used. Infrared radiation is detected by the skin and is, therefore, only a hazard in unconscious persons. Ultraviolet light, on the other hand, is not detected by the skin; everyone is familiar with resultant burns due to excessive sunbathing while extreme exposure undoubtedly predisposes to cancer of the skin (particularly of basal cell or 'rodent ulcer' type and the malignant melanomas). Ionising radiations are clinically more important and owe their biological effects to their ability to alter the chemical properties of 'ionised' cells. The original unit of measurement of X-rays

16 Some 50,000 times that of the Earth's magnetic field, which is 5×10^{-5} T (T = tesla or the unit of measurement of magnetic flux density).

17 Ad hoc Advisory Group on Nuclear Magnetic Resonance Clinical Imaging 'Revised Guidance on Acceptable Limits of Exposure during Nuclear Magnetic Resonance Clinical Imaging' (1983) 56 Brit J Radiol 975. Subject to that, there is no evidence of abnormality in children who had been exposed in utero: H Clements, K R Duncan, K Fielding et al 'Infants Exposed to MRI *in utero* have a Normal Paediatric Assessment at 9 Months of Age' (2000) 73 Brit J Radiol 190.

18 For a précis of guidelines, see F Godlee 'Warning over Magnetic Resonance Imaging' (1991) 303 BMJ 205.

19 The suggestion that electromagnetic fields associated with power lines cause leukaemia and other cancers has been discussed at p 306. Modern work confirms the very doubtful basis for this assertion; for references, see D Spurgeon 'Link between Magnetic Fields and Cancer is Weak' (1999) 319 BMJ 10.

was the roentgen but, from the point of view of the biological effect, it is the energy absorbed, rather than the dose, that is significant. Ionising radiations were originally measured in 'rads', one rad closely corresponding to the energy absorbed when one roentgen is received by 1 g of tissue. There are, however, variations in response to radiation and, accordingly, the biological effect on man was measured as 'rems' (rem being the acronym for roentgen equivalent for man); rads and rems are numerically equal for X-rays, gamma rays and beta particles but, for alpha particles and neutrons, 1 rad is equivalent to 10 rems. These units have been replaced in the International System of Units (SI) by the gray (Gy; 1 Gy = 100 rad) and the sievert (Sv; 1 Sv = 100 rem). The important unit for man is, therefore, the Sv.[20] The effect of radioactivity is to produce electromagnetic radiation in the tissues. The unit of radioactivity was originally the curie but this is a massive number; the new SI measure is the becquerel (Bq; 1 Bq = 1 disintegration per second)—this is about one 4000 millionth of a curie!

Table 26.1 Types of electromagnetic radiation

Very	1 MHz	Radio	
low	1 GHz	Radar or microwave	
	10^3 GHz	Infrared	Non-ionising
Frequency	10^5 GHz	Light	
	10^7 GHz	Ultraviolet	
	10^9 GHz	X-rays	
Very	10^{10} GHz	Gamma rays	Ionising
high	10^{12} GHz	Cosmic rays	

NB 1 Hz = 1 cycle per second. For an explanation of SI units see Appendix S.

For ease of description it can be taken that rapidly growing and multiplying cells are the most sensitive to ionising radiation. The organs within the body most easily damaged are the bone marrow, the epithelium of the bowel, the testes or ovaries and the lymphatic glands. Similarly, children, because they are growing faster than adults—and this includes, especially, the fetus at the time the organs are being formed (ie from 3–18 weeks after conception)—are generally more sensitive to radiation. External sources of radiation, other than those of natural origin, act in a relatively transient fashion—most can either be avoided or switched off. But a source of radiation that is bound to the tissues will exert a continuous influence until it decays. Such foci of radiation can come from radioactive substances deliberately introduced into the body—almost invariably for medical diagnostic purposes.[1] It is imperative that such substances decay rapidly, the rate

20 The average person in the United Kingdom receives about 2 mSv annually from background, natural radiation. The dose received from a normal chest X-ray is of the order of 0.01–0.04 mSv.

1 Authorisation is required before a doctor or a dentist can administer radioactive medicinal products for diagnosis, treatment or research: Medicines (Administration of Radioactive Substances) Regulations 1978, SI 1978/1006, as amended by SI 1995/2147 and associated regulations.

being dependent upon the 'half-life' of the radioactive element; the half-life is defined as the time taken for half the available radioactive atoms to disintegrate. An alternative source of internal radiation is food that has itself been contaminated by external sources of abnormal radioactivity. The half-life of such radioactive elements may be long and in certain cases, notably strontium 90 (which is chemically similar to calcium), the element is stored in the body; this type of radiation therefore constitutes a serious health hazard.

The results of radiation will vary from person to person but, in general, it can be said that high doses, of the order of 5–10 Sv and above, will kill within a matter of weeks; medium doses (1–5 Sv) will increase the risk of later malignant disease, particularly of the blood, several years after exposure; and low doses may cause genetic damage to future generations. It is small wonder that radiation hazards at work are strongly controlled by legislation.[2]

Industrial hazards

The effects of exposure to neutrons and alpha particles are, to an extent, of all or nothing type, whereas those of exposure to X-rays and gamma rays are cumulative. Thus, the amount of radiation sustained by workers in occupations associated with this hazard must be carefully controlled and is monitored by sensitive devices such as film badges or thermoluminescent dosimeters and by periodic blood tests.[3] The maximum permissible dose for adult workers is set by international regulations at 20 mSv per year with a degree of flexibility allowing for a maximum of 50 mSv in any one year.[4] The corresponding recommended permissible dose for the public at large is 1 mSv per year with a maximum 0.5 mSv per year emanating from a single source; the accepted limits exclude exposure for the purposes of medical diagnosis or treatment. The difference between occupational and public levels is accepted as a safe compromise that allows for the use of radiation in an advantageous way—cost and social benefit being taken into account. In practice, very few radiation workers receive a dose above 15 mSv in a year; levels above this dictate an investigation to ensure that exposure is, in fact, as low as is reasonably possible.

As indicated above, the ill effects of radiation are of two types. First, disease may result either from the destructive effect of ionising radiations or from their capacity to stimulate cells into abnormal activity and, thus, predispose to cancer.

2   The Euratom Council Directive 80/836 (amended by Directive 84/467) on radiological protection is mandatory. There is a mass of UK legislation relevant not only to the individual worker but also to the environment. The major regulations are to be found in the Ionising Radiations Regulations 1999, SI 1999/3232, which are designed to implement, in part, Council of Europe Directives 96/29/Euratom, 90/641/Euratom and 97/43/Euratom. The more important statutes include the Nuclear Installations Acts 1965 and 1969 as amended by the Energy Act 1983, the Radiological Protection Act 1970 (which established the National Radiological Protection Board), the Radioactive Material (Road Transport) Act 1991 (see Radioactive Material (Road Transport) (Great Britain) Regulations, SI 1996/1350) and the Radioactive Substances Act 1993 (which deals especially with the registration of those allowed to keep radioactive material (s 6) and the disposal of radioactive waste (s 13)).
3   A minimal decrease in the blood lymphocyte count might be appreciated after a dose of 0.1–0.2 Sv.
4   The limit for trainees under the age of 18 is set at 6 mSv in any year. But the general rule is that all doses should be kept as low as is reasonably practicable. See R J Berry 'Ionizing Radiations' in P A B Raffle et al (eds) *Hunter's Diseases of Occupations* (8th edn, 1994) ch 17.

The tissue most commonly harmed is the bone marrow, a process that leads to severe anaemia; the lymphoid tissue is also sensitive to radiation and its destruction results in an increased susceptibility to infection. Acute damage of this type is limited to the levels of exposure sustained following survival from an atomic bomb explosion or during the treatment of cancer; more subtly, however, there is an increased statistical risk of disease of those systems that are most sensitive that is proportional to the degree of exposure to radiation. Radiation can provoke cancer in many sites—particularly in the blood (leukaemia), lungs and thyroid gland. Symptoms and signs of the disease may be delayed for many years after exposure and this may make the establishment of a cause-and-effect relationship very difficult. The evidence for an occupational association is, however, sometimes irrefutable. Classic examples include cancer of the lung occurring in miners in radioactive mines, particularly in Central Europe, and the malignancies induced in the early painters of luminous dials; there is little doubt that a high incidence of malignancy is to be found among those who are employed as uranium miners. Short of such obvious exposures, the difficulty in assessing risk lies in the fact that the common sites of radiation-induced cancers are those in which cancer is common in the general population. It is currently estimated that the long-term risk of developing a radiation-induced cancer is around 4×10^{-2} per Gy of cumulative exposure. Thus, if 10,000 workers are exposed to the working dose limit of 20 mSv per year for 40 years, they will each have received 800 mSv and the likelihood is that 320 will die of radiation induced cancer; but this is against the background that, in the same population not exposed to industrial radiation, some 3,000 would develop cancer anyway and between 2,000–2,500 would die from cancer.[5] It is easy to see what a complex matter it may be to prove an association between industrial exposure and a given malignancy—and this is irrespective of whether one is thinking in terms of a legal or an epidemiological standard.

The second group of adverse effects results from genetic damage; alternation of the chromosomes in the gonads may be caused by direct ionising damage or by an increase in the rate at which spontaneous changes occur—the process of mutation. The dose of radiation required to produce genetic change is certainly less than that needed to provoke cancer and, for all that is known, it may be very small. The effects of abnormal gene changes are also problematical. Most harmful genes are eliminated naturally and those that survive will almost certainly be recessive. But an increase in homozygous, clinically abnormal persons would follow should there be a sudden widespread increase in altered genes—the elimination of the harmful genes might then be difficult; it is encouraging that, if there has been any increase in genetically controlled abnormalities in the cities of Hiroshima and Nagasaki since 1945, it has been slight.

The general public

Mention of which serves to remind us that, of all the artificial sources of radiation, the most dramatic is that derived from the detonation above ground of nuclear bombs or test devices. The explosion of a nuclear bomb results in a central zone of massive destruction surrounded by a wide area of lethal heat; beyond this is a

5   This illustration is taken from Berry, fn 4 above.

circle of radiation which falls off in intensity from an original area in which a rapidly fatal dose is sustained. Additionally, radioactivity is displaced into the upper atmosphere, returning to earth with rainfall over a prolonged period; it is this type of radiation fall-out that gives rise to a persistent hazard as the radioactive elements, being taken up by plant life, become a source of internal radiation to animals and humans. The particular importance of strontium 90, which is stored in bone, has been mentioned above.

Turning to more prosaic considerations, the level to which the general public is exposed to preventable radiation has to be considered in the context of overall exposure including that due to natural causes. The average annual dose per person in the United Kingdom is 2.5 mSv. Diagnostic radiology accounts for some 12% of this but the more significant figure is that it constitutes 90% of exposure from man-made sources.[6] A very considerable responsibility thus rests on health services to reduce this figure.[7] A sizeable proportion of the unavoidable exposure results from the inevitable presence in the body of radioactive isotopes of normal body components—notably potassium. The remainder of the background exposure stems from the ground and buildings—which is very geographically dependent; from cosmic rays—which increase at altitude and, incidentally, are a limiting factor in supersonic air travel;[8] and from ingested substances. It seems that the greater part of radiation associated with housing is due to emanation of radon—some 1 in 200 homes have been said to show levels at which action should be taken or higher.[9]

The theoretical possibility of dangerous leaks of radioactivity from nuclear power stations is always with us. Fortunately, theory has turned into practice very rarely and, in these accidents, a significant dose was sustained only by those working close to the plant—it has, for example, been pointed out that the annual exposure of the British population from diagnostic radiology is eight times the exposure it received from Chernobyl in the year after the accident.[10] The risk from a nuclear power plant can, therefore, be looked at in two ways. Either it may be seen as a permanent potential disaster situation, or one could compare the total adverse effect of even an occasional accident with the amount of disease and suffering resulting from the production of other sources of power, especially coal and coal burning (see page 304). A far more worrying aspect of nuclear power is the ultimate effect on world-wide natural radiation of the disposal of waste products in increasing quantities—a problem that is beyond the scope of discussion here.

The individual patient

We have seen that exposure to a diagnostic X-ray constitutes very little hazard to the individual patient, particularly when this is balanced against the advantages derived. Nevertheless, there are certain circumstances in which a decision to

---

6 See D Gifford 'Reducing Radiation Exposure of Patients' (1990) 301 BMJ 451.

7 Attention is drawn to Ionising Radiation (Protection of Persons Undergoing Medical Examination or Treatment) Regulations 1988, SI 1988/778. It is noteworthy that computed tomography accounts for only 2% of the total X-ray examinations but for about 20% of the collective dose.

8 Although the risk of significant exposure of crew or passengers is negligible save during the cyclical spasms of solar hyperactivity.

9 National Radiological Protection Board *Radon in Dwellings in England* (1992).

10 Gifford, fn 6 above.

make such an examination would be taken only after careful consideration, the absence of which might well constitute negligence. These mainly concern pregnant women and the possible effect on the fetus. There can be very few circumstances in which a diagnostic pelvic X-ray would be justified when a woman was known to be in the early stages of pregnancy. The mature fetus, on the other hand, is little different from a child in this respect and is, moreover, shielded by its mother's tissues;[11] nevertheless, mere 'safety-first' principles would suggest that the apparently innocuous imaging by ultrasonography should be used in the presence of a fetus whenever practical in preference to X-rays. It has been the practice in the past to refuse to make an X-ray examination below the waist of a woman who had her last menstrual period more than ten days previously—the so-called '10 day rule'. This policy has been discontinued. Women of child-bearing age who are referred for X-ray of the lower abdomen or upper thigh region—eg for radiography of the lumbar spine and pelvis—are now asked if they are pregnant. If they are, or are unsure, the examination is deferred whenever possible. At times, however, the clinical requirement takes precedence over the small risk from radiation. Rather more concern now attaches to the possibility that the ovum is unduly sensitive to radiation in the last seven weeks before it is discharged from the ovary. There seems little positive that can be done about this, short of exhorting a woman not to become pregnant during the seven weeks after examination. Speaking passively, it raises the question 'is this investigation really necessary?' in stark form; non-essential X-rays of all types are always to be deprecated.

There remains the problem of women at work which carries a hazard or exposure to radiation—the radiographer is a good example. Special dose limits are imposed in respect of women of reproductive capacity;[12]any discrimination resulting from compliance with these provisions is not unlawful under the Sex Discrimination Act 1975.[13] Any risk to a fetus is, thus, essentially limited by the good working practices which should be operating as a routine—and the pattern of work can be altered to accommodate the pregnancy. The suggestion that the resulting financial loss to a woman who stops work to avoid radiation in pregnancy could be more harmful to the fetus than the ionising radiation that has been avoided[14] seems to capture the situation well.

---

11 Something which would not apply were the woman treated with or examined using radionuclides. For permissible concentrations of radionuclides, see Ionising Radiations Regulations 1999, SI 1999/3232, Sch 8.
12 For women of child-bearing age, the limit is 13 mSv in any consecutive three-month period (SI 1999/3232, reg 11, Sch 4, para 11). Pregnant women must not be exposed to more than 10 mSv during their declared term of pregnancy.
13 By virtue of the Employment Act 1989, s 4, Sch 1.
14 J G B Russell 'Pregnancy and Ionising Radiation' (1992) 305 BMJ 1172.

27

Forensic psychiatry

Derek Chiswick

Forensic psychiatry is concerned with the assessment and treatment of mentally disordered offenders, the provision of psychiatric evidence to the criminal and civil courts and the application of the law to psychiatric practice. In this chapter we will consider the relationship between psychiatric disorder and crime, the ways in which the criminal justice system may deal with mentally disordered offenders, the facilities available for the treatment of mentally disordered offenders and the measures available for compulsory admission and detention of people with mental disorders. There is also consideration of some civil issues.

Psychiatrists

Psychiatrists are medical practitioners who specialise in the diagnosis and treatment of psychiatric disorders. They have special obligations when acting as responsible medical officers under the Mental Health Act 1983.[1] Most psychiatrists and some other medical practitioners are likely to be approved by the Secretary of State as having special experience for the purpose of applying s 12 of the Mental Health Act 1983;[2] only approved doctors can carry out certain tasks under the Act. Forensic psychiatrists specialise in the assessment and treatment of mentally disordered offenders. They are likely to have clinical responsibilities within a forensic psychiatry service, secure psychiatric hospital or prison.

Range and classification of psychiatric disorders

Psychiatric disorders are common and account for significant morbidity; 14% of certificated sickness absence is due to mental illness. Patients referred to specialist

---

1   Separate legislation exists for Scotland and Northern Ireland (see p 411). This chapter will
    refer to details in the English statute only, except when there is a specific point of difference.
2   Similar approval is granted by a health board under the Mental Health (Scotland) Act
    1984, s 20.

psychiatric services represent less than a third of patients who attend general practitioners with mental symptoms.[3] Psychiatric illness varies enormously in type and severity.[4] Even minor forms of disorder may significantly limit aspects of daily living: severe forms may be completely disabling such that the sufferer is dependent on others for the most basic activities of daily living.

Given the range and diversity of mental illnesses, some form of classification is necessary if we are to make any attempt to research the causes of an illness or to investigate the efficacy of different treatments. That is not to infer that all patients with the same mental illness are alike; they are not. The particular manifestation of the illness is unique to an individual, but he or she will share some features with others who have the same illness.

The current system of classification of mental illnesses is based mainly, but not exclusively, on the symptoms and signs of individual illnesses rather than on their cause or causes. With some important exceptions, we do not know the cause of most major mental illnesses, although we know a good deal more than we did 25 years ago. New knowledge about brain chemistry has emerged from investigations such as magnetic resonance imagery, while studies of molecular genetics have pinpointed the genetic basis of many psychiatric conditions. Like physical disorders, most mental disorders are probably due to a combination of inherited constitutional (or biological) factors and, as yet poorly understood, life events or influences (eg the early loss of a parent or even prenatal intrauterine factors)—that is to say, to a combination of nature, nurture and beyond.

Classically, mental disorders have been divided into psychotic and neurotic categories and these two terms remain in clinical use. The psychoses are serious disorders in which there is loss of contact with reality, a lack of appreciation of the illness by the sufferer and abnormalities of thinking and perception—eg delusions (false beliefs) and hallucinations (false perceptions). The neuroses are less serious disorders in which contact with reality is maintained and the sufferer is normally aware, at least partially, of the fact of the illness.

The accurate diagnosis of psychiatric disorder is a skilled task. It depends on listening carefully to the patient's account (of his symptoms and their development, his background, his family and relationships), examining special features in his mental functioning and obtaining additional information from others, eg family members. It is never based on a snapshot view of one piece of behaviour or one symptom; it requires global consideration of many factors. In current practice the most widely accepted classifications of mental disorders are known as 'ICD-10', prepared under the aegis of the World Health Organisation[5] and 'DSM-IV', published by the American Psychiatric Association.[6] The following list of eight psychiatric disorders is modified from ICD-10 and covers the most important conditions for the purpose of this discussion:

3   Department of Health *The Health of the Nation, Key Area Handbook: mental illness* (1993).
4   90% of people who commit suicide have some form of mental disorder.
5   World Health Organisation *The ICD-10 Classification of Mental and Behavioural Disorders* (1992).
6   American Psychiatric Association *Diagnostic and Statistical Manual of Mental Disorders* (4th edn,1994).

1. schizophrenia;
2. disorders of mood;
3. organic mental disorders;
4. disorders due to psychoactive substances;
5. neurotic disorders;
6. behavioural syndromes;
7. personality disorders;
8. mental retardation.

Nearly all psychiatric disorders are associated with increased mortality rates involving both natural and unnatural death, particularly death by suicide. It cannot be overemphasised that the great majority of people who suffer from any of these disorders is unlikely to come into contact with the criminal justice system but some will do so. We will now consider how each disorder may lead to criminal behaviour. How the courts may deal with such cases is a separate matter for consideration later in this chapter.

Crime and psychiatric disorder

1. Schizophrenia

Schizophrenia is a grave mental illness affecting 1% of the world population. It causes enormous suffering to patients and their families and approximately 10% of those with schizophrenia die by suicide. It affects people in early adult life and, thus, creates a major economic cost to the state in terms of the provision of care and in loss of normal productivity. It is characterised by gross disturbance of thinking and perception with 'blunting' of mood. There is no significant effect on intellect. The course of the disorder varies from single episodes with recovery to life-long disease producing complete disintegration of the previous personality and major disability.

Symptoms are commonly divided into positive and negative features. The former occur in the acute phase of the illness and consist of disturbances in thinking and perception. Negative features are associated with the chronic condition and are manifested by aimlessness, self-absorption and social withdrawal. In the face of these serious features, it is unsurprising that they are commonly associated with a generalised deterioration in personal functioning.

Criminal acts by people with schizophrenia are common but are usually minor, eg damage to property or assault on an arresting officer. Rarely, there is a grave act of violence driven by paranoid delusions or hallucinations. In a comprehensive study of 500 homicides, there were 30 perpetrators who had been diagnosed as schizophrenic at some time in their lives.[7] The victim of homicide is most likely to be a family member or carer but, occasionally, he or she is a random stranger; these cases understandably cause major public concern.[8] Delusions involving bodily interference, or of impending cataclysmic happenings or of poisoning, are

---

7   National Confidential Inquiry into Suicide and Homicide by People with Mental Illness *Safer Services* (1999).
8   North East Thames and South East Thames Regional Health Authorities *Report of the Inquiry into the Care and Treatment of Christopher Clunis* (1994); L Blom-Cooper, H Hally and E Murphy *The Falling Shadow: One Patient's Mental Health Care 1978-1993* (1995).

seen commonly in homicides. Criminal acts may be related to negative symptoms—eg stealing to survive, or breaking and entering to obtain shelter. Sometimes fire-raising may occur, this often involving places of worship.

Schizophrenia may not always provide the complete explanation for a crime; there may be a significant contextual or situational element—for example, a stormy relationship with a family member, particularly a parent, since young people with schizophrenia often remain dependent on parents well into adulthood. Finally, alcohol and/or drug misuse commonly makes a significant contribution to disturbed behaviour, as it may do in any person. Substances such as cannabis, LSD, Ecstasy and amphetamines have an aggravating effect on schizophrenia.

2.   Disorders of mood

Disorders of mood (also known as affective disorders) range from mild, or neurotic, disorders to severe psychotic illness. The most common disorder is depressive in type, in which low mood, loss of interest and enjoyment in life and reduced activity are the predominant features. Loss of a sense of personal worth and nihilistic ruminations are features that indicate why suicidal ideation and behaviour are so common in depressive disorders. Mortality by suicide is in the order of 15%.

Sometimes the disorder of mood may be the complete opposite: pathological elation or mania. Here there is a feeling of boundless energy, uncontrollable excitement, and overactivity with grandiose but unrealistic ideas. Manic patients are overactive, over-talkative and have a decreased need for sleep. Their intrusiveness and overbearing manner quickly leads them into difficulties. Some patients experience both types of episode and may do so in a cyclical pattern. This is known as manic depressive disorder or by the more modern term—bipolar affective disorder.

The extent of offending by people with mood disorder is difficult to establish with any degree of certainty. There were 53 people with a lifetime diagnosis of mood disorder in the sample of 500 homicides reported in the Confidential Inquiry; it was more often present in women than in men.[9] The person most at risk of harm in depression is the sufferer. However, sometimes the despair extends so that the depressed person imagines they must spare his or her nearest and dearest any more 'suffering'. The tragic killing of one or more family members may then follow in a so-called altruistic homicide. This is frequently accompanied by the suicide or attempted suicide of the subject. The victim is usually the infant or young child (or children) of the sufferer or the spouse or an elderly parent. Some depressed women, driven to desperation by years of physical abuse from violent partners, may kill them, not for reasons of altruism but in order to end an intolerable situation (see also page 252).

The relationship of other forms of criminal behaviour to depressive disorder is contentious. It is often suspected as a factor in otherwise inexplicable accidents, particularly those involving drivers of public transport vehicles which crash 'for no reason'. Shoplifting, occurring for the first time in a middle-aged person, should arouse the suspicion of a depressive illness. Typically, depressed shoplifters steal goods they do not need and can afford to buy. The theft is carried out with no attempt to conceal the stolen item and they readily admit their behaviour when

9   Fn 7 above.

apprehended. It may represent the equivalent of a suicide attempt or some form of cry for help. Depressed patients receiving antidepressant medication may shoplift due to absentmindedness.

Offending is more likely to occur during a manic illness than in depression. Aggression is never far from the surface in severe mania, particularly when the sufferer's wishes or demands are thwarted. Sometimes they may spend beyond their means and thereby commit fraud or theft; hotels and restaurants are likely locations for such behaviour. Dangerous driving by manic patients is a serious problem; they may drive the wrong way down a motorway, insisting that it is of no consequence, or become involved in a dramatic police car chase. Finally, the degree of disinhibition and failed judgment involved may lead them to sexual indiscretions or worse; manic men may commit rape or other sex offences and manic women may become dangerously promiscuous.

3. Organic mental disorders

These are characterised by having a demonstrable cause based on disease of, or injury to, the brain. They are commonly divided into acute conditions (such as delirium) and chronic conditions (known as dementia). Delirium is an acute disturbance of consciousness, usually sudden in onset, in which the patient shows abnormalities of orientation, perception and thinking, with impaired recent memory and disturbance of the normal sleep-wake cycle. It indicates an underlying physical disorder and is a medical emergency requiring treatment as such. A specific form of delirium associated with alcohol withdrawal is known as delirium tremens (or in common parlance the 'DTs' or 'the shakes'). Patients with delirium tremens are terrified owing to their disturbed perceptions—particularly visual hallucinations. They may be convinced they are under threat and hence act recklessly—eg by jumping from a building or attacking an imagined enemy, sometimes with fatal consequences.

Dementia refers to a progressive, and usually irreversible, loss of mental functions associated with deterioration in behaviour and personal functioning. Dementia is common in the elderly, where it may result from Alzheimer's disease or from hardening of the arteries in and supplying the brain. In the early stages of dementia, impaired judgment, impulsiveness, sudden displays of anger and paranoid beliefs may lead to assaultive behaviour or inappropriate sexual acts. A particular form of dementia is associated with a rare inherited brain disease— Huntington's disease (or Huntington's chorea). Criminal behaviour is common in the prodromal or early stages of this devastating condition. Personality is commonly affected by the results of serious brain injury, eg following assault, accident or insult to the brain from any other cause. Disinhibition, aggression and impulsivity may manifest themselves, particularly in combination with substance abuse.

Epilepsy is a physical (not mental) disorder of the brain in which sudden episodic losses of consciousness, or epileptic seizures, occur. It is a common condition in which there is a disputed association with criminal behaviour. Certainly prison populations contain an excess of people with epilepsy, though there is no relationship with prisoners convicted of violent crimes. The excess of prisoners with epilepsy may be accounted for by associated factors which, in themselves, strongly correlate with offending, eg generalised brain damage, social and economic disadvantage, substance abuse or an unstable family background.

Violent behaviour by someone with epilepsy before, during or after an epileptic seizure is rare. It would be even rarer for epilepsy first to manifest itself by an act of criminal violence. Unusual behaviour can occur during an epileptic seizure but it is likely to be purposeless, not sustained, and of brief duration (ie lasting seconds rather than minutes). Any element of preconception, planning or motivation generally rules out epilepsy as an explanation for criminal behaviour. Normally there is amnesia for the duration of the seizure.

The search for organic abnormalities in general criminal populations has been a recurring activity in criminological research over the years; it is one of many 'biological markers' that have been sought in order to explain criminality. Some authorities think that subtle abnormalities in brain function may contribute to criminality but the evidence is not convincing.

4.   *Disorders due to psychoactive substances*

The association between substance misuse, in its various forms, and offending behaviour is strong, although it usually operates in combination with other elements such as the personality of the offender, social and family influences and situational factors. The nature of the offending may vary from minor crimes involving public disorder or prostitution to fire-raising and the most grave homicidal or sexual assaults. Two-thirds of men and a third of women in prison have alcohol problems. More than half of all prisoners (male and female) have abused drugs in the year before their imprisonment.[10] Finally, substance misuse is a major factor in domestic violence and in crimes of dishonesty.

Offences may be committed in states of intoxication, in order to acquire funds to sustain a habit, or in association with a psychiatric disorder related to substance misuse; these categories are not mutually exclusive. Alcohol dependence may also cause organic diseases of the brain such as delirium tremens (see page 395 above) and alcoholic dementia. Drugs can induce dangerous psychotic states, particularly of a paranoid type, which may lead to violence. Infection with human immunodeficiency virus (HIV) and AIDS are unlikely, in themselves, to contribute to offending behaviour but they are now significantly present in populations of imprisoned drug misusers.

5.   *Neurotic disorders*

This is a huge category of disorders in ICD-10 and DSM-IV, and includes anxiety disorder, panic disorder, reactions to stress and various conditions in which the patient makes persistent complaints of innumerable physical symptoms for which no cause can ever be found (formerly referred to as hypochondriasis). Although many offenders have neurotic symptoms, it is uncommon to find a diagnosable neurotic disorder as a major component of offending.

Some would argue that depressive symptoms, which commonly co-exist with neurotic complaints, play a large part in crime (eg in acquisitive crimes) but the argument is contentious. Some shoplifters, who do not seem to be clinically depressed, are recidivist offenders who neither use nor sell their acquisitions but hoard them. They can amass huge quantities of stolen goods and seem to derive comfort from looking at and handling them from time to time. People (usually men)

---

10 Office for National Statistics *Psychiatric Morbidity Among Prisoners in England and Wales* (1998).

who present to agencies claiming a complete loss of memory for their identity and past have often recently committed offences (or personal indiscretions). This type of memory loss, known as a dissociative condition, is a form of neurotic disorder.

6. Behavioural syndromes

These comprise a miscellaneous collection of syndromes in which there is associated altered body functioning. Included here are eating disorders such as anorexia and bulimia nervosa. The latter is characterised by repeated bouts of over-eating and a preoccupation with control of body weight. Some patients with these disorders, unable to afford the vast quantities of food they eat, resort to stealing it.

7. Personality disorders

This is a group of disorders in which there is severe disturbance in character and behavioural tendencies, in several areas of personality, that result in significant personal and social disruption. The behavioural abnormalities generally appear in late childhood or adolescence and persist into adult life. The diagnosis is often made incorrectly and is sometimes missed. Both errors can have serious consequences in medical and psychiatric practice. Although personality disorders are classified into sub-types, there is much overlap between categories. People with personality disorders may (and frequently do) develop other psychiatric and medical conditions.

Among offenders, it is common to find abnormal personality traits (eg irresponsibility, egocentricity or impulsivity) that may not fully amount to a disorder. Some offenders of this type seem to maintain interpersonal relationships which may be surprisingly stable. However, the constellation of features which make for an antisocial personality is well recognised in clinical practice. The descriptive terms that have been applied have changed over time, some being enshrined in legislation. Thus the 'moral imbecile' of the early twentieth century became the 'psychopathically disordered' of today—but probably not for much longer. 'Psychopathic disorder' is found in statute (see page 412 below) but the clinical terms in current use are 'dissocial personality disorder' in ICD-10 and antisocial personality disorder in DSM-IV.

People with dissocial personality disorder come to attention because of the gross disparity between their behaviour and social norms. There is callous unconcern for others, major disregard for social obligations, an inability to maintain enduring relationships and a low threshold for aggression. Such aggression may be callous and sadistic. The disorder is serious for the person, his family, potential victims and for society. The diagnosis requires a longitudinal appraisal of the person including, for example, early development and childhood: it should never be made solely on the basis of a single episode of violence, however extreme in nature. The pathological process, possibly in the brain, causing this disorder is unknown but heredity and early childhood experiences both have a part in aetiology.

A significant proportion of the prison population demonstrates personality disorder – up to 64% of sentenced men.[11] Their offences include the complete calendar of crime. Substance misuse is a common contributory factor, since

11 Fn 10 above.

personality disordered people frequently have alcohol and drug habits. Most offending is impulsive, with loss of control in situations they find 'provocative'. Others are premeditated and sometimes carefully planned. Sadistic offenders, serial rapists and serial killers are rare, though their crimes receive disproportionate media coverage. Some of these offenders have complex personalities in which they are able to maintain an outward semblance of normality (often holding down a job and engaging in relationships) while having a secret inner life.

Dissocial personality disorder is seen less often in females, although other types of personality disorder are common. Affected women may drift into petty recidivism, substance abuse, prostitution and unstable relationships with violent men. Some women, often with backgrounds of serious sexual abuse, show behaviour characterised by repeated acts of self-harm, bouts of despair, and impulsive acts which may include serious violence or fire-raising. The term 'borderline personality disorder' is sometimes applied.

8. Mental retardation

This is the term found in ICD-10, although favoured practice is to use the term 'learning disability'; the latter should not be confused with 'learning difficulty', which does not imply any disorder. Learning disability is a condition of arrested or incomplete development of the mind. There is reduced intellectual functioning, together with a diminished ability to adapt to the daily demands of normal life. It should never be established solely on the basis of an intelligence test or intelligence quotient (IQ), but as a rough guide it is divided into mild (IQ 50-69), moderate (IQ 35-49) and severe (IQ 20-34) forms. There are likely to be associated major physical abnormalities or deformity in the severe forms. People with severe learning disability require to be cared for by others.

The great majority of people with mild and moderate learning disability lead stable lives with their families or other carers. Only a minority come into conflict with the law and, when they do, it is usually in association with those factors that contribute to offending in the population at large, ie unstable family backgrounds, inadequate child-rearing and socio-economic disadvantage.

Property offences are the most common types of crime committed by the learning disabled but sex offences and arson are over-represented in captive populations of such people (in prisons and hospitals). These crimes vary widely in their gravity. Minor sex offences may be a clumsy attempt at sexual behaviour by an inexperienced adolescent or something much more serious. Common features in such offenders include distinctive physical disability, other criminal convictions and a history of residential care. Crimes of arson may be accounted for by a persistence of the normal childhood interest in setting fires. The learning disabled who function in the borderline between disability and normality pose problems. They are expected to compete in society on normal terms but are significantly disadvantaged. They are at risk of committing crimes if they have other major disadvantages (eg incompetent parenting).

Summary

The relationship between crime and psychiatric disorder is complex and difficult to establish by research. Much depends on the nature of the sample studied and how entities such as 'crime' and 'mental disorder' are defined. Research findings tend to concentrate on samples that may be misleading, for example captive populations rather than community samples, and detected, arrested and convicted criminals rather than the majority of criminals who remain undetected, unprosecuted and unconvicted. In addition, researchers may take a broad or narrow definition of mental disorder and diagnostic criteria based on standardised assessments introduced only recently.

The criminal justice system and mentally disordered offenders

Special provisions exist within the criminal justice system for dealing with mentally disordered offenders. There is discretion in decision-making at all stages—arrest, prosecution, trial, conviction and sentencing. Practices may also show wide geographical variation reflecting, among other factors, the availability, or otherwise, of an effective clinical service for dealing with mentally disordered offenders. It is government policy for such persons to be removed, where possible, from the criminal justice system and to have their needs met by health and social care agencies.[12] This statement of principle is often unrealised due to a lack of service provision. There is good evidence that the resources and infrastructure necessary to provide accommodation and support in the community for those with severe mental illness is woefully inadequate. Mentally disordered people, particularly those suffering from illnesses such as schizophrenia, are likely to 'surface' through the criminal justice system if their needs are not adequately met in the community. The situation has become more acute with the transfer of resources from hospital-based to community-based services.

Police and arrest

The police have authority under the Mental Health Act 1983, s 136 to remove from a public place a person they believe to be suffering from mental disorder to a place of safety, usually a hospital. Detention is permissible for up to 72 hours pending further psychiatric and social work assessment. The extent to which this power is exercised will depend largely on local arrangements for dealing with mentally disturbed people coming to the attention of the police. In practice, extensive use of the section appears to be confined to the Greater London area, and there is some evidence of disproportionate rates of use in respect of ethnic minorities, particularly black men.[13]

A mentally disordered suspect in police custody is vulnerable. First, he is at risk of injury if the police use excessive or inappropriate physical force to control his disturbed behaviour. Secondly, his impaired capacity to understand his situation may cause him to incriminate himself. Suspects who have a learning disability may admit to offences they have not committed, particularly if they are unfamiliar with police procedure. Anxiety, fear, confusion, eagerness to please and a sense of excitement at being 'centre-stage' may all play a part. Questioning of suspects must conform with the Code of Practice as laid down in s 66 of the Police and

12 Department of Health and Home Office *Review of Health and Social Services for Mentally Disordered Offenders and Others Requiring Similar Services* (Reed Report) (Cm 2088, 1992).
13 J Dunn and T A Fahy 'Police admissions to a psychiatric hospital: demographic and clinical differences between ethnic groups' (1990) 156 Brit J Psychiat 373.

Criminal Evidence Act 1984 (PACE). This includes a requirement for the presence of an appropriate adult.

Some recent miscarriages of justice have been based on unreliable confessions made by mentally disordered suspects, eg Engin Raghip in the 'Tottenham three' case.[14] The extent to which a person is suggestible can be measured by expert psychological assessment and such testimony may be persuasive in court. The Court of Appeal has recently defined the limits on the use of expert testimony with regard to unreliable confessions; there must be evidence of a wider abnormality than simply one that might cause a confession to be regarded as unreliable, and juries are not obliged to accept this type of expert testimony.[15]

Prosecution

The decision to prosecute rests with the Crown Prosecution Service (CPS) guided by the Code for Crown Prosecutors[16] and by government policy to the effect that mentally disordered offenders should not be prosecuted unless there is a clear public interest in doing so.[17] The CPS will consider whether difficulties during any period of police custody might lessen the likelihood of conviction and also whether the ordeal of court proceedings may have an aggravating effect on the mental condition of the arrested person. These must be balanced against other aspects of public interest.

Decision-making can be assisted where the court has access to early psychiatric assessment of the arrested person. The development of court liaison or court diversion schemes has been encouraged.[18] Assessment by a psychiatrist at this stage might effect removal of mentally disordered, and often petty, offenders from the criminal justice system, provided there exist appropriate facilities to which the offender can be diverted. Diversion schemes vary in their degree of sophistication. Some are well resourced with regular attendance at the court of a psychiatrist and an approved social worker, so that admission to hospital under the civil provisions of the Mental Health Act can be implemented. Others may depend on preliminary screening of cases by a community psychiatric nurse who is then able to seek advice from a psychiatrist. If properly resourced and supported, court diversion schemes should bring about the removal of mentally disordered people from the criminal justice system at an early stage. Research suggests that the most effective diversion schemes are: police station liaison; liaison linked with community mental health teams and covering both courts and police stations; and inner city schemes with access to hospital beds.[19]

Pre-trial matters

The court may seek a psychiatric report on a defendant, who may be remanded in custody, placed on bail or sent to a hospital for this purpose. There are problems associated with all three mechanisms. A remand in custody (ie to prison) is

14 J Rozenburg 'Miscarriages of Justice' in E Stockdale and S Casale (eds) *Criminal Justice under Stress* (1992) pp 91-117.
15 *R v O'Brien, R v Hall, R v Sherwood* [2000] Crim LR 676.
16 Prosecution of Offences Act 1985, s 10.
17 *Provision for Mentally Disordered Offenders* Home Office Circular 66/90 (1990).
18 See fn 12 above.
19 D James 'Court diversion at 10 years: can it work, does it work and has it a future?' (1999) 10 J Forens Psychiat 507.

administratively easy for the court to order. It requires neither medical authorisation nor a requirement to ensure that a place in prison is available. However, remands in custody solely for the purpose of obtaining a medical report are to be deprecated. Remands on bail for medical reports enable the defendant to be examined by a psychiatrist at an out-patient clinic. However, there are problems in the availability of bail accommodation for the homeless, and some bailed defendants fail to keep their appointment with the doctor. In any event, bail is unlikely to be granted for a defendant facing grave charges.

Remand to hospital for a report is possible both at the pre-trial and post-conviction stages (Mental Health Act 1983, s 35); the person can also be remanded to hospital for treatment (s 36). The former requires a medical recommendation that the defendant may suffer from a mental disorder and that a bed is available in hospital. However, in the case of untried defendants, the court must be satisfied that the person committed the offence or, alternatively, that he consents to admission to hospital. It is, therefore, not suitable for the unwilling mentally disordered defendant. Section 35 gives no authority to treat the patient in hospital. That power is available under s 36 but can be invoked only by a Crown Court; it requires two medical recommendations and it applies only to people with mental illness or severe mental impairment (see page 412 below).

Prison is not the appropriate place for a prisoner who is suffering from any significant degree of psychotic mental illness. The conditions in most prison hospitals bear little resemblance to modern psychiatric facilities; there are unlikely to be sufficient trained staff to manage such prisoners and many are detained in insanitary 'strip cells', ie cells from which all furniture has been removed leaving an (often dirty) mattress on the floor. Transfer to hospital of untried mentally disordered prisoners is available under the Mental Health Act, s 48 and is encouraged by government policy. These patients can be treated in hospital so that they are usually improved by the time they go to trial.

Fitness to plead

A fair trial requires that the defendant should be able to understand his situation and instruct his lawyer. This general capacity is colloquially known as 'fitness to plead', a phrase which appears as a marginal note to the Criminal Procedure (Insanity) Act 1964, s 4(1); the text refers to a defendant being 'under any disability such that apart from this Act it would constitute a bar to his being tried'. Prior to 1991 (see below), findings of 'under disability' were rare, approximately 20 being recorded per year in England and Wales. The Criminal Procedure (Insanity) Act 1964 does not specify the criteria for fitness to plead. These are derived from a nineteenth-century case involving a deaf mute.[20] They depend on the defendant's capacity to:

• understand the charge;
• distinguish between a plea of guilty and not guilty;
• instruct a lawyer;
• challenge a juror to whom he might object;
• understand the evidence.

20 *R v Pritchard* (1836) 7 C & P 303. The history of fitness to plead is bound up with the way courts dealt with defendants who failed to plead due to mutism; an authoritative account is given in N Walker *Crime and Insanity in England, Vol 1: The Historical Perspective* (1968).

A finding of 'under disability' can only be returned by a jury and is therefore a matter for determination in a Crown Court. Psychiatrists should always indicate in their court reports that they have considered the matter of fitness to plead— which depends on the mental condition of the defendant at the time of his trial; his mental condition at the time of the alleged offence is of no relevance. In practice, the psychiatrist takes a broad view: does the defendant know what is going on and can he instruct his lawyer? Only the most serious of psychiatric disorders, such as a psychotic state, organic brain disease or severe learning disability, are likely to affect fitness to plead. Early transfer to hospital (eg under ss 35, 36 or 48 of the 1983 Act) has probably helped to reduce the frequency of such findings.

Before 1991, defendants who were unfit to plead had no trial and there was a fixed court disposal—automatic detention in hospital with restrictions on discharge (see page 407 below). This represented a denial of natural justice, since it was, in effect, detention without trial; sometimes detention could last for many years.[1] The Criminal Procedure (Insanity and Unfitness to Plead) Act 1991 introduced major changes. First, defendants who are found to be under disability now have a trial of the facts. If the facts are not found the defendant walks free; if the facts are found there is a range of flexible disposals including community-based care (either under guardianship or a supervision and treatment order), as well as detention in hospital. The defendant may also be discharged absolutely. This flexibility applies to all charges except murder, where there remains mandatory committal to hospital under a hospital order with restrictions on discharge. The House of Lords has recently made two important decisions. First, the defence of diminished responsibility is not available in a trial of the facts on a charge of murder. Secondly, the defence may not be based on the absence of mens rea, other than by way of mistake, accident or self-defence.[2] There has been a substantial increase in the number of under disability findings since introductions of the 1991 Act. This legislation, of course, opened a potential route to freedom that is, not surprisingly, being vigorously explored by defence lawyers.

In Scotland, unfitness to plead results in the finding of insanity in bar of trial.[3] The criteria are those laid down in *HM Advocate v Brown*.[4] The finding can be made under both summary and solemn procedure. Legislation for an examination of the facts and for flexible disposals is contained in the Criminal Procedure (Scotland) Act 1995, ss 55–57.

Responsibility

The verdict of 'not guilty by reason of insanity' or the 'special verdict'[5] is even more rare than is a finding of under disability. It is returned in barely a handful of cases each year but its jurisprudential implications are of profound importance. It has a dramatic history which reached a high point of fevered debate in 1843 when the then Prime Minister's private secretary, William Drummond, was murdered by Daniel M'Naghten in what was an attempt on the life of the Prime Minister. Much

---

1   For full discussion, see Home Office and Department of Health and Social Security *Report of the Committee on Mentally Abnormal Offenders (Butler Report)* (1975, Cmnd 6244).
2   *R v Antoine (a juvenile)* [2000] 2 WLR 703, HL.
3   Criminal Procedure (Scotland) Act 1995, s 54.
4   1907 SC 67.
5   Criminal Procedure (Insanity) Act 1964, s 4.

the same passions were aroused in 1982, when President Ronald Reagan's would-be assassin, John Hinckley, escaped conviction on the grounds of insanity. Indeed, cynics might say the insanity defence only becomes an issue when public figures are assassinated—or when lawyers and psychiatrists attend medico-legal conferences.

The special verdict depends on the demonstration of legal insanity at the time of the act and, therefore, requires a retrospective assessment to be made. It results in acquittal, though the fixed disposal was similar to that for those found unfit to plead until it was changed for both categories of offender by the Criminal Procedure (Insanity and Unfitness to Plead) Act 1991.

The legal criteria remain those laid down in the M'Naghten Rules,[6] which were drawn up by the Law Lords after the furore occasioned by the acquittal of M'Naghten. The relevant part states:

> 'to establish a defence on the grounds of insanity, it must be clearly proved that, at the time of the committing of the act, the party accused was labouring under such a defect of reason, from disease of the mind, as not to know the nature and quality of the act he was doing, or if he did know it, that he did not know that what he was doing was wrong.'

Thus, there must be a disease of the mind, causing a defect of reason such that the offender does not know what he is doing or that it is wrong. The rules have been criticised since their inception and they still present problems to psychiatrists today. The 'mind' is not a medical concept and the phrase 'disease of the mind' has been given wide interpretation:

> '. . . any mental disorder which has manifested itself in violence and is prone to recur is a disease of the mind. At any rate it is the sort of disease for which a person should be detained in hospital . . .'[7]

Aside from the difficulty of applying the legal concept of a disease of the mind, psychiatrists have problems in opining on what a person does, or does not, know. It is relatively easy to give an opinion on what the defendant was thinking when he committed the act but very difficult to say what he knew at the time. Special verdicts have usually depended on the presence of psychotic illnesses due to schizophrenia, depressive disorder, epilepsy or in association with substance abuse—although not on simple intoxication by alcohol.

In assessing a defendant's probable mental condition at the time of the crime, the psychiatrist is making a retrospective judgment. This depends on 'reconstructing' the mental state from all the available information and not simply using the account of the defendant. Thus, it is usually essential to have access to tape recordings of police interviews with the accused, the statements of witnesses and, often, a face-to-face interview with relevant family members or work colleagues.

Two factors have had a profound effect on the use of the special verdict—first, the introduction of the concept of diminished responsibility (see below) in 1957 and, second, the abolition of the death penalty in 1965. When a plea of insanity represented one of the few ways a killer might hope to escape with his life (as it

6   *R v MacNaughten* (1843) 4 State Tr (NS) 847.
7   *Bratty v A-G for Northern Ireland* [1963] AC 386 at 412, HL, per Lord Denning.

still does in some states of America), it was, not surprisingly, a plea to be entered in desperation. The situation has changed and, today, alternative routes to mitigation exist.[8]

Diminished responsibility and infanticide

Nearly all the difficulties associated with the special verdict can be avoided by use of the plea of diminished responsibility. Introduced into England and Wales by the Homicide Act 1957, diminished responsibility is a mitigating plea which, when successful, reduces a charge of murder to one of manslaughter. Whereas murder carries a fixed penalty (life imprisonment), manslaughter gives the sentencing judge complete flexibility in disposal. Diminished responsibility applies only to a charge of murder. There are approximately 70 successful pleas per year; it is the most common way of dealing with mentally disordered defendants who commit homicide. However, a psychiatric disposal is not invariable; nearly half the people found to be of diminished responsibility are imprisoned, some receiving a life sentence.

The definition of diminished responsibility is that the accused:

> 'was suffering from such an abnormality of mind (whether arising from a condition of arrested or retarded development of mind or any inherent causes or induced by disease or injury) as substantially impaired his mental responsibility for his acts and omissions in doing or being a party to the killing.'[9]

Diminished responsibility is not a mental disorder. It is a legal invention, the purpose of which is to circumvent the mandatory life sentence in cases seen as deserving; there would be little need for diminished responsibility if the latter were abolished. Proof is required on a balance of probabilities that there is an abnormality of mind, that it arises from one of the specified causes and that it substantially reduces mental responsibility. Only the first two are psychiatric matters.

In practice, there must be a specific psychiatric condition, not simply anger or jealousy or impulsiveness. Nearly all the commonly recognised psychiatric conditions have been accepted—eg depression, schizophrenia, learning disability and also psychopathic disorder and the premenstrual syndrome. In *R v Byrne*[10] the phrase 'abnormality of mind' was given the widest of interpretations: 'a mind so different from that of ordinary human beings that the reasonable man would term it abnormal.' It is, however, by no means true that a particular diagnosis, once accepted, will always be regarded as satisfying the conditions. Most diminished responsibility pleas are uncontested; failure is the usual outcome in the small number that are contested in a jury trial. Much seems to depend on the global features of the case rather than the niceties of psychiatric diagnosis— ie whether or not there is compassion for the defendant. In the trial of Peter Sutcliffe (the 'Yorkshire Ripper'), unanimous psychiatric opinions from Crown

---

8 In Scotland, acquittal on the grounds of insanity is governed by the charge to the jury in *HM Advocate v Kidd* 1960 JC 61. Flexible disposals are now available (Criminal Procedure (Scotland) Act 1995).
9 Homicide Act 1957, s 2.
10 (1960) 44 Cr App Rep 246.

and defence to the effect that Sutcliffe was suffering from schizophrenia were subjected to two weeks of intense cross-examination by the Crown and were rejected by the jury.[11]

The concept of infanticide was a forerunner of the doctrine of diminished responsibility.[12] It is, again, not a clinical entity but a device for dealing compassionately with mothers who kill an infant child of their own under the age of one year. The Infanticide Act 1938, s 1 provides that, if a woman causes the death of her child when under the age of 12 months, and the court is satisfied that the balance of her mind was disturbed by reason of her not fully having recovered from the effect of giving birth to the child or by reason of the effect of lactation consequent upon the birth, she is guilty of infanticide. The range of court disposals is exactly as for manslaughter. The wording of the 1938 Act is now outdated but is sufficiently vague to bring about the desired objective. Mothers who killed their babies prior to infanticide legislation were sentenced to death and were then reprieved.[13]

Mothers committing neonaticide—here defined as killing the baby within 24 hours of birth—are almost invariably convicted of infanticide even though there may be no significant psychiatric disorder. Most other killings in the first year are dealt with similarly, the exception being killings which bear the hallmarks of baby-battering. Most mothers convicted of infanticide are placed on probation and a few are sent to hospital.[14]

Automatism

In English law, mens rea is a necessary ingredient for finding a person guilty of a crime: *actus non facit reum nisi mens sit rea*—the deed does not make a man guilty unless his mind is guilty. The act is automatic where the mind is absent when the act is carried out and the defence of automatism may apply. The legal definition is given in *Bratty*:[15]

'the state of a person who, though capable of action is not conscious of what he is doing . . . it means unconscious involuntary action and it is a defence because the mind does not go with what is being done.'

The defence is used exceedingly rarely. Major problems for psychiatrists arise for two reasons. First, there is confusion between legal automatism and a clinical condition of the same name; the latter is a much broader concept. Secondly, legal automatism has been traditionally divided into insane automatism and sane automatism (the latter being automatism simpliciter). This division has no clinical basis. In practice the distinction depends on the court's view of whether it considers the defendant is likely to repeat his act and, therefore, whether the public needs

---

11 B Jones *Voices from an Evil God* (1992).
12 Diminished responsibility was established by case law in Scotland in *HM Advocate v Dingwall* (1867) 5 Irv 466. It is now governed by *HM Advocate v Savage* 1923 JC 49. It results in a conviction for culpable homicide in place of murder.
13 The crime of infanticide has never existed in Scotland; infant killings by mothers have, nearly always, been indicted as culpable homicide.
14 For a general discussion of killing within the family, see J K Mason *Medico-legal Aspects of Reproduction and Parenthood* (2nd edn, 1998), ch 14.
15 *Bratty v A-G for Northern Ireland* [1963] AC 386.

protecting. Such cases are called insane automatism, are attributed to a disease of the mind, and led formerly to a special verdict and committal to hospital; now, there are flexible disposals under the Criminal Procedure (Insanity and Unfitness to Plead) Act 1991.

Insane automatisms have included behaviour attributable to brain diseases, tumours, epilepsy and, most recently, sleep-walking.[16] By contrast, sane automatisms are regarded as once-only events, are attributed to an 'external cause' and result in acquittal and freedom for the accused. Cases have included concussion, confusional states, reflex actions following a bee sting and hypoglycaemia.[17]

Post-conviction disposals

The great majority of psychiatric disposals take place at the post-conviction stage—ie after guilt has been established. The court has available a menu of disposals by which psychiatric treatment can be obtained.[18] At this stage the psychiatrist is applying himself to clinical questions. First, does the convicted person have a mental disorder? second, does it require treatment? and third, under what legal conditions?

Hospital order

Under the Mental Health Act 1983, s 37, the court may order a mentally disordered offender to hospital for treatment. It must be satisfied that there is a mental disorder of a nature and degree which make it appropriate for him to be detained in hospital for treatment. The treatability criteria apply (see page 413 below) if the disorder is psychopathic disorder or mental impairment. Two medical recommendations are necessary and a hospital bed must be available within 28 days.

A hospital order lasts for up to six months and is then renewable. Discharge is at the discretion of the responsible medical officer or through a mental health review tribunal (see page 418 below). The criminal court has no further interest in the case. Approximately 1,000 hospital orders are made each year and more than 90% are for people in the legal category of mental illness. A small number are made for people with psychopathic disorder or mental impairment (see page 412 below).

Interim hospital order

This is similar to a hospital order, with the important distinction that the interim hospital order—made under s 38 of the 1983 Act—provides for a trial period of hospital admission to test the appropriateness of treatment in hospital. It lasts for 12 weeks but is renewable for up to 12 months. The person must then return to the court for sentencing—which could be by way of a hospital order or by a penal disposal. The interim hospital order is useful for testing the treatability of offenders with psychopathic disorder.

---

16 *R v Burgess* [1991] 2 QB 92, CA.
17 The defence of sane automatism has become available in Scotland only recently: *Ross v HM Advocate* 1991 SLT 564.
18 There are equivalent post-conviction disposals available in Scotland under summary and solemn procedures. See the Criminal Procedure (Scotland) Act 1995, ss 57–59.

Restriction order

The patient under a hospital order is essentially in the hands of the consultant in charge of the case. Where the court does not wish to leave discharge decisions to the consultant but wishes to impose some executive control, it may do so by making an order restricting discharge; this is known as a restriction order and is made under s 41 of the 1983 Act. Approximately 250 such orders are made each year.

A restriction order can only be made in the Crown Court and is at the discretion of the judge. He must be satisfied that it is necessary in order to protect the public from serious harm. He must consider the nature of the offence, the antecedents of the offender and the risk of further offences being committed. He is obliged to hear oral psychiatric evidence before making the order. Restriction orders are made without limit of time—ie they are of indefinite duration.

A hospital order with restrictions on discharge is in effect 'the psychiatric life sentence'. Indeed, discharge is at the discretion of the Home Secretary, although it can also be ordered by a mental health review tribunal. Most orders are made in respect of men who have committed grave offences. In making his decisions about discharge, the Home Secretary may seek the advice of the Advisory Board on Restricted Patients. This was established in 1972 after the case of Graham Young, a poisoner released from Broadmoor Hospital who, within a short time, killed again by poisoning his victims.[19]

Hospital direction

The Crime (Sentences) Act 1997 and the Crime and Punishment (Scotland) Act 1997 both introduced a range of measures designed to strengthen the law in respect of serious offenders. These included the hospital direction (Crime (Sentences) Act 1997, s 46 (inserting s 45A into the 1983 Act) and Crime and Punishment (Scotland) Act 1997, s 6). The hospital direction is available for all indictable crimes, with the exception of murder for which the sentence is fixed by law. It is a hybrid court disposal combining a prison sentence of any length (including a life sentence) with an order for initial treatment in hospital. The patient is transferred to prison to complete his sentence when treatment is concluded. In England and Wales, the hospital direction may be made only in cases of psychopathic disorder although the Crime (Sentences) Act 1997, s 10 gives the Home Secretary power to extend the legislation to cover other categories of mental disorder. In Scotland, a hospital direction may be made for any type of mental disorder.

The introduction of the hospital direction broke the well-established principle of clearly separating punishment from treatment. Psychiatrists were strongly opposed to this blurring of disposal and saw few benefits from the hospital direction.[20] Their evidence is required for making the order and, thus, they are drawn in to advise on punishment, a role that is both inappropriate and unethical. Only a tiny number of hospital directions have been imposed. It may have some value in cases where there appears to be little relationship between the commission

---

19 *Report on the Review of Procedures for the Discharge and Supervision of Psychiatric Patients subject to Special Restrictions* (Aavold report) (1973, Cmnd 5191).
20 D Chiswick 'Sentencing Mentally Disordered Offenders' (1996) 313 BMJ 1497.

of a dangerous crime by a defendant and his requirement for treatment of a mental disorder, particularly where the latter is likely to improve quickly.

Guardianship order

The court may make a guardianship order under s 37(1) of the 1983 Act. This places the offender under the care of local authority social services or of an approved person. It is intended to provide care and supervision in the community. Guardianship may be useful for some offenders with mental impairment.

Probation with a condition of treatment

If an offender is suffering from a mental condition which does not require compulsory treatment in hospital and the court wishes to make a probation order, then it may include a condition of psychiatric treatment under the Powers of Criminal Courts Act 1973, s 3, as amended by the Criminal Justice Act 1991, s 9(3) and Sch 1A. The order requires the agreement of the individual. Treatment may be as an outpatient, day patient or inpatient. It cannot be enforced, but an offender in breach of the conditions of probation can be returned to court for further sentencing. Probation orders of this type are useful for people with less severe psychiatric conditions that would benefit from treatment.

Mentally disordered offenders in prisons

A person with a mental disorder who is sentenced to imprisonment may or may not receive treatment in prison. Most large prisons have programmes for assisting prisoners with alcohol and drug problems. Some (such as Grendon Underwood, Buckinghamshire) provide special facilities for sex offenders. But services for prisoners with any significant degree of mental illness such as schizophrenia are limited. A rise in the rate of suicides in prison has engendered a series of reviews; the causal factors are complex and are not simply related to the presence of a possible mental illness in the prisoner.[1] Mentally disordered offenders serving sentences may be transferred to a psychiatric hospital by order of the Home Secretary under s 47 of the 1983 Act. An order restricting discharge is usually included (s 49). The prisoner may return to prison after treatment or, if suffering from continuing mental illness, may remain within the hospital system.

Commissioning psychiatric reports in criminal cases

Preparing psychiatric court reports is likely to form part of the day-to-day work of most general psychiatrists. Reports may be commissioned by the Crown Prosecution Service, by defence solicitors or through a medical officer in a prison. Not all psychiatrists are equally familiar with the procedures and issues within the criminal justice system—indeed, some positively dislike 'getting involved'. Lawyers tend to request reports from psychiatrists who have previously been of help. Forensic psychiatrists have special knowledge of the

---

1   HM Inspectorate of Prisons for England and Wales *Suicide is Everyone's Concern* (1999).

criminal justice system and of services for mentally disordered offenders. Some have particular expertise on certain subjects—eg unreliable confessions or epilepsy. Telephone discussion with a psychiatrist before asking for a report is often helpful.

Some simple ground rules make for a better relationship between psychiatrist and lawyer:

- It is helpful to have as much notice as possible; it is rarely possible to drop everything to see a defendant in custody.
- Psychiatrists like to be told the reason for seeking the report. Matters that are obvious to the lawyer may not be so to the psychiatrist. It is helpful if the psychiatrist is informed even if the only reason for the request is 'a hunch that things don't seem right' with the mental condition of the accused.
- A good report will deal with all relevant issues but the psychiatrist may need to be told if there are particular issues—eg fitness to plead or diminished responsibility.
- The psychiatrist should be provided with as much background information as is available.
- Court appearances are time-consuming and disruptive. The clearer the report, the less likely it is that oral evidence will be required. Where it is unavoidable (eg when diminished responsibility is contested), as much notice as possible is helpful.
- Finally, psychiatrists like feedback and should therefore be informed if the result of the report is particularly good or bad.

Facilities for mentally disordered offenders

Mentally disordered offenders may receive treatment in the community, as ordinary inpatients in psychiatric units, in medium secure units or in high security hospitals; all these facilities lie within the National Health Service. There is also growing provision for secure care within the independent sector.

Medium secure units provide a regional service for catchment populations of between two and five million people and are usually linked to aftercare services in the community. Security is such that escape is difficult but not impossible. There is emphasis on good quality staffing and on a range of therapeutic activities. High (or maximum) security is currently provided by the three special hospitals, namely Broadmoor in Berkshire, Rampton in Nottinghamshire and Ashworth on Merseyside. There are proposals to reduce the size but increase the number of high security hospitals.[2] They are (or should be) escape-proof, with security equivalent to that of a maximum security prison. Services in the special hospitals have improved enormously following a series of inquiries and reviews. In Scotland, a specialist forensic psychiatry unit providing some security is shortly to open in Edinburgh. High security care is provided at the State Hospital, Carstairs.

---

2   Department of Health *Report of the Working Group on High Security and Related Psychiatric Provisions* (chairman Dr J Reed) (1994).

Compulsory admission and treatment

Principles of legislation

A cardinal principle of medical practice is that treatment can only proceed with the consent of the patient. However, for over 200 years there have been special laws relating to those who suffer from mental disorders whereby they may be admitted to hospital, detained, and treated without their consent. These laws have combined protective functions for both the patient and society. They flow from the premise that psychiatric disorders can affect the judgment of the mentally disordered person in such a way that he may be incapable of making a rational decision about the need for treatment. In common with other social welfare legislation, laws that permit the compulsory detention of people in hospital can, at times, be misused and even abused. There has been acknowledged abuse of psychiatric laws which have been used to detain political dissidents in the former Soviet Union and in other police states on the spurious ground of mental illness.[3] Nearer home, there is much concern that the potential of mental health law to provide indefinite incarceration is about to be exploited by the introduction of new laws for those who are said to have 'dangerous severe personality disorder', whether or not they have offended and whether or not their condition is treatable.[4]

Mental health law must be framed such as to strike the correct balance between three important rights. These are:

1. the right of the individual to liberty and other freedoms (now enshrined in the European Convention on Human Rights and the Human Rights Act 1998);
2. the right of the individual to receive treatment for mental disorder, if necessary against his will, where his safety or that of others is at risk;
3. the right of society to be protected from the acts of mentally ill people.

Striking the appropriate balance between these conflicting rights is a task for government; not surprisingly, political and public policy considerations are more likely to drive the agenda than are ethical concerns and clinical realities. Recurrent problems in meeting the needs of mentally disordered people usually result from deficiencies and failings in services. It seems unlikely that changes in mental health legislation will do much to remedy these serious problems of service quality and provision. The government intends to reform mental health law. Having established an expert committee, chaired by an academic lawyer, it has produced for consultation a White Paper[5] that differs substantially from the proposals of the expert committee.[6] An outline of current legislation is given below, followed by the government's main proposals.

3   See A A Stone *Law, Psychiatry and Morality* (1984).
4   Dangerous People with Severe Personality Disorder Bill 2000; Mental Health (Public Safety and Appeals) (Scotland) Act 1999—which is said to be something of an interim measure.
5   Department of Health *Reform of the Mental Health Act 1983: Proposals for Consultation* (Cm 4480, 1999).
6   Department of Health *Report of the Expert Committee: Review of the Mental Health Act 1983* (1999).

Mental Health Act 1983

British mental health law has been something of a model for other nations[7] and has undergone regular revision at approximately 25-year intervals. The Mental Health Act 1983 applies to England and Wales. There is separate legislation for Scotland and for Northern Ireland which is similar to, but not identical with, the 1983 Act.[8] Current legislation reflects the importance of patients' rights and of correct legal process in compulsory detention and treatment, the so-called 'shift to legalism' in the 1980s. The 1983 Act introduced:

- a requirement to inform patients of their rights under the Act;
- shorter periods of detention;
- increased opportunities for appeal against detention;
- completely new laws relating to consent to treatment;
- new powers in respect of offender patients;
- a Mental Health Act Commission;
- a Code of Practice.

The Code of Practice, produced by virtue of s 118 of the Act, is an important document with which all users of the Act should be familiar.[9] It includes the cautionary note that 'the Act does not impose a legal duty to comply with the Code, but failure to follow the Code could be referred to in evidence in legal proceedings'.

Civil powers: Part II of the Mental Health Act 1983

There are three crucial criteria which must be met in order to effect compulsory admission to hospital:

1. the presence of a mental disorder which warrants detention in hospital;
2. an element of risk to the health or safety of the patient or of others;
3. no alternative to detention in hospital as a way of safeguarding the risk.

It cannot be over-emphasised that subjective judgment plays a significant role in identifying each of these criteria.

Mental disorder

'Mental disorder' is a legal term defined in s 1(2) as:

> 'mental illness, arrested or incomplete development of mind, psychopathic disorder and any other disorder or disability of mind.'

It is sometimes known, for obvious reasons, as the 'broad definition' of mental disorder. Admission for assessment (s 2) (or, in an emergency, s 4) depends on this

---

7   In 1998–99, there were 27,000 compulsory admissions under the Mental Health Act 1983, a rise of 69% in ten years.
8   Mental Health (Scotland) Act 1984; Mental Health (Northern Ireland) Order 1986.
9   Department of Health *Revised Code of Practice: Mental Health Act 1983* (1999).

broad definition of mental disorder. Admission for treatment (s 3), however, requires the identification of one of four specific categories of mental disorder. These are:

1. mental illness;
2. psychopathic disorder;
3. mental impairment;
4. severe mental impairment.

These four[10] legal terms do not equate with any specific psychiatric disorder. Three of them are further defined in the 1983 Act but the term 'mental illness', which accounts for 98% of compulsory admissions, remains undefined.[11] It presumably has the legal meaning given to the term by Lawton LJ in *W v L*.[12]

In practice, 'mental illness' is usually interpreted by clinicians as a psychotic or severe mental illness—eg schizophrenia, manic depressive disorder, organic brain disease or anorexia nervosa. While it could apply to neurotic illnesses such as an anxiety disorder or a phobic condition, it is unlikely that such a condition would be of a nature or degree warranting detention in hospital. The 1983 Act excludes the compulsory treatment of a person by reason only of promiscuity or other immoral conduct, sexual deviancy or dependence on alcohol or drugs. Detention and treatment under the Act is, however, permissible when these features exist in addition to a mental disorder, such as schizophrenia or psychopathic disorder.

Psychopathic disorder

The term 'psychopathic disorder' causes enormous confusion, since it has a legal definition, an increasingly outdated clinical meaning and a lay use, all of which differ. The legal definition is discussed below. In clinical use, psychopathic disorder is a pejorative term implying therapeutic nihilism and often rejection by psychiatric services. Today we recognise that there are those among the range of people with personality disorders in whom aggression and other antisocial behaviours are a recurrent feature. However, the existence of this form of personality disorder as a discrete clinical entity is not reliably established.[13] Lay people, including the media, often use the term 'psychopath' as a description of the perpetrator (actual or imagined) of any particularly hideous or brutal crime.

The legal definition is:

> 'a persistent disorder or disability of mind (whether or not including significant impairment of intelligence) which results in abnormally aggressive or seriously irresponsible conduct on the part of the person concerned.'[14]

---

10 The term 'psychopathic disorder' does not appear in the Mental Health (Scotland) Act 1984. Instead, s 17(1) includes a mental disorder which 'is a persistent one manifested only by abnormally aggressive or seriously irresponsible conduct'. However, personality disorder is now included as a form of mental disorder in s 1(2) by virtue of Mental Health (Public Safety and Appeals) (Scotland) Act 1999, s 3(1).

11 The only definition in United Kingdom legislation appears in the Mental Health (Northern Ireland) Order 1986, SI 1986/595 (NI 4), art 3(1).

12 A mental illness 'should be construed in the way that ordinary sensible people would construe the words': *W v L* [1974] QB 711 at 719, per Lawton LJ.

13 B Dolan and J Coid *Psychopathic and Antisocial Personality Disorders: Treatment and Research Issues* (1993).

14 Mental Health Act 1983, s 1(2).

This definition has long been criticised on the grounds of its circularity—the disorder is defined in terms of abnormal aggression and simultaneously regarded as the cause of that aggression. It is theoretically possible for any person who has a history of persistent abnormal aggression to be regarded as having a psychopathic disorder in legal terms. In practice, only a small number of patients in the category psychopathic disorder are sent by courts (or transferred from prisons) to hospitals for treatment.[15] Detention in hospital for such offender-patients may be for substantially longer than would be likely under the criminal justice system. Decisions as to the discharge of psychopathic disorder patients pose serious difficulties for psychiatrists. The government has proposed new measures in respect of those it considers to have a 'dangerous severe personality disorder'. The matter is discussed below.

Mental impairment and severe mental impairment

These are the two legal categories of mental handicap or learning disability; they have no clinical equivalent. They are defined as:

> 'a state of incomplete or arrested development of mind which includes significant [or "severe" in the case of severe mental impairment] impairment of intelligence and social functioning and is associated with abnormally aggressive or seriously irresponsible conduct on the part of the person concerned.'[16]

Thus, only those people whose mental handicap is associated with abnormally aggressive or seriously irresponsible conduct can be detained under the Act. This reasonably excludes the great majority of mentally handicapped people, for whom compulsory admission is rarely an appropriate clinical step.

For two categories of mental disorder (psychopathic disorder and mental impairment), admission for treatment under the Act must satisfy the treatability criteria—that is, treatment must be likely to alleviate or prevent a deterioration of the condition.[17]

It may have been Parliament's intention[18] in 1983 that untreatable psychopaths should not be detained indefinitely in hospital, but patients in the category of psychopathic disorder who put forward 'untreatability' as grounds for discharge, met with little success in the courts. Medical treatment has a broad statutory definition ('nursing, . . . and care, habilitation and rehabilitation under medical supervision')[19] and has been interpreted widely in the courts.[20] In *Canons Park* the court confirmed that a mental health tribunal is not bound to have regard to the treatability test in determining whether a psychopathically disordered patient is entitled to discharge.[1] In the same judgment, Roch LJ stated that the alleviation or prevention of deterioration need not be immediate, and that nursing care aimed at encouraging a reluctant patient to accept therapy was, of itself, treatment.

---

15 50 patients, from a total of 1,655, were transferred from courts and prisons to hospital in 1998/99.
16 Mental Health Act 1983, s 1(2).
17 Mental Health Act 1983, s 3(2)(b).
18 Department of Health and Social Security *Reform of Mental Health Legislation* (1981, Cmnd 8405).
19 Mental Health Act 1983, s 145(1).
20 *R v Mersey Mental Health Tribunal, ex p Dillon* (1987) Times, 13 April.
 1 *R v Canons Park Mental Health Review Tribunal, ex p A* [1995] QB 60, CA.

However a ground-breaking decision of the House of Lords in 1999[2] effectively overturned *Canons Park*. In *Reid* the House of Lords declined to follow *Canons Park* and determined that an application for discharge by a restricted patient must be construed by reference to the same criteria as are necessary for hospital detention. Thus, in the case of a patient with psychopathic disorder, failure to fulfil the treatability criteria requires discharge of the psychopathically disordered patient.

Reid's application was not successful because the House of Lords ruled that his condition was in fact treatable. But, subsequently, a restricted patient (convicted of shooting a man with a rifle seven years earlier) relied on the Reid decision and was successful in his application for discharge; a sheriff ruled that his psychopathic disorder was not treatable and ordered his discharge.[3] The case caused public uproar and resulted in the newly constituted Scottish Parliament passing its first piece of legislation, the Mental Health (Public Safety and Appeals) (Scotland) Act 1999. This brief Act prevents the discharge of any restricted patient if the effect of his mental disorder is such that detention is necessary in order 'to protect the public from serious harm', whether or not there is any medical treatment. It is, of course, not surprising that issues of public protection weigh so heavily with governments; indeed, these issues are driving current proposals for mental health law reform generally (see below). Compliance of the 1999 Act with art 5 of the European Convention on Human Rights was quickly tested in the Court of Session by three detained patients at the State Hospital.[4] The court ruled that detention on the grounds of public protection was compatible with art 5, notwithstanding any issues of treatability. The retrospective nature of the legislation was also held to be lawful, taking into account the public interest considerations.

Grounds for admission and treatment

Health/safety of the patient or protection of others This phrase forms one of the conditions for compulsory admission; it is often incorrectly paraphrased as 'dangerous to self or to others'. The Mental Health Act 1983 does not contain the word 'dangerous' in this context, and the Department of Health has emphasised that the phrase 'interests of the health or safety of the patient' may be given a wide interpretation. It clearly covers the risk of suicide or self-harm but it also includes the impaired capacity to exercise self-care—eg to obtain and maintain food, shelter, warmth and organised life. Some psychiatric patients (not solely those with eating disorders) may refuse food or fluids and put their lives at risk. Psychiatric patients may pose a risk to the safety of others—eg where paranoid delusions or hallucinations 'drive' a person to act violently against another or threaten to do so.

No alternative to detention Admission for treatment (s 3) requires that treatment cannot be provided unless the patient is detained. In other words, alternative forms of care, including informal (or voluntary) admission are not possible.

Length of detention

Shorter periods of detention are associated with:

---

2   *Reid v Secretary of State for Scotland* [1999] 1 All ER 481.
3   *Ruddle v Secretary of State for Scotland* (1999) 29 GWD 1395.
4   *A v Scottish Ministers* (2000) Times, 21 June.

- the broad definition of mental disorder;
- ease of application;
- fewer safeguards for patients.

Thus, emergency admission for assessment (s 4) requires only one doctor's recommendation, there is no appeal and detention is for up to 72 hours. This section may also apply to patients already in hospital who require detention. Admission for assessment (s 2) requires two medical recommendations, lasts for 28 days and there is right of appeal to a mental health review tribunal (MHRT). Admission for treatment (s 3) requires two medical recommendations in which the category of mental disorder must be stated. It allows detention for six months and is renewable; there are opportunities for appeal to a MHRT.[5] Compulsory treatment in hospital is only permissible for patients detained for more than 72 hours.

Social workers who are approved to carry out duties under the Act must be involved in all compulsory admission procedures. They are required to undergo training and assessment organised by the Central Council for Education and Training in Social Work.

Guardianship under s 7 of the Act is a method of providing care and supervision in the community. The method of application is similar to that for compulsory admission. It does not allow for compulsory treatment with medication in the community.

Consent to treatment

The introduction of law for consent to treatment, detailed in Part IV of the Act, was a major innovation. It applies only to treatment for mental disorder and, with one important exception, only to detained patients. It strikes a balance between two equally unattractive theoretical positions: on the one hand, the doctor having no authority to treat and, on the other, the patient having no power to refuse treatment. In practice this is achieved by grading psychiatric treatments into what might be called degrees of seriousness or irreversibility and by involving more persons than the treating doctor in decision-making. For descriptive purposes, we may call the treatments 'most', 'moderate' and 'least serious'; these terms do not appear in the Act.

Most serious treatments

These treatments come within s 57 of the Act and, at present, only two are included[6]—brain surgery for mental disorder (sometimes called psychosurgery) and the surgical implantation of anti-male sex hormones to reduce male sexual drive. These are rare treatments. In England and Wales in 1997–99 there were 17 referrals for psychosurgery and in all cases certificates of treatment were issued by the Mental Health Act Commission (MHAC).

Because of the serious and irreversible nature of these treatments, the most stringent criteria apply to their use. The patient must give real consent and there

5   In Scotland, detention for more than 28 days (Mental Health (Scotland) Act 1984, s 18) requires application to, and approval by, a sheriff.
6   Section 57 applies to *all* patients, whether informal or detained; the equivalent legislation (Mental Health (Scotland) Act 1984, s 97) applies only to detained patients.

is independent complex decision-making. First, an independent doctor and two lay members appointed by the MHAC must certify that the patient is capable of giving, and has given, real consent. Secondly, the independent doctor must certify that the treatment is necessary.

The surgical implantation of anti-male sex hormones is an exceedingly rare treatment. An important test case—and the only one in this category of treatment that was referred to the MHAC—involved the use of goserelin, a synthetic hormone analogue. The court ruled that goserelin was not a hormone—it was produced in a laboratory, not in the human body—and that an injection was not surgical implantation. The treatment did not therefore come under s 57.[7]

Moderately serious treatments

At present, only two treatments are in this category (s 58), namely electroconvulsive treatment (ECT) and medication for mental disorder given for more than three months. The requirement for either of these two treatments is the real consent of the patient or a certificate issued by an authorised second opinion doctor that the treatment should be given. Treatments are common under s 58, the practical implication of which is that detained patients can be treated with medication for mental disorder, whether or not they consent, for the first three months of admission.

Least serious treatment

All treatments for mental disorder not included in ss 57 and 58 may be given to detained patients without their consent (s 63). In practice, this includes nursing care, habilitation, rehabilitation and psychological therapies. In fact, few of them would be possible without the patient's co-operation. Tube feeding was held by the Court of Appeal to be lawful under s 63.[8]

Treatment of patients who lack capacity

Consent to treatment in respect of informal patients is governed by exactly the same standards that apply in general medical practice (see page 455). When the patient lacks capacity to consent (referred to as being incompetent or incapable) and the treatment is for mental disorder, it has generally been practice to distinguish 'passive acceptors' from 'active resistors'. The former are generally regarded as informal patients and given treatment under the common law on the basis of 'necessity' and their 'best interests'. Patients in the 'active resistor' group are usually detained under the Mental Health Act and Part IV of the Act, as outlined above, is implemented to give treatment.

This situation was dramatically challenged in 1998 in the case of *R v Bournewood Community and Mental Health Trust, ex p L*.[9] Mr L was an autistic man with a severe learning disability. He was admitted informally to a learning disability unit using common law authority of necessity. His carers challenged this decision. Initially, the Court of Appeal ruled that the comprehensive powers of the Mental Health Act 1983 superseded common law authority; if incompetent patients required admission to a psychiatric hospital, it could only take place under the provisions of

7   *R v Mental Health Act Commission, ex p X* (1988) 9 BMLR 77.
8   *B v Croydon Health Authority* [1995] 1 All ER 683.
9   [1998] 1 All ER 634.

the 1983 Act. The decision would have had major implications for the inpatient care of thousands of incompetent patients with, for example, learning disability or dementia, who hitherto were treated on the basis of common law necessity. Contingency plans were drawn up for the mass implementation of compulsory detention of such patients. However, the House of Lords reversed the Court of Appeal decision citing unnecessary formal detentions, a waste of resources and increased stigmatisation of a vulnerable group of people among their reasons for so doing. However, their Lordships noted that compliant incapacitated patients were left without the protective benefits of the 1983 Act while they remained in informal status.

The Act says nothing about the treatment of physical disorders. What, for example, is the position of the incompetent mentally disordered patient who requires surgical removal of a malignant tumour? Here, the common law principles apply. These were reaffirmed in *Re F (mental patient: sterilisation)*[10] and permit treatment that is in the best interests of the patient and is provided by a doctor who is acting in accordance with a responsible body of medical opinion. It is good practice to consult relatives of the patient, but they have no power to consent on behalf of an adult and the decision to proceed is one for the doctor to make. However, a declaration from the court is needed in the case of certain special treatments.

Reports from the Law Commissions of both England[11] and Scotland[12] proposed entirely novel procedures depending on the gravity of the treatment under consideration. Scotland has gone further and the Adults with Incapacity (Scotland) Act 2000 will be implemented in phases in 2001-02. The 2000 Act affects up to 100,000 adults in Scotland who lack capacity to manage their financial and personal affairs or to make decisions about their health. In relation to the latter, a key role will be played by the medical practitioner primary responsible (MPPR) for treatment. He may issue a time-limited certificate authorising treatment appropriate for promoting the physical or mental health of the adult, except for compulsory admission to a psychiatric hospital against the will of the adult (here mental health legislation will apply). The Act also allows for the appointment of a guardian or welfare attorney who, when so appointed, must be consulted by the MPPR. Treatment may be undertaken if they agree, subject only to a right of appeal to the Court of Session by 'any person having an interest in the personal welfare of the patient'. In the event of disagreement, the doctor must ask the Mental Welfare Commission to appoint an independent practitioner to give an opinion as to whether or not the treatment should be given.[13]

In England and Wales, the Law Commission's proposals[14] have been amended for the purposes of consultation by the Lord Chancellor's Department.[15] The proposals for health-care decision making are wide-ranging and exceed those in the Scottish Act in that they include decisions involving procedures that are not immediately to the advantage of the incapacitated person. No definitive action has, however, been taken yet.[16]

---

10 [1990] 2 AC 1.
11 *Mental Incapacity* Law Commission Paper 231 (1995).
12 *Report on Incapable Adults* Scottish Law Commission Report 151 (1995).
13 The complexities of the Act are discussed in G T Laurie and J K Mason 'Negative Treatment of Vulnerable Patients: Euthanasia by any other Name?' (2000) Juridical Rev 159.
14 Law Com 231 (1995).
15 Lord Chancellor's Department *Who Decides?* (Consultation Paper 1997) (Cm 3803).
16 For criticism of some proposals, see J Keown and L Gormally 'Human Dignity, Autonomy and Mentally Incapacitated Patients: A Critique of *Who Decides?*' [1999] 4 Web JCLI.

Mental health review tribunals

Mental health review tribunals are established on a regional basis in England and Wales; tribunal members are appointed by the Lord Chancellor. A lawyer is appointed chairman in each of the 15 regions; his task is to convene panels of tribunal members to hear applications from patients, relatives, hospital managers and, in certain cases of restricted patients, the Home Secretary. A panel consists of a lawyer as chairman, a medical member and a lay member. The chairman must be a specially approved judge when cases concerning patients detained under restriction orders are being considered.

Tribunals are governed by the Mental Health Review Tribunal Rules 1983.[17] They normally convene at the hospital and patients may be represented by solicitors and, in some cases, by counsel. Proceedings may be informal or formal, according to the rules, and, if formal, may be held in public. There are no mental health review tribunals in Scotland, where broadly equivalent functions are exercised by a sheriff.

The essential consideration for the MHRT is to be satisfied as to whether or not the patient has a mental disorder or whether or not it is appropriate or necessary for him to be detained for treatment. It has absolute authority to direct either discharge or a delayed discharge to enable arrangements to be made. It can recommend, but not direct, leave of absence or transfer to another hospital or to guardianship. For restricted patients it can order discharge or conditional discharge; it has no other powers in these cases.

Mental Health Act Commission

The establishment of the Mental Health Act Commission (MHAC) under the 1983 Act represented a return of the hospital inspectorate which had existed previously from 1774 until being disbanded by legislation in 1959. The task of the MHAC is to visit hospitals and review the powers of detention, to appoint doctors for providing second opinions under Part IV of the Act, to keep under review the long-term treatment of detained patients and to prepare a code of practice for the Secretary of State. It does not have authority to order the discharge of patients. It has a chairman and nearly 100 part-time members, mostly professionals from the fields of medicine, nursing, social work, psychology and law. There are also academic and lay members. It is required to produce biennial reports.[18]

Compulsory treatment in the community

Patients who have enduring illnesses such as schizophrenia may improve with treatment in hospital. On discharge they may cease to take medication, relapse and need readmission—often on a compulsory basis. Ensuring continuing care in the community for such patients is a profound challenge facing, not just health services and local authorities, but also the public and its politicians. Delivering effective community care to patients suffering from severe and

---

17 SI 1983/942.
18 In Scotland, the Mental Welfare Commission has wide powers in relation to all psychiatric patients: see Mental Health (Scotland) Act 1984, Pt II.

enduring mental illness depends more on resources, recruitment and training of staff, and on sound organisation than it does on legislation. None the less some commentators focus on the law as the underlying problem.[19]　While it is true that legislation has been totally focused on hospital rather than community care, the issues are too complex to be addressed solely by way of passing new laws.

At present, detained patients may proceed on leave of absence under s 17 of the 1983 Act and are obliged to continue to receive medication in the community; this is, however, only until the section lapses and, in any event, for not more than 12 months. The practice—now rendered historical—of admitting such patients 'overnight' in order to renew the authority for detention was declared to be unlawful under the 1983 Act.[20]

The Mental Health (Patients in the Community) Act 1995 introduced a supervised discharge order for England and a community care order for Scotland. Both of these may be applied at the point of discharge of a previously detained patient. These measures do not provide for the forcible use of medication in the community. Such treatment, even were it legal, would not be desired by professionals, since it is both practically and professionally unacceptable. The desirable elements of an order for treatment in the community are:

- requirement to reside at an agreed address;
- requirement to give access to visiting professional staff;
- requirement to attend at a place of treatment;
- requirement to accept prescribed medication;
- early re-admission to hospital in the event of failure to comply.

No existing measure (eg leave of absence, supervised discharge order, community care order or guardianship) meets all these requirements. All have defects and all face the insoluble question, namely 'how do you enforce a requirement?' other than by swift re-admission to hospital. The law, however, is of secondary importance in all this discussion. Two factors make continued care of mentally ill patients in the community so problematical: first, these are difficult illnesses to treat even with sufficient resources; secondly, the current resources are inadequate. Psychiatry faces a huge challenge in its attempt to deliver care in the community to patients who do not want to receive it.

Government proposals on mental health legislation

In its proposals for mental health reform[1] the government has relied on the risk presented by mentally disordered patients, either to themselves or to others, as its principle on which to base law reform. This is in stark contrast to the views of the expert committee,[2] which recommended that non-discrimination and autonomy should be the basis of new legislation. The essential government proposals are as follows:

---

19 See fn 8, p 393 above.
20 *R v Hallstrom, ex p W (No 2); R v Gardiner, ex p L* [1986] 2 All ER 306.
　1 See fn 5, p 410 above.
　2 See fn 6, p 410 above.

- *Mental disorder*: to be given a broad definition without categories—'any disability or disorder of mind or brain, whether permanent or temporary, which results in an impairment or disturbance of mental functioning'. Personality disorder and learning disability are not excluded.
- *Criteria for compulsory care*: mental disorder of such seriousness that care and treatment under specialist mental health services is required. Such care cannot be implemented without compulsion and is necessary either for the health/safety of the patient or the protection of others, or to protect the patient from serious exploitation. It should be provided in the least restrictive setting possible.
- *Initial formal assessment*: may be made in the hospital or the community and is to be carried out according to specified standards.
- *Compulsory care and treatment*: may be in hospital or in the community. Compulsory care beyond a defined maximum period will require a decision taken by an independent judicial body.
- *Discharge*: in most cases by the clinical supervisor but with reference to a tribunal where there is a history of non-compliance with treatment or of risk to others.

Most observers will welcome the attempt to end the rigid distinction between inpatient and community-based care. But there is concern that legislation previously regarded as protective of the patient has shifted to a position of control. Complex issues, such as compulsory care depending largely on a test of capacity, as suggested by the expert committee, have been avoided in the consultation paper. Governments like to appear in control. Mental health law reform, previously seen as a somewhat non-political issue, has become a 'law-and-order' subject with all the inevitable politicisation. It remains to be seen whether new legislation based on the consultation paper will, first, deliver the public safety the government wishes to see and, secondly, whether it will clear the hurdles of the Human Rights Act 1998 now in force. The Council of Europe has published a consultation paper that requires member countries to ensure that their mental health legislation complies with the European Convention on Human Rights.[3]

Separately from general issues of mental health law reform, governments both north and south of the border have been examining the problems of dangerous offenders and, in England, of a specific group identified as having 'dangerous severe personality disorder' (DSPD).[4] Proposals in relation to the latter are aimed at identifying such individuals in advance of their offending and detaining them on the grounds of preventive detention. The proposals have caused widespread concern to clinicians, academics and others.[5] The category, DSPD, is government-created. This is not a group that can be said to share common clinical characteristics and, therefore, the afflicted people cannot be medically identified. Even if they were identifiable, according to the government's own figures, they make a tiny contribution to the overall crime figures. In terms of current legislation, there already exists the power to impose indeterminate (life) sentences for a wide range

3 Council of Europe *CM(2000)23, Addendum*, 10 February 2000.
4 Home Office and Department of Health *Managing Dangerous People with Severe Personality Disorder* (1999).   Interim legislation is already in place in Scotland (see fn 4, p 410 above).
5 P E Mullen 'Dangerous People with Severe Personality Disorder' (1999) 319 BMJ 1146; J K Mason 'The Legal Aspects and Implications of Risk Assessment' (2000) 8 Med L Rev 69.

of crimes apart from murder where it is mandatory.[6] The courts seem reluctant to exercise these sentencing powers that are already available to them.

However, the most fraught issue is that of detention on the basis of the crimes that DSPD individuals might commit at some unspecified time in the future. This is envisaged whether or not treatment is available or beneficial. It remains unclear exactly what professional group is likely, or willing, to provide care for such people. Appropriate psychiatric facilities for personality disordered people are in short supply and the history of attempting to provide appropriate clinical centres is littered with crisis and scandal.[7] In current practice, as described above, compulsory powers to detain personality disorder people in hospital are rarely used, principally because of the lack of success in treatment. Creating a new law does not create a new treatment, and it is clear that that the psychiatric profession will not become involved in providing preventive detention of suspected cases of DSPD.[8]

In Scotland, an independent committee has reviewed the sentencing of dangerous violent and sexual offenders including those who may have a personality disorder.[9] The approach of the MacLean Committee was based on the proper assessment of risk in offenders perceived by the court to require such an assessment. The committee recommended that there should be agreed standards of risk assessment and that it should only be carried out by appropriately trained staff in designated centres. In cases assessed as high risk, the judge would be required to pass an order for lifelong restriction. This would be a reviewable prison sentence during which time the authorities will be required to address those factors in the prisoner contributing to the high risk. Release, subject to stringent conditions, would be determined by a judicial body.

Civil issues

Psychiatric injury

Criminal or negligent acts may cause psychiatric injury just as they may cause physical injury. The person who is psychiatrically damaged may seek compensation from the negligent party or, where there has been a crime of violence, from the Criminal Injuries Compensation Authority. Usually, the negligent act causes a road traffic, industrial or medical accident and there is physical injury together with a psychiatric injury—eg mental incapacity secondary to a head injury or depression in association with deformity or scarring. In these cases, the psychiatric injury is considered in the same way as the physical injury. The plaintiff must show that the defendant owed him a duty of care, that the defendant's conduct breached that duty, that psychiatric injury was reasonably foreseeable and that the breach caused the plaintiff's psychiatric disorder.

---

6   Criminal Justice Act 1991.
7   Department of Health *Report of the Committee of Inquiry into the Personality Disorder Unit, Ashworth Special Hospital* (1999, Cm 4195).
8   For discussion, see N Eastman 'Who Should Take Responsibility for Anti-Social Personality Disorder?' (1999) 318 BMJ 206.
9   Scottish Executive *Report of the Committee on Serious Violent and Sexual Offenders* (Lord MacLean, chairman) (2000) (SE/2000/68).

It is common for psychiatrists to be instructed to provide reports in these cases, perhaps by both plaintiff and defendant. The psychiatrist should carefully peruse all the relevant documents, including any medical records from before the accident, examine the plaintiff and interview a spouse or other close relative so that a full clinical picture is obtained. The psychiatric report should answer the following questions:

- is there a psychiatric disorder?
- if so, what is its nature and extent?
- was it caused, or contributed to, by the accident?
- what are the effects and prognosis?

Nervous shock

Problems arise in two circumstances, both of which are of great current interest. First are those cases in which there is *only* psychiatric injury—so-called 'nervous shock'—and, second, are cases where the plaintiff is not the primary victim of the negligence but is a third party, eg a relative, witness, rescuer or bystander. 'Nervous shock' is a crude term, without clinical meaning, but still in legal use; a better term is 'psychiatric illness'. Normal mental distress is not usually compensatable; there must be a recognised psychiatric illness. In theory, almost any psychiatric illness, or its worsening, could be related to a traumatic event, but the conditions which are commonly implicated in nervous shock are: post-traumatic stress disorder (PTSD), adjustment disorder, depressive illness, pathological grief, anxiety states and phobias (pathological fear), somatoform disorders (physical complaints not attributable to physical illness or injury), enduring personality change and accident neurosis. More than one of these may present in an individual, and alcohol or drug misuse is a common complicating factor. The recognition of PTSD as a psychiatric disorder which may sometimes follow a traumatic event has been of profound medico-legal importance.[10] Key features include general nervousness, preoccupation with the accident, disturbed sleep and distressing mental images of the accident known as 'flashbacks'.

Sudden trauma causing a reasonable fear of physical injury is generally a necessary prerequisite to establishing nervous shock. However, non-sudden events have also been the basis of successful litigation, including intentional acts (eg harassment, discrimination and dismissal), professional negligence and, recently, stress at work in the case of a social worker who claimed that an excessive workload caused a mental breakdown.[11]

The victim's previous mental health is relevant in respect of foreseeability. The negligent act must be such as would cause psychiatric injury in a person of ordinary fortitude. Once this is established, the eggshell skull (or 'eggshell personality') rule applies; particularly *severe* psychiatric illness in someone with a pre-existing mental condition is compensatable, provided an 'ordinary' person would have developed a psychiatric illness due to the same event. The House of Lords (in a majority decision) ruled that even though a plaintiff had not been

10 The *Herald of Free Enterprise* arbitration awards. Personal and Medical Injuries Law Letter, London, Legal Studies and Services (1989).
11 *Walker v Northumberland County Council* [1995] 1 All ER 737.

physically injured in a relatively trivial road accident, the foreseeability of such injury was sufficient to recover damages in nervous shock.[12]

What is the position of a plaintiff who, though not negligently injured or imperilled, develops foreseeable shock-induced psychiatric illness? The law is more restrictive in relation to these secondary victims for fear of opening the floodgates to vast numbers of potential claimants. It has been tested in two important cases. The first concerned the Hillsborough football ground tragedy in 1989, in which 95 spectators were killed, and which was broadcast live by television to a national audience of viewers, many of whom had friends and relatives at the match. In the legal action for negligence against the police that followed, plaintiffs included relatives who had been at, or near to, the ground and others who had watched the tragedy unfold on television. The House of Lords identified the crucial issue of proximity of the plaintiff and defined it in terms of: (1) relationship with the primary victim—a tie of love and affection is necessary; (2) closeness in time and space to the accident—the plaintiff must be present at the accident or its immediate aftermath; (3) the means by which the accident is perceived—it must be through the plaintiff's own unaided senses.[13]

In the second case, the Court of Session in Scotland interpreted the criterion of relationship as 'the closest ties of friendship or family' in rejecting claims by two long-standing colleagues of a work-mate whom they saw blown to his death when crossing the Forth road bridge in a strong wind. It was held that neither had the necessary close tie of love and affection to the deceased. The claim also failed on the grounds that they were not participants in the accident.[14] These decisions have raised many concerns and the Law Commission has produced a consultation paper on liability for psychiatric illness which advocates a more liberal interpretation.[15]

Mental disorder and financial matters

Testamentary capacity

Testamentary capacity is the ability to make a valid will. It requires that the testator is of 'sound disposing mind and memory'; he must understand the nature and purpose of making a will, know in broad terms the extent of his property and possessions and the people who might reasonably be expected to benefit. If there is any doubt about a testator's capacity to make a will, it is wise to arrange a psychiatric evaluation before he does so. Capacity does not depend on the presence of any particular disorder but on the criteria outlined above. Psychiatrists are sometimes instructed to perform a 'psychiatric post-mortem' to assess testamentary capacity when a will is challenged after death. It is a difficult task, requiring perusal of papers, medical records, and interviews with relatives and friends of the deceased.

Managing property and affairs

There are three legal structures by which the property and affairs of mentally incapable persons may be protected and managed.

12 *Page v Smith* [1995] 2 All ER 736, HL.
13 *Alcock v Chief Constable of the South Yorkshire Police* [1992] 1 AC 310.
14 *Robertson v Forth Road Bridge Joint Board* 1996 SLT 263, IH.
15 Law Commission *Liability for Psychiatric Illness* (1995) Consultation Paper No 137.

Court of Protection. The Court of Protection is an office of the Supreme Court whose functions are defined in Part VII of the Mental Health Act 1983. It currently manages the affairs of approximately 28,000 people, the majority of whom are elderly women suffering from dementia. Application to the court is normally made by a relative, solicitor or social worker with supporting medical evidence that the person is incapable, by reason of mental disorder, of managing and administering his or her property and affairs. The court appoints a receiver and has total control of all the property and affairs of the patient. It may sell or acquire new property, make financial settlements, make a will and conduct legal proceedings on behalf of the patient.

Appointeeship. Appointeeship is a method of dealing with social security and other benefits for those who are unable to act for themselves.[16] It is widely used, with approximately 47,000 appointees created each year. The appointee is normally a close relative.

Enduring power of attorney. The Enduring Powers of Attorney Act 1985 enables a person, when capable, to make plans for the management of his property should he, at a future time, become mentally incapable. He does this by appointing an attorney. If, later, the attorney believes that the donor is becoming mentally incapable, he must inform the donor and register the power of attorney with the Court of Protection. The latter has a supervisory role in relation to the attorney, but does not have direct authority over the donor's assets. There are currently approximately 15,000 powers of attorney registered with the Court of Protection.

Until recently, the property and financial affairs of an incapacitated person in Scotland have been managed by a curator bonis or tutor-at-law appointed by the courts. Such appointments will, however, be incompetent in the case of persons aged over 16 years once the Adults with Incapacity (Scotland) Act 2000 comes into force (2000 Act, s 80).

The rather complex arrangements for dealing with the affairs of an incompetent adult that are detailed in the 2000 Act derive, on the one hand, from the office of the Public Guardian, with whom all guardianships must be registered, and, on the other, from the duties of the Mental Welfare Commission. Both these bodies may, acting either alone or in concert, supervise the guardianship of and protect the interests of a person who is subject to an intervention or guardianship order. Similar co-operative functions are laid on the local authority. In the event of a power of attorney having been granted while capable, a continuing power of attorney persists into incapacity (s 15). The Act also allows for the appointment of a welfare attorney who may act in support of the subject's personal welfare (s 16). Otherwise, given that it is necessary for the protection of the subject, the sheriff may make an intervention order or a guardianship order on the application of any person having an interest in the financial affairs or welfare of an incapable adult— any person, in this context, includes the adult him- or herself and the local authority. An intervention order persists for three months or until the appointment of a guardian. An appointed guardian may be given very wide powers over the financial and welfare aspects of the subject's life but, specifically, he or she cannot place the subject in a hospital for the treatment of mental disorder against the

16 Social Security (Claims and Payment) Regulations 1987, SI 1987/1968, n 33.

latter's wishes or consent to any of the restricted therapies outlined above at page 415.[17]   We have already noted that the authority to provide reasonable treatment without the subject's valid consent that is granted to his or her primary medical practitioner by virtue of s 47(2) ceases once an intervention or guardianship order has been granted or initiated (s 49).

17 Covered in Part X of the Mental Health (Scotland) Act 1984.

28

Forensic odontology

Human dentition[1]

Human dentition is of two types—the deciduous of infancy and the permanent; the former consists of 20 and the latter of 32 teeth. The permanent dentition comprises four symmetrical quadrants each containing two incisors, one canine, two premolar and three molar teeth. Although the differentiation of individual molars, premolars and lower incisors presents some complications, it is generally not difficult for a dental practitioner to identify an individual tooth on the basis of its size and shape; for court purposes, however, the opinion of a specialist dental anatomist might be sought in cases of special importance.

Several systems for recording the dentition are current. That attributed to Zsigmondy has been used in the National Health Service for many years and, as a result, has been regarded as the standard method in the United Kingdom. In this, the teeth in each quadrant are numbered consecutively from the midline in the front; the second molar tooth in the right lower jaw thus becomes lower right 7 or, in common dental notation, $\overline{7|}$. The five deciduous teeth are annotated A–E in a similar fashion. It is clear, however, that this annotation sits uneasily within the computer and the fax machine and an alternative system, which is being lobbied at an international level is being introduced with this in mind. This method, which is known as Viohl's Two Digit System,[2] substitutes the prefix 1 for right upper, 2 for left upper, 3 for left lower and 4 for right lower quadrants; using this notation the second molar in the right lower jaw would be designated 47. The deciduous teeth are prefixed 5–8 according to quadrant.[3] An understanding of the notations is important as all types may be encountered in the circumstance in which dental identification is of greatest value—the international airline disaster (see Figure 28.1).

If one considers a tooth for descriptive purposes as a cube projecting from the jaw, it has five surfaces. The surface that is opposed to its fellow in the other jaw

---

1   This section has been kindly reviewed by Mr and Mrs Y Maidment.
2   The commonest notation in the USA numbers the upper right third (back) molar tooth as 1. Each tooth is then numbered consecutively, the upper back molar on the left side being 16. The lower left back molar is then numbered 17 and the process continued to 32 which represents the lower right back molar.
3   The British Dental Journal has intimated that it favours this system for publication.

is called the occlusal surface (O in shorthand); except in unusual circumstances, such as the loss of rear teeth, there is no occlusal surface on the incisor and canine teeth which are sharp. The surface nearest the anterior midline is called the mesial surface (M), and that furthest away the distal (D). The surface contacting the cheek is called buccal (B), and the inner surface is designated palatal (P) in the upper and lingual (L) in the lower jaw. Thus, the common massive filling that involves the biting surface and the mesial and distal walls of a tooth would be noted as MOD.

The lower right canine may be:

$\overline{3|}$	Zsigmondy
43	Viohl
3 –	Haderup
27	Parreidt
RLT	Haines

Figure 28.1 An example of how the position of a tooth may be described. The first two are described in the text. Hadup's system was in vogue some 25 years ago but is now rarely used outside Scandinavia; Parreidt's (or Cunningham's) system is that described in footnote 1; Haine's system was devised simply to get round the difficulties of sending numbers by telex— it is, now, probably of historic interest only.

Any tooth may be unerupted, it may be normal, it may contain a cavity caused by caries or a lost filling or a cavity may have been restored. The restoration may be by synthetic porcelain or resin complexes, by a silver/tin amalgam or by gold; the tooth may have been crowned and there is the possibility of dental implants. A tooth may have been extracted and, if so, been replaced by a partial denture, or bridge, or there may be a complete denture; the dentures may be made of plastic or of metal, they may be deliberately coloured, marked or even numbered and national practices lead to characteristic designs. Add to all these variables the possibilities of removable or fixed mechanical devices to straighten the teeth (orthodontic appliances) or of obvious deformities together with characteristics associated with race or with occupation, not forgetting changes due to age, and it will be appreciated that the potential variations in the mouth are so great in number that the dentition could provide as personal a method of identification as can fingerprints.

The relative merits of odontology and dactylography as identification methods have been mentioned in Chapter 3 and are amplified here. Odontology scores in two main areas. First, in a country provided with a National Health Service, it is at least probable that a record of the dentition of a missing person will be available somewhere—either in the files of a practitioner or at the Dental Estimates Boards where records of treatment are maintained for up to four years.[4] By contrast, permanent records of fingerprints are maintained in the United Kingdom only

---

4   The quality of dental record keeping should not be compromised in the private sector. But, for an interesting self-audit, see V F Delattre and P G Stimson 'Self-assessment of the Forensic Value of Dental Records' (1999) 44 J Forens Sci 906.

rarely (see page 54); there is no way of tracing a *completely* unknown body through its fingerprints although, given some clue to identity, a match may be made with impressions obtained from selected personal possessions. It should be noted, however, that these limitations would not apply, say, in the United States where filed fingerprints are commonplace throughout the population. Secondly, the teeth are very resistant to fire. Odontology therefore becomes the method of choice for identification of a major group of bodies that is unsuitable for visual recognition.[5]

On the other hand, although developmental differences between two persons are almost always demonstrable by X-rays etc, the dentition can only become 'personalised' if abnormalities have arisen or have been induced. The fewer the deviations from the normal, the less precise can be the identification and it is difficult to identify, with certainty from the mouth alone, someone who has had no treatment or dental investigations; it may be hard even to distinguish between two persons of similar age and race with such an unblemished dental history. Fingerprints, on the other hand, are personalised from birth and remain so until death. It follows that odontological identification finds its greatest use either in confirming or denying an identification suspected in an individual on other grounds or in discriminating between the bodies of a large number of known but individually unrecognisable persons. The reasons why dental identification of, say, a completely unknown skeleton discovered in a wood is generally disappointing will become clear later.

Estimation of age from the teeth

Four observations can be made on the teeth with relative ease. In chronological order of appearance these are: mineralisation, formation of the crown, eruption of the tooth and completion of the root of the tooth.[6] This applies both to the deciduous and to the permanent dentition and observations may be made on two or more changes at the same time; one can, for example, estimate the eruption of the deciduous teeth and their degree of root development at the same time as assessing the state of completion of the crowns of the following permanent teeth embedded in the jaw.

These variables are shown in diagrammatic form in Figure 28.2.[7] There is considerable variation in the appearance of each characteristic. For example, the range of eruption of the first lower deciduous incisors is from four to ten months and, although the remaining deciduous teeth behave more regularly than this, the 'scatter' in the permanent teeth is far greater; in addition, the teeth generally develop rather earlier in girls than in boys. The more characteristics that are examined and taken into account, the more accurate will be the final assessment of age. In brief, the dental practitioner will utilise X-ray or microscopic evidence

---

5   For a variation on the aircraft disaster, see S Chapenoire, Y Schuliar and J M Corvisier 'Rapid, Efficient Dental Identification of 92% of 13 Train Passengers Carbonized during a Collision with a Petrol Tanker' (1998) 19 Amer J Forens Med Pathol 352.
6   Age and dentition is well overviewed by B G Sims 'Paediatric Forensic Odontology' in J K Mason (ed) *Paediatric Forensic Medicine and Pathology* (1989) ch 7(i).
7   G Gustafson *Forensic Odontology* (1966) remains the classic work on the topic.

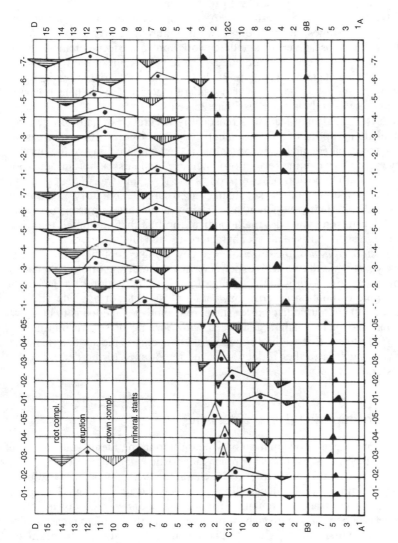

Figure 28.2 Schematic representation of tooth formation and eruption. A–B = intrauterine life; B–C = first year of life; C–D = 2–16 years. Upper and lower teeth are represented by + and – signs, respectively. Deciduous tooth numbers are prefixed by 'O'. The apex of each triange indicates the average value and the spread of the base the earliest and the latest occurrence of the several features. (Reproduced by kind permission of Dr Gosta Gustafson from his book *Forensic Odontology* (1966); London; Staples Press.)

of early tooth development in the fetus or neonate; up to the age of one year the eruption of the deciduous teeth combined with an evaluation of the oncoming permanent teeth will give a most useful assessment of age. Following this—up to the age of about two and a half years—age can be estimated from the state of tooth eruption, always accepting the proviso in each case of a 'bracket of probability'. Eruption of the permanent teeth generally begins between six and seven years. Eruption proceeds in a fairly standard order in each individual but the range among different persons may be up to ± two years; it is of some interest that Gustafson's *average* ages for eruption shown in Figure 28.2 are, in many cases, rather higher than those given in standard works on forensic medicine—much depends on the phase of eruption intended. The development of the third molar or wisdom tooth is not shown in Figure 28.2; its eruption is variable but its roots are important in the young adult—if its roots are incompletely formed it can at least be said that the body is aged less than 25 years.

Characteristics that may lead to a reasonably accurate estimate of age may still be found after eruption of the permanent teeth. These are attrition, or wearing down of the teeth; paradentosis, or loosening of the teeth; infilling of the normal root cavity (secondary dentine formation); increase in the tissue holding the root in place (cementum apposition); resorption of the root; and transparency of the root.[8] All but the first two of these six changes need careful laboratory preparation of the material and their assessment is certainly a process requiring previous experience. Gustafson evolved a mathematical formula that attempted to arrive at a nominal age on the basis of all six characteristics and this still gives acceptable results in *specialised hands*; the order of accuracy, using computer techniques, is about ± five years.[9] It is this writer's experience that a dental practitioner interested in the subject can give a very fair estimate of age—in the region of a decade— from the simple estimation of attrition, paradontosis, mouth hygiene and the like;[10] certainly the odontologist's assessment of a subject's age tends to be more accurate than that of the pathologist faced with burning or severe mutilation. Perhaps it is fair to say that odontology as an aid to ageing is most valuable in the comparative context, a further reflection of the importance of the dentist at the major disaster.

Racial and occupational characteristics

The assessment of race or occupation may be of help in the identification of the single unknown body. A few traits approach diagnostic value but most are, again, of greatest use in a comparative role; racial characteristics may be very useful in a preliminary sorting of multiple casualties from, say, an air accident. Except in such a circumstance, when the tentative isolation of a *known* group of negroids from a *known* group of caucasoids may be relatively easy, the problem is essentially one for the specialist anthropologist. Three lines of observation might be

---

8 Unnatural changes, such as chemical erosions due to overuse of carbonated drinks may also be noted.
9 It is difficult to improve on this figure: Y K Kim, H S Kho and K H Lee 'Age Estimation by Occlusal Tooth Wear' (2000) 45 J Forens Sci 303.
10 The dental hygienist may also have a role to play: R B Brannon and C M Connick 'The Role of the Dental Hygienist in Mass Disasters' (2000) 45 J Forens Sci 381.

followed—the size and shape of the teeth themselves, the extent and nature of any restorations and the quality of prostheses (bridges or dentures).

The size of the teeth, which are generally large in non-industrialised peoples, is so variable as to be virtually useless save at extremes of the scale. Mention may be made of the high incidence of so-called shovel-shaped upper incisors in mongoloid and eskimo races. Subtle differences in the premolar and molar teeth are also to be found in these groups. The arch of the jaw is wide in negroid persons and the teeth are usually in good alignment and occlusion; this is in general contrast to the European caucasoid, in whom a narrow arch predisposes to crowding and misplacement of teeth—the wisdom teeth are very commonly unerupted or are extracted.

As to the recognition of restorations and prostheses, it has been pointed out that it is far easier to say that a given piece of work was unlikely to have been done in a certain place rather than to identify the area in which it was performed; moreover, the place of treatment is not necessarily the same as the homeland of the person treated. There are, nevertheless, some interesting geographical variations in dental restoration. Certain nationals, in particular Africans, have remarkably good teeth requiring virtually no restorative treatment; they are therefore very difficult to identify individually from their dentition. The use of gold is far less common in the United Kingdom than elsewhere; it is particularly prevalent in southern Europe and in the mongoloid races. Silver alloys for fashioning false tooth crowns are common in eastern Europe. Composite resins are generally used in Great Britain for restoring front teeth but porcelain, which was once more likely to be used in the United States, is now readily available in this country.

Such findings are, however, no more than guides to identification and the same is true of bridges and dentures. Certain types of work may be more common in one country than another but to make an 'exclusion' type of identification solely on this basis would be a hazardous undertaking.

Occupational stigmata can arise from mechanical or chemical injury. Classic mechanical injuries are said to be found in the form of notches in the incisors of those who grasp nails or twine in the mouth—shoemakers, upholsterers and seamstresses—but such persons are unlikely to present in large numbers as subjects for identification. Gustafson has also described changes in the front teeth of musicians, those working in dusty environments and in miners; most of these changes can now be relegated to historical interest. Chemical stains are most often due to the use of tobacco which, in pipe smokers, may also produce highly personalised mechanical injury, but chemical injury due to occupation is most common in those whose work involves the use of strong acids; this last effect is more commonly due to drinking fluids containing a high concentration of citric acid. Such observations must, however, be of forensic significance only very rarely.

Practical dental identification

Dental identification of the dead at the personal rather than exclusion level depends almost entirely on the availability of ante-mortem records. Figure 28.3 shows how this operates in practice. It follows that nothing can be done in the absence of a retrieval service for these records and it is this which so severely limits the

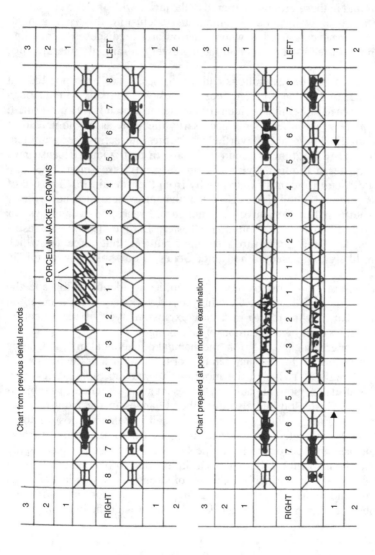

Figure 28.3 Dental identification in practice. The lower chart shows the teeth as recorded in the cadaver; the upper is prepared from previous dental records. Note that the lower 6 is charted as missing at post-mortem examination with a drift of lower 7 and 8 on each side to close the spaces; the lower 8 on each side is charted as missing in the dental records. The cavity recorded in the dental records in the lower right 5 was found to have been filled at post-mortem. A new cavity, not previously recorded, was found in the lower left 5 at post-mortem. Such inconsistencies are compatable with a positive identification which can be made despite the loss of much of the anterior jaw during the accident. (The example was kindly contributed by Dr Keith Ashley.)

value of the method in the case of the wholly unknown body. It is certainly true that, in cases of major importance, a description of a cadaver's teeth can be sent to every practising dentist and hospital, but the process is time consuming and expensive; success generally attends only when there is *some* other indication as to identity.

This is largely because dental charts are seldom absolutely correct even when they are available. Some dentists record only the work that they have done, others are not so thorough as perfection would demand, while many persons undergo emergency treatment which may not appear in their records until noted at a later date. The Dental Estimates Board keeps records only of extractions or major work. For all of these reasons, dental identification is at its most useful in a comparative or exclusive role and has been most used in the mass disaster, in particular the aircraft accident, in which an especially good indication of the group identity of the dead is available through the list of passengers. Effectively, in such a situation, one is searching for the best-fitting charts among a known population rather than perfect matches. It is this which those accustomed to the mathematical accuracy of fingerprinting find hard to understand.

Dental identification in the major disaster

The essence of rapid dental identification in the mass lies in the efficiency of retrieval of the records of the missing persons—the conventional methods of the International Police Organisation are generally too slow to satisfy public demand for rapid restitution of the dead. British airlines are given service by a firm of funeral directors who maintain a control room for this purpose and whose facilities are at the disposal of the police wherever the accident occurs; the use of electronic and facsimile communication is an essential element in the rapid provision of information and has minimised the difficulties in the transmission of records—although, as already pointed out, the system of notation must be compatible with the technology in use.

Dental identification then depends mainly upon comparison between the records of the missing persons and the findings in the bodies in relation to:

- Restorative work: Teeth may require treatment, have been filled, have been extracted or replaced by prostheses.
- Unusual features: Important features may include absence, persistence, malformation or discoloration of teeth; malocclusion of the jaws; and abnormalities of the mouth or lips.
- X-rays: if ante-mortem X-rays are available, matching radiographs taken post mortem may provide unequivocal evidence of identification.[11]

A comparison of restorations may result in inconsistencies which can be either compatible or incompatible with a positive identification. Comparison in any form may be affected by trauma—the possibility of fillings having been dislodged, teeth lost and the like must always be considered. From the technical aspect, a compatible inconsistency is one that can be explained either by the failure of the dental practitioner to record what he has done or by the treatment having been

---

11 For review, see C J McKenna 'Radiography in Forensic Dental Identification' (1999) 17 J Forens Odonto-stom 47. The increasing use of digital dental radiographic superimposition is also to be noted: R E Wood, N J Kirk and D J Sweet 'Digital Dental Radiographic Identification in the Pediatric, Mixed and Permanent Dentitions' (1999) 44 J Forens Sci 910.

given subsequent to the last recording. Thus, a filling discovered in a tooth of a cadaver that is not shown in the chart of a missing person need not necessarily exclude a match. An incompatible inconsistency is one that involves deletion of a recorded treatment. Thus, the absence of a filling in a tooth said to have had three treatments would normally exclude identification. Even so, very occasionally an identification is so certain on other grounds that it must be accepted despite the presence of an incompatible inconsistency. Such a situation is usually attributed to clerical error or slipshod record keeping. The phenomenon of tooth migration, which occurs particularly in the molar region, may pose real problems both for the recorder and observer. Identifications allowing for such anomalies must, however, be accepted only after careful analyses by competent authorities of all the relevant factors.

Strong confirmatory evidence of identification can also be provided by dentures. As discussed previously, many of these may have national characteristics. Different colours are used and the majority of laboratories incorporate some mark by which they can identify their work. Observations such as these are particularly useful, say, in separating the last three bodies from a large number of casualties. There is also a growing habit of including a number in the denture; once the laboratory performing the work for the deceased has been identified, this number may be as certain evidence of identification as is the use of identification discs. Increasingly often, the patient's name is incorporated.[12]

Just how the matching is performed depends very much on the facts of the individual case. The use of large numbers of different forms with subsequent visual analysis and association smacks of a by-gone age and methods involving computerisation of the available data has worked well in a number of cases.[13] The use of computers and the like depends, however, upon the sophistication of the investigative base. They may well be invaluable when it has been possible to return the bodies to a major centre[14] but the majority of investigations will be undertaken in primitive conditions where there is no alternative to hand-sorting of data—which, in its turn, depends for success upon a co-operative dental team.

But, no matter how it is organised, there can be no comparative identification in the absence of available data to compare.[15] Dental identification of mass casualties is doomed to failure if there has been no dental work on the casualties or if there are no records of such work as has been performed.[16]

12 For international standards, see H I Borrman, J A DiZinno, J Wasen and N Rene 'On Denture Marking' (1999) 17 J Forens Odonto-stom 20.
13 See, for example, the accident in Antarctica reported by F J Cairns, P B Herdson, G C Hitchcock et al 'Air Crash on Mount Erebus' (1981) 21 Med Sci Law 184 or, more recently, B Ludes, A Tracqui, H Pfitzinger et al 'Medico-Legal Investigations of the Airbus A320 Crash upon Mount Ste-Odile, France' (1994) 39 J Forens Sci 1147.
14 Even then, consideration has to be given to the degree of interference with the normal working of, say, a district general hospital. See C T Doyle and M A Bolster 'Medico-legal Organization of a Mass Disaster—the Air India Crash' (1992) 32 Med Sci Law 5.
15 This is one of the main difficulties in the genocidal situation: H Brkic, D Strinovic, M Slaus et al 'Dental Identification of War Victims from Petrinja in Croatia' (1997) 110 Internat J Leg Med 47.
16 See D H Clark 'Dental Identification Problems in the Abu Dhabi Air Accident' (1986) 7 Amer J Forens Med Pathol 317; P Nambiar, N Jalil and B Singh 'The Dental Identification of Victims of an Aircraft Accident in Malaysia' (1997) 47 Internat Dent J 9. For a review of the limitations, see R B Brannon and H P Kessler 'Problems in Mass-Disaster Dental Identification: A Retrospective Review' (1999) 44 J Forens Sci 123.

Accident reconstruction

A large proportion of persons killed in automobile or aircraft accidents sustain maxillofacial injuries. The precise distribution of these when correlated with the crash environment and the safety harness in use may give invaluable information as to the direction and strength of the deceleration forces; the observations made may also have a profound influence on the design of equipment, instrument panels and the like. This aspect of forensic odontology does not receive the attention it deserves.

Bite marks

Animals may bite humans either in life or after death. However, such injuries are not the concern of this chapter,[17] which deals solely with human/human bites and bites in food.

The main values of bite-mark evidence lie in two fields of examination:

* Of the skin of a person assaulted, a prime objective being to identify or exclude the assailant.
* Of food and other inanimate objects in an attempt to prove the presence of someone at the locus at some time.

In either case, the evidence must be of a comparative nature—the dentition of a person must be examined and compared with the mark before he or she can be identified or excluded as a suspect.

Human/human bites are most commonly associated with sexually motivated assault and with non-accidental injury inflicted on children. The examinations may, therefore, be required in both the living and the dead and, while the majority of evidence is likely to be derived from an examination of the victim, the reverse might hold if biting has formed part of a defence reaction to assault.

The comparison of records falls into two phases. The first, recording the bite mark, is a matter of urgency in the living person as the mark may alter in intensity and definition with time; indeed, such alterations may also occur in the dead body even before putrefaction intervenes.

In instances of recent biting, say within five hours, the first stage of recording should be to swab the mark for saliva; this must not be delayed as previous physical examination, or interference by other investigators or mortuary technicians, may remove a large proportion of the saliva available and may contaminate the area with the examiner's own secretions. DNA can be extracted from the buccal cells in saliva and will provide the best evidence of identification when the method can be used. However, the amount of DNA is small and there is almost inevitable contamination by cells from the victim's skin. Recourse to standard serological methods may, therefore, be needed. Approximately 76% of people secrete readily recognisable amounts of either A, B or O ('H') antigens in

17 This does not exclude the fact that the distinction of animal bites as such—and, particularly, those inflicted post-mortem— may be of extreme importance in the investigation of suspicious deaths. See J H Davis 'Injuries due to Animals' in J K Mason (ed) *The Pathology of Trauma* (2nd edn, 1993) ch 18.

their saliva and these antigens correspond to the person's blood group (see Chapter 31). Saliva is best obtained from the skin by swabbing the area with damp cigarette papers which can then be preserved individually between glass slides. The examinee's own sweat may contain her or his water-soluble antigens. Control specimens taken from elsewhere—ideally, from the same area on the other side of the body—are, therefore, essential, as is a 'negative control' containing no more than the water used to dampen the papers; for the same reason, the examiner's hands should be gloved. Discovery of an antigen incompatible with the suspect's blood group may positively exclude a him or her as having inflicted a bite. Alternatively, a match of antigens may add further to the evidence giving rise to suspicion—but no more; the finding, say, of water soluble antigen A means, by itself, no more than that any suspect of blood group A is one of the 31% of Caucasians who could have provided the specimen. In either event, it is clear that, for any useful result to emerge, the blood group of the suspect must be known. Failure to identify water soluble antigens may be due to one or more of several causes —to the absence of saliva, to the saliva coming from a 'non-secretor'—ie something in the region of 24% of the population—or to poor collection technique.

Following attempted salvage of saliva, the bite is photographed both in black and white and in colour. Both sets of prints must incorporate a suitable linear scale following the natural curves of the part bitten, and the latter should also show a colour comparison chart; this has special importance in that repetitive colour photography is useful to follow the changes in the appearance of a bite mark and it is important to ensure a standard colour balance. The photographs should be supported by a sketch or tracing showing the actual measurements between landmarks. Useful landmarks are variable but would normally include such items as the distance between the canine teeth and the width of or between any clear individual tooth marks. Obvious abnormalities of size or position will be of major importance and it is a general rule that the more unusual is an abnormality, the more useful it is as evidence of positive identification. It is probably true that no two persons have *exactly* the same tooth characteristics when these are expressed as a bite impression; the disappointing feature of bite mark evidence is, however, that such is the variation in shape and elasticity of the skin bitten, that it is difficult to reproduce perfectly a bite mark even when made under experimental conditions by the same participant. Thus, while removal of post-mortem specimens in toto may be found useful for further study, it must be remembered that tissues shrink in preserving fluids even if pinned on a board; moreover, flattening the specimen alters the alignment of a mark made originally on, say, the curve of an arm.

Recognisable marks on the skin may not be due only to direct pressure by the teeth. Scrape marks may provide valuable information in demonstrating characteristic contours of the cutting surface of the front teeth. The combination of suction and pressure by the tongue may result in bruises derived from parts of the mouth other than the teeth or from the surfaces of the teeth in contact with the tongue. The result of such a bite resembles an archer's target; the finding is strongly suggestive of a 'love-bite' rather than aggression.[18] Consideration should

---

18 Which is not to say that an apparently aggressive bite could not also be part of consensual love-making.

also be given to the possibility of self-infliction—the rapist may force a woman's arm into her mouth or the child may deliberately stifle its cries in order to avoid further punishment. If there is any doubt, evidence that might be needed—ie models of the victim's teeth—should be made available.

The second phase of comparison requires the recording of, and obtaining impressions from, the teeth of a suspect and the law in this respect has been clarified. The powers of the police to fingerprint, to take swabs from the hand and body and from the orifices of an arrested person are laid down in the Police and Criminal Evidence Act 1984, ss 61–65 and have been discussed in Chapter 20. Subsequent legislation has defined the previously anomalous position as to dental impressions. Saliva is now classified as a non-intimate sample as is a swab taken from the mouth,[19] while a dental impression is included by name as an intimate specimen; moreover, such an impression can only be taken by a registered dentist.[20] A clear distinction is thus made between the non-specific assessment of, say, a person's secretor status and his specific identification from his dentition. The dentist must have the consent of the subject and, for practical purposes, it can be said that the taking of a dental impression can only be authorised if the subject is in police detention.[1] As discussed at page 298, the situation in Scotland is rather less precise. The provision of specimens is governed by the Criminal Procedure (Scotland) Act 1995, s 18 which empowers a constable to take such relevant personal data—defined as fingerprints, palm prints and such other prints and impressions of an external part of the body—as he reasonably considers it appropriate to take 'having regard to the circumstances of the suspected offence in respect of which the person has been arrested or detained'.[2] It is difficult to see how this could include a dental impression but there is no doubt that a sheriff's warrant would be available and this common law power is preserved in the 1995 Act.[3]

Having obtained impressions of a suspect's dentition, the next step is that of modelling and subsequent comparison with the bite mark. If a match be obtained, the presentation of the case in court in an acceptable fashion is likely to follow. There is no 'minimum number of points of conformity' required to prove the identity of a biter—it is simply a matter of the skill of the advocate and of the credibility and weight to be attached to the evidence of the expert witness. This is primarily because, in contrast to fingerprinting, the possible configurations in bite marks are less systematised. Similarly, there is no standard system of notation or presentation of the results, various experts having their own chosen methods. Certainly, photography must play an important part; superimposition techniques involving the use of transparencies are very convincing when they can be used but, unfortunately, the elasticity of the skin and the distortion introduced by

19 Criminal Justice and Public Order Act 1994, s 58.
20 Police and Criminal Evidence Act 1984, s 62(9) inserted by the 1994 Act, s 54.
1 Intimate specimens can be taken when not in detention but only if two previous specimens have been found to be inadequate (1984 Act, s 62(1A) inserted by the 1994 Act, s 54). Such a situation could hardly arise in the case of dental impressions.
2 Note that the Scottish statute makes no distinction as to intimate and non-intimate samples.
3 1995 Act, s 18(8)(c). The clear precedent lies in the widely publicised case of *H M Advocate v Hay* 1968 JC 40 where a warrant obtained to make impressions from the mouth of a close suspect, who happened to be detained in an approved school, was held to be valid or, at least, granted in accordance with the overriding public interest. The case was very fully reported from the dental aspect in (1968) 8 J Forens Sci Soc 156.

contours often makes the method self-defeating. The criteria to be met are that the deductive processes should be easily demonstrable to and understandable by a jury and that the method should be free from attack on the grounds of unwitting distortion of the evidence. It is again emphasised that individual, distinctive abnormalities are of greater evidential value than is the general configuration of the mouth.

Compared with those in flesh, bite marks in food are stable evidence and, while it is possible to take impressions from marks in the former using, say, rubber-based impression material, they are not nearly so satisfactory as those that can be obtained from apples, cheese and the like. Nevertheless, all foodstuffs lose moisture and become deformed as they decay and this process must involve any tooth marks present. From the evidential aspect, therefore, impressions must either be taken with a reasonable sense of urgency or it must be established that the specimen was preserved in a solution known to preserve the original size and shape of the material. Within these limitations there is no doubt that models made from foodstuffs can provide positive comparisons with those made from the teeth which are easily understood by juries. What seems less credible is the likelihood of criminals leaving such evidence at the locus in any but extraordinary circumstances—but it does occur with surprising frequency.

The science of bite-mark investigation has developed rapidly over the last quarter of a century; even so, few dentists can claim to be experts and, as a result, it may be difficult for the police to obtain the essential expertise at short notice. The situation probably remains that bite-mark evidence is of firmer value in excluding suspects when there are several rather than in confirming the identity of an assailant.

29

Legal aspects of medical practice

The General Medical Council

Medical registration

A registered medical practitioner is one who is registered with the General Medical Council. While anyone may practice his 'healing art', it is an offence in doing so to pretend to be properly registered. A person who has passed the necessary examination and who has received the relevant diploma (Appendix Q) will be duly qualified but this is, effectively, meaningless without registration.[1] The unregistered person is denied certain privileges and protection and is disqualified from holding medical office under the Crown, from holding medical appointments in the public services and from practising under the aegis of the National Health Service Acts.[2] An unregistered practitioner cannot prescribe or supply certain poisons (see Chapter 22) nor sign valid medical certificates required under many statutes.[3]

This supervision is based on sequential Medical Acts, of which the first was passed in 1858 and the most recent is dated 1983. The principal cumulative effect of these has been to establish the General Medical Council.[4] Similar councils are established for the dental profession, nursing and allied professions, pharmacists, opticians and makers of hearing aids;[5] it is to be noted that so-called 'alternative medicine' is also gaining increasing official recognition.[6] We are,

---

1 Medical Act 1983, ss 15, 16, 56.
2 National Health Service (General Medical Services) Regulations 1992, SI 1992/635, reg 2.
3 Eg Births and Deaths Registration Act 1953, ss 22, 41.
4 As at 1998, the General Medical Council consisted of 107 members. Membership included the President and 52 elected members together with 25 members appointed by the universities having medical schools and by the Royal Colleges and Faculties; the majority of professional members must be elected. Twenty-five members of the public were nominated by the Queen in Council; the majority of nominated members must be lay persons (General Medical Council (Constitution) Order 1979, SI 1979/112, as amended). The four Chief Medical Officers of the UK filled the remaining places. Current plans are to increase the number of lay persons on the Council.
5 Dentists Act 1984; Pharmacy Act 1954; Opticians Act 1989; Hearing Aid Council Acts 1968 and 1969. Health Act 1999, s 60 and Sch 3, replaces the previous council with the Nursing, Midwifery and Health Visiting Council. The Professions Supplementary to Medicine Act 1960 is repealed.
6 Eg Osteopaths Act 1993; Chiropractors Act 1994.

however, here concerned in the main with the General Medical Council which has the following major functions:

- To maintain the official list of medical practitioners.
- To supervise standards of medical education.
- To exercise discipline over the medical profession and to lay down standards of fitness to practise.

In addition, the Council is responsible for supervising the employment and registration of overseas doctors.

The official register

The register contains the names of all fully and provisionally registered practitioners on 1 January of the year in question. Entries in the main register for those practitioners undergoing a compulsory year of postgraduate training are marked by an asterisk; during this time of provisional registration their practice is limited to their appointment. Those who have completed specialist training are now annotated as specialists in the register.[7]

An annual retention fee of £135 is currently levied and it is within the powers of the registrar to erase a practitioner's name by reason of non-payment of this fee; there is a £120 charge for reinstatement. Erasure may follow loss of contact with the practitioner or as a result of disciplinary action.[8] Reinstatement involves a charge of £135 in the former case; in the latter, provision is made for suspension as an alternative to erasure.

Doctors who have qualified overseas may obtain full British registration if they have qualifications approved for the purpose by the General Medical Council,[9] if they have held a year's appointment as a resident house officer in an approved hospital or institution and if they have an adequate command of English. Provisional registration can be granted to overseas practitioners with recognised qualifications on the same basis as it is available to United Kingdom graduates— that is, their practice is limited to resident posts in hospitals or institutions approved for the purpose of pre-registration service. Limited registration, for which a separate register is kept, is granted in respect of practice only under the supervision of a fully registered practitioner. It is available for a maximum of five years to doctors with a wide range of qualifications outwith the United Kingdom who have already been offered an appointment. To be registered, the practitioners must have undertaken an internship of at least one year and have passed a test in English. Before proceeding to full registration they must either pass a test of professional knowledge and competence or satisfy the General Medical Council in another way. In the event of refusal of full registration or of extension of limited registration, there is a right of appeal to a review board for Overseas Qualified Practitioners.[10]

---

7 European Specialists Medical Qualifications Order 1995, SI 1995/3208, art 3.
8 Voluntary erasure is also possible on application.
9 Medical Act 1983, s 19. Currently, the qualifications relate to specified universities in Australia, New Zealand, South Africa, Hong Kong, Singapore, Malaysia (limited registration only) and the West Indies.
10 General Medical Council (Review Board for Overseas Qualified Practitioners) Rules Order of Council 1979, SI 1979/29.

Doctors who are nationals of and qualified in states of the European Economic Area are entitled to full registration as of right.[11]

Supervision of educational standards

The Education Committee which, alone of the Council's committees, contains a majority of appointed members, can look into the courses given by, and the methods of examination practice in, the universities and other bodies empowered to grant qualification for registration. The Committee oversees the training given in the pre-registration year and has the power to visit any approved hospital or institution to assess the tuition provided. There is also a responsibility for advising on continuing postgraduate education. The competent authority overseeing specialist training—and the subsequent issue of the certificate of completion of specialist training—is, however, the newly formed Specialist Training Authority of the Medical Royal Colleges.[12]

Professional conduct and performance

Although the General Medical Council may itself instigate actions against doctors on information received, it most commonly acts only in the event of an allegation being made as to the conduct of a registered medical practitioner. There are two main ways in which the Council may become aware of matters needing their attention in a disciplinary role:

1. On a doctor's conviction of a criminal offence by a court in Great Britain and Ireland (including Eire) or in the Isle of Man or the Channel Islands, the Clerk of the Court will inform the Council of the fact. This applies also to courts martial. A doctor justifiably cited as co-respondent in the Family Division of the High Court in a case involving a patient would also be reported but the number of such cases has greatly reduced since divorce laws were revolutionised in 1969.
2. Complaints against a doctor's conduct may be made by members of the public, including other doctors acting in a private capacity, or by such bodies as a Health Authority (Health Board in Scotland), a Hospital Trust or the relevant Department of Health. An individual complaint must be supported by one or more statutory declarations which must include the name and description of the complainant.

Until 1995, the remit of the Council's disciplinary tribunal was to decide whether a doctor was or was not guilty of 'serious professional misconduct', which is to say that his conduct was such 'as would reasonably be regarded as disgraceful or dishonourable by his professional brethren of good repute and competency'.[13] Thus, to a large extent, serious professional misconduct was a matter of professional

---

11 Medical Act 1983, ss 3, 17.
12 Established under European Specialist Medical Qualifications Order 1995, SI 1995/3208. The Authority consists of 21 members of which four are appointed by the Secretary of State and two by the GMC; the remainder are appointed by the Colleges and their Faculties. The list of recognised specialities has been amended (SIs 1997/2928, 1999/1373, 1999/3154) but the amendments are, generally, of a semantic nature only.
13 *Allinson v General Council of Medical Education and Registration* [1894] 1 QB 750 at 763 per Lopes LJ.

behaviour to be judged on current public attitudes. As a result, the tribunal's power was seriously deficient in that no allowance was made for control of the incompetent rather than the dishonourable doctor; undoubtedly, the public expected that it would be protected from the frankly bad practitioner and was, at the same time, ignorant of the vacuum that existed. This was rectified by the Medical (Professional Performance) Act 1995. It will be convenient to discuss the Council's resulting two major powers separately.

Professional misconduct

In the usual and traditional case, information is first laid by the registrar before the person, or screener, who is nominated by the President to undertake the initial consideration of cases. He or she will reject complaints that are obviously insignificant. The remainder of those that are concerned with professional misconduct will be passed to the Preliminary Proceedings Committee, who may invite the doctor to explain his behaviour.[14] A number of options are then open. In an emergency, the Preliminary Proceedings Committee may itself order an interim suspension or conditional registration for a period not exceeding six months. Otherwise, the case may be dismissed or it is referred either to the Professional Conduct Committee or to the Health Committee.[15]

The Professional Conduct Committee is advised on questions of law by an Assessor of at least ten years' general qualification and the hearings conform to the practices of a court of law.[16] The respondent may be represented, usually through his protection or defence society, and there is provision in all parts of the United Kingdom for appeal to the Privy Council against suspension or erasure (see below). A similar right of appeal applies to a dentist appearing before the General Dental Council and to those arraigned before other comparable paramedical councils.[17] Findings in a previous court of law are accepted as factual and may not be argued. The hearings are public, this being a source of justifiable complaint—no matter what his innocence in relation to professional conduct, a doctor's standing in a community can seldom be unaffected by sensational reportage of his private life. The Committee has discretion to hear parts of the evidence in camera if so requested by any party to the case;[18] the Committee can, itself, make such a direction in the

14 General Medical Council Preliminary Proceedings Committee and Professional Conduct Committee (Procedure) Rules Order of Council 1988, SI 1988/2255 as amended. The role of the screener has recently been criticised: *R v General Medical Council, ex p Toth* (2000) unreported. As a result, relevant materials will be disclosed to a complainant in order to comply with the Human Rights Act 1998, Sch 1, arts 6 and 10.

15 The Professional Conduct Committee consists of 30 persons composed of the President and his two nominees, 16 elected members, seven appointed members and seven lay members. Eleven members are invited to attend the hearing of any case and these must include at least six elected, two appointed and two lay members in addition to the chairman or deputy chairman. A quorum consists of five members of which at least one must be a lay member (General Medical Council (Constitution of Fitness to Practise Committees) Rules Order of Council 1996, SI 1996/2125).

16 But although exercising judicial powers, the GMC is not part of the judicial system of the state: *General Medical Council v British Broadcasting Corpn* [1998] 3 All ER 426.

17 The conduct of the GMC is subject to judicial review both as to the advice which it may now give and to the actions of the PCC: *R v General Medical Council, ex p Colman* [1990] 1 All ER 489; *R v General Medical Council, ex p Gee* [1987] 1 All ER 1204.

18 General Medical Council Preliminary Proceedings Committee and Professional Conduct Committee (Procedure) Rules Order of Council, SI 1988/2255, r 48.

absence of a request. The Professional Conduct Committee has only two courses open to it—to dismiss the complaint or to find the allegations proved and amounting to serious professional misconduct.

After a finding of proven 'serious professional misconduct',[19] the Professional Conduct Committee may postpone sentence, in which case the practitioner is, in effect, put on probation, or it may suspend the doctor's registration for a period not exceeding 12 months, which can be extended. In addition, the Committee may make a doctor's registration conditional upon compliance with such requirements as the Committee may impose for the protection of members of the public or in his own interest. The most severe penalty is that of erasure from the register. Apart from the general right to appeal to the Privy Council,[20] applications for restoration to the register may, in this case, be made at any time after ten months have elapsed and thereafter at intervals of 11 months.[1]

In general, there is no delimiting definition of serious professional misconduct, but the Committee is likely to regard as most serious any misconduct that implies that the doctor has taken advantage of his privileges and of his special training and position as a professional man. Thus, false certification and the improper prescription of—or self-indulgence in—drugs are bound to be censured; in the latter case, further action may be taken by the Secretary of State under the Misuse of Drugs Act 1971[2] (see Chapter 22).

Several of the traditional reasons for erasure are no longer significant. We have already seen (Chapter 18) that the very wide terms of the amended Abortion Act 1967 make it very difficult to perform an illegal termination in Great Britain provided that the necessary documentation is completed; there simply is no need for the doctor to undertake such a procedure. Similarly, a combination of permissive legislation and increasingly liberal public attitudes has greatly reduced the number of cases of adultery that are reported; the PCC would, however, take a very serious view of a doctor who abused his privileges so as to obtain consensual sexual intercourse with a member of his patient's household. Other manifest criminal abuses of position, such as indecent assault or attempted rape, will be likely to reach the Committee by virtue of notification from a criminal court and will, then, be irrebuttable.[3]

There has, in fact, been something of a sea-change in what constitutes professional misconduct. Advertising is a case in point. On the one hand, the age

---

19 The standard of proof normally required is that applicable to civil proceedings: *McAllister v General Medical Council* [1993] 1 All ER 982, PC.

20 The Privy Council will be very reluctant to interfere with a Council's 'professional' findings: see eg *Carmichael v General Dental Council* (1989) 4 BMLR 80. The Council has, however, recently drawn attention to a possible distinction to be made between sentencing for professional misconduct and sentencing where the offence was based on proof of conviction: *Dad v General Dental Council* [2000] 1 WLR 1538.

1 This is, currently, a major bone of contention. It has been authoritatively suggested that the minimum period for erasure should be five years: L Beecham 'UK Government Wants GMC to be given Stronger Powers' (2000) 320 BMJ 890.

2 Although, alternatively, the doctor may be judged by the Health Committee (see below).

3 The most frequent cause for notification following conviction stems from the abuse of alcohol, particularly in association with the more mundane Road Traffic Acts. Most first offences are dealt with by warning letter, but repeated convictions will attract more serious action in the end—often by way of the Health Committee (see below).

of 'instant television' and the widespread interest in medical matters have dictated a relaxation of the old—and very strict—rule of professional anonymity in public. The current view seems to be that, as long as a doctor is already a recognised authority in the field under discussion, the public have a reasonable right to know his name and its publication would not constitute an offence provided the doctor was not using a television interview to raise his professional reputation or to attract patients. Criticism of a fellow practitioner, whether unwitting or intended, would also attract censure unless it could be justified in the public interest—and, in this respect, doctors are now encouraged to report instances of inadequacy in their colleagues directly to the Council.[4] From the other aspect, the rules as to 'pure' advertising of services on offer have also been revolutionised since a ban on so doing was referred to the Monopolies and Mergers Commission, which held it to be improper. The current position is that: 'Doctors may provide factual information about their professional qualifications and services . . . in any form to the public or other members of the profession.'[5] It is, however, to be noted that the courts are sympathetic to the General Medical Council's antagonism to advertising in the newspapers.[6]

The main driving force behind the changing pattern of what is regarded as serious professional misconduct lies, however, in the increasing acceptance of what might be called 'patients' rights'. Thus, the majority of referrals to the Professional Conduct Committee now relate to matters such as rudeness to patients, failure to visit and the like.[7] In fact, the somewhat aloof and introspective attitude of the General Medical Council—and its apparent concern for the good of the profession rather than that of its patients—is coming under increasing attack.[8] For example, no mention has yet been made of professional negligence. This is because, except in unusual circumstances, medical negligence is a matter of civil litigation, as is any other tort or delict, rather than one for the GMC, and is discussed under that heading in the following chapter.

Deficiency in standards of performance

We have, however, noted that the General Medical Council is now empowered to review the general professional performance of registered medical practitioners. This is a matter for the Committee on Professional Performance.

If the doctor's standard of professional performance is in issue, the medical screener may reject the application, but only if he or she has consulted a lay screener who agrees. Otherwise, he or she will direct the case to the Assessment

---

4   The employment status of health care workers who report their colleagues is now protected: Public Interest Disclosure Act 1998.

5   For a history of this change in attitude, see D H Irvine 'The Advertising of Doctors' Services' (1991) 17 J Med Ethics 35.

6   *R v General Medical Council, ex p Colman* [1990] 1 All ER 489. A subsequent claim to European recognition of a right to advertise was rejected by the European Commission on Human Rights.

7   Twenty-six out of 53 cases of alleged serious professional misconduct heard by the Professional Conduct Committee in 1993 related to disregard of professional responsibilities to patients. All resulted in a verdict of guilty and the doctor's name was erased from the register in 12 instances. Similar breakdowns are not now available.

8   Possibly since the major critical review by M Stacey *Regulating British Medicine* (1992). At the time of writing, the media are exposing 'medical scandals' on a regular basis. It is customary to blame the GMC but the Council has, in fact, been powerless to act under existing legislation.

Referral Committee, which, after consideration, may pass it to the Committee on Professional Performance. By contrast with the basically punitive function of the Professional Conduct Committee, that of the Committee on Professional Performance (CCP) is essentially remedial and protective of the public against bad doctoring rather than against bad doctors. The intention is that this should be achieved in a four-step fashion—screening, assessment, remedy and, in the last resort, sanctions. Thus, the greater part of the CPP's work is conducted on a voluntary basis with the co-operation of the doctor concerned and consists of providing advice and retraining.[9] The 1983 statute, as amended, is, however, concerned with the last eventuality and, here, the Committee's powers are severe but, at the same time, also limited.

Essentially, s 1 of the 1995 Act inserts s 36A to the Medical Act 1983 and this allows the CPP to suspend an incompetent doctor's registration for up to 12 months or to permit him or her to practice subject to compliance with such conditions as the Committee requires. Failure in the latter circumstance can result in suspension for a further 12 months. The Committee can extend a period of suspension or it can add a period of up to three years' conditional registration to a suspension that has expired—but it can do this only on a yearly basis. A period of suspension that has lasted for more than two years can be extended indefinitely should the Committee find it necessary for the protection of the public but an indefinite suspension must be reviewed at two-yearly intervals at the request of the doctor concerned.

Section 2 of the 1995 Act inserts s 31A to the Medical Act 1983, under which the doctor who feels he has lost his ability to perform adequately can apply for voluntary removal of his name from the register. His name can be restored at his request subject to the Committee's approval. A 'seriously deficient standard of performance' is not defined in the Act. Rather as in the case of professional misconduct, it is left to the Committee on Professional Performance to establish its own standards and to judge each case on its own merits.

Fitness to practise

The Medical Act 1978 established a Health Committee of the General Medical Council. A doctor's fitness to practise may be questioned by individuals or official bodies. Such doubts as appear to have substance are referred to the Preliminary Proceedings Committee, which, again, has the authority to order an interim suspension or conditional registration for up to six months. The Preliminary Proceedings Committee may take expert medical opinion before deciding whether to refer the case to the Health Committee, which consists of the President or his appointee, a member of the General Medical Council, and seven other members; the total membership must include five elected members, two appointed and two lay members.[10] The question to be put to the Health Committee is whether the

---

9 Hearings before the CPP are, currently, in private. A number of doctors have been referred for retraining but suspension or striking-off under the General Medical Council (Professional Performance) Rules Order of Council 1997, SI 1997/1529 is rare: S Kirwin 'First Doctor Suspended under GMC Performance Procedures' (1999) 318 BMJ 10. Five performance assessments were completed in 1999: GMC *Changing Times, Changing Culture* (1999).
10 General Medical Council (Constitution of Fitness to Practise Committees) Rules Order of Council 1996, SI 1996/2125.

practitioner is seriously impaired by reason of his or her physical or mental condition. The Committee must arrange for an examination by two independent practitioners and the subject under review may have an examination by a doctor of his or her own choice. The hearings are in private and legal representation is allowed. The Health Committee may, if they find the case proved, order conditional registration or suspension for not more than 12 months. The President must confer with two other Council members before taking action. An appeal to the Privy Council against a ruling of the Health Committee can be made only on a point of law.

Further control in the interests of patients

The traditional clinical freedom accorded to the medical profession is now being controlled in other ways both in the general public interest and following the demands of modern health economics. Two new organisations have been established with these in mind. The Committee for Health Improvement (CHIMP) was set up by the Health Act 1999, s 19 and underpins the duty of National Health Trusts and Professional Care Trusts to ensure the quality of care that they are providing. CHIMP is essentially an enforcement agency and will visit all trusts periodically to ensure that clinical governance arrangements meet the national standards. CHIMP's inspectors will also monitor the implementation of the recommendations made by the parallel National Institute for Clinical Excellence (NICE). NICE was established as a special health authority[11] within the National Health Service with an educative role. It will produce and disseminate clinical guidelines based on evidence as to the best practices in clinical audit; clearly, it will be a brave or foolhardy doctor who ignores such advice as is given. NICE will offer guidance and will be able to report individuals and organisations that are failing in their task. In addition to these organisations, the Department of Health will, itself, produce National Service Frameworks, which will outline policies based on clinical and cost effectiveness that are to be adopted in major care areas and disease groups. Clearly, the next few years will see increasingly centralised control not only of the doctor's conduct but also of his or her clinical activities.

The doctor and the National Health Service

The practice of medicine in the National Health Service is currently managed by way of health authorities (health boards in Scotland), NHS trusts and primary care trusts. The sharp distinction which had developed between services provided by hospitals and those provided in the community has been softened by the Health Authorities Act 1995, which made the health authorities responsible for primary care and hospital and community services (as Scottish health boards always have been), and by the National Health Service (Primary Care) Act 1997, which advocated a more diverse approach to management. Even so, the contrasting

11 National Institute for Clinical Excellence (Establishment and Constitution) Order 1999, SI 1999/220. Under an amendment order, SI 1999/2219, meetings of NICE must be open to the public.

concepts of doctors being servants of the hospital in which they serve but contractors in general practice remain. There is no doubt that hospital authorities— the great majority of which are now self-accountable National Health Service trusts—are liable for the actions of all their staff irrespective of their seniority and their consequent freedom to adopt working methods of their own choice. The liability of a master (ie the hospital) for the wrongful or negligent acts of his servants extends throughout the hospital hierarchy from non-medical staff to senior consultants.[12] At one time, all hospital medical staff in the National Health Service were required to belong to a defence society. Costs have escalated to such an extent that they are now protected by the centrally funded Clinical Negligence Scheme;[13] general practitioners are specifically excluded from this indemnity but they must now provide private cover.[14]

The general practitioner is not a servant of the health authority or board, but, in providing his services, he accepts certain terms of contract which have been drawn up in the interests of the patients who depend upon the service. Breach of responsibility in relation to contracts may be the subject of complaint either by the administration itself or by the patient, or by the patient's spouse or (if the patient is deceased, ill or young) by any person; the practitioner is also liable for lapses by his nursing or secretarial staff and by any registered medical practitioner acting as his deputy.[15]

The terms of contract accepted by a practitioner in the Health Service[16] include that he is obliged to take medical responsibility for patients on his list and for certain other relatively minor categories which include any person in need of emergency treatment. A patient may leave the list of a doctor immediately if he obtains that doctor's signature on his medical card and another practitioner accepts him; without the doctor's signature, he must give notice to the health authority and must wait 14 days before he can register with another doctor.[17] The practitioner can ask the relevant Committee to remove the name of a patient from his list in which case he must inform the Committee if he is treating him or her once a week or more often. Transfer can still take place immediately upon acceptance by another doctor but, in the absence of such acceptance, the doctor must inform the Committee when he ceases to treat the patient at intervals of seven days or less.

---

12 The case law on vicarious liability has shown a logical progression and now includes responsibility for the whole staff including those temporary or part time (*Roe v Minister of Health, Woolley v same* [1954] 2 QB 66; *Razzell v Snowball* [1954] 1 WLR 1382) and visiting consultants (*Higgins v North West Metropolitan Hospital Board and Bach* [1954] 1 WLR 411). Scots practice was brought into line with that of England in *McDonald v Glasgow Western Hospitals and Hayward v Board of Management of Royal Infirmary Edinburgh* 1954 SC 453.

13 National Health Service (Clinical Negligence Scheme) Regulations 1996, SI 1996/251. Department of Health *Claims of Medical Negligence against Hospital and Community Doctors and Dentists* HC (89) 34. Responsibility passes to NHS trusts where appropriate: NHS Management Executive EC (90) 195 and EC (91) 19.

14 Health Act 1999, s 9 inserts s 43C into the National Health Service Act 1977. The hospital doctor would be well advised to do so also as the scheme covers work done for the NHS only.

15 The practitioner must now set up a 'practice based complaints procedure' and must inform his patients of its existence; he must specify a person, who may be unconnected with the practice who will be responsible for receiving and investigating all complaints: para 47A is added to the National Health Service (General Medical Services) Regulations 1992 , SI 92/635) Sch 2.

16 Fn 2 above, p 439, Sch 2.

17 National Health Service (Choice of Medical Practitioner) Regulations 1998, SI 1998/668.

Inevitably, conflict must occasionally arise as to the interpretation of the terms of contract, the commonest source of complaint being from those patients who believe they have received inadequate consideration; these are mainly dealt with by way of the practice-based complaints procedure.[18] However, every health authority must now establish discipline committees[19]—related to doctors, dentists, pharmacists, etc and including a joint discipline committee—the basic function of which is to investigate allegations that a practitioner is failing to comply with his or her terms of service.

Discipline committees consist of a chairman, who must be a solicitor or barrister, appointed by the health authority, together with not more than three lay persons appointed by the health authority and not more than three professionals also appointed by the health authority but from a list provided by the local representative committee.[20] Having received an allegation, the health authority can:

- take no further action; or
- refer the matter to another health authority for investigation; and/or
- refer it to the tribunal (see below), to the relevant professional body (eg the GMC, GDC etc),[1] or the local police authority as considered appropriate.

The independent health authority will investigate such a referral through its own discipline committee and must inform the practitioner as to the nature of its case within 28 days of the referral.

Hearings before the discipline committee are of little interest to the legal profession, as they are held in private and the practitioner can be represented only by a friend—a legally qualified friend cannot examine witnesses or address the committee. The discipline committee will report to the appropriate health authority as to its findings of fact and the inferences it has drawn, together with recommendations as to action that should be taken. The health authority can, as a result, take no action or can fine the practitioner by way of a deduction from his or her remuneration.

In the latter event, there is provision for appeal within 30 days—including an appeal on the findings of fact—to the Secretary of State who, if he does not dismiss the appeal on documentary evidence, can call for an oral hearing by an Appeal Body consisting of a lawyer and two relevant professionals. The hearing is, again, in private but legal representation is permitted on both sides.

Allegations that the inclusion of a practitioner's name in the appropriate list is prejudicial to the welfare of the service (efficiency cases) or that the practitioner is guilty of fraud (fraud cases) carry with them the possibility of disqualification. In such an event, the health authority may refer the matter to the NHS Tribunal.[2]

---

18 Fn 15 above.
19 National Health Service (Service Committees and Tribunal) Regulations 1992, SI 92/664, as substantially amended by the Amendment Regulations 1996, SI 1996/703.
20 A body of professionals who are recognised by the health authority as representative of the professionals in the area.
 1 National Health Service (Service Committees and Tribunal) Regulations 1992, SI 1992/664, reg 37, added by Amendment Regulations, SI 1996/703, reg 11.
 2 National Health Service Act 1977, s 46, as substituted by the Health Act 1999, s 40.

The tribunal is chaired by a solicitor or barrister of at least ten years' standing and contains two persons nominated by the Secretary of State, one of whom is a professional. The practitioner may be represented before the tribunal which normally sits in private unless the respondent wishes it to be in public.[3] Should the tribunal find the conditions in the allegation proved, it must disqualify the practitioner from inclusion in the list to which the case relates and may impose a national disqualification—effectively finding the respondent unfit to practise (1977 Act, s 46B). The tribunal can also impose a conditional disqualification. There is a right of appeal to the Secretary of State, who will be represented by a single relevant professional and the tribunal itself may review a disqualification on request.

It will be seen that there is something of a contrast between the publicity afforded to hearings before the General Medical Council and the privacy of investigations under the National Health Service Act. The latter processes are, however, cumbersome and lengthy; they also lead to considerable individual stress and are extravagant of public money.

Discipline in the hospital service

The maintenance of discipline within NHS hospitals is a complicated process which is specifically allowed for in the doctors' or dentists' contracts of employment. Different procedures apply according to whether the case is one of personal conduct[4] or is an issue of professional conduct or competence[5]—a distinction that is often hard to define. The former cases are investigated by the chief executive or his deputy, subject to an appeal to a committee consisting of three appropriate authority members; the doctor or dentist may state his or her case at this hearing, may call and cross-examine witnesses and may be represented.

Cases relating to professional competence are, again, dealt with in different fashion according to their seriousness.[6] The less serious accusations are dealt with through two external assessors nominated by the Joint Consultative Committee of the region, who interview willing witnesses of their choosing— including the practitioner concerned—in private. They report to the Chief Administrative Medical Officer and Director of Public Health, who decides on the action to be taken. The more serious cases are, first, dealt with by the chairman of the health authority—at which stage the practitioner may be suspended from duty as a precautionary measure. Given that a prima facie case has been established, a full inquiry may be mounted[7] and conducted by a legal chairman with either two professional members in cases involving competence

---

3   National Health Service Act 1977, s 49(a).
4   *Whitley Councils for the Health Services of Great Britain, Conditions of Service*, s 40.
5   *Disciplinary Proceedings in Cases Relating to Hospital Medical and Dental Staff* (1990) Department of Health Circular HC (90) 9. Somewhat surprisingly, the recommendations have not been substantially changed in the last decade.
6   The health authority or board may take immediate action against a practitioner when this is required in cases of a very serious nature.
7   But it might well not be called if the facts have been established by another inquiry or tribunal. For a full analysis, see B Raymond 'The Employment Rights of the NHS Hospital Doctor' in C Dyer (ed) *Doctors, Patients and the Law* (1992).

or a professional and a lay member in issues of conduct; the hearing is adversarial and the practitioner may be represented. The panel report to the health authority, whose decision is subject to an appeal to the Secretary of State; the Secretary of State must then, himself, set up an advisory professional committee which may or may not hear witnesses as it chooses. It is to be noted that these highly stylised procedures apply only to consultants and those of equivalent status. Objectionable or incompetent juniors are subject to justice of a far more summary nature.

Discipline in the future

The reader will have noted that the functions of the various committees overlap in ways that may, at times, appear illogical.[8] A prime example is that of the so-called 'Bristol heart cases' of 1998, in which 29 babies died following heart surgery.[9] Three doctors, including the Chief Executive of the NHS trust concerned were charged before the PCC. All were convicted of serious professional misconduct but only two were erased from the register; these included the one in an administrative position.[10] None was brought before the CPP and none were investigated under the disciplinary codes of the National Health Service. Compounding the confusion, a ministerial public inquiry was set up as soon as the proceedings within the General Medical Council were completed—and the possibilities of both civil and criminal litigation remain open.

A number of 'scandals' related to substandard treatment have been publicised both politically and in the popular press during the preparation of this edition and a feature common to all has been the tendency to place the blame on the General Medical Council. We have seen, however, that the Council's powers are strictly limited by statute and, in many of the cases, direct pre-emptive action would have been impossible. What the cases have, in fact, demonstrated is not so much that the General Medical Council is an incompetent anachronism, as that its powers need to be brought into line with modern concepts and expectations. This has received some recognition in what can often be seen as 'knee-jerk' legislative responses—the government, for example, can now make major changes to the professional Councils without having to lay their proposals before Parliament.[11] This reactive approach can, perhaps, be best seen in the case of Dr Shipman, who, as the prototype medical multiple murderer, surely merits his place in a book on forensic medicine.[12] In this author's view, the blame for Dr Shipman's long immunity to justice lies in the regulations for death certification and cremation (for which see page 75), which are the responsibility of the Home Office rather than the Department of Health. The case, at the time of writing is the

---

8 For little more than the sake of completeness, it might be mentioned that excessive prescribing may, within a time-span of two years, be referred to the professional committee consisting of three doctors, one of whom is selected by the Secretary of State as having substantial experience of clinical pharmacology.

9 C Dyer 'Bristol Doctors Found Guilty of Serious Professional Misconduct' (1998) 316 BMJ 1924.

10 *Roylance v General Medical Council (No 2)* [2000] 1 AC 311. The Privy Council appreciated the anomaly but would not alter the decision of the PCC.

11 Health Act 1999, s 60 and Sch 3.

12 B O'Neill 'Doctor as Murderer' (2000) 320 BMJ 329. Dr Shipman was found guilty of the murder of 15 patients and it is widely conjectured that this is an underestimate.

subject of another ministerial inquiry; meantime, regulations that are of a predominantly medical nature have been rushed through in order to plug what one would hope to be a very rare gap in the defences of the public health.[13]

The doctor outwith the Health Service

Doctors working wholly in private practice have similar responsibilities to their patients, which are based not only on medical ethics but also on the law of contract between provider and consumer. The aggrieved private patient has little recourse other than through the courts, where he could bring an action either in tort or in contract. Even then, in the event of treatment being considered to be of inadequate quality as, for example, by failure to make a home visit when asked, the patient would probably need to show that damage had resulted before an action taken against the doctor would succeed; a complaint could, however, be laid before the General Medical Council. Such conditions must be rare in private practice, where economic laws operate as effectively as do the statutory rules of the Health Service.

Employment in industry carries some ethical difficulties. If employed as a Health Officer, the doctor still must base his professional conduct on a doctor-patient relationship; the acceptance of a contract involving disclosure of confidential information to employers against the wishes of the persons in medical care would certainly lead to a charge of unethical conduct against which there would be no defence. The factory doctor should firmly dissociate his function from that of an employee's regular medical attendant. Other problems in industry—for example, those associated with research, advertising and the like—might arise and are dealt with below.

On the face of things, the position of medical officers in the armed forces is equivocal, in that they are the regular medical practitioners of the service personnel and yet at the same time are paid by and clearly owe an allegiance to the Crown which also employs their patients. The principle governing medical practice in relation to servicemen—but not their dependants—must be modified to some extent in favour of the need to benefit the specialised 'community' as a whole. Two main factors work to minimise difficulties which are often the subject of ill-informed exaggeration. In the first place, by accepting service in the armed forces, the patients appreciate that they have accepted both the advantages and disadvantages of a corporate system while, secondly, the service authorities themselves are only too anxious to preserve a normal doctor-patient relationship in all matters that do not directly and adversely affect the efficiency of a fighting unit.

Complaints procedures in the National Health Service

It is to be noted that internal discipline and matters for complaint by patients or their representatives are very firmly dissociated within the NHS. None the less,

---

13 National Health Service (General Medical Services) Amendment Regulations 2000, SI 2000/220. A doctor applying for a position must now declare his or her criminal history and the health authority must remove from their list any doctor they know to have been sentenced to more than six months' imprisonment. For Scotland, see SI 2000/28.

this is an appropriate point at which to outline the statutory remedies open to the dissatisfied patient.[14]

A complaint against an NHS organisation or an individual health carer, whether of a clinical or an administrative nature, is dealt with under the umbrella of the Hospital Complaints Procedure Act 1995— in fact, the procedures adopted are the same whether the complaint arises within a hospital setting or in general practice.[15] A hospital or primary care trust[16] or health authority must nominate, and publicise the name of, a complaints manager, who will 'screen' the complaint for validity. Normally, and in virtually every case in which there is a written complaint, an internal inquiry will then be carried out by a member of the staff. In the event that a complainant is dissatisfied, the case is referred to an appointed convenor, who may set up an inquiry by an independent review panel. This consists of three lay persons who will, in the event that the complaint refers to clinical matters, be assisted by professional assessors. The panel meets in private but both the complainant and the person complained about must have access to the proceedings and must be allowed to plead their case; professional legal representation is not, however, allowed. Following the review, the report is distributed to all the principals including the chairman and the chief executive of the trust or authority concerned. The chief executive will then inform the complainant of the outcome and also of his or her right to complain to the Health Service Commissioner. In very serious cases, the minister may order a public inquiry under the National Health Service Act 1977, s 84—and, indeed, a number of such inquiries related to mass patient protests are sitting at the time of writing.

The Health Service Commissioners

The functions of the Health Service Commissioners for England and Scotland are now consolidated in the Health Service Commissioners Act 1993.[17] The Commissioners are empowered to investigate complaints made directly by individuals or bodies of persons other than a public authority (s 8)—subject to a general one-year limitation period. The complaints can relate to failures in the service provided, failure to provide a service, maladministration and to allegations that a person has sustained injustice or hardship in consequence of their provision by a number of bodies including health authorities (or health boards in Scotland), NHS trusts and primary care trusts or other facilities that are contracted to provide services for the NHS. The inquiries are private; the Commissioners can decide

---

14 There is, of course, nothing to prevent, and a great deal to commend, a health trust or authority setting up an internal inquiry of their own in the event of a mishap (NHS Circular 1977 (GEN) 13). However, evidence given to such an investigation is not necessarily privileged: *Lask v Gloucester Health Authority* [1991] 2 Med LR 379. The use of such a report in disciplinary proceedings is strictly limited.

15 National Health Service Executive *Guidance on Implementation of the NHS Complaints Procedure* (1996). The details are to be found in *Directions to NHS Trusts, Health Authorities and Special Health Authorities for Special Hospitals on Hospital Complaints Procedures* (March, 1996).

16 Section 1A, inserted by the Health Authorities Act 1995, Sch 1, art 109; s 1B inserted by the Health Care Act 1999, Sch 4, art 71(c).

17 As amended by the Health Service Commissioners (Amendment) Act 1996. A further amendment Bill is currently going through Parliament. The functions of the Health Service Commissioner for Wales are now stated in the Government of Wales Act 1998, Sch 10.

themselves whether there is a case for investigation and can regulate their own procedure—the latter can, however, include representation by legal professionals. The Commissioners cannot investigate any action taken by the health authority when acting in its disciplinary capacity (s 6(3)) and, of greatest importance, they are specifically excluded from action in any case in which the complainant has a remedy available through a court of law or other statutory process (s 4(1)). It is to be noted that they now have jurisdiction to examine the merits of clinical decisions (s 3(7)). In the event that a claim is substantiated and has not been remedied, the report can be sent to each House of Parliament.

Section 4(5) of the 1993 Act specifies that the Commissioner shall not conduct an investigation unless satisfied that other remedies have been invoked and exhausted including those that have been discussed above. Complaints to the Health Service Commissioner can be distinct from those investigated under the Hospital Complaints Procedure Act 1985 although, as we have seen, the Commissioner is as, or more, likely to serve as an appeal from what is, in effect, a local Health Service Commission.

30

Medical ethics

One aspect of medical practice that has become increasingly obvious over the last two to three decades is that medical law and medical ethics are indivisible. The classic dictum of Lord Chief Justice Coleridge sums it up:

> 'It would not be correct to say that every moral obligation involves a legal duty; but every legal duty is founded on a moral obligation.'[1]

It follows that forensic medicine must consider medical matters that are not, as yet, covered by established law but for which the law is currently seeking a consensus given the pluralistic nature of modern society. The legal answers to such problems are to be found in the courts; as a result, the lawyer's contact with medicine is likely to be greatest in the minefields of the ethics of modern medicine; the purpose of this chapter is to take a brief look at some of these areas. At the same time, it has to be admitted that much of the ethos of medical practice represents a purely intraprofessional code of conduct; this used to be described as medical ethics but, today, it is far better regarded as medical etiquette. The maintenance of good professional relations devolves mainly on the professional associations, whether they be of an academic or a political nature, and seldom involves the lawyer. Ethics and etiquette often intermix but, here, we will avoid the latter save where it has a strong influence on the former.

The medical code

It is doubtful whether any universities now require the recitation of the 'Hippocratic Oath' at graduation, though a shortened *sponsio academica* is acknowledged by graduands at, at least, the Universities of Edinburgh and Glasgow. None the less, even when there is no such requirement, it is a reasonable assumption that the act of qualifying for registration implies acceptance of a code that has been fashioned over centuries of development; it is worth reiterating the main components of what is held to be the original work.[2]

---

1   *R v Instan* [1893] 1 QB 450 at 453.
2   For this and other medical declarations, see J K Mason and R A McCall Smith *Law and Medical Ethics* (5th edn, 1999) Appendices A–F.

The primary consideration is the welfare of the patient; not only is a general affirmation given to apply one's skills to his or her benefit but it is positively declared to be improper to do anything that might be expected to harm the patient. Euthanasia and abortion are specifically condemned and, by implication, so is exceeding one's skill in undertaking specialist treatment. Improper association with patients or their families is barred and, finally, much importance is attached to what is now known as professional confidence.

These principles, together with those arising from many barbarities peculiar to the twentieth century, are restated in the Declaration of Geneva, which was approved by the World Medical Association and was last amended in Stockholm in 1994.

It is surprising that a declaration approved so recently as 1994 is directed almost entirely to standards applicable to the medical profession itself—the interests of the patient are considered only indirectly. In practice, the major change in medical ethics in the later parts of the last century can be summarised as the wide acceptance of the patient's autonomy as the driving force in the doctor-patient relationship. Consent has become the cornerstone of modern ethical medical treatment; it is also possibly the most important single cause of contentious medical litigation. Some general principles follow.

Consent to examination and treatment

The examination or treatment of a patient without his or her consent may constitute an assault unless it can be justified under the legal doctrine of necessity. The form of consent is, however, not uniform, and special difficulties may arise in relation to medico-legal examinations that may be positively to the subject's detriment.

There is adequate general judicial comment to make it clear that consent to a routine examination may be taken as implied when the patient presents himself or herself to the surgery or out-patients' department. Even so, the implication only pertains to what the patient would reasonably expect—a patient does not expect a vaginal examination if she complains of a cough, although a really dedicated physician might contend that a *full* examination of every patient is necessary for accurate diagnosis. In this case, he should obtain specific consent to unusual clinical methods and it is well to have such consent given in front of a witness. Examinations of the opposite sex, particularly of women patients by male doctors, should ideally always be chaperoned; unfortunately, the current shortage of nursing staff makes this a counsel of perfection which it is almost impossible to observe.

Minor invasive investigations—such as withdrawal of blood from a vein—which might cause pain and have a very small morbidity can, as a matter of practicality, be undertaken on the basis of oral consent; they are no more than part of the normal practice of patient care. Yet, while any invasion of the patient's privacy is technically an assault which is actionable both in the criminal and civil courts, it should be equally clear that valid consent to medical procedures intended for the benefit of the patient absolves the doctor from blame. The important word here is 'valid' and it is now well established that, to be valid, consent must be in the nature of what is popularly known as 'informed consent'.[3] To achieve this,

---

3 This primarily American expression is now firmly established in United Kingdom medical jurisprudence despite the fact that we have, inter alia, Dunn LJ saying: 'The concept of informed consent forms no part of English law': *Sidaway v Board of Governors of the Bethlem Royal Hospital* [1984] QB 493 at 517.

there must be understandable communication between the doctor and the patient.[4]
The underlying principle is that a patient must be free to make a choice or decision
when such a choice exists; it follows that the wider the choice or the greater the
risks involved in one or other course, the greater must be the communication.[5] For
these reasons, the problems of 'informed consent' are best discussed in relation to
major surgical procedures (see Chapter 31).

The statutory legal age above which valid consent to medical treatment can
be given is now 16 in England.[6] It is the same in Scotland but, there, the minor
below the age of 16 is specifically empowered to consent provided that he or she
fully understands the implications.[7] In England and Wales, the capacity of the
minor below the age of 16 to consent to treatment is governed by *Gillick v West
Norfolk and Wisbech Area Health Authority,*[8] in which case it was held that,
again, the minor's understanding of the proposed procedure is the determinant
factor. *Gillick* was concerned specifically with the issue of contraceptive advice
to minors; nevertheless, the principles established have been widely extrapolated
to medical decisions of all types and the phrase '*Gillick*-competence' is now in
common use.[9] There is no doubt that a competent adult has an absolute right to
refuse treatment but, in the event that the patient is rendered incompetent, the
doctor may have to decide whether, at the time a refusal was expressed, it was
intended by the patient to apply in the changed situation.[10] The position as to the
minor who refuses treatment is a trifle uncertain. The general academic view is
that there is a right to refuse treatment which parallels that to consent.[11] The legal
position is that, even if this is so, a parent, and the court, retains the right to
consent to treatment of a minor who refuses it—and this right persists until the
minor is aged 18. This, however, merely relieves the doctor who feels that treatment
is essential of a charge of assault; it by no means determines that treatment *will* be
given and the fact that the minor had refused would be a very important factor
influencing the doctor's decision.[12]

Any consent to examination or treatment of a person below the age of '*Gillick*-
competence' must be obtained from a parent or guardian. The doctor is in a

---

4 Using the present example, a consent to the taking of blood might well not be valid if the
  patient did not know it was for the purpose of testing for HIV infection. For discussion, see
  J Keown 'The Ashes of AIDS and the Phoenix of Informed Consent' (1989) 52 MLR 790.
5 The test of adequacy in the United Kingdom is based on a 'professional standard' set by
  Bolam v Friern Hospital Management Committee [1957] 2 All ER 118 or *Hunter v Hanley*
  1955 SC 200 (see Medical Negligence, below).
6 Family Law Reform Act 1969, s 8.
7 Age of Legal Capacity (Scotland) Act 1991, s 2(4). The terms of the Scottish Act are also
  wider than those of its English counterpart as the former refers to consent to a medical
  procedure while the latter is confined to medical treatment.
8 [1986] AC 112.
9 Introduced by Lord Donaldson in *Re R (a minor) (wardship: medical treatment)* [1992]
  Fam 11 at 23.
10 A rather obscure explanation given by Lord Donaldson in *Re T (adult: refusal of medical
  treatment)* [1992] 4 All ER 649 at 662. The general rule as to refusal applies throughout
  the common law countries.
11 The author believes that, while there is an undoubted right to refuse treatment, the degree
  of understanding needed to validate refusal is greater than that needed in consent to
  treatment. This, however, is a minority opinion. See J K Mason 'Master of the Balancers:
  Non-voluntary Therapy under the Mantle of Lord Donaldson' [1993] JR 115.
12 *Re R (a minor)* [1992] Fam 11, confirmed in *Re W* [1992] 4 All ER 627. In the author's
  view, this is a reasonable interpretation of the Family Law Reform Act 1969, s 8(3).

dilemma if this is not forthcoming, say on religious grounds, and each such case must be decided, first, on the doctor's assessment of the importance of the matter and, secondly, on the chance of mishap; any decision to override parental opposition must be justified on the legal basis of necessity. The more assured alternative would be to institute care proceedings, in the course of which the local authority could apply to the court for a specific order under the Children Act 1989, s 8.[13] Such situations often stem from parental resistance to blood transfusion when the court's attitude tends to be rigid—even to the extent of overriding an admittedly '*Gillick*-competent' child's refusal.[14]

Adult patients who are unconscious or who are incapable of understanding for other reasons cannot give consent—treatment is then described as non-voluntary. In such cases, the consent of a relative—which is commonly sought—has no legal force but would be valuable support for the doctor who treats by way of the doctrine of necessity. As things stand at present, the High Court has lost its parens patriae jurisdiction and, with it, the power to consent to treatment on behalf of the incompetent adult.[15] However, if approached in a difficult case, the court can make a declaration that treatment will not be unlawful; even so, the courts are increasingly taking the view that doctors should depend upon their common law right—or even duty—to treat incompetent patients according to their best interests.[16]

In dire circumstances, such as a road-traffic accident, it is reasonable for a doctor to give treatment that he knows to be inadequate—for example, in the absence of sterile gauze, it would be quite proper to use unsterile material to stop lethal bleeding. Such treatment must be confined to the actual emergency; any that could be postponed pending admission to hospital should be left aside. It is difficult to believe that opprobrium would attach to the roadside doctor save in very exceptional circumstances.[17] The problems of consent to procedures that bear upon others, especially a husband or wife, are considered elsewhere (see Chapter 17).

Examinations for legal purposes, the results of which may be damaging to the patient, constitute a special category but, again, a general rule is that, with a few well-defined exceptions, consent is necessary to eliminate any suspicion of assault. The most obvious examples of such examinations are those requested by the police, the conditions for which are codified in England and Wales in the Police and Criminal Evidence Act 1984.[18] In Scotland, a sheriff's warrant would be acceptable to the courts in the absence of consent. These problems have been discussed already at page 297.

---

13 *Re R (a minor)* [1993] 2 FLR 757. A 'back-up' procedure would be to invite the High Court to exercise its inherent jurisdiction under the 1989 Act, s 100: *Re O (a minor) (medical treatment)* [1993] 2 FLR 149.
14 *Re E (a minor)* (1990) 9 BMLR 1.
15 G T Laurie 'Parens Patriae in the Medico-legal Context: The Vagaries of Judicial Activism' (1993) 3 ELR 96. The jurisdiction is still available in Scotland.
16 *Re F (mental patient: sterilisation)* [1990] 2 AC 1. This has been followed in a long line of cases covering many varied circumstances.
17 By contrast, it is an offence, for example, in France for a doctor *not* to stop at an accident (Decree 79-506 of 28th June 1979, art 4). Several US states have passed 'Good Samaritan' laws to regularise the position.
18 But evidence which is obtained without consent may still be admissible: (*R v Apicella (Alfred Robert)* (1986) 82 Cr App Rep 295.

Professional secrecy

It is an accepted legal principle that the patient, in confiding in the medical practitioner, can expect that confidence to be sustained.[19] The moral obligation is clear and extends, save in well-defined circumstances, to include the rights of maturing children to secrecy in relation to their parents. Parental rights are not, however, to be lightly undermined and decisions in such cases must rest with the individual doctor—guided by the principles laid down by Lord Fraser in *Gillick*.[20] The results of any subsequent action based on a breach of professional secrecy would be decided largely on the qualification of the party to whom the information was given.[1]

Legally, the doctrine of medical confidentiality is founded on the law of contract and of equity. There is surprisingly little direct case law but there can be no doubt that the law acknowledges a public interest in a legally enforceable protection of confidences received under notice of confidentiality.[2] Nevertheless, a duty of confidence is certainly not absolute and the fact that some qualification exists has been recognised for a long time. The classic reference is that of Lord Riddell who, describing the necessity and importance of medical confidence, said that:

> 'We must recognise also that the rules regarding them exist for the welfare of the community . . . [T]hey must be modified to meet the inevitable changes that occur in the necessities of various generations.'[3]

From the point of view of the doctor, the General Medical Council imposes a strict duty on registered medical practitioners to refrain from disclosing voluntarily to any third party information which they have learned directly or indirectly in a professional capacity—and this duty persists after the death of the patient. Certain exceptions have, however, been effectively codified.[4] In addition to any obvious judicial or statutory requirements, these include:

* when the patient consents to publication—in which case he or she must be fully informed as to what is being disclosed and to whom;
* when a breach is justified in the interests of the patient—an exception which clearly calls for a well-considered professional opinion;
* for research purposes—which would normally be undertaken anonymously;[5]
* when the public interest demands disclosure.

---

19 *Stephens v Avery* [1988] Ch 449, quoting *Coco v A N Clark (Engineers) Ltd* [1969] RPC 41 for the necessary elements of a confidential relationship.
20 [1986] AC 112 at 174. In an interesting Scottish Fatal Accident Inquiry, the doctor's decision not to inform the parents of a 14-year-old girl without her consent that she was taking anti-depressant drugs was considered to be professionally correct: *Inquiry into the Death of Emma Jane Hendry* (1998) Glasgow Sheriff Court, unreported.
 1 In *General Medical Council v Browne* (1971) Times, 6 and 8 March, a doctor who reported to her parents that a minor had been prescribed contraception was found not guilty of serious professional misconduct. The outcome would be far less certain today.
 2 *A-G v Guardian Newspapers Ltd (No 2)* [1990] 1 AC 109. The assumption that an actionable breach of confidence must involve detriment to the party imparting that confidence may not be necessary: *X v Y* [1988] 2 All ER 648 at 657, per Rose J.
 3 *Medico Legal Problems* (1929).
 4 General Medical Council *Duties of a Doctor: Confidentiality* (1995).
 5 Disclosure of properly anonymised information does not necessarily breach the duty of confidentiality: *R v Department of Health, ex p Source Informatics Ltd* [2000] 1 All ER 786, CA.

The public interest exception is the most important in the present context and has been subject to close judicial scrutiny—two cases are of particular interest. In the first, *X v Y*,[6] the confidentiality of the HIV status of two doctors with AIDS was discussed. The court considered the public interest in knowing that specific health carers were carriers of the virus and found that this was outweighed by the public interest in the success of the campaign against the acquired immune deficiency syndrome—in which a guarantee of non-disclosure of status was regarded as an essential element. The delicacy of this balance has been demonstrated by the fact that, subsequently, it has been found impossible to preserve the anonymity of infected doctors—in effect, the public demand to be informed of what they see, although certainly in error, as a serious hazard; it is possible to imagine that the decision in *X v Y* was influenced by the fact that the doctors concerned were general practitioners and, as a result, very unlikely to pose a threat to their patients.

The second case[7] concerned a patient in a special hospital who wished to be transferred to a regional secure unit and who, to this end, sought an opinion from a consultant psychiatrist. This proved adverse to his case and the patient asked that it be suppressed. The psychiatrist, however, believing W to be still dangerous, published his report to the responsible authorities. The Court of Appeal found that the public interest in the availability of all the facts concerning the health of a convicted killer was to be preferred to the public interest in maintaining medical confidentiality. This outcome is, in many ways, disturbing—not least because of the comment of Scott J in the court of first instance:

'The question in the present case is not whether Dr Egdell was under a duty of confidence; he plainly was. The question is as to the breadth of that duty.'

which suggests that patients—and, particularly, psychiatric patients—may be running a risky gauntlet in depending upon the doctor's appraisal not only of their medical but also their social condition. There is, indeed, a suggestion that the courts are less concerned for the patient's private rights of confidentiality than some might wish.[8]

The cases discussed so far, however, relate to the relatively relaxed conditions of the civil legal process. The doctor is in a rather different position when confronted with an immediate threat to public order—but, even then, his position can be uncertain. There is no problem if only the doctor and his patient are concerned, as in a case of self-induced abortion. But what if third parties are involved? Should the doctor provide or offer information disclosed in consultation that he knows will lead to the arrest of his patient as a multiple rapist? In failing to do so, he is no longer guilty of 'misprision of felony' (Criminal Law Act 1967) but this merely places the burden of disclosure more firmly upon his own conscience. In such an extreme case, it is probable that most doctors would opt for disclosure and, it is thought, would be supported in the General Medical Council. Not every decision would be so clear-cut and the magistrate cannot

6   [1988] 2 All ER 648.
7   *W v Egdell* [1990] Ch 359.
8   In *R v Crozier* (1990) 8 BMLR 128, the court approved the action of a doctor who, when called for the defence, ensured that his opinion would be available by handing a copy to the prosecution.

issue a warrant for the police to search for 'excluded material'—which includes medical records held in confidence.[9] However, a circuit court judge can order the production of such material in defined circumstance.[10]

On a more mundane note, considerable interest attaches to the medical role in the prevention of road-traffic accidents. Thus, it now seems clear that a doctor who is aware that a driver is subject to epilepsy has a right, if not a duty, to report the case to the licensing authority—although, as a prelude to any intended breach of confidence, every effort should be made to induce the patient to disclose the matter himself. The GMC is, however, obviously uneasy on the point in respect of the private driver and advises an intricate system of avoidance of official disclosure, including the possibility of informing the next of kin.[11] An ethical duty certainly lies on the doctor when the patient is in a position to injure many people as, for example, in the case of a driver of public transport; moreover 'it is not out of the question that a doctor who knew an unsafe patient of his was continuing to drive and yet did nothing about it might be liable to damages for negligence to anyone harmed by his patient on the roads'.[12] The important principles lie, first, in the degree of public risk involved and, more importantly, in the 'right to know' of the person informed. In a most instructive case from New Zealand, a doctor who advised potential passengers not to accept a driver who had undergone cardiac surgery was found guilty of professional misconduct by the equivalent of the GMC. On judicial review, the interests of the public were acknowledged but, in confirming the verdict, it was stated: 'A doctor who has decided to communicate should discriminate and ensure that the recipient is a responsible authority.'[13]

In general, issues as to confidentiality arise only when the doctor is providing care for his patient. A person submitting to examination for, say, life insurance purposes or for obtaining a pilot's licence is not 'in care' and consents to disclosure of the result of his examination to the appropriate body by virtue of his signature on the document. In default of such consent, insurance companies are not entitled to medical information as of right; the results of a post-mortem examination, for example, would not necessarily be subject to disclosure without the consent of the next-of-kin. It is also doubtful whether such consent is implied when the examination is carried out at the request of an employer;[14] if the doctor fails to persuade the person examined either to report an abnormality himself or to change his occupation, the need for breach of confidence must be carefully balanced against any public hazard.

Many such breaches of confidentiality are dictated by statute, generally related to public health, eg the notification of infectious disease or of abortion. The

---

9   Police and Criminal Evidence Act 1984, s 9(1). Excluded material is defined in ss 11 and 12.
10 1984 Act, Sch 1. In *R v Cardiff Crown Court, ex p Kellam* (1993) 16 BMLR 76 the court was forced to set aside an order to produce documents relating to a potentially dangerous patient's whereabouts 'with considerable reluctance'.
11 General Medical Council *Duties of a Doctor: Confidentiality* (1995). The regulations for epileptic driving are described above at p 144.
12 Legal Correspondent 'Doctors, Drivers, and Confidentiality' (1974) i BMJ 399. The proposition seems doubtful as the individual at risk would be unidentifiable. There is some evidence from the USA, however, that negligence could be based on a general risk: *Durflinger v Artiles* 673 P 2d 86 (Kan, 1983); affd 727 F 2d 888 (1984).
13 *Duncan v Medical Practitioners' Disciplinary Committee* [1986] 1 NZLR 513 at 521, per Jeffries J.
14 Certainly, the doctor owes no duty of care to the examinee: *Kapfunde v Abbey National plc* (1999) 45 BMLR 176.

important principle that obligatory transmission of medical information should be only from doctor to *doctor* is gaining ground.

There is no doubt that, in both English and Scots law, the doctor cannot refuse to give evidence in court simply because such evidence is based on information received in the course of a professional relationship.[15] The courts normally exercise great care in enforcing this doctrine and devices for satisfying the ends of justice and the doctor's conscience—such as passing information on paper—may be used; in the end, however, the implications of Lord Denning's opinion must apply—that judges have the power to direct a doctor to answer a question that is not only relevant but is also a proper and necessary question to be put in the course of justice.[16] Absolute immunity from allegations of breach of contract then follows and this applies also to statements made to lawyers during preparation of a case prior to hearings; Scottish precognitions are similarly privileged. A doctor is not excluded when there is a statutory obligation for 'any other person' to disclose information to the police.[17] The general access to medical records by the police is now governed by the Police and Criminal Evidence Act 1984.[18] Medical records come within the compass of excluded material to which, as a general rule, the police have no right of access.[19] When engaged in the investigation of a serious arrestable offence, they can search for such confidential documents only on the order of a circuit judge who must be satisfied of the need for access; moreover, there must have been some statutory authority passed before the 1984 Act which would have authorised such a search.[20] However, the records remain the property of the doctor concerned, who is empowered to disclose them should he so wish.[1]

The provision of confidential medical records for use in litigation is also controlled by statute. Only the order of a court can give absolute justification for their publication in advance of trial.[2] A potential plaintiff or pursuer can now obtain medical records from a defendant at an early stage—even before proceedings have been started. Furthermore, in cases in which a claim in respect of personal injuries is made, either party can demand a sight of a doctor's or hospital's records once proceedings have started, even if the doctor or institution is not concerned in the action.[3] Beyond this, such records should not be disclosed without the specific consent of the patient or of his guardians or next-of-kin. Good sense must, however, prevail—consent unreasonably withheld can only

---

15 J McHale and M Fox *Health Care Law* (1997) quote *Duchess of Kingston's case* (1776) 20 State Tr 355 as the basic authority of this.

16 In *A-G v Mulholland, A-G v Foster* [1963] 2 QB 477 at 489. Relevance is the only consideration in Scots Law (*H M Advocate v Airs* 1975 SLT 177) except where it is a matter of disclosing an informant (Contempt of Court Act 1981, s 10).

17 Road Traffic Act 1988, s 172; see *Hunter v Mann* [1974] QB 767; Terrorism Act 2000, s 19. See also Road Traffic Regulation Act 1984, s 112 (2)(b).

18 Police and Criminal Evidence Act 1984, s 9(1). Excluded material is defined in ss 11 and 12.

19 Specimens provided at the request of solicitors would also be confidential within the meaning of the 1984 Act, s 10: *R v R* [1994] 4 All ER 260, CA .

20 1984 Act, Sch 1, art 3.

 1 *R v Singleton* (1994) Times, 22 June, CA.

 2 Supreme Court Act 1981, ss 33 and 34; Administration of Justice (Scotland) Act 1972, s 1. The court order may stipulate that the documents must be produced either to the applicant, his legal advisers or his medical advisers.

 3 Social work documents also have no absolute immunity from disclosure in England: *Re M (a minor)* [1990] 2 FLR 36.

provoke an adverse reaction and it is now clear that reports on medical examinations made for the purpose of litigation must be exchanged if so requested in the interests of justice.[4] Experts' reports prepared for use in the criminal courts must also be exchanged when so requested.[5]

Since the client must have unfettered access to his legal adviser, communication between the two is covered by what is known as 'legal professional privilege'. The secrecy thus secured is, however, not absolute and is certainly likely to be questioned when later proceedings are conducted in an inquisitorial forum.[6] Of greater importance in the present context is the somewhat arcane statement that an important distinction is to be made between the instructions given to an expert, which are subject to privilege, and the responses to those instructions, which are not;[7] medical experts should be made fully aware of this important exception.

Medical research and experimentation

A discussion of the ethics of research in medicine need only be brief, as the lawyer will seldom be involved.

Some human research and experimentation is essential if medical knowledge is to advance to the good of the community; much preliminary work can be done on animals,[8] but, ultimately, it is the effect of the procedure upon human beings in controlled circumstances that will determine its use in practice.

It is convenient to isolate experimentation from research, as the former implies treatment given in an experimental fashion rather than in accordance with a pre-ordained protocol. Uncontrolled experimental treatment of the individual is ethical only provided that there is no recognised alternative or that the recognised treatments have failed and the patient is seriously ill; the situation must always be explained and specific consent obtained. The additional consent of a spouse or a close relative would be desirable if the treatment might possibly shorten life still further, though, as will be discussed later, such consent has no legal significance.

Research involves foresight and a rigid protocol which must be followed strictly if the results are to be meaningful. Medical research may be designed to increase academic knowledge with little prospect of immediate practical application; more commonly, it will be required to test the efficacy of an innovative or modified treatment or to study the spread of disease. The research subjects may be the researchers themselves, healthy volunteers or sick patients. Internationally accepted guidelines are detailed in the Declaration of Helsinki, which emphasises the distinction to be made between therapeutic and non-therapeutic investigation.[9]

The introduction of new treatments for general use is ethically more complicated because a controlled experiment dictates that one group of patients

4   *Naylor v Preston Area Health Authority* [1987] 2 All ER 353.
5   Police and Criminal Evidence Act 1984, s 81.
6   *Oxfordshire County Council v M* [1994] 1 FLR 175.
7   *W v Egdell* [1990] Ch 359 at 396, per Scott J. He was fully supported in the Court of Appeal.
8   And *should* be according to the Declaration of Helsinki, para I.1. For the 1996 revision of which, see J K Mason and R A McCall Smith *Law and Medical Ethics* (5th edn, 1999) Appendix F.
9   The Declaration is in the process of yet more revision where the suggested distinction is made between 'all medical research' and 'research combined with medical care'.

must be maintained on the old, and potentially less useful, regimen; if the untried treatment is quite novel, it may be necessary to include a 'placebo group'—that is, one that is effectively being deluded as to therapy. Again, the lawyer's only concern lies in the importance of fully informed consent in a research ambience—there can be no place for 'therapeutic privilege' such as may be available in ordinary medical practice.[10] All such investigations now have to be approved by Ethical Research Committees, which include lay and paramedical members.[11]

Experiments designed mainly for academic advancement of knowledge do not involve patients and are the prerogative of dedicated research workers and their assistants; much heroic work of this type is undertaken by physiologists—it is doubtful, for example, whether modern air travel would have been possible in its absence. Two points of medico-legal importance arise. First, the head of department must ensure that the risks taken are calculated to eliminate so far as is possible any serious danger to health. Secondly, the problem of the use of students as volunteer subjects often arises; such students will generally be of adult status but most teaching organisations are conscious of some responsibility in loco parentis and formulate very stringent rules.

Much ethical interest centres around the use of disinterested groups who are easily controlled—prisoners, soldiers, etc. Research using such persons can only be justified provided that it does no significant harm to the subjects and that the results are likely to be generally beneficial. Yet again, valid consent is at issue. It must be freely given and not associated with unreasonable reward—it is at least arguable whether prisoners can ever meet these requirements.[12]

The fundamental nature of consent is the same irrespective of the group involved—the exact nature of and the discomfort associated with the experiment must be explained; withdrawal must be possible at any time; and the subjects must be capable of consent—this being a matter of mental capability and of age. The use of children for medical research is a particularly emotive subject and one that has medico-legal implications in that it is doubtful whether a parent or guardian has the right to consent to a technical assault on a child unless the procedure is of positive benefit to that individual child.[13] The position of the minor above the age of 16 is similarly ambiguous. The Family Law Reform Act 1969, s 8(1) empowers a person over that age to consent to medical treatment as if he or she were an adult. The section, however, says nothing about research and it may well be that the common law rights of minors who are capable of understanding what is proposed are wider in this respect than are those conferred by statute[14]—much would depend on the severity of the procedure to which 'consent' was given. The researchers' legal position is apparently easier in Scotland, where a minor of any age who is considered capable of understanding may give valid consent to any

10 The classic case is *Halushka v University of Sasketchewan* (1965) 53 DLR (2d) 436.
11 National Health Service Management Executive *Local Research Ethics Committees* HSG (91) 5.
12 But the *fact* that a man is a prisoner does not make it impossible for him to give valid consent: *Freeman v Home Office (No 2)* [1984] QB 524.
13 For a recent example of doubtfully ethical research, see *Report of the Review into the Research Framework in North Staffordshire* (R Griffiths, chairman), reproduced in *Bulletin of Medical Ethics* (2000) no 158.
14 See *Re W (a minor) (medical treatment)* [1992] 4 All ER 627 at 635, 639, per Lord Donaldson. Lord Donaldson was discussing transplantation of organs but his reasoning can be transferred to research procedures.

surgical, medical or dental *procedure* (my emphasis).[15]   Despite the properly cautious attitude taken by the legal and medical professions, advances in paediatric medicine must be made—and this entails some research on children.   Clearly, however, there can be no 'blanket' approach to a subject that is governed, in the end, by humane pragmatism.[16]

Medical negligence

The lawyer may well become involved in cases of medical negligence, which is a subject so wide that it cannot possibly be covered fully.   Only an outline of the principles involved will be attempted.

Criminal negligence cannot now be dismissed as rapidly as it was a decade ago—a number of prosecutions have been mounted recently and some have been successful.   Prosecutions have been limited to charges of manslaughter and have been based on the assessment of criminality in terms of gross negligence—or negligence going:

> 'beyond a mere matter of compensation between subjects and [showing] such disregard for the life and safety of others as to amount to . . . conduct deserving punishment.'[17]

It is arguable that incompetence should not attract criminality in the absence of subjective wrongdoing and that the better test would be that of recklessness.   The two young doctors in the seminal case,[18] who wrongly injected cytotoxic drugs, were relatively unsupervised and can hardly be supposed to have acted in a criminal fashion—and their convictions were duly overturned in the Court of Appeal.   None the less, the Court of Appeal confirmed that the legal test was that of gross negligence.[19]   Perhaps the British doctor is still at less risk than his New Zealand counterpart—it was held in New Zealand that a doctor who 'fails to show reasonable knowledge, skill and care in the treatment of his patients' can be held to be criminally liable[20] and this was upheld in the Privy Council.   As a result of the public response, the government itself brought in an amendment to the Crimes Act 1961 and effectively raised the standard to that of gross negligence which is now the norm.

The vast majority of actions for negligence are civil actions for tort or delict and certain well-known facts must be proved for the action to succeed.

First, the doctor must have owed a duty of care to the complainer or plaintiff. This, as has been seen, may not always exist despite the fact that an examination

15 Age of Legal Capacity (Scotland) Act 1991, s 2(4).
16 For analysis in depth see R H Nicholson (ed) *Medical Research with Children: Ethics, Law and Practice* (1990).   See also R J Robinson 'Ethics Committees and Research on Children' (1987) 294 BMJ 1243.
17 *R v Bateman* [1925] All ER Rep 45.
18 *R v Prentice, R v Adomako, R v Holloway* [1993] 4 All ER 935.   For extended discussion, see A McCall Smith 'Criminal Negligence and the Incompetent Doctor' (1993) 1 Med L Rev 336.
19 Following *Andrews v DPP* [1937] AC 576.   Dr Adomako's anaesthetic lapse was of a different nature and his conviction was upheld in the House of Lords: *R v Adomako* [1995] 1 AC 171.
20 *R v Yogasakaran* [1990] 1 NZLR 399.

has taken place as, for example, in relation to fitness for employment. On the other hand, no bilateral agreement is needed to establish a duty of care. The essential feature is the intention of the doctor to treat or to heal; once the intent is established, the duty continues until the need for care is past or until alternative arrangements have been willingly made. Secondly, it must be shown that the doctor failed in his duty of care. Failure is a relative term; its degree must be measured against the skill that might reasonably be expected of a responsible doctor. Much will depend upon the diagnostic and therapeutic aids available at the time; a doctor would be expected to be more efficient in an intensive care unit than by the roadside. The acceptance of such common-sense principles in British law makes it unnecessary to pass 'Good Samaritan' protective legislation as has been required under many other jurisdictions. Provided he has executed reasonable skill and care, a doctor cannot be held negligent for a mistake in diagnosis or treatment. The classic authority for this is Lord Clyde who, when Lord President, stated:

> 'In the realm of diagnosis and treatment, there is ample scope for genuine difference of opinion, and one man clearly is not negligent merely because his conclusion differs from that of other professional men, nor because he has displayed less skill or knowledge than others would have shown.'[1]

The test, in short, is that of the standard of the ordinary skilled man exercising and professing to have that special skill[2] and, while an error of clinical judgment need not necessarily be negligence, it can be so if it is reached in a manner falling below the test standard.[3]

Lord Clyde's judgment in *Hunter* also introduced the concept of 'accepted medical practice', giving his opinion that, having shown that there was an accepted practice and that the doctor failed to follow that practice, the plaintiff in an action for medical negligence must further show that the course the doctor adopted was one that no professional man of ordinary skill would have taken had he been acting with ordinary care. Accepted practice may differ from hospital to hospital; the important question is whether an approach to diagnosis and therapy was or was not reasonable—and the decision is one that is open to the courts.[4] On the other hand, it has been authoritatively stated that allegations of negligence against medical practitioners should be regarded as serious and that the standard of proof

---

1   In *Hunter v Hanley* 1955 SLT 213 at 217.
2   *Bolam v Friern Hospital Management Committee* [1957] 2 All ER 118 at 121, per McNair J. *Bolam* was approved in the Privy Council in *Chin Keow v Government of Malaysia* [1967] 1 WLR 813 and has since been applied across the board in England extending to the provision of information and warnings: *Maynard v West Midlands Regional Health Authority* [1985] 1 All ER 635. It is accepted in parallel with *Hunter v Hanley* 1955 SLT 213 in Scotland—*Moyes v Lothian Health Board* 1990 SLT 444—but there are strong moves to limit its application in the Commonwealth: *Rogers v Whitaker* (1992) 109 ALR 625. Similarly, the English courts are taking the view that the *Bolam* principle is subject to the court's approval in individual cases: *Bolitho v City and Hackney Health Authority* [1998] AC 232. For a very full discussion, see M Brazier and J Miola 'Bye-Bye Bolam: A Medical Litigation Revolution?' (2000) 8 Med L Rev 85.
3   *Whitehouse v Jordan* [1981] 1 All ER 267 at 276, per Lord Edmund-Davies.
4   See, for example, the Master of the Rolls in *Sidaway v Board of Governors of the Bethlem Royal Hospital and Maudsley Hospital* [1984] QB 493 and the important Canadian case of *Reibl v Hughes* (1980) 114 DLR (3d) 1.

should, therefore, be a high degree of probability.[5] It is widely claimed that medical negligence is more difficult to establish than is negligence in other fields and empirical evidence suggests that this may well be so.

Thirdly, the patient must have suffered damage. The definition of 'damage' is certainly widening, and, when extended to mental distress, is almost all-embracing. It is, however, a function of the court to measure the loss or damage in terms of money and, as the costs involved in caring for a disabled person escalate, so do the sums of money awarded. Compensation may be paid in a lump sum; the court may, however, order that damages should be paid as periodical payments.[6] The courts cannot take into account the free medical attention available under the National Health Service when assessing the quantum of damages.[7] At the same time, the courts are now bound to consider whether the imposition of a duty of care, with all that it implies, is fair, just and reasonable.[8]

A doctor may be liable for the negligence of his subordinates, stand-ins and other members of staff—including, particularly, receptionists who are sometimes forced into making medical decisions.[9] The vicarious responsibility of hospitals for members of staff has been discussed in the previous chapter.

In certain circumstances, negligence as defined above is self-evident. For example, there has clearly been negligence if a pair of forceps is left in the abdomen and the patient is thereby subjected to a second operation. The doctrine of *res ipsa loquitur* might then operate and would give rise to an inference of negligence on the defendant's part; Denning LJ has summarised it: '. . . that should not have happened if due care had been used. Explain it if you can.'[10] Such cases are commonly settled but the courts are reluctant to accept the plea in the event of their being contested. Almost invariably, it is for the plaintiff or pursuer to prove the fact of negligence.[11]

The doctor, generally in concert with the hospital or other employing authority, may claim that no negligence existed in the true sense; he may defend himself on the grounds that his course of action carried well-known risks that were fully explained to the patient and which the patient accepted; or he may assert that the patient himself contributed to his own disability.[12] It is apparent that two patients can leave hospital each with a disability of comparable gravity and each deriving from the treatment received; yet one may receive substantial damages while the other is not compensated, depending on whether 'fault' was proved. There is much to be said for the introduction of a 'no fault' scheme of compensation operated by some form of compulsory insurance. As Lawton LJ said: 'As long as

5 Lawton LJ in *Whitehouse v Jordan* [1980] 1 All ER 650 at 659. But see the contrary view in *Ashcroft v Mersey Regional Health Authority* [1983] 2 All ER 245 at 247.
6 Damages Act 1996, s 2. Alternatively a 'structured settlement' may be arranged between the plaintiff and the defendant's insurers (s 5).
7 *Lim Poh Choo v Camden and Islington Area Health Authority* [1979] 2 All ER 910 at 914, per Lord Scarman, commenting on Denning, MR in the Court of Appeal [1979] 1 All ER 332 at 341, 344.
8 *Caparo Industries plc v Dickman* [1990] 2 AC 605, applied in the very interesting medical case *McFarlane v Tayside Health Board* [1999] 4 All ER 961, HL.
9 The doctor may, of course, also be liable in his obligations as a citizen—eg to keep his surgery in a safe condition (Occupier's Liability Act 1957).
10 In *Cassidy v Ministry of Health* [1951] 2 KB 343 at 365.
11 See, for example, *Wilsher v Essex Area Health Authority* [1988] AC 1074.
12 The acceptance of contributory negligence would not affect the fact of negligence but would alter the damages awarded.

liability in this type of case rests on proof of fault, judges will have to go on making decisions which they would prefer not to make. The victims of medical mishaps should, in my opinion, be cared for by the community not by the hazards of litigation.'[13] There is much practical difficulty in the application of such a policy but further discussion is beyond the scope of this book.[14]

Euthanasia

Euthanasia is now one of the most burning issues in medical jurisprudence. The traditional medical ethos of 'the sanctity of life', implying the unqualified duty to preserve life, has come under increasing challenge. Modern technology has now transformed the struggle to survive into a 'right to die' movement which has achieved such strength that it cannot be ignored—an assessment of the legal and medical implications of 'allowing to die' must now be an essential feature of forensic medicine. The problem presents at three main points in time—at the beginning and at the end of natural life, and during life when an individual is severely impaired as a result of brain damage.

The last situation has been partly discussed in Chapter 13. Here, it is sufficient to re-emphasise again the essential difference between brain-stem death on the one hand and irreversible brain damage on the other. Understanding is not helped by semantic confusion such as derives from the use of the phrase 'irreversible coma' in the United States,[15] which is synonymous with brain-stem death and not, as might be expected, with the persistent vegetative state. There is a growing movement to do away with a distinction between the two conditions and to establish a state of 'cognitive death'[16] but, whatever may be the philosophical position, the law in the United Kingdom is quite clear—a person in the persistent vegetative state is not legally dead and to actively induce cardio-respiratory death in such a person could amount to unlawful homicide. None the less, the House of Lords has accepted that the persistent vegetative state is a unique condition and has established that, within strictly confined conditions, it is lawful to withdraw artificial feeding from such cases.[17] Their Lordships acknowledged

---

13 In *Whitehouse v Jordan* [1980] 1 All ER at 661. See also *Ashcroft v Mersey Regional Health Authority* [1983] 2 All ER 245.

14 The archetypal scheme is to be found in the consolidating Accident Compensation Act 1982 of New Zealand. In fact, problems over the definition of the word 'accident' led to supplementary legislation following the original 1972 Act and the scope of the legislation has been restricted in the Accident Compensation (Amendment) Act 1992. See Mahoney 'New Zealand's Accident Compensation Scheme: A Reassessment' (1992) 40 Amer J Comp Law 159.

15 H K Beecher (Chairman) 'A definition of irreversible coma. Report of the ad hoc Committee of the Harvard Medical School to Examine the Definition of Brain Death' (1968) 205 J Amer Med Ass 337.

16 For a useful review of attitudes, see R J Devettere 'Neocortical Death and Human Death' (1990) 18 J Law Med Hlth Care 96.

17 *Airedale NHS Trust v Bland* [1993] AC 789. For an incremental shift from a rigid position, see *Frenchay Healthcare NHS Trust v S* [1994] 2 All ER 403. By the end of 1998, some 18 cases had been considered in the courts since *Bland* and there is little doubt that the conditions needed to support withdrawal of nutrition have been relaxed. See D A Cusack, A A Sheikh and J L Hyslop-Westrup 'Near PVS: A New Medico-legal Syndrome?' (2000) 40 Med Sci Law 133; G T Laurie and J K Mason 'Negative Treatment of Vulnerable Patients; Euthanasia by any Other Name?' [2000] JR 159.

in *Bland* that there was no logical distinction between active intervention and withdrawal of feeding in such cases but emphasised the profound legal difference. Somewhat unsatisfactorily, it was concluded that the original cerebral insult, rather than the therapeutic intervention, should be regarded as the cause of death in these circumstances.

The problems at the end of life are summed up in the current phrase 'death with dignity', the present trend being to move away from the obligation to preserve life and towards a duty to prevent suffering. Terminal illness is considered best treated by providing the optimum conditions for death rather than by the use of increasingly invasive techniques to prolong some sort of existence. The incapable patient is presumed to agree to this and many persons now affect an 'advance directive' or 'living will' in which this course is specifically directed. Currently, the advance directive has no legal status in the United Kingdom but can be regarded as a strong guideline for those having to make a therapeutic decision.[18] The conscious dying patient can, of course, make his own decision; patients' autonomy is now a cornerstone of ethical medical practice and to continue to treat in the face of contrary instructions could constitute either a criminal or civil assault.[19] But the position is not completely clear cut. The doctor must still ensure that the patient's refusal of treatment was valid—that is, uncoerced—and that it was intended to apply in the particular circumstances,[20] both of which obligations seem to place the doctor in a well-nigh insoluble dilemma.

Absent any indication from the patient, the moral justification for elective non-treatment (or what is more often called passive euthanasia) is commonly based on the doctrine of 'ordinary' and 'extraordinary' means of treatment. This moral doctrine, which attempts to distinguish between what treatment a doctor *need* or need not give is not, however, to be construed as relating to particular techniques. In making a decision, the distinction must rather be between productive and non-productive treatment, the response of the individual patient being the ultimate determinant of the definition. Thus, there is no moral obligation on the doctor to preserve life at the expense of suffering and, if, in the course of good terminal care, the use of drugs actually hastens death, this is ethically acceptable within the concept of 'double effect'; this, basically, states that an ill effect is morally acceptable as long as there is a greater, and intended, good effect from an action—it is thus directly comparable to the legal doctrine of necessity. If this is agreed, it is reasonable to ask why passive euthanasia as a means of alleviating an otherwise intolerable condition should be any less objectionable than would be the active ending of life—something which, as discussed above in *Bland*, is indefensible. Justification can only lie on the grounds that the former is allowing nature to take its course; the latter implies a positive, extraneous intervention which not even a British jury will tolerate.[1]

---

18 *Practice Note* [1994] 2 All ER 413. The UK adopts what is, perhaps, a minority position. The advance directive is a legally binding document in a majority of the American states and is statutorily binding in Victoria by way of the Medical Treatment Act 1988.
19 *Airedale NHS Trust v Bland* [1993] AC 789. For a rigid approval of patient autonomy in the face of death, see *St George's Healthcare NHS Trust v S* (1998) 44 BMLR 160, CA.
20 *Re T (adult) (refusal of medical treatment)* [1992] 4 All ER 649.
 1 *R v Cox* (1992) 12 BMLR 38. Dr Cox injected a suffering patient with potassium chloride and was convicted of attempted murder—murder was not charged due to the precipitate disposal of the body.

These considerations are, in some ways, more complex when applied to the beginning of life. Here the problem is whether to assist or obstruct the physically or mentally defective infant in its struggle for life. Such choices are undoubtedly made as a matter of routine; their morality and legality depend on anticipating the 'quality of life' for the neonate.

The situation here is different from the end of life in so far as the person most intimately concerned, the infant, is never able to make an autonomous decision— this must be surrogate and made by the parents and the doctor aided, or confused, by the law. While some support an absolute adherence to the 'sanctity of life', most would now agree that a case exists for balancing the possible blessing of an early, painless death against the probable sufferings of a 'fruitless' life—suffering not being measured solely from the point of view of the principal but also from that of the parents and, indeed, of society. First, however, we must accept that we are judging the 'fruitfulness of life'—or the futility of medical or surgical treatment—through the subjective eyes of adults who have experienced a 'normal' life; as a result, we can understand physical pain and can, to an extent, share that understanding with the physically defective child. By contrast, we have no common experience with the mentally handicapped neonate of whom it has been said:

'. . . he would not compare his life with that of a person enjoying normal advantages. He would know nothing of a normal life having never experienced it.'[2]

Thus, it is essential to consider the management of the physically defective and the mentally handicapped infant as separate entities—and even more so because, whereas the former may have a condition which is incompatible with life unless treated, the latter must be helped on its way if it is to die. In 1981, a paediatrician, confronted with an apparently physically normal Downs' syndrome neonate which was unwanted by its parents, prescribed 'nursing care only' and large doses of dihydrocodeine; he was charged with murder on the baby's death and was subsequently acquitted of both murder and attempted murder.[3] The case had unusual features and is of little value as a precedent; it is, however, unlikely that such a tolerant attitude would be adopted today. The far more useful determination lies in the civil case of *Re B (a minor) (wardship: medical treatment).*[4] In that instance, a Downsian child was born with an intestinal obstruction and it was left to the Court of Appeal to arbitrate between conflicting views as to whether or not the deformity should be corrected. In opting for operation, it was said:

'. . . it devolves on this court . . . to decide whether the life of this child is demonstrably going to be so awful that in effect the child must be condemned to die or whether the life of this child is still so imponderable that it would be wrong for her to be condemned to die . . . Faced with [the] choice, I have no doubt that it is the duty of this court to decide that the child must live.'[5]

---

2   *Re Superintendent of Family and Child Service and Dawson* (1983) 145 DLR (3d) 610 at 621, per McKenzie J.
3   *R v Arthur* (1981) 12 BMLR 1.
4   (1981) 1 WLR 1421.
5   (1981) 1 WLR 1421 at 1424, per Templeman LJ.

There is, thus, a clear indication that mental handicap per se does not constitute a reason for lawful passive euthanasia of the newborn.

Re B was later cited by the Master of the Rolls as being near to a binding authority for the proposition that there is a balancing exercise to be performed in assessing the course to be adopted in the best interests of a disabled child.[6] Since then, there have been a series of cases which clearly demonstrate the current judicial attitude to selective non-treatment. In *Re C*,[7] the balancing act led to the conclusion that it is not necessary to needlessly prolong the suffering of a dying child. *Re J*[8] extended the reasoning to the severely handicapped infant who was not in immediate danger of death. It was held, first, that there was no obligation to resuscitate a child whose quality of life was abysmally low; secondly, that, while there was a strong presumption in favour of action that would prolong life, the decision must be taken from the assumed view of the patient and exclusively in the patient's best interests; thirdly, that the decision is a co-operative effort between the health carers and the parents; and, finally, it was emphasised that the debate was not about terminating life—which would be unlawful—but was about withholding treatment which was designed to prevent death from natural causes. In a later but parallel case[9] it was held that doctors were under no obligation to provide intensive care when to do so was against their better judgment—and to do so was, incidentally, a misuse of scarce resources.

The law in England (and almost certainly throughout the United Kingdom) is, therefore, now clear. Elective non-treatment of physically defective infants is lawful provided the decision is taken in the best interests of the subject. Active steps designed to terminate the child's life or accelerate its death remain unlawful. The last vestiges of *R v Arthur* as a possible legal precedent have been removed.

Physician assisted suicide

The legal position of physician assisted suicide (PAS)—which, morally, lies somewhere between suicide, which is legal, and active euthanasia, which is unlawful homicide—merits a brief word in view of its current interest and its forensic implications.

On the face of things, there is little that is problematic—while suicide is no longer proscribed, aiding or abetting suicide remains an offence carrying serious

---

6   *Re J (a minor) (wardship: medical treatment)* [1990] 3 All ER 930. These cases have been discussed at length in J K Mason 'Master of the Balancers: Non-voluntary Therapy under the Mantle of Lord Donaldson' [1993] Juridical Rev 115.

7   *Re C (a minor) (wardship: medical treatment)* [1989] 2 All ER 791. These cases involve infants but the reasoning is immediately applicable to neonates. For a practical review, see I M Balfour-Lynn and R C Tasker 'Futility and Death in Paediatric Medical Intensive Care' (1996) 22 J Med Ethics 279.

8   [1990] 3 All ER 930.

9   *Re J (a minor) (medical treatment)* [1992] 2 FLR 165. Note that there is a divergence here between practice in the UK and the USA; parents in the latter jurisdiction may demand treatment from a reluctant doctor. See F H Miller 'Infant Resuscitation, A US/UK Divide' (1994) 343 Lancet 1584 discussing *Re Baby K*. Even so, the doctor's clinical autonomy has been reaffirmed recently; elective non-treatment has also been held not to be contrary to the European Convention for the Protection of Human Rights (shortly to be enforced by the Human Rights Act 1998, which is in force in Scotland at the time of writing): *A National Health Service Trust v D* [2000] 2 FCR 677.

penalties.[10] The Act contains no exception in the case of medical practitioners who may be asked to provide assistance in dying by those in intolerable pain, as from malignant disease, or by those who are physically unable to end their own lives, of whom those suffering from progressive neurological degenerative conditions, such as motor neurone disease, provide the most vivid examples. Either might claim that, in being denied medical assistance they are being deprived of the care that is their due and that, at the same time, their autonomy is being compromised—in a survey undertaken in Scotland, 55% of the adult population thought that physician assisted suicide should be made legal.[11]

One of the major difficulties is to define PAS. Is the doctor who disconnects the ventilator at the request of a sufferer from motor neurone disease assisting suicide or complying with the patient's refusal of treatment? Is he or she acting positively in so doing or merely withdrawing treatment? Is the doctor who performs a venepuncture, so that the patient may inject a lethal drug, assisting suicide or engaged in active euthanasia? Is he, in any case, acting in his or her patient's 'best interests'?[12] There are no British cases in point but we have already noted two important Commonwealth cases (at page 191) in which the principle of PAS was accepted.[13] By contrast, the Supreme Court of the United States has held that there is no fundamental right to PAS and that the distinction between assisting suicide and withdrawing life sustaining treatment is 'logical, widely recognised and endorsed by the medical profession'.[14] Would that it was always so simple!

The present author suggests that there is a case for lifting the ban on physician assisted suicide but that the complexities are such that positive legislation would be unlikely to succeed. A fair compromise would be to do no more than exclude medical practitioners, when acting in good faith and within controlled parameters, from the conditions of the Suicide Act 1961, s 2.[15] It is probable, however, that PAS will remain a criminal offence for the foreseeable future.

---

10 Suicide Act 1961, s 2. Suicide has never been an offence in Scotland and it is at least doubtful if there is, as a result, an offence of abetting suicide; an abettor might, however, be charged with, say, recklessly endangering life.
11 S A M McLean and A Britton *Sometimes a Small Victory* (1996). This is not an overwhelming majority and a House of Lords Select Committee has rejected the need for a change in the law: House of Lords Paper HL21-1 (1994).
12 For discussion, see D W Meyers and J K Mason 'Physician Assisted Suicide: A Second view from Mid-Atlantic' (1999) 28 Anglo-Amer L Rev 265. There is no doubt that the doctor who actually injects the drug is at risk of a charge of murder: *R v Cox* (1992) 12 BMLR 38.
13 *Nancy B v Hôtel-Dieu de Québec* (1992) 15 BMLR 95; *Auckland Area Health Board v A-G* [1993] 4 Med LR 239. In a third case, the right to have the respirator disconnected was refused but it is understood that no action was taken against the doctor who subsequently did so: *Rodriguez v A-G of Canada* (1999) 50 BMLR 1.
14 *Washington v Glucksberg* (1997) 117 S Ct 2258; *Vacco v Quill* (1997) 117 S Ct 2293.
15 J K Mason and D Mulligan 'Euthanasia by Stages' (1996) 347 Lancet 810.

31

Deaths associated with medical and surgical care

Medico-legal procedure

Medico-legal interest focuses on deaths occurring during or as a result of surgical operations for several reasons. First, a thorough investigation of fatalities is one means by which surgical treatment can be improved and unsatisfactory techniques can be eliminated. Secondly, the patient undergoing elective surgery is not expected to die; such deaths, therefore, cause considerable concern to those directly and indirectly affected and actions for negligence may result. Related to both these considerations is the availability of major surgical procedures to patients in increasingly 'high-risk' categories; forensic medicine has a part to play in maintaining a balance between advances in treatment and the associated increase in risk.[1]

Deaths associated with surgery are often loosely referred to as 'anaesthetic deaths'. This is a misnomer which, apart from its undeserved professional implications, may, by limiting the field of investigation, be positively detrimental to progress. The term should be reserved for those deaths that can properly be attributed to the anaesthetic *only after full investigation*; phrases that presuppose this conclusion should be avoided.

Deaths following medical mishap—and, in particular, deaths associated with surgery—figure prominently among those which are reportable both to the coroner and to the procurator fiscal. A special procedure has, however, been developed in the latter case. The following categories of death, which are not intended to be exhaustive, are specified as being reportable to the fiscal by the doctor concerned in the care of the patient or by the doctor called in at the time of death:

* deaths which occur unexpectedly having regard to the clinical condition of the deceased prior to his receiving medical care;
* deaths which are clinically unexplained;

---

1 The reader will be reminded of the concern expressed some years ago at the poorly controlled introduction of minimal access surgery. See *Silverman v Singer and Macdonald* unreported in C Dyer (1995) 310 BMJ 551.

- deaths seemingly attributable to a therapeutic or diagnostic hazard;
- deaths which are apparently associated with lack of medical care;
- deaths which occur during the actual administration of a general or local anaesthetic;
- deaths which may be due to an anaesthetic.

A particular format is followed in their investigation.[2] Having reported the death informally, the doctors concerned are required to complete a standard questionnaire (Appendix R) which is then forwarded to the fiscal. The fiscal will then obtain a report from a forensic pathologist and/or an independent consultant in the specialty concerned or an appropriate general practitioner—appropriate, in this connection, implying that he is qualified to act as a police surgeon; this report will be based on the questionnaire and on discussions with the doctors concerned. A decision as to the need for a post-mortem dissection rests with the fiscal but, in reaching such a decision, he will be heavily influenced by his advisers. The one-time anachronism of isolating death associated with anaesthesia has, thus, now been removed in Scotland but still persists in England, where the registrar is required to report to the coroner any death appearing to have occurred during an operation or before recovery from the effects of an anaesthetic;[3] many coroners, acting on a purely local basis, insist that deaths occurring within 24 hours of the administration of an anaesthetic should be reported by the hospital authority.

Hazards of surgical operations

All surgical operations, whether accompanied by local, regional or general anaesthesia, have some morbidity and mortality. Efficient surgical practice is based on accurate clinical judgment as to whether the risks of surgery and anaesthesia outweigh the dangers or discomfort to the patient of withholding the operation.

'Informed' consent

Consent to operation is mandatory. The situation is summed up in the now immortal words of Cardozo J:

> 'Every human being of adult years and sound mind has a right to determine what shall be done with his own body; and a surgeon who performs an operation without the patient's consent commits an assault.'[4]

Thus, the wide-ranging 'consent to operation' form, which patients are invited to sign, protects the surgeon against allegations of battery or assault[5] (see page 455). Consent to a 'touching' does not, however, necessarily include consent to a risk

2 'Medical care' includes surgical, anaesthetic, nursing or any other kind of medical care and these deaths may be the result of medication (oral or parenteral and including inhalation) or of diagnostic or therapeutic procedures (operations, investigations, X-ray procedures, etc).
3 Registration of Births and Deaths Regulations 1987, SI 1987/2088, reg 41(1)(e).
4 *Schloendorff v Society of New York Hospital* 105 NE 92 (NY, 1914).
5 *Chatterton v Gerson* [1981] QB 432.

and it is this distinction that underlies the concept of what is commonly referred to as 'informed consent'.

It is clear that the patient, in consenting to operation, does not consent to a negligent performance on the part of the surgeon. The critical issue is that of consent to the risks that are *inherent* to the proposed procedure. Should such a risk materialise, the patient who was unaware of the possibility can rightly say: 'But for the fact that I did not know of the risk, I would not have had the operation. The risk has materialised and I am suffering a disability due to an operation which I would not have undergone had I known of the risk. Thus, my disability is *caused* by your failure to inform me of the risk.' The surgeon who fails to *inform* of a risk is, therefore, liable to an action in negligence.

In general, the patient must be given sufficient information to enable him or her to make an autonomous decision as to an assumption of the risks involved. What constitutes *sufficient* information is, however, still in dispute. Briefly, there are two ways of measuring the requirement. Either one can consider what the patient wishes to know—and this could be either the average or reasonable patient (the *objective patient* standard) or the particular patient (the *subjective patient* standard); or one could base one's assessment on what the doctor felt was appropriate information (the *professional* standard). By and large, the trend in the United States has been towards use of the patient standard[6]—and often to the subjective patient standard which is bound to be clouded by the wisdom of hindsight.[7] The courts in the United Kingdom have, however, opted for the professional standard.[8] The corollary to this is that, since the issue is one of negligence, disputes will be settled on the *Bolam* principle,[9] which is that a doctor will not be considered negligent if he acts in accordance with a practice accepted at the time as proper by a responsible body of medical opinion. The *Bolam* test greatly biases any debate in favour of the doctor in that it effectively allows the medical profession to set its own standards; moreover, it is at least arguable that giving information on which someone else will act is different from the provision of medical treatment.[10] As a consequence, there is a current move away from *Bolam* in common law countries in relation to consent to treatment. The principle was significantly modified in favour of the patient in *Sidaway* and has almost

---

6 *Canterbury v Spence* 464 F 2d 772 (DC, 1972) is the leading case.

7 A library of literature has grown up around the topic of informed consent. The seminal work is that of S A M McLean *A Patient's Right to Know* (1989). A very readable account, easily accessible to the British lawyer, is M Brazier 'Patient Autonomy and Consent to Treatment: The Role of the Law' (1987) 7 LS 169. Times are, however, changing—for a modern review, see J K Mason and R A McCall Smith *Law and Medical Ethics* (5th edn, 1999) ch 10.

8 The leading case in England is *Sidaway v Board of Governors of the Bethlem Royal Hospital* [1985] AC 871, HL; for Scotland, see *Moyes v Lothian Health Board* 1990 SLT 444. An unfortunate result has been some confusing judicial statements such as: 'The concept of informed consent forms no part of English law' (per Dunn LJ in *Sidaway* [1984] QB 493 at 517, CA) or 'English law does not accept the transatlantic concept of informed consent' (per Lord Donaldson MR in *Re T (adult) (refusal of medical treatment)* [1992] 4 All ER 649 at 663). Such remarks clearly pertain only to consent based on the subjective patient standard.

9 *Bolam v Friern Hospital Management Committee* [1957] 2 All ER 118. The Scottish equivalent is *Hunter v Hanley* 1955 SC 200.

10 Though this was specifically denied in *Gold v Haringey Health Authority* [1988] QB 481, CA.

been abandoned in the Commonwealth.[11] The English courts have made sporadic attempts, mainly in those of first instance, to shake off the chains of *Bolam*[12] and the House of Lords has indicated that, in limited circumstances, the court might find that 'medical opinion' could not survive the test of logical analysis.[13] Nevertheless, we are unlikely to see any marked change in the United Kingdom in the near future and whether or not a patient has consented to the risks of an operation will be judged, as before, on a professional standard.[14] In general, the extent of necessary disclosure will be regarded as being proportional to the understanding of the patient, the questions he or she asks, the extent of the risk, the availability of alternatives, any element of experimentation and the effect on the patient of imparting the knowledge; but, at the end of the day, the question of whether any failure to disclose was negligent will be determined by current medical opinion.[15] The position is probably best summarised in the words of Lord Templeman:

> 'The duty of a doctor is to provide the patient with information that will enable the patient to make a balanced judgment if the patient chooses to make a balanced judgment.'[16]

Finally, it is to be noted that the patient's consent is, in general, specific to a stated intended course of action; whether an operation can be extended beyond that consented to depends on the urgency and relevance to the primary treatment and on the additional effects of the secondary procedure.[17] An interesting variation on this theme arose in a recent case in which an anaesthetist inserted an analgesic rectal suppository into a dental patient for the purpose of alleviating post-operative pain; the patient contended she had not consented to the procedure and the GMC found the anaesthetist guilty of serious professional misconduct by reason of assaulting the patient.[18]

Consent is of special importance when it is being given on behalf of another— eg a minor—or when an operation attended by some risk, such as the examination of an organ by biopsy, is performed mainly or partly as a research procedure. The subject has been addressed in Chapter 30; here, it is sufficient to say that, in such

---

11 The first major attack came in the Canadian case *Reibl v Hughes* (1980) 114 DLR (3d) 1. Virtually a knock-out blow was administered in Australia in *Rogers v Whitaker* (1992) 109 ALR 625. For most interesting criticism, see H Teff *Reasonable Care* (1994) pp 34–38, 184–187.

12 Eg *Smith v Tunbridge Wells Health Authority* [1994] 5 Med LR 334; *Newell v Goldenberg* (1995) 6 Med LR 371.

13 *Bolitho v City and Hackney Health Authority* [1998] AC 232.

14 How *Bolam* will fare in a human rights context is discussed in M Earle 'The Future of Informed Consent in British Common Law' (1999) 6 Euro J Hlth Law 235.

15 And the judge cannot prefer one body of medical opinion to another: *Maynard v West Midlands Regional Health Authority* [1985] 1 All ER 635.

16 In *Sidaway v Board of Governors of the Bethlem Royal Hospital* [1985] AC 871 at 904.

17 Compare, for example, *Marshall v Curry* [1933] 3 DLR 260, where a hernia operation could not be completed without removal of a testis, with *Murray v McMurchy* (1949) 2 DLR 442, where a sterilisation coincidental to Caesarian section was regarded as beyond the surgeon's discretion. For a recent case, see *Williamson v East London and the City Health Authority* [1998] Lloyd's Rep Med 7 (removal of an unwanted implant *and* the associated breast tissue).

18 See J Mitchell 'A Fundamental Problem of Consent' (1995) 310 BMJ 43. The case was complicated by the fact that the suppository was inadvertently placed in the vagina rather than the rectum. In the absence of a full report, it is not easy to see how the GMC could find the anaesthetist guilty of a criminal action for which he had not been tried.

circumstances, explanation must be particularly full and that there is no place for withholding information purely on the grounds that the *doctor* believes that to do so is in the interests of the patient.[19]

The decision to operate

The correctness of the decision to proceed has to be considered whenever a death occurs during—or is obviously referable to—an operation.

No one would question the validity of an operation of even heroic proportions undertaken to save a life that would otherwise undoubtedly be lost. Very few would dispute the need for an admittedly palliative procedure designed to alleviate the pain of a terminal illness. But what if the disease underlying severe pain has a negligible mortality in relation to suppressive surgery? Or what if the risks to life of undertaking an operation can be assessed as greater than those of inaction? It could be argued that a large proportion of operations undertaken, such as virtually all plastic surgery, much of ENT surgery and many general surgical operations (hernias, varicose veins) come into this category.

Obviously, no general ruling can be given and each case must be assessed by the surgeon and the anaesthetist acting together. The risk/benefit ratio for the particular operation in that particular patient must be assessed. Balanced decisions must be based on full preoperative information and must take into account what measures are available to counteract difficulties that are reasonably foreseeable. It might, for example, be justifiable to perform an operation that would be expected to result in severe blood loss; it would be unjustifiable to do so without previously arranging for a readily available supply of replacement blood known to be compatible with the recipient (see below, page 489).

The choice of patient

Recent advances in anaesthesia, particularly the introduction of muscle relaxants, now allow for a relatively low level of narcosis in major surgery. As a result, patients in an older age group and less physically fit can be anaesthetised with increasing confidence and safety—there are few occasions on which age per se is a contraindication to surgery.[20] However, the physiological upset to patients, although less than would have been experienced a decade ago, can still be significant and, while surgical techniques are continually improving, the physical damage resulting from a given operation must affect the infirm more adversely than those who are otherwise healthy. On the other hand, an implication of negligence based on the death of a patient in a suspect category might well have the effect of depriving elderly patients of a potentially fuller remaining life simply because of apprehension of the consequences of failure. There are, therefore, very

---

19 *Halushka v University of Saskatchewan* (1965) 53 DLR (2d) 436. For general discussion, see A Herxheimer 'The Rights of the Patient in Clinical Research' (1988) 2 Lancet 1128.
20 There is an ethical dimension here as well. Currently, there is something of a groundswell which see 'ageism' as covert rationing of resources, including operating theatre time: A Tonks 'Medicine Must Change to Serve an Ageing Society' (1999) 319 BMJ 1450. A Health Care Standards for Elderly Persons Bill 2000 is currently before Parliament.

good reasons for dispensing with public inquest in all cases in which there is no evidence of avoidable mishap.[1]

The problems facing the investigating pathologist are often formidable and are certainly greatest in relation to the hazards specific to anaesthetics. These must be considered separately—but still without prejudice to the thesis that they are only one aspect of the whole spectrum of the risks of major surgery.

Anaesthesia[2]

Anaesthesia is the largest clinical specialty in the National Health Service—it is also one of the most rapidly advancing and, as already pointed out, the emphasis laid on 'anaesthetic deaths' by coroners and procurator fiscals is now something of an anachronism. Whereas it may be practised in many countries by nurses or others similarly trained, an anaesthetic in Britain may be administered only by a registered medical practitioner. General anaesthesia has three components— hypnosis, analgesia and muscular relaxation—which implies that the patient is rendered unconscious and all sensation is lost. In the past, all three aims were achieved by administering a single drug, such as chloroform. The introduction of agents which did no more than produce muscle relaxation, such as curare, gave anaesthetists an opportunity to select specific drugs to produce the individual effects separately. Complicated anaesthetics may now entail the administration of ten or more different drugs. Hence, the individual components can be altered to meet the demands of the surgeon in relation to the particular operation and to the particular patient. In essence, therefore, no two modern 'anaesthetics' are the same.

The responsibilities of anaesthetists in the operating theatre include:

- To prepare the patient for theatre. This will usually involve recommending various pre-operative investigations to assess the patient's fitness for the operation and also the prescribing of premedication drugs given to allay anxiety in the run up to the operation.
- To enable the surgeon to perform his function. This will entail administering the appropriate anaesthetic drugs and maintaining the patient's physiological function. The anaesthetist has available a large number of monitors and equipment with which to control anaesthesia safely. Routine minimum monitoring today entails measurement of the patient's blood pressure at regular intervals, a continuous recording of the electrocardiogram (ECG), capnography[3] and pulse oximetry. This last monitor indicates the level of oxygen in the patient's blood and is fundamental to the now remarkable safety

---

1   While the Brodrick Committee could not agree with this entirely, there is a clear indication from their report that they favoured some form of selection in relation to the type of inquiry (*Report of the Committee on Death Certification and Coroners* (1971) pp 57, 207). In any event, the coroner has the option to regard such a death as natural and to dispense with an inquest under the Coroners Act 1988, s 19. The problem does not, of course, obtain in Scotland, where there would have to be a suspicion of serious negligence to precipitate a Fatal Accident Inquiry.

2   This section has been kindly reviewed by Dr A S Buchan.

3   This measure of ventilation of the lungs is also of major value in confirming the correct emplacement of the endotracheal tube.

record of anaesthesia. More sophisticated and, at times, invasive monitoring is available for the more complicated case. The use of such techniques may require a judgment of the balance between the benefits that would accrue from their use and the increased risks in using them. This is not necessarily straightforward and each case has to be assessed individually.

- To ascertain at the end of surgery when the patient is ready for discharge back to the ward. In some serious cases this may require transfer to an intensive care unit whereas in simple cases it may mean the patient is allowed to be discharged home—as occurs in the day treatment centre.

It is convenient to discuss individually local, regional and general anaesthesia.

Local anaesthetics

These agents, which may be given by infiltration of an area or by blocking specific nerves, act by paralysing the sensory nerves with which they come in contact. Thus, a localised area can be made pain free without narcotising the whole patient, an obvious advantage when only minor surgery is to be performed or when the subject is unfit for a general anaesthetic.

All these drugs are absorbed to some extent and a maximum therapeutic dose is established for each agent on the assumption that absorption and detoxication will be normal. The old and debilitated may destroy the drug less efficiently but, young or old, the major hazard lies in rapid absorption through widely dilated vessels in the part injected. Absorption is notoriously rapid from some areas—eg the nose and throat—and these are well known to anaesthetists. In order to reduce the size of the available vessels and thus decrease absorption, it is common practice to inject a vasoconstrictive agent such as adrenaline at the same time as the anaesthetic. However, although rare, adrenaline, of itself, may produce adverse reactions. Moreover, the possibility of accidental injection directly into a major vessel— which will result in the sudden absorption of the whole dose—still remains.

The hazards of local anaesthesia can, therefore, be summarised as:

- Overdosage of either the anaesthetic or vasoconstrictive agent, the total quantity and concentration of which must be related to the age, stature and fitness of the patient.
- Rapid absorption from highly absorptive areas or as a result of local vasodilatation.
- Accidental injection into a vessel.
- Hypersensitivity reactions to the drug.
- Injection of adrenaline close to an end artery.

In the event of serious error, there may be a general excitory effect on the central nervous system—in which case convulsions may occur—or there may be rapid cardiac arrest. Less commonly, the heart may be directly affected. It is to be noted that modern local anaesthetics have been introduced which are far less toxic than the old when, for example, injected into a blood vessel.

Very occasionally, there may be local residua that result in long-term damage to the patient. Thus, an abnormally high concentration of drug injected directly into a nerve may lead to a permanent loss of function. As with any injection, there is also the remote possibility of needle breakage.

Regional anaesthesia

Whole areas of the body can be rendered insensitive if the local anaesthetic is applied to nerves remote from the site of the operation. Thus, injection of drug close to a nerve or nerve bundle (eg block of the brachial plexus by injection above the clavicle) allows surgery to be undertaken at a site far distant from the injection —in this case, in the hand.

Spinal anaesthesia (see Figure 31.1)

A more dramatic effect can be achieved by injecting local anaesthetic very close to the spinal cord by way of the cerebrospinal fluid (CSF). A major advantage of the technique is that, by withdrawing CSF through the injection needle, the operator knows that the drug has been correctly placed. Despite the best precautions, however, spinal anaesthesia has a definite morbidity and mortality. The reasons for this are various. Since the nerves that supply the life-support functions are placed high in the cord, the dangers of spinal anaesthesia increase if the anaesthetic is allowed to rise too high in the CSF. This may happen because

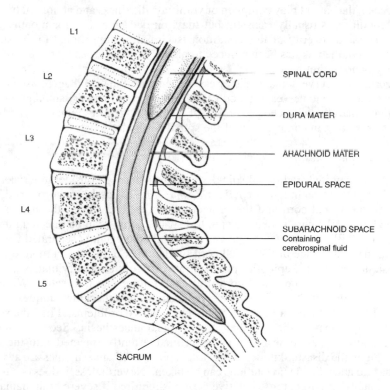

Figure 31.1 The terminal spinal column and spinal cord. The spinal cord is covered exteriorly by the dura mater. The space outside this—the epidural space—is filled mainly with liquid fat. There is, effectively, no subdural space as the arachnoid membrane is closely applied to the inner surface of the dura. The subarachnoid space is filled with cerebrospinal fluid. The spinal cord ends higher in the spinal column than where the arachnoid membrane closes; there is, thus, a large space which can be entered without risk of damage to the cord.

too large a volume of drug is injected or because of an unexpectedly high spread. There are other unwanted effects on the nerves, the main one being that, in addition to paralysing the sensory nerves, the anaesthetic has an action on the sympathetic nerves that control the strength or tone of the blood vessels; a fall in blood pressure is the almost invariable result unless remedial action is taken. A moderate fall in a healthy person is of little significance but the effect may be severe if it occurs in the elderly, in those with pre-existing heart disease or in association with haemorrhage. The result may be disastrous if some degree of respiratory hypoxia is added; true coronary artery insufficiency may be precipitated and there may be either cardiac or respiratory arrest if it becomes impossible to maintain the circulation. Recovery following prolonged hypotension may be accompanied by acute renal failure or, even more importantly, by a varying degree of brain damage.

The introduction of sepsis into the spinal canal presents a further problem. This is a hazard peculiar to the method but, fortunately, it has been almost eliminated by modern techniques of sterilisation.

Leakage of CSF through the hole made by the needle in the dura mater, which covers the spinal cord, results in the so called 'spinal headache'. In addition to headache, the patient may complain of vomiting, dizziness and abnormal hearing. The condition is usually transient but may, on occasion, last for months. The incidence and severity of this condition is virtually proportional to the size of needle used; the risk has been reduced to about 1–2% of cases by the use of very fine or pencil-point needles.

Permanent nerve damage, either associated with the actual agent used or due to direct damage to nerves or blood vessels, may occur in a very small proportion of spinal anaesthetics. The possibility of haemorrhage after puncture of a blood vessel, resulting in compression of the spinal cord, also exists.

Epidural anaesthesia

It will be seen that traditional spinal anaesthesia carries considerable risks and, accordingly, the technique of *epidural anaesthesia* has been introduced. On leaving the spinal cord and the protection of the dura mater, the nerves pass through a small cavity called the epidural space. Drugs can be injected into this space and will, thus, affect the nerve roots while the agent is separated from the central nervous tissue of the spinal cord by the thick dura. It is a more difficult technique because the epidural space is more difficult to identify than is the fluid filled space around the spinal cord; thus, the failure rate is greater. While the epidural method is theoretically far safer than the intrathecal technique, a larger dose of anaesthetic must be given. This leads to two problems. First, the spread of the drug is less predictable than it is in spinal anaesthesia. Secondly, serious complications may arise if the agent is inadvertently injected into the CSF, resulting in the disaster known as the 'total spinal'. All anaesthetists are aware of the hazard and suitable precautions can be taken. Nevertheless, it does occur very occasionally and urgent resuscitative action is required if severe brain damage is to be avoided.[4]

A major advantage of the epidural technique is that a catheter can be introduced and left in the space. Thereafter, regular injections of the analgesic drug through

4   For an example, see *Ritchie v Chichester Health Authority* [1994] 5 Med LR 187.

the catheter will greatly prolong the duration of pain relief. This principle is regularly employed to provide pain relief during the labours of childbirth.

The recently introduced practice of injecting drugs such as morphine together with reduced doses of local anaesthetic into the two spaces has led to even greater prolongation of pain relief; equally importantly, it allows the sensory nerves to be inactivated while not, at the same time, paralysing the motor system. However, the technique also introduces a potential for serious side effects, such as delayed respiratory depression. Regular and prolonged monitoring of the patient is essential.[5]

There are a number of contraindications to both techniques which should be well known to those practising them. As a result, the incidence of severe adverse reactions is very low but the risks certainly increase with infirmity—so much so that many anaesthetists may prefer to use a modern, relatively non-toxic general anaesthetic in 'high-risk' patients.

General anaesthesia

General anaesthetics may be given by inhalation, intravenously or even by intramuscular injection. Intriguingly, the exact method by which the various drugs produce their effect is at present unknown and is still a subject of research throughout the world—in practice, the efficiency of an inhalation anaesthetic agent depends largely on its insolubility in blood and this property is a feature of the more modern agents. By any definition, inhalation anaesthetics are toxic substances and it is remarkable that pharmacological and medical skills have combined to limit the mortality from a deliberate interference with the patient's physiological balance to miniscule proportions.

Children and the very aged are rather more susceptible to general inhalation anaesthetics than are adults in the middle age range; there is some suggestion that Afro Caribbeans are more susceptible to their ill effects, particularly those with sickle-cell trait (see page 9). As mentioned before, 'death under anaesthesia' is not the same as 'death due to anaesthesia'. The number of cases of the former vastly outnumber the latter. The 1987 Confidential Enquiry into Perioperative Deaths[6] revealed a 0.7% mortality from all causes within 30 days of surgery. The estimated mortality resulting from purely anaesthetic causes is now less than 1 in 200,000. Unexpected occurrences do occur, despite the most meticulous preparation and conduct.

The two most likely causes of death due to anaesthesia are lack of oxygen (hypoxia) and cardiac arrest. The hazards of general anaesthesia can be summarised as being due to complications arising from:

- airway maintenance;
- the patient's breathing;
- problems with the circulation;
- the drugs used;
- anaesthetic equipment;
- fires and explosions;
- inhalation of gastric contents.

5   It would seem that the misuse of this technique was responsible for the conviction for manslaughter of a doctor in Zimbabwe in 1995.
6   N Buck, H B Devlin and J N Lunn *Report of a Confidential Enquiry into Perioperative Deaths* (1987).

Airway maintenance

The unconscious patient poses special problems because he is unable to take corrective reflex action if an adverse situation arises. One of the main problems is that the patient's tongue may fall back, obstruct the airway and cause suffocation. This requires prompt recognition and remedy. Various simple manoeuvres such as lifting the patient's chin are available. More complicated techniques, such as endotracheal intubation, in which a plastic tube is inserted into the patient's trachea, need to be learned. Such manoeuvres often form an integral part of the anaesthetic technique and failure to perform them adequately can lead to the patient becoming hypoxic.

The technique of endotracheal intubation also carries the risk of damage to the patient's teeth or lips, due to pressure from the laryngoscope during intubation.

The patient's breathing

By far the greatest risk of anaesthesia lies in the provocation of hypoxia. The skill of anaesthesia lies in preventing this while, at the same time, achieving unconsciousness in the patient; this is done by the addition of oxygen to the anaesthetic mixture. It is essential, therefore, for the patient's breathing to be satisfactory. Severe shortage of oxygen during deep anaesthesia may be due to inadequate ventilation and can result in sudden death on the table due to heart failure. Conditions such as anaemia, haemorrhage or lung disease may have an important synergistic action and the patient's breathing may need to be supplemented by assisted ventilation. The experience of the anaesthetist guards the patient; warning signs may be missed by the inexperienced or even by the consultant if he is required to supervise more than one operating theatre.

The maintenance of adequate oxygenation is fundamental to the safe practice of anaesthesia. The patient may suffer long-term effects if the lack of oxygen is not corrected quickly. The margin of safety is low as there are only four to five minutes before significant hypoxia results in permanent brain damage or even death.[7] There are particular hazards in dental practice in which, although anaesthesia is generally of short duration, cerebral hypoxia may be exaggerated by the sitting position.

Severe long-term effects may be seen in the lungs after general inhalation anaesthesia of any type—generally in the form of collapse of portions of the lung (usually due to faulty intubation techniques) or of pneumonia.

Problems with the circulation

It is essential that adequate circulation of blood around the body is maintained. Stimulation of the respiratory lining by a high concentration of irritant gas, the passing of a tube through an inadequately anaesthetised larynx, or certain surgical manoeuvres such as pulling on the peritoneum or eyeball may each result in sudden arrest of the heart. Cardiac failure of a rather different type (ventricular fibrillation) can result from excessive secretion of adrenaline by patients who have been inadequately anaesthetised; dental patients are particularly susceptible by reason of their generally ambulant treatment.

---

7   Failure in this respect has led to convictions for manslaughter: see, for example, *R v Adomako* [1995] 1 AC 171.

The drugs used

Ill-effects from the actual anaesthetics depend upon their toxicity; this may be selective as to organ and some agents—eg the now obsolete agents chloroform and cyclopropane—were particularly cardiotoxic. This, however, is not to say that similar toxic drugs should not be used by competent practitioners if they have other advantages; the delicate balance upon which good medical practice depends is well illustrated in this context.

Fatal disease of the liver may be attributed to the anaesthetic agent. Chloroform was especially implicated in the past; any toxic effect of an anaesthetic on the liver is greatly potentiated by associated hypoxia and this was especially true of that old agent which was used when anaesthetic techniques were rudimentary. Therapeutic dilemmas also arise using modern drugs and, in certain cases, the doctor must balance the advantage to the patient of a good anaesthetic agent against the possibility of subsequent damage; the important point is that this is a legitimate decision which becomes unacceptable only if the judgment is unconsidered. For example, halothane was judged by most practitioners to be the best 'general' anaesthetic agent available in the later twentieth century. Its repeated administration, however, can load the liver with metabolic problems to which it may succumb—particularly if the anaesthetics are repeated at very short intervals and the liver was previously unhealthy, for example, due to the effects of alcoholism. The availability of newer inhalational agents such as enflurane, isoflurane and sevoflurane has, in fact, led to a marked decrease in the use of halothane.

Some patients are unduly susceptible to particular anaesthetics and may react abnormally. A patient may be allergic to a particular drug, resulting in severe, potentially fatal, anaphylaxis. Malignant hyperpyrexia—or a rapid and severe rise in body temperature accompanied by convulsions— is another example which can be associated with most anaesthetic drugs—including newer introductions such as enflurane. Susceptibility to malignant hyperpyrexia, and probably to other forms of hypersensitivity, is genetically controlled; the importance of taking a good preoperative history is emphasised.[8]

The use of relaxant drugs, which has opened up major surgery to a wide group of patients who might well have died under a comparably effective unassisted general anaesthetic, is not without hazard—mainly because of concurrent paralysis of the respiratory muscles. Thus, the patient is unable to breath following their administration; breathing must be maintained by the anaesthetist who must have equipment available for artificial respiration. Nevertheless, such equipment occasionally fails or the anaesthetist is unable to implement its use because of a failure on his part, such as inability to pass an endotracheal tube.

An increasingly recognised hazard associated with relaxant drugs is that of awareness. In the past, an inadequately anaesthetised patient moved in response to surgical stimulation. However, the use of these drugs has led to situations where the patient is not fully asleep and yet is paralysed and unable to alert the anaesthetist to his or her condition. The stress engendered has led to actions for negligence.[9]

---

8   W A Macrae, K M Miller and A A Watson 'Malignant Hyperpyrexia' (1979) 19 Med Sci Law 261.
9   Eg *Ackers v Wigan Area Health Authority* [1991] 2 Med LR 232; *Phelan v Cumbria Health Authority* [1991] 2 Med LR 419; *Early v Newham Health Authority* [1994] 5 Med LR 214.

The equipment

The apparatus itself may deliver an inadequate oxygen supply. Murder mysteries have been written around mistaken colouring or filling of gas cylinders—and it can happen accidentally. Cylinders may run dry or taps may be inadvertently turned off—or may not turn on in an emergency. Responsibility for the apparatus is clearly vested in the anaesthetist and the prevention of catastrophe due to malfunction depends on his vigilance.

Fires and explosions

The spectacular nature of fires and explosions leads to an exaggeration of their frequency. In the past, very considerable effort was put into their prevention and this was one reason for the increasingly widespread use of halothane once it was introduced. The use of explosive gases is now virtually eliminated in the United Kingdom.

Inhalation of gastric contents

As mentioned earlier, one of the results of anaesthesia is the abolishment of protective reflexes. A common danger lies in failure to protect the air passages against inhalation of foreign material. This is especially so in the emergency case where there is insufficient time to fast the patient preoperatively and the stomach is not empty at the time of operation. Stomach contents may flow back into the mouth and air passages of a supine patient or the patient may vomit—particularly if there has been no preoperative sedation. Blood, swabs or even teeth may be inhaled without reflex coughing—there is an obvious potential association with dental surgery.[10] An acute asphyxial death may follow aspiration but survival can also be accompanied by an inflammatory process in the lungs which is particularly severe due to the acidity of the inhaled stomach contents; the aspiration of a solid object will cause collapse of a part of or the whole of the lung, which will then be particularly susceptible to infection. The danger of inhalation of regurgitated stomach contents is increased by using muscle relaxants.

Occasionally, patients who have been operated upon may appear well for several days until, quite unheralded, sudden death occurs. The cause is nearly always pulmonary embolism—a clot of blood, usually forming in a leg or pelvic vein, detaches and lodges in the pulmonary artery. The formation of such clots is naturally associated with immobility in bed and, while every prophylactic care such as stockings and anticoagulants may be taken, occasional instances are unfortunately inevitable; death is effectively due to natural causes.

Special factors relating to intravenous anaesthesia

Although one of the major advantages of the new generation of anaesthetic agents, such as sevoflurane, is that they can be used to induce anaesthesia in a pleasant way, the majority of inhalation anaesthetics are preceded by the injection of short-acting drugs called induction agents. There is a wide selection and each has

10 A problem which was, at one time, exacerbated by the practice of single-handed dental surgery and anaesthesis. The General Dental Council have now condemned the procedure in very certain terms. See *Abrol v General Dental Council* (1984) 156 Brit Dent J 369.

its own advantages and side effects. Occasionally, the whole surgical procedure may be covered by this method, which is known as total intravenous anaesthesia. It is, indeed, possible that automated intravenous anaesthesia may become widely used in the future. So-called target controlled infusion involves computerised control of the blood level of the drug in use and the system may also include an automatic warning of awareness in a paralysed patient as discussed above.

Such things are, however, for the future and probably also depend on the development of new agents—such as those based on the opioids. Meantime, it should be noted that many of the current induction drugs, especially if given in too great a dose, have a profound effect on the blood pressure and on the action of the heart; as a result, they must be used with particular care in the elderly and unfit. Many intravenous drugs of this type also act on the respiratory centre, which may be so affected by overdose that the breathing becomes ineffective. Moreover, a tendency to uncontrolled reflex spasm is especially marked under barbiturate anaesthesia; any irritation of the throat may result in spasm of the glottis and suffocation of the patient. It has to be remembered that there is no physiological control over the absorption of a substance injected into a vein; the whole dose is instantly available for transmission to the tissues and it can only be excreted from the body over a period of time—everything depends, therefore, on the skill of the injector.

The hazards of anaesthesia have been most dramatically illustrated in the field of dental surgery. Apart from the problems associated with the single-handed anaesthetist/surgeon, coincidental complications with resuscitative apparatus have also been described. Coroners' inquests have revealed some dramatic examples of hazards related to the maintenance of apparatus or the training of assistants, including unnoticed breakage of the tap on the oxygen cylinder or lack of oxygen dictating the summoning of help from the fire brigade; one assistant was reported as stating that she 'had not been on any course but had trained by watching others'.[11] From the medico-legal aspect, conditions of this type are of far greater significance than are the physiological problems of anaesthesia. Such practises are now, happily, obsolete. Since 1998, general anaesthesia in the dental surgery has had to be administered by an individual who is on the specialist register of the General Medical Council as an anaesthetist or who is a supervised trainee. The dentist must be assisted by an appropriately trained nurse and the anaesthetist must be supported by a specifically trained person who has the skills to assist in monitoring the patient's condition and in any emergency. All those involved must train as a team to deal with an emergency.[12] Anything less is unacceptable— failure to comply will lay the practitioner open to a charge of serious professional misconduct.

The expert witness

The pathologist's evidence in a case of death during an operation may well be limited. There will be little difficulty if death has resulted from a frank surgical

---

11 See Legal Correspondent 'Another Death during Dentistry' (1974) ii BMJ 352.
12 General Dental Council *General Anaesthesia in Dentistry: Maintaining Standards (Amendment)* (1998).

mishap—the result, say, of failing to secure adequately an artery of moderate size is very obvious. Beyond this, the findings and interpretations become progressively less dogmatic. Thus, the presence of a tooth or a swab in the main air passages may be simple to demonstrate, but to state with certainty that death resulted from their presence is very much harder. Vomit may be found in the trachea but it may be extremely difficult to decide whether this was the cause of, or the result of, a hypoxic death.

The pathologist will seek and demonstrate any pre-existing disease. But having done so, the standard dilemma of the interrelationship of disease with any accident remains to be solved—was it causative, contributory to or incidental to the death? It is seldom easy to make the choice with certainty and a cautious approach by the witness may be a sign of experience rather than of indecisiveness. If disease discovered is considered significant, further consideration must be given as to whether it was noted or, if not, whether it should have been noted before the operation.

The fundamental problem lies in the fact that the majority of operation deaths, and certainly most of those correctly regarded as 'anaesthetic deaths', will be due to a physiological abnormality. There will be no anatomical evidence available to the pathologist and much of his opinion must be based on exclusion and reasoning. One cannot do better than quote the late Keith Simpson:[13]

> 'The pathologist is bound to rely in part on what he is told of the events leading to death, for functional lapses like fall in blood pressure, cardiac arrhythmia, spasm of the glottis, or vagal inhibition leave no trace at autopsy. A candid review of the circumstances by clinician, anaesthetist, and pathologist is most likely to elucidate the truth.'

The post-mortem examination in such cases is incomplete without toxicological analyses designed to disclose a positive overdose of anaesthetic or other therapeutic agent, and it is important that both the pathologist and the analyst be properly informed as to the drugs that have been administered. Specimens should also be taken to assess any biochemical or enzymatic abnormalities that may have caused the catastrophe or that may indicate its mechanism; due regard, must, however, be paid to post-mortem changes which may affect the analytical results. But even with maximum investigation, the pathologist is often able to do little more than decide 'death was due to operation under anaesthesia but there is no [*or*, and there is] evidence that the anaesthetic was given incorrectly'.

In eliciting expert evidence, the advocate should remember that the pathologist is seldom an expert clinician. He is often pressed to state whether an operation or anaesthetic procedure was good or proper; his correct attitude is to refuse to be drawn unless he has a special knowledge or unless the matter is of great simplicity.

Responsibility for the patient at operation

It is almost impossible to lay down dividing lines of responsibility between the surgeon and the anaesthetist that can be applied as a generalisation. Decisions taken can only be assessed in the light of the particular circumstances. The operating theatre in some ways resembles the flight deck of an aircraft—the captain

---

13 In *Forensic Medicine* (8th edn, 1979) p 155.

is in command and takes ultimate decisions but it would be an unusual man who disregarded the advice of the flight controller without careful consideration.[14]

On this analogy, the surgeon is the captain and is ultimately responsible for the decision to operate, the extent of the operation and for any decisions as to whether to complete or abort his intended routine. But in making these, he will be advised by the anaesthetist as to the patient's preoperative physical state and his condition during the operation. The anaesthetist is responsible for the functioning of the anaesthetic apparatus, for maintaining adequate anaesthesia and adequate cardio-respiratory function during the operation and for ensuring that the patient is fit to be returned to the ward. It is also the anaesthetist's responsibility to maintain or resuscitate the patient by means of intravenous fluid replacement therapy, including blood, during the operation. Afterwards, the anaesthetist usually recommends a post-operative fluid regime but this may be changed by the surgical team if the patient's condition changes.

The most 'twilight' area of authority lies in the administration of antibiotics. Surgeons frequently request their administration at the start and during the operation. It would be unreasonable to expect a member of the surgical team to unscrub just to administer these drugs. On the other hand, they have nothing to do with the anaesthetic. A commonsense approach is recommended. It is the surgeon's responsibility to prescribe the required antibiotic and ensure the patient is not allergic to it. On the other hand, the anaesthetist carries some responsibility for injecting the drug and would be wise to double check the drug against any possible patient allergy.

The patient in intensive care

Special considerations apply to the intensive care unit (ICU). Few of these will have any direct bearing on the pathologist but they fall within the remit of forensic medicine and merit brief mention.

Almost by definition, the patient admitted to the ICU will be incapable of consenting to treatment. It should be noted that a relative cannot 'consent' on behalf of an incompetent adult patient;[15] the intervention of the intensivist is justified by the legal principle of necessity. It follows that the decision to remove the patient from care can be justified in the same way, supported by the assumption of good medical practice. Clearly, removal can be effected without qualm when, either, the patient has improved sufficiently or when he or she has been declared brain-stem dead—there is no obligation to continue to ventilate a corpse.[16] The difficult decision arises when the patient is not dead but further treatment is considered futile. There is little doubt that, given good faith on the part of the doctor, the courts would support him or her in his or her clinical judgment. Moreover, the cause of death would be the cause of admission to the ICU—not the removal of support.[17]

14 And he cannot simply rely on his 'crew'—eg the theatre nurses. See the *locus classicus* of the law: *Mahon v Osborne* [1939] 2 KB 14, where it was said: '[The surgeon] cannot absolve himself, if a mistake has been made, by saying, " relied on the nurse"'(per Goddard LJ at 47).
15 *Re T (adult) (refusal of medical treatment)* [1992] 4 All ER 649 at 653, per Lord Donaldson MR.
16 *Re A* (1992) 3 Med LR 303. It might be *desirable* to do so in the context of transplantation therapy.
17 *R v Malcherek, R v Steel* [1981] 2 All ER 422; *Finlayson v HM Advocate* 1978 SLT 60. See also the very apposite New Zealand case: *Auckland Area Health Board v A-G* [1993] 1 NZLR 235.

The corollary is that cases should or should not be reported to the coroner or procurator fiscal on similar criteria; the mere fact that treatment is withdrawn from a patient in intensive care does not dictate that the medico-legal authorities should be involved. It is the *reason for admission* that is significant.

Fluid replacement therapy

The body subjected to operation may be deficient in fluid for two reasons:

- The condition requiring treatment may have precipitated fluid loss— eg haemorrhage from a ruptured vessel in a stomach ulcer.
- The operation itself may lead to significant loss of fluid. All operations incur some blood loss and it is the mark of the good surgical team to reduce this to a minimum. But fluid loss is to be anticipated even in the best of hands in many procedures.

The condition of hypovolaemic shock may be present before, or arise during or after, the operation. It may result from active blood loss, from burning, from crushing, from circulating toxins or, indeed, from any condition in which the body's physiological defences are overstretched. Whatever the precipitating cause, fluid is removed from the circulation and is either lost to the exterior or left stagnant in the tissues; the effective volume of the blood is reduced. If whole blood is lost, there is reduction in the number of oxygen-carrying cells; if only plasma is lost, the blood thickens and the red cells circulate inadequately.[18] In either case, oxygenation of the tissues is impaired and fluid loss from the consequently damaged capillaries is accentuated. The vicious cycle is aggravated by increasing failure of the heart to cope with the excessive demands imposed upon it; so-called 'compensated shock' becomes 'irreversible shock' and death follows. Prolonged shock is often complicated by acute renal failure or, in the more severe case, by multi-organ failure.

Treatment or prevention of the 'spiral' lies mainly in replacing the volume of circulating blood by the intravenous infusion of artificially prepared solutions of electrolytes, of simulated or natural plasma or of blood.

Infusion of fluids other than blood

The choice of fluid for infusion depends on careful biochemical monitoring. This will indicate the degree of fluid loss, the particular electrolytes required and the efficacy of treatment. There is no purpose in detailing the methods involved, save to say that they are complicated and ideal surveillance in very ill patients may well be beyond the capabilities of a small hospital; in such circumstances, the control of fluid balance has to depend on clinical judgment aided by a fluid balance chart which must be kept to give some quantitative, albeit rough, guide.

Subsequent problems arise from the possibilities that the infusion given contained the wrong electrolytes or that either electrolytes or fluid were given in inadequate quantity to achieve cure. An equally important error is to use too much fluid so that the heart is embarrassed by hypervolaemia—too *great* a circulating blood volume. Such a condition can readily occur in the elderly and in

18 Indeed, the condition known as 'disseminated intravascular coagulation' may be established.

patients who have poor heart function. More fluid then escapes into the tissues and, in particular, into the lungs—the patient is effectively drowning in his own fluid.

Several viruses are transmitted, either in the main or largely, through blood plasma. These include the hepatitis B virus (HBV), the hepatitis C virus (HCV) and the human immunodeficiency virus (HIV). Very large numbers of people have been infected due to the transfusion of contaminated blood and lawsuits against the transfusion authorities have either succeeded or are pending in many parts of the world including the United Kingdom and other countries of the European Community.[19] The major problem for both producers and litigants is that viruses tend to appear spontaneously and can be spread widely before an efficient diagnostic test is developed or prophylactic measures can be introduced. All blood products that are to be used for transfusion are, however, now tested for the three main viral contaminants and/or are heat treated to destroy them. Artificial plasma expanders, of which dextran is a typical example, are also used widely and are equally, if not more, effective as natural human plasma in the treatment of shock.

Hazards particular to blood transfusion

Most readers will be familiar with the well-demarcated blood group systems related to the red cell. Even so, an understanding of the hazards of blood transfusion will be simplified if a brief recapitulation of the main facts is provided. Each 'system' contains a minimum of two alleles—or antigenic alternatives—and, in most, there are considerably more. The chances of transfused blood containing a 'foreign' antigen are, therefore, high. The concept of rejection of non-self by the formation of antibodies has been discussed in Chapter 1. In general, the strength of the rejection reaction depends on the 'strength' of the antigen; from the point of view of blood transfusion reactions, the antigens of the ABO and Rhesus (CDE) systems are by far the most important.[20] Nevertheless, repetitive exposure to the same foreign antigen of any 'strength' leads, in the end, to antibody production so that the effect of the lesser antigens increases as more transfusions are given; clinically, it becomes increasingly difficult to find donor blood that is fully compatible with the recipient of multiple transfusions.

The nature of antibodies differs. Those of the ABO system are of 'naturally occurring' type and are present normally as antitheses to the antigens. The four basic blood profiles can be summarised:

Blood Group	Antigen present on cell	Antibodies present in plasma
A	A[1]	Anti-B
B	B	Anti-A
AB	AB	None[1]
O	O	Anti-A and Anti-B

19 Though the majority of those infected are being treated for blood disorders: *Re HIV Haemophiliac Litigation,* CA (1990) Independent, 2 October; *AB v Glasgow and West of Scotland Blood Transfusion Service* (1989) 15 BMLR 91; *X (haemophiliac-HIV) v France* (1992) 14 EHHR 483. See C Zinn et al 'Countries Struggle with Hepatitis C Contamination' (1995) 310 BMJ 417.
20 Others which may appear in medical reports include the MNS, Kidd, Duffy and Kell systems.
 1 The A antigen can appear in a number of variants known as A_1 (which is the common presentation), A_2, etc. This is of practical importance as the plasma of patients of blood group A_2, and particularly of A_2B, may contain anti-A_1 in their plasma.

Not only are the antigens and antibodies particularly reactive but, since the antibodies are already present, an incompatible ABO transfusion—for example, transfusing group A blood to a group B recipient—will result in an immediate reaction.

The Rhesus system is very much more complicated and, essentially, consists of three allelic pairs—Dd, Cc and Ee—of which D is by far the most powerful;[2] hence, in common parlance, a Rhesus-positive person is one who carries the D antigen (whether in the paired form DD or Dd—some 85% of the British population) while the Rhesus-negative person carries no D and is, therefore, of the genotype dd (15% of the population). However, the three antigens can be combined in eight different ways[3] and are always transmitted as a group. The MNS group is also complicated but, for practical purposes, we can regard all the other significant groups as consisting of single allelic pairs.

All blood group antibodies other than those in the ABO system are of simple 'immune' type which come into being only as a result of active stimulation by the specific antigen. The effect, say, of transfusing Rhesus-positive (D+) blood into a Rhesus-negative (dd) person will be to alert the body's defensive mechanism and to lay down the template of antibody production in preparation for a second attack. In all probability, there will be no clinical effect from the first 'incompatible' transfusion. Nevertheless, the body has been sensitised, antibody is now circulating and the next similar transfusion may result in an immediate reaction. The word 'may' is used advisedly, as antibody production depends on the ability of the recipient to do so and on the 'strength' of the foreign donor antigen; a number of incompatible transfusions may be required to stimulate sufficient antibody to provoke a reaction to the lesser antigens.

In passing, it is to be noted that fetal blood cells will pass across the placenta and enter the mother's blood stream. Thus, in some blood group systems, bearing a fetus of a different group from the mother is similar to a transfusion of equivalently different blood. Thus, if a Rhesus-negative mother (dd) carries a fetus that is Rhesus-positive by virtue of inheriting the D antigen from its father, she will form anti-D antibodies which will pass back to the fetus whose D-positive cells will be destroyed.[4] This is the basis of the potentially lethal condition of haemolytic disease of the newborn. One medico-legally important aspect of the condition is that, nowadays, it would certainly be negligent to fail to identify the possibility and to take the necessary steps to protect the fetus and the mother.[5] The effect may be additive—ie the first 'incompatible' pregnancy may do no more than sensitise the mother, while subsequent fetuses will be increasingly affected. It is here that an association with blood transfusion becomes apparent, for it will be seen that a mismatched transfusion can be equivalent to an 'incompatible' pregnancy. Thus, such a transfusion may have a profound effect on a woman's future child-bearing

---

2   By contrast, d is so weak as to be incapable of producing antibodies. Variants on the standard antigens occur; the most common of these is designated Cw.

3   Ie CDE, CDe, cDE, cDe, CdE, Cde, cdE and cde. 98% of the groups in Great Britain consist of CDe, cDE or cde. If we include the antigen Cw, the groups s a whole can be combined to form 78 genotypes.

4   The genotype of the father is, then, very important. If he is homozygous DD, all the children of the union will be affected; only half will be at risk if he is heterozygous Dd.

5   And this might extend to protection of later fetuses. See the American case *Yeager v Bloomington Obstetrics and Gynecology Inc* 585 NE 2d (Ind, 1992).

capacity and accurate matching of blood is particularly important in the case of female patients.

An incompatible transfusion may, as described, give no clinical signs but simply set the scene for the future. A mild antigen/antibody reaction will produce a rise in temperature, a 'rigor' and varying constitutional upset. A severe reaction, and particularly one associated with ABO incompatibility, will result from massive destruction of blood within the vessels, the condition of shock will develop and the patient may die. Recovery from this, as from shock of any origin, may well be followed by acute renal, or even multi-organ, failure.

The prevention of transfusion reactions depends on compatibility testing in the laboratory. The techniques are immaterial here but the lawyer should understand the general principles.

The cells of the recipient are irrelevant in the context of transfusion reactions—their importance lies in indicating the group of the donor to be chosen. The plasma of the donor is similarly irrelevant because any contained antibodies are rapidly diluted in the recipient's body. Thus it is possible, and reasonable in an emergency, to transfuse group O blood (the so-called universal donor blood) to a male recipient irrespective of his blood group. If the O blood is also D- negative, it could be used for a female recipient, the calculated risk being the provocation of a transfusion reaction due to the presence in the recipient of an immune antibody other than anti-D. Such emergency practice is rarely undertaken; the delay due to testing introduces less risk than does an unmatched transfusion and full compatibility is almost always assured.

This is done in two stages. First, the donor cells are selected as being similar in ABO and CDE groups to those of the recipient. Compatibility of the recipient's plasma is then ensured by 'cross-matching'—the effect of mixing the actual donor cells with the actual recipient plasma (in practice, serum) is studied in the laboratory. Each donor unit (ie bottle or bag of blood) must be tested separately. This method does not exclude the possibility of sensitising the recipient to one of the less important blood group antigens but testing for complete similarity of all blood group factors would be technologically impossible; provided cross-matching is undertaken regularly, the danger to the patient approximates to zero.

In practice, transfusions that are given and prove to be incompatible by reason of inaccuracy of cross-matching are extremely rare; faults are far more often organisational in nature. The commonest mistakes include errors in transcription—due simply to clerical error or to the introduction of confusing terms such as 'group A serum' rather than 'anti-B serum'. Failure of the nursing staff to check the reference on the bag or bottle against the actual laboratory report on compatibility is another potent source of error which may have serious results. The presence of similarly named patients in the ward may be disastrous if the donor blood is not checked against the patient's notes. Such errors are compounded by the use of the telephone combined with trusting the delivery of messages to intermediates—conditions that commonly obtain in an emergency. A famous instance, probably apocryphal, was quoted concerning a telephone message to the effect. 'We are sending up the blood for the melaena patient'—meaning 'for the patient with bowel haemorrhage'; the blood was transfused into a child with the first name 'Melina'.

Not all reactions are due to antigen/antibody incompatibility. Some are due to infection of the unit of blood. It is most important that the storage cabinet be maintained at constant optimal temperature—cabinets should be fitted with alarm systems that operate if the temperature range is exceeded. Similarly, expiry dates must be scrupulously observed, as blood that has degenerated may cause considerable disability in its own right due to leakage of electrolytes from damaged red cells. Finally, the blood may have contained transmissible pathogenic organisms other than the viruses mentioned; the best known are malaria and syphilis but these will have been screened out by any competent transfusion service.

The expert witness

Much as in the case of deaths associated with anaesthesia, the investigation of transfusion reactions requires the co-operation of all concerned and, again, the primary object must be to prevent similar mistakes in the future.

Inquiries must be made as to the method of cross-matching, the documentation, and the chain of orders by which the transfusion was given and as to the precise clinical presentation. A full investigation of the remaining blood in the container, including a bacteriological analysis, must be made and correlated with the serum obtained from the patient either while living or, if death occurs, at autopsy.

The anatomic pathological evidence will be directed to demonstrating signs of blood destruction. At the same time, the contribution of the condition requiring transfusion to the death has to be assessed and, of course, the presence of unsuspected disease must be sought. In general, the precise cause of death is likely to be elucidated and suitable remedial measures can be introduced.

Appendix A

A guide to medical terminology

Prepositional prefixes

Prefix	Meaning	Example
A- or An-	Without	Anoxia = without oxygen
Ante-	Before	Ante-mortem = before death
Anti-	Against	Antiseptic = prevents sepsis
Circum-	Around	Circumoral = around the mouth
Contra-	Against, opposite	Contralateral = on the other side
De-	Away from	Dehydrate = remove water
Dia	Through	Dialyse = to pass through a membrane
Dys-	Abnormal	Dysfunction = abnormal function
En- or Endo-	Within	Endotracheal = within the trachea
Epi-	Outside	Epidermis = outermost part of the skin
Extra- or Exo-	Outside	Extradural = outside the coverings of the brain
		Exogenous = produced from outside
Hetero-	Different	Heterotopic = in the wrong place
Homo-	Similar	Homozygous = similar genes combined
Hyper-	Excessive	Hypertrophy = overgrowth
Hypo-	Too little	Hypotension = low blood pressure
Infra-	Below	Infraorbital = below the eye
Inter-	Between	Intercostal = between the ribs
Intra-	Within	Intrahepatic = within the liver
Juxta-	Beside	Juxtaposition = closeness together
Para-	Close to, around	Paravertebral = near the spine
Per-	Through	Percutaneous = through the skin
Poly-	Many	Polymorphic = many-shaped
Post-	After	Post-traumatic = after injury
Pre-	In front of	Prepatellar = in front of the knee cap
Proto-	First	Prototype = the original of the form
Retro-	Behind	Retrosternal = behind the sternum
Sub-	Beneath	Subcutaneous = beneath the skin
Supra-	Above	Supralabial = above the lip

493

| Syn- | Together | Syndactyly = web fingers |
| Trans- | Through, across | Transplacental = across the placenta |

Some suffixes

Suffix	Meaning	Example
-aemia	In or of the blood	Anaemia = no (or less than normal) blood
-algia	Pain	Neuralgia = pain in a nerve
-ectomy	Removal	Prostatectomy = removal of the prostate
-genic	Producing	Pathogenic = causing disease
-itis	Inflammation of	Laryngitis = inflammation of the larynx
-logy	Study of	Pathology = study of disease
-megaly	Enlargement of	Splenomegaly = enlargement of the spleen
-oma	Tumour	Adenoma = a tumour of glands
-osis	Abnormal process other than inflammation	Fibrosis = proliferation of fibrous tissue (scarring)
-pathy	Abnormal structure	Myopathy = abnormal muscle
-plasia	Growth	Hyperplasia = excessive growth
-stomy	Making a hole	Tracheostomy = artificial opening in trachea

Anatomic prefixes

Prefix	Relating to	Example
Aden(o)-	Glands	Adenitis = inflammation of glands
Angio-	Blood vessels	Angiospasm = spasm of the arteries
Arthr(o)-	Joints	Arthralgia = pain in the joints
Cardio-	Heart	Cardiomyopathy = abnormality of the heart muscle
Cerebro-	Brain	Cerebrospinal fluid = fluid surrounding the brain and spinal cord
Chol(o)- or (e)-	Bile	Cholecystitis = inflammation of the gall bladder
Chondro-	Cartilage	Chondroma = a tumour of cartilage
Colo-	Large bowel	Colostomy = making an opening in the colon
Costo-	Ribs	Costochondral = of the rib cartilages
Encephal(o)-	Brain	Encephalitis = inflammation of the brain
Enter(o)-	Intestines	Enteritis = inflammation of the intestine

Prefix	Relating to	Example
Gastr(o)-	Stomach	Gastroenterostomy = making a connecting hole between stomach and intestine
Haem(o)-	Blood	Haemothorax = blood in the thoracic cavity
Hepat(o)-	Liver	Hepatomegaly = enlargement of the liver
My(o)-	Muscle	Myesthenia = wasting of the muscle
Nephr(o)-	Kidney	Nephrosis = an abnormal process in the kidney
Neur(o)-	Nerve	Ncurotoxic = poisonous to nerves
Pneumo-	Lung (or simply air)	Pneumoconiosis = an abnormality of the lung associated with dust
		Pneumothorax = free air in the thoracic cavity
Oste(o)-	Bone	Osteology = the study of bones

Note: American medical writing does not usually use diphthongs. Hence anaemia becomes anemia; tumour becomes tumor; oesophagus becomes esophagus.

Registrar's duty to report deaths to the coroner

The registrar shall report the death to the coroner if the death is one:

a) in respect of which the deceased was not attended during his last illness by a registered medical practitioner; or
b) in respect of which the registrar—
    i) has been unable to obtain a duly completed certificate of cause of death, or
    ii) has received such a certificate with respect to which it appears to him . . . that the deceased was not seen by the certifying medical practitioner either after death or within 14 days before death; or
c) the cause of which appears to be unknown; or
d) which the registrar has reason to believe to have been unnatural or to have been caused by violence or neglect or by abortion or to have been attended by suspicious circumstances; or
e) which appears to the registrar to have occurred during an operation or before recovery from the effects of an anaesthetic; or
f) which appears to the registrar . . . to have been due to industrial disease or industrial poisoning.

In addition, if the registrar has reason to believe . . . that the circumstances of the death were such that it is the duty of some person or authority other than himself to report the death to the coroner, he shall either satisfy himself that it has been reported or report it himself.[1]

---

1   The Registration of Births and Deaths Regulations 1987, SI 1987/2088, r 41.

Duty of the doctor to report a death to the coroner

There is no official list to guide the doctor other than the guidelines given on the reverse of the English Medical Certificate of Cause of Death. These are insufficiently comprehensive and most coroners provide their own guide. The following is taken from *Reportable Deaths: A Brief Guide for Doctors* issued by HM Coroner for South Yorkshire (West):

A death should be reported to HM Coroner if:

a) it cannot readily be certified as being due to natural causes;
b) the deceased was not seen by a doctor within the last 14 days prior to death;[1]
c) there is any element of suspicious circumstances;
d) there is any history of violence;
e) the death may be linked to an accident (whenever it occurred);
f) there is any question of self neglect or neglect by others;
g) the death has occurred or the illness arisen during or shortly after detention in police or prison custody (including voluntary attendance at a police station);
h) the deceased was detained under the Mental Health Act;
i) the death is linked with abortion;
j) the death may have been contributed to by the actions of the deceased himself (eg overdose, alcoholism, self-injury, history of drug addiction or solvent abuse);[2]
k) the deceased was receiving any form of war pension or industrial disability pension unless the death can be shown to be wholly unconnected;
l) the death could be due to industrial disease or related in any way to the deceased's employment;

---

1   This is an example of coroners requiring more than the minimum (cf Appendix B, item b(ii)).
2   There are obvious grey areas in such categories. A heavy smoker who dies from carcinoma of the lung has clearly contributed to his own death but it is very unlikely that the coroner would wish to investigate the death.

m) the death was during an operation or before full recovery from the effects of the anaesthetic or was in any way related to the anaesthetic (in any event, a death within 24 hours should normally be referred);

n) the death may be related to a medical procedure or treatment whether invasive or not;

o) the death may be due to lack of medical care;

p) there are any other unusual or disturbing features to the case;

q) it may be wise to report any death where there is an allegation of medical mis-management.

NB   Other coroners might well include other categories—eg deaths of foster children, obscure infant deaths, doubtful stillbirths, etc.

Conclusions of the jury/coroner as to the death

Killed unlawfully[1]
Killed himself [whilst the balance of his mind was disturbed]
Attempted/Self-induced abortion
Accident/Misadventure[2]
Execution of sentence of death
Killed lawfully
Natural causes*
Industrial disease*
Want of attention at birth*
Dependence on drugs/non-dependent abuse of drugs*
[Died in the . . . . disaster (insert name of disaster which was subject
of a public inquiry)][3]
Stillbirth
Open verdict

---

* In these cases, and in no others, the words 'the cause of death was aggravated by lack of care[4]/self neglect' may be added.

(Coroners Rules 1984, SI 1984/552, Sch 4 (as amended).)

---

1 See, for example, the jury verdict in *Inquest on Conrad Cole, Oxford, May 1992* (1992) Times, 19 May, p 1. (See also p 80).
2 But this distinction has been deprecated: *R v Coroner for City of Portsmouth, ex p Anderson* [1988] 2 All ER 604.
3 Inserted by SI 1999/3325.
4 In *R v HM Coroner for North Humberside and Scunthorpe, ex p Jamieson* [1994] 3 All ER 972, it was hoped that 'lack of care' would be replaced by 'neglect'—the obverse of 'self-neglect'. 'Lack of care' in the coroner's verdict was to be distinguished from what amounted to a claim in negligence at common law. See also *R v HM Coroner for Surrey, ex p Wright* [1997] 1 All ER 823.

Deaths reportable to the procurator fiscal

1. Any uncertified death.
2. Any death that was caused by an accident arising out of the use of a vehicle including an aircraft, a ship, or a train. This category will now include a hovercraft.
3. Any death of a person while at work.
4. Any death resulting from an accident in the course of work or arising out of industrial disease or poisoning.
5. Any death due to poisoning.
6. Any death where the circumstances indicate that suicide may be a possibility.
7. Any death under medical care.
8. Any death resulting from an accident.
9. Any death following an abortion or an attempted abortion.
10. Any death where the circumstances seem to indicate fault on the part of another person (ie a person other than the deceased).
11. Any death occurring while the deceased was in legal custody.
12. Any death of a new-born child whose body is found.
13. Any death (occurring not in a house) where deceased's residence is unknown.
14. Any death by drowning.
15. Any death of a child from suffocation, including overlaying.
16. Any death which may be due to sudden death in infancy syndrome.
17. Any death occurring as a result of food poisoning or infectious disease.
18. Any death by burning or scalding or as a result of fire or explosion.
19. Any death of a foster-child.
20. Any death possibly linked to defects in medicinal products.
21. Any other death due to violent, suspicious or unexplained cause.
22. Any other death which comes in circumstances when its immediate arrival is unexplained or sudden.

This list is taken from I H B Carmichael *Sudden Deaths and Fatal Accident Inquiries* (2nd edn, 1993) para 1.07. There is no statutory basis for the list, which can be altered at any time by the Crown Office. It is emphasised that it is not exhaustive—the procurator fiscal has the right and duty to inquire into any death if he thinks it necessary to do so.

Deaths reportable after investigation by the procurator fiscal to the Crown Office

1. Where there are any suspicious circumstances.
2. Where the procurator fiscal considers that a crime has been committed and where there is a possibility that criminal proceedings may be instituted.
3. Where the circumstances point to suicide.
4. Where the death occurred in circumstances, the continuance of which, or the possible recurrence of which, is prejudicial to the health and safety of the public.
5. Where the death is due to medical mishap.
6. Where there has been a request by a person having an interest that a public inquiry should be held into the circumstances of the death.
7. Where a public inquiry has been held under the Fatal Accidents and Sudden Deaths Inquiry (Scotland) Act 1976.
8. Any death of a police officer or member of the armed forces, including visiting forces.
9. Any death as a result of fire or explosion.
10. Any death resulting from the use of volatile substances.
11. Any death in which the circumstances are such that in the opinion of the procurator fiscal the death should be brought to the notice of Crown counsel.

From I H B Carmichael *Sudden Deaths and Fatal Accident Inquiries* (2nd edn, 1993) para 1.19.

Approximate times of appearance of some centres of ossification

---

Intrauterine

$1^1/_2$ months—clavicle.
2 months—shafts of long bones.
3 months—ischium.
5 months—calcaneus.
6 months—manubrium sterni.
7 months—talus.
8 months—all segments of sternum.
9 months—lower end of femur, cuboid, head of humerus.

After birth

---

1 month—head of tibia.
3 months—head of femur, lower end of tibia.
6 months—lower end of fibula.
7 months—lower end of radius, greater tuberosity of humerus.
10 months to 3 years—many of the small bones of hands and feet.
3 years—head of fibula, patella, greater trochanter of femur.
4 years—head of radius.
5 years—lower end of ulna.

Later life

---

8 years—olecranon.
9 years—lesser trochanter of femur.

Later life

10 years—tibial tuberosity.
13 years—anterior spine of ilium, iliac crest.
15 years—ischial tuberosity, medial end of clavicle.

Note: While all these appearances are very variable, females are advanced compared with males throughout.

Adapted from W M Krogman *The Human Skeleton in Forensic Medicine* (1962).

Union of epiphyses

Union	Earliest age (years)	Latest age (years)
Humerus/lower end	15	18
Ulna/upper end	15	21
Ischial tuberosity	15	25
Radius/upper end	16	20
Scapula/acromion	16	25
Tibia/lower end	17	25
Fibula/lower end	17	25
Iliac crest	17	25
Radius/lower end	18	25
Ulna/lower end	18	25
Femur/head of femur	18	25
Tibia/upper end	18	25
Clavicle	18	25
Femur/lower end	19	24
Fibula/upper end	19	25
Humerus/head	20	25

Adapted from W M Krogman *The Human Skeleton in Forensic Medicine* (1962).

Appendix I

Death certificates

SB

COUNTERFOIL

For use of Medical Practitioner or
Midwife, who should complete
in all cases.

Name of mother ....

Date of still-birth ....

Place of still-birth ....

Post mortem†   1   2   3

Weight of fetus .... grams

Duration of pregnancy .... weeks

Death occurred
before labour/during labour/not known*

Cause of death

   a

   b

   c

   d

   e

Date of certification ....

Certificate issued to
(name) ....

of (address) ....

*Strike out the words which do not apply
†Ring appropriate digit

SB

MEDICAL CERTIFICATE OF STILL-BIRTH

(Births and Deaths Registration Act 1953, S 11(1), as amended by the Population (Statistics) Act 1960)
(Form prescribed by the Registration of Births and Deaths Regulations 1987)

Registered at
Entry No.

To be given only in respect of a child which has issued forth from its mother
after the 24th week of pregnancy and which did not at any time after being
completely expelled from its mother breathe or show any other signs of life.

*I was present at the still-birth of a *male / *female child born

*I have examined the body of a *male / *female child which I am informed and believe was born

on .... day of .... 19........ to .... (NAME OF MOTHER)

at .... (PLACE OF BIRTH)

Weight of fetus .... grams

Estimated duration of pregnancy ....

State (a) the number of weeks of delivery
(b) When the child died   (i) before labour*
   (ii) during labour*
   (iii) not known*

*Strike out the words which do not apply.
†Ring appropriate digit.

CAUSE OF DEATH

a.   Main diseases or conditions in fetus

b.   Other diseases or conditions in fetus

c.   Main maternal diseases or conditions affecting fetus

d.   Other maternal diseases or conditions affecting fetus

e.   Other relevant causes

I hereby certify that (i) the child was not born alive, and
(ii) to the best of my knowledge and belief the cause of death and the estimated duration of
pregnancy of the mother were as stated above.

Signature .... Date ....

Qualification as registered by General Medical Council, or }
Registered No. as Registered Midwife.

Address ....

For still-births in hospital: please give the name of the consultant responsible for the care of the mother ....

THIS IS NOT AN AUTHORITY FOR BURIAL OR CREMATION [SEE OVER]

SPECIMEN

Certificate of stillbirth—England and Wales (the Scottish certificate differs only as to layout).

NOTE TO INFORMANT

Under Section 11(1) of the Births and Deaths Registration Act 1953, this certificate must be delivered to the Registrar of Births and Deaths by the person attending to give information of the particulars required to be registered concerning the still-birth. The persons qualified and liable to give such information include:

(1) the mother;
(2) the father (of a legitimate child only);
(3) the occupier of the house in which to the knowledge of that occupier the still-birth occurred;*
(4) any person present at the still-birth;
(5) any person in charge of the still-born child;
(6) in the case of a still-born child found exposed, the person who found the child.

The still-birth is required to be registered within 42 days of its occurrence.

*Occupier in relation to a public institution includes the governor, keeper, master, matron, superintendent, or other chief resident officer.

Certificate of stillbirth—England and Wales (reverse).

MED A
20

COUNTERFOIL

For use of Medical Practitioner, who should complete in all cases.

Name of deceased

Date of death

Age

Place of death

Last seen alive by me

Post-mortem?*   1   2   3   4

Coroner

Whether seen after death*   a   b   c

Cause of death:—

I   (a)

   (b)

   (c)

II

Employment?   ☐ *Please tick where applicable*

B. Further information offered?

Signature

Date

Ring appropriate digit(s) and letter.

MED A
20

Register number
No. of Death Entry ☐

BIRTHS AND DEATHS REGISTRATION ACT 1953

(Form prescribed by the Registration of Births and Deaths Regulations 1987)

MEDICAL CERTIFICATE OF CAUSE OF DEATH

For use only by a Registered Medical Practitioner WHO HAS BEEN IN ATTENDANCE during the deceased's last illness, and to be delivered by him forthwith to the Registrar of Births and Deaths.

Name of deceased

Date of death as stated to me .... day of .... Age as stated to me

Place of death

Last seen alive by me .... day of

1   The certified cause of death takes account of information obtained from post-mortem.   a   Seen after death by me.

2   Information from post-mortem may be available later.   b   Seen after death by another medical practitioner but not by me.

3   Post-mortem not being held.   c   Not seen after death by a medical practitioner.

4   I have reported this death to the Coroner for further action.

Please ring appropriate digit(s) and letter

[See overleaf]

CAUSE OF DEATH

The condition thought to be the 'Underlying cause of death' should appear in the lowest completed line of Part I.

These particulars not to be entered in death register

Approximate interval between onset and death

I (a) Disease or condition directly leading to death†

(b) Other disease or condition, if any, leading to I(a)

(c) Other disease or condition, if any, leading to I(b)

II   Other significant conditions CONTRIBUTING TO THE DEATH but not related to the disease or condition causing it.

The death might have been due to or contributed to by the employment followed at some time by the deceased.   ☐ *Please tick where applicable.*

†*This does not mean the mode of dying, such as heart failure, asphyxia, asthenia, etc: it means the disease, injury, or complication which caused death.*

I hereby certify that I was in medical attendance during the above named deceased's last illness, and that the particulars and cause of death above written are true to the best of my knowledge and belief.

Signature ....

Residence ....   Qualifications as registered by General Medical Council }   Date ....

For deaths in hospital: Please give the name of the consultant responsible for the above—named as a patient. ....

MED A
20

(Form prescribed by the Registration of Births and Deaths Regulations 1987)

NOTICE TO INFORMANT

I hereby give notice that I have this day signed a medical certificate of cause of death of

....

Signature ....

Date ....

This notice is to be delivered by the informant to the registrar of births and deaths for the sub-district in which the death occurred.

The certifying medical practitioner must give this notice to the person who is qualified and liable to act as informant for the registration of death (see list overleaf).

DUTIES OF INFORMANT

Failure to deliver this notice to the registrar renders the informant liable to prosecution. The death cannot be registered until the medical certificate has reached the registrar.

When the death is registered the informant must be prepared to give to the registrar the following particulars relating to the deceased:

1. The date and place of death.

2. The full name and surname (and the maiden surname if the deceased was a woman who had married).

3. The date and place of birth.

4. The occupation (and if the deceased was a married woman or a widow the name and occupation of her husband).

5. The usual address.

6. Whether the deceased was in receipt of a pension or allowance from public funds.

7. If the deceased was married, the date of birth of the surviving widow or widower.

THE DECEASED'S MEDICAL CARD SHOULD BE DELIVERED TO THE REGISTRAR

Certificate of cause of death as used in England and Wales.

Complete where applicable

A	B
I have reported this death to the Coroner for further action.	I may be in a position later to give, on application by the Registrar General, additional information as to the cause of death for the purpose of more precise statistical classification.
Initials of certifying medical practitioner.	Initials of certifying medical practitioner. ....

The Coroner needs to consider all cases where:

The death might have been due to or contributed to by a violent or unnatural cause (including an accident);

or the cause of death cannot be identified;

or the death might have been due to or contributed to by drugs, medicine, abortion or poison.

or there is reason to believe that the death occurred during an operation or under or prior to complete recovery from an anaesthetic or arising subsequently out of an incident during an operation or an anaesthetic;

or the death might have been due to or contributed to by the employment followed at some time by the deceased.

LIST OF SOME OF THE CATEGORIES OF DEATH WHICH MAY BE OF INDUSTRIAL ORIGIN

MALIGNANT DISEASE Causes include:

(a) Skin — radiation and sunlight
— pitch, tar, mineral oils

(b) Nasal — wood, leather work
— nickel

(c) Lung — asbestos
— nickel
— radiation

(d) Pleura — asbestos

(e) Urinary Tract — benzidine
— dyestuff
— chemicals in rubbers

(f) Liver — PVC manufacture

(g) Bone — radiation

(h) Lymphatics and haematopoietic — radiation
— benzene

POISONING

(a) Metals e.g. arsenics, cadmium, lead

(b) Chemicals e.g. chlorine, benzene

(c) Solvents e.g. trichlorethylene

INFECTIOUS DISEASES Causes include:

(a) Anthrax — imported bone, bonemeal, hide or fur

(b) Brucellosis — farming or veterinary

(c) Tuberculosis — contact at work

(d) Leptospirosis — farming, sewer or under-ground workers

(e) Tetanus — farming or gardening

(f) Rabies — animal handling

(g) Viral hepatitis — contact at work

BRONCHIAL ASTHMA AND PNEUMONITIS

(a) Occupational asthma — sensitising agent at work

(b) Allergic Alveolitis — farming

PNEUMOCONIOSIS — mining and quarrying
— potteries
— asbestos

NOTE:—The Practitioner, on signing the certificate, should complete, sign and date the Notice to the Informant, which should be detached and handed to the Informant. The Practitioner should then, without delay, deliver the certificate itself to the Registrar of Births and Deaths for the sub-district in which the death occurred. Envelopes for enclosing the certificates are supplied by the Registrar.

PERSONS QUALIFIED AND LIABLE TO ACT AS INFORMANTS

The following persons are designated by the Births and Deaths Registration Act 1953 as qualified to give information concerning a death:—

DEATHS IN HOUSES AND PUBLIC INSTITUTIONS

(1) A relative of the deceased, present at the death.

(2) A relative of the deceased, in attendance during the last illness.

(3) A relative of the deceased, residing or being in the sub-district where the death occurred.

(4) A person present at the death.

(5) The occupier* if he knew of the happening of the death.

(6) Any inmate if he knew of the happening of the death.

(7) The person causing the disposal of the body.

DEATHS NOT IN HOUSES OR DEAD BODIES FOUND

(1) Any relative of the deceased having knowledge of any of the particulars required to be registered.

(2) Any person present at the death.

(3) Any person who found the body.

(4) Any person in charge of the body.

(5) The person causing the disposal of the body.

*"Occupier" in relation to a public institution includes the governor, keeper, master, matron, superintendent, or other chief resident officer.

Certificate of cause of death as used in England and Wales (reverse).

MED B
1

COUNTERFOIL

For use of Medical Practitioner, who should complete in all cases.

Name of child

Date of death

Sex

Age at death

Place of death

Last seen alive by me

Post-mortem/* Coroner | 1 2 3 4

Whether seen after death* | a b c

Cause of death:—

a

b

c

d

e

B. Further information offered?

Signature

Date

Ring appropriate digit(s) and later.

MED B
1

BIRTHS AND DEATHS REGISTRATION ACT 1953

(Form prescribed by the Registration of Births, Deaths and Marriages (Amendment) (No. 2) Regulations 1985)

MEDICAL CERTIFICATE OF CAUSE OF DEATH OF A LIVE-BORN CHILD DYING WITHIN THE FIRST TWENTY-EIGHT DAYS OF LIFE

For use only by a Registered Medical Practitioner WHO HAS BEEN IN ATTENDANCE during the deceased's last illness, and to be delivered by him forthwith to the Registrar of Births and Deaths.

Register to enter
No. of Death Entry

Name of child

Date of death .... day of .... 19 .... Sex

Age at death .... days (complete period of 24 hours) .... hours

Place of death

Place of birth

Last seen alive by me .... day of 19

1 The certified cause of death has been confirmed by post-mortem.
2 Information from post-mortem may be available later.
3 Post-mortem not being held.
4 I have reported this death to the Coroner for further action.
[See overleaf]

Please ring appropriate digit and later.

a Seen after death by me.
b Seen after death by another medical practitioner but not by me.
c Not seen after death by a medical practitioner.

CAUSE OF DEATH

a. Main diseases or conditions in infant

b. Other diseases or conditions in infant

c. Main maternal diseases or conditions affecting infant

d. Other maternal diseases or conditions affecting infant

e. Other relevant causes

I hereby certify that I was in medical attendance during the above named deceased's last illness, and that the particulars and cause of death above written are true to the best of my knowledge and belief.

Signature

Address

Qualifications as registered by General Medical Council

Date

For deaths in hospital: Please give the name of the consultant responsible for the above-named as a patient

---

MED B
1

(Form prescribed by the Registration of Births, Deaths and Marriages Regulations 1968)

NOTICE TO INFORMANT

I hereby give notice that I have this day signed a medical certificate of cause of death of

Signature

Date

This notice is to be delivered by the informant to the registrar of births and deaths for the sub-district in which the death occurred.

The certifying medical practitioner must give this notice to the person who is qualified and liable to act as informant for the registration of death (see list overleaf).

DUTIES OF INFORMANT

Failure to deliver this notice to the registrar renders the informant liable to prosecution. The death cannot be registered until the medical certificate has reached the registrar.

When the death is registered the informant must be prepared to give to the registrar the following particulars relating to the deceased:

1. The date and place of death.
2. The full name and surname.
3. The date and place of birth.
4. The names and occupations of the parents.
5. The usual address.

IF THE CHILD WAS ISSUED WITH A MEDICAL CARD, THE CARD SHOULD BE DELIVERED TO THE REGISTRAR.

Certificate of neonatal death—England and Wales.

Complete where applicable

A

I have reported this death to the Coroner for further action.

Initials of certifying medical practitioner. ....

The Coroner needs to consider all cases where:

The death might have been due to or contributed to by a violent or unnatural cause (including an accident);

or the cause of death cannot be identified;

or the death might have been due to or contributed to by drugs, medicine, abortion or poison;

B

I may be in a position later to give, on application by the Registrar General, additional information as to the cause of death for the purpose of more precise statistical classification.

Initials of certifying medical practitioner. ....

or there is reason to believe that the death occurred during an operation or under or prior to complete recovery from an anaesthetic or arising subsequently out of an incident during an operation or an anaesthetic.

NOTE:—The Practitioner, on signing the certificate, should complete, sign and date the Notice to the Informant, which should be detached and handed to the Informant. The Practitioner should then, without delay, deliver the certificate itself to the Registrar of Births and Deaths for the sub-district in which the death occurred. Envelopes for enclosing the certificates are supplied by the Registrar.

PERSONS QUALIFIED AND LIABLE TO ACT AS INFORMANTS

The following persons are designated by the Births and Deaths Registration Act 1953 as qualified to give information concerning a death:—

DEATHS IN HOUSES AND PUBLIC INSTITUTIONS

(1) A relative of the deceased, present at the death.

(2) A relative of the deceased, in attendance during the last illness.

(3) A relative of the deceased, residing or being in the sub-district where the death occurred.

(4) A person present at the death.

(5) The occupier* if he knew of the happening of the death.

(6) Any inmate if he knew of the happening of the death.

(7) The person causing the disposal of the body.

DEATHS NOT IN HOUSES OR DEAD BODIES FOUND

(1) Any relative of the deceased having knowledge of any of the particulars required to be registered.

(2) Any person present at the death.

(3) Any person who found the body.

(4) Any person in charge of the body.

(5) The person causing the disposal of the body.

**Occupier" in relation to a public institution includes the governor, keeper, master, matron, superintendent, or other chief resident officer.

Certificate of neonatal death—England and Wales (reverse).

MEDICAL CERTIFICATE OF CAUSE OF DEATH   FORM 11

This certificate is intended for the use of the Registrar of Births, Deaths and Marriages, and all persons are warned against accepting or using this certificate for any other purpose. See back of this form for notes about registration of a death.

To the Registrar of Births, Deaths and Marriages

Name of deceased . . . .

	Day	Month	Year
Date of death			

Time of death . . . . hours
(Enter approximate time if exact time not known)

Place of death . . . .

I hereby certify that to the best of my knowledge and belief, the cause of death and duration of disease were as stated below.

Registrar to enter
District no . . . .
Year . . . .
Entry no . . . .

Not to be entered in register

Approximate interval between onset and death

CAUSE OF DEATH *(PLEASE PRINT CLEARLY)*		years	months	days
I	**I**			
Disease or condition directly leading to death*	a . . . . *due to (or as a consequence of)*			
Antecedent causes Morbid conditions, if any, giving rise to the above cause, the **underlying** condition to be stated **last**	b . . . . *due to (or as a consequence of)* c			
II	**II**			
Other significant conditions contributing to the death, but not related to the disease or condition causing it	. . . .			

* *This does not mean the mode of dying such as heart failure, asthenia, etc; it means the disease, injury or complication which caused death.*

Please ring the appropriate letter and appropriate figures:—

Certified cause takes account of post-mortem information . . . . . . .A
Information from post-mortem may be available later . . . . .B
Post-mortem not proposed C

Seen after death by me 1
Seen after death by another medical practitioner but not by me 2
Not seen after death by a medical practitioner 3

The deceased woman died during pregnancy
or within six weeks thereafter 1
The deceased woman died between six weeks
and twelve months after pregnancy 2

Please tick box if appropriate

I may be in a position later to give, if asked by the Registrar General, additional information as to the cause of this death for the purpose of more precise statistical classification ☐

Procurator Fiscal has been informed ☐

Signature . . . .

Date . . . . 19 . .

Name in BLOCK
CAPITALS . . . .

Registered medical qualifications . . . .

Address . . . .
. . . .

For a death in hospital
Name of consultant responsible
for deceased as a patient . . . .

NOTES ABOUT REGISTRATION OF A DEATH

A death may be registered either in the registration district where it takes place (the district of its occurrence) or in such other registration district in Scotland where the deceased person had his usual residence immediately before his death.

Usual residence for this purpose means the deceased person's permanent home and not an address (e.g. a holiday address) at which he may have been staying temporarily at the time of his death.

Persons required to give information for the registration of a death are:

a   any relative of the deceased;

b   any person present at the death;

c   the deceased's executor or other legal representative;

d   the occupier, at the time of death, of the premises where the death took place;

e   if there is no such person as aforesaid, any other person having knowledge of the particulars to be registered.

N.B.   The word "occupier" includes the governor, keeper, matron, superintendent or other person in charge of a prison, hospital or other institution, and, in relation to a house, includes any person residing therein.

The Scottish death certificate.

Control of infectious diseases in England and Wales

The following diseases are affected by the Public Health (Control of Disease) Act 1984, section 10. Not all the sections of the Act apply to all diseases. The following is not a full list of application but relates to a selected number of sections listed below. The full list is to be found in Public Health (Infectious Diseases) Regulations 1988, SI 1988/1546, Schedule 1.

The whole of Part II of the Act
Cholera	Smallpox
Plague	Typhus
Relapsing fever	

Sections 35, 37, 38, 44
Acquired immune deficiency syndrome

Sections 11, 17, 19, 20, 21 35*, 37 38, 44
Acute encephalitis	Meningitis
Acute poliomyelitis	Meningococcal septicaemia
Anthrax	(without meningitis)

Sections 11, 17, 19, 20, 21, 35, 36, 37, 38, 44
Diphtheria	Paratyphoid fever
Dysentery	Typhoid fever
(amoebic or bacillary)	Viral hepatitis

Sections 11, 17, 19, 20, 21, 35* 37, 38, 44
Leprosy	Mumps
Leptospirosis	Rubella
Measles	Whooping cough

Sections 11, 35*
Malaria	Yellow fever
Tetanus	

Sections 11, 17
    Ophthalmia neonatorum

Sections 11, 17, 19, 20, 21, 35, 36, 37, 38
    Rabies

Sections 11, 17, 19, 20, 21, 35, 36, 37, 38, 44
    Scarlet fever

Sections 11**, 17, 19, 20, 21, 35*, 37***, 38***, 44
    Tuberculosis

Sections 11, 17, 19, 20, 21, 35, 36, 37, 38, 44, 48
    Viral haemorrhagic fever

The following are brief descriptions of the various sections:
- 11 Notification to local authority required
- 17 Offence of exposing others to risk of infection
- 19 Restriction of trading
- 20 Stopping the infected person working
- 21 Children's schooling affected
- 35 Medical examination empowered
- 36 Groups of persons may be examined
- 37 Admission to hospital
- 38 Detention in hospital
- 44 Isolation of dead body
- 48 Removal of body to a mortuary for immediate disposal

*   Infection in the carrier state excluded (reg 4)
** Not when the diagnosis is solely on the basis of a tuberculin test
*** When the condition is respiratory and in an infective state

Notification of infectious disease in Scotland

Notifiable by virtue of Infectious Disease (Notification) Act 1889

Smallpox	Typhus
Cholera	Typhoid
Diphtheria	Other enteric fevers
Membranous croup	Relapsing fever
Erysipelas	Continued or puerperal fever
Scarlet fever	Any other disease notifiable locally

Notifiable under Public Health (Notification of Infectious Disease) (Scotland) Regulations 1988, SI 1988/1550.

Anthrax	Plague
Bacillary dysentery	Poliomyelitis
Chicken pox	Rabies
Food poisoning	Rubella
Legionellosis	Tetanus
Leptospirosis	Tuberculosis
Malaria	Viral haemorrhagic fever
Measles	Viral hepatitis
Meningococcal infection	Whooping cough
Mumps	

Notifiable under Public Health (Notification of Infectious Disease) (Scotland) Amendment Regulations 1989, SI 1989/2250.

Lyme disease	Toxoplasmosis

Prescribed diseases

Prescribed disease or injury	Occupation
A. *Conditions due to physical agents*	Any occupation involving:
[A1 Leukaemia (other than chronic lymphatic leukaemia) or cancer of the bone, female breast, testis or thyroid.	Exposure to electro-magnetic radiations (other than radiant heat) or to ionising particles where the dose is sufficient to double the risk of the occurrence of the condition.]
A2 . . . cataract.	[Frequent or prolonged exposure to radiation from red-hot or white-hot material.]
A3 Dysbarism, including decompression sickness, barotrauma and osteonecrosis.	Subjection to compressed or rarefied air or other respirable gases or gaseous mixtures.
A4 Cramp of the hand or forearm due to repetitive movements.	Prolonged periods of handwriting, typing or other repetitive movements of the fingers, hand or arm.
A5 Subcutaneous cellulitis of the hand (beat hand).	Manual labour causing severe or prolonged friction or pressure on the hand.
A6 Bursitis or subcutaneous cellulitis arising at or about the knee due to severe or prolonged external friction or pressure at or about the knee (beat knee).	Manual labour causing severe or prolonged external friction or pressure at or about the knee.
A7 Bursitis or subcutaneous cellulitis arising at or about the elbow due to severe or prolonged external friction or pressure at or about the elbow (beat elbow).	Manual labour causing severe or prolonged external friction or pressure at or about the elbow.
A8 Traumatic inflammation of the tendons of the hand or forearm, or of the associated tendon sheaths.	Manual labour, or frequent or repeated movements of the hand or wrist.
A9 Miner's nystagmus.	Work in or about a mine.

[A10 Sensorineural hearing loss amounting to at least 50 dB in each ear, being the average of hearing losses at 1, 2 and 3 kHz frequencies, and being due in the case of at least one ear to occupational noise (occupational deafness).]

[(a) The use of powered (but not hand powered) grinding tools on [metal (other than sheet metal or plate metal)] . . . , or work wholly or mainly in the immediate vicinity of those tools whilst they are being so used; or

(b) the use of pneumatic percussive tools on metal, or work wholly or mainly in the immediate vicinity of those tools whilst they are being so used; or

(c) the use of pneumatic percussive tools for drilling rock in quarries or underground or in mining coal [or in sinking shafts or for tunnelling in civil engineering works], or work wholly or mainly in the immediate vicinity of those tools whilst they are being so used; or

[(ca) the use of pneumatic percussive tools on stone in quarry works, or work wholly or mainly in the immediate vicinity of those tools whilst they are being so used; or]

(d) work wholly or mainly in the immediate vicinity of plant (excluding power press plant) engaged in the forging (including drop stamping) of metal by means of closed or open dies or drop hammers; or

(e) work in textile manufacturing where the work is undertaken wholly is undertaken wholly or mainly in rooms or sheds in which there are machines engaged in weaving man-made or natural (including mineral) fibres or in the high speed false twisting of fibres; or]

(f) the use of, or work wholly or mainly in the immediate vicinity of, machines engaged in cutting, shaping or cleaning metal nails; or

(g) the use of, or work wholly or mainly in the immediate vicinity of, plasma spray guns engaged in the deposition of metal; or

(h) the use of, or work wholly or mainly in the immediate vicinity of, any of the following machines engaged in the working of wood or material composed partly of wood, that is to say: multi-cutter moulding machines, planing machines, automatic or semi-automatic lathes, multiple cross-cut machines, automatic shaping machines, double-end tenoning machines, vertical spindle moulding machines (including high speed routing machines), edge banding machines, bandsawing machines with a blade width of not less than 75 millimetres and circular sawing machines in the operation of which the blade is moved towards the material being cut; or

(i) the use of chain saws in forestry[; or]

[(j) air arc gouging or work wholly or mainly in the immediate vicinity of air arc gouging; or

(k) the use of band saws, circular saws or cutting discs for cutting metal in the metal founding or forging industries, or work wholly or mainly in the immediate vicinity of those tools whilst they are being so used; or

(l) the use of circular saws for cutting products in the manufacture of steel, or work wholly or mainly in the immediate vicinity of those tools whilst they are being so used; or

(m) the use of burners or torches for cutting or dressing steel based products, or work wholly or mainly in the immediate vicinity of those tools whilst they are being so used; or

(n) work wholly or mainly in the immediate vicinity of skid transfer banks; or

(o) work wholly or mainly in the immediate vicinity of knock out and shake out grids in foundries; or

(p) mechanical bobbin cleaning or work wholly or mainly in the immediate vicinity of mechanical bobbin cleaning; or

(q) the use of, or work wholly or mainly in the immediate vicinity of, vibrating metal moulding boxes in the concrete products industry; or

(r) the use of, or work wholly or mainly in the immediate vicinity of, high pressure jets of water or a mixture of water and abrasive material in the water jetting industry (including work under water); or

(s) work in ships' engine rooms; or

(t) the use of circular saws for cutting concrete masonry blocks during manufacture or work wholly or mainly in the immediate vicinity of those tools whilst they are being so used; or

(u) burning stone in quarries by jet channelling processes, or work wholly or mainly in the immediate vicinity of such processes; or

(v) work on gas turbines in connection with—
   (i) performance testing on test bed;
   (ii) installation testing of replacement engines in aircraft;
   (iii) acceptance testing of Armed Service fixed wing combat planes; or

(w) the use of, or work wholly or mainly in the immediate vicinity of—
  (i)   machines for automatic moulding, automatic blow moulding or automatic glass pressing and forming machines used in the manufacture of glass containers or hollow ware;
  (ii) spinning machines using compressed air to produce glass wool or mineral wool;
  (iii) continuous glass toughening furnaces.]

A11 Episodic blanching, occurring throughout the year, affecting the middle or proximal phalanges or in the case of a thumb the proximal phalanx, of—

(a) the use of hand-held chain saws in forestry; or

(a) in the case of a person with 5 fingers (including thumb) on one hand, any 3 of those fingers, or

(b) the use of hand-held rotary tools in grinding or in the sanding or polishing of metal, or the holding of material being ground, or metal being sanded or polished, by rotary tools; or

(b) in the case of a person with only 4 such fingers, any 2 of those fingers, or

(c) the use of hand-held percussive metal-working tools, or the holding of metal being worked upon by percussive tools, in riveting, caulking, chipping, hammering, fettling or swaging; or

(c) in the case of a person with less than 4 such fingers, any one of those fingers or, as the case may be, the one remaining finger (vibration white finger).

(d) the use of hand-held powered percussive drills or hand-held powered percussive hammers in mining, quarrying, demolition, or on roads or footpaths, including road construction; or

(e) the holding of material being worked upon by pounding machines in shoe manufacture.

[A12 Carpal tunnel syndrome.

The use of hand-held powered tools whose internal parts vibrate so as to transmit that vibration to the hand, but excluding those which are solely powered by hand.]

B. *Conditions due to biological agents*

Any occupation involving

B1 Anthrax.

Contact with animals infected with anthrax or the handling (including the loading or unloading or transport) of animal products or residues.

B2 Glanders.

Contact with equine animals or their carcases.

B3 Infection by leptospira.

(a) Work in places which are, or are liable to be, infested by rats, field mice or voles, or other small mammals; or

(b) work at dog kennels or the care or handling of dogs; or

(c) contact with bovine animals or their meat products or pigs or their meat products.

B4 Ankylostomiasis.

Work in or about a mine.

B5 Tuberculosis.

Contact with a source of tuberculous infection.

B6 Extrinsic allergic alveolitis (including farmer's lung).

Exposure to moulds or fungal spores or heterologous proteins by reason of employment in:—

(a) agriculture, horticulture, forestry, cultivation of edible fungi or malt-working; or

(b) loading or unloading or handling in storage mouldy vegetable matter or edible fungi; or

(c) caring for or handling birds; or

(d) handling bagasse.

B7 Infection by organisms of the genus brucella.

Contact with—

(a) animals infected by brucella, or their carcases or parts thereof, or their untreated products; or

	(b) laboratory specimens or vaccines of, or containing, brucella.
B8 Viral hepatitis.	Any occupation involving: Contact with—
	(a) human blood or human blood products; or
	(b) a source of viral hepatitis.
B9 Infection by Streptococcus suis.	Contact with pigs infected by Streptococus suis, or with the carcases, products or residues of pigs so infected.
[B10 (a) Avian chlamydiosis	Contact with birds infected with chlamydia psittaci, or with the remains or untreated products of such birds.
B10 (b) Ovine chlamydiosis	Contact with sheep infected with chlamydia psittaci, or with the remains or untreated products of such sheep.
B11 Q fever	Contact with animals, their remains or their untreated products.]
[B12 Orf.	Contact with sheep, goats or with the carcasses of sheep or goats.
B13 Hydatidosis.	Contact with dogs.].

C. *Conditions due to chemical agents*

C1 Poisoning by lead or a compound of lead.	The use or handling of, or exposure to the fumes, dust or vapour of, lead or a compound of lead, or a substance containing lead.
C2 Poisoning by manganese or a compound of manganese.	The use or handling of, or exposure to the fumes, dust or vapour of, manganese or a compound of manganese, or a substance containing manganese.

C3 Poisoning by phosphorus or an inorganic compound of phosphorus or poisoning due to the anti-cholinesterase or pseudo anti-cholinesterase action of organic phosphorus compounds.

The use or handling of, or exposure to the fumes, dust or vapour of, phosphorus or a compound of phosphorus, or a substance containing phosphorus.

C4 Poisoning by arsenic or a compound of arsenic.

The use or handling of, or exposure to the fumes, dust or vapour of, arsenic or a compound of arsenic, or a substance containing arsenic.

C5 Poisoning by mercury or a compound of mercury.

The use or handling of, or exposure to the fumes, dust or vapour of, mercury or a compound of mercury, or a substance containing mercury.

C6 Poisoning by carbon bisulphide.

The use or handling of, or exposure to the fumes or vapour of, carbon bisulphide or a compound of carbon bisulphide, or a substance containing carbon bisulphide.

C7 Poisoning by benzene or a homologue of benzene.

The use or handling of, or exposure to the fumes of, or vapour containing benzene or any of its homologues.

C8 Poisoning by a nitro- or amino- or chloro- derivative of benzene or of a homologue of benzene, or poisoning by nitrochlorbenzene.

The use or handling of, or exposure to the fumes of, or vapour containing, a nitro- or amino- or chloro- derivative of benzene, or of a homologue of benzene, or nitrochlorbenzene.

C9 Poisoning by dinitrophenol or a homologue of dinitrophenol or by substituted dinitrophenols or by the salts of such substances.

The use or handling of, or exposure to the fumes of, or vapour containing, dinitrophenol or a homologue or substituted dinitrophenols or the salts of such substances.

C10 Poisoning by tetrachloroethane.

Any occupation involving: The use or handling of, or exposure to the fumes of, or vapour containing, tetrachloroethane.

C11 Poisoning by diethylene dioxide (dioxan).

The use or handling of, or exposure to the fumes of, or vapour containing, diethylene dioxide (dioxan).

C12 Poisoning by methyl bromide.

The use or handling of, or exposure to the fumes of, or vapour containing, methyl bromide.

C13 Poisoning by chlorinated naphthalene.

The use or handling of, or exposure to the fumes of, or dust or vapour containing, chlorinated naphthalene.

C14 Poisoning by nickel carbonyl.

Exposure to nickel carbonyl gas.

C15 Poisoning by oxides of nitrogen.

Exposure to oxides of nitrogen.

C16 Poisoning by gonioma kamassi (African boxwood)

The manipulation of gonioma kamassi or any process in or incidental to the manufacture of articles therefrom.

C17 Poisoning by beryllium or a compound of beryllium.

The use or handling of, or exposure to the fumes, dust or vapour of, beryllium or a compound of beryllium, or a substance containing beryllium.

C18 Poisoning by cadmium.

Exposure to cadmium dust or fumes.

C19 Poisoning by acrylamide monomer.

The use or handling of, or exposure to, acrylamide monomer.

C20 Dystrophy of the cornea (including ulceration of the corneal surface) of the eye.

(a) The use or handling of, or exposure to, arsenic, tar, pitch, bitumen, mineral oil (including paraffin), soot or any compound, product or residue of any of these substances, except quinone or hydroquinone; or

(b) exposure to quinone or hydroquinone during their manufacture.

C21
(a) Localised new growth of the skin, papillomatous or keratotic;

The use or handling of, or exposure to, arsenic, tar, pitch, bitumen, mineral oil (including paraffin), soot or any compound, product or residue of any of these substances, except quinone or hydroquinone.

(b) squamous-celled carcinoma of the skin.

C22
(a) Carcinoma of the mucous membrane of the nose or associated air sinuses;

Work in a factory where nickel is produced by decomposition of a gaseous nickel compound which necessitates working in or about a building or buildings where that process or any other industrial process ancillary or incidental thereto is carried on.

(b) primary carcinoma of a bronchus or of a lung.

C23 Primary neoplasm (including papilloma, carcinoma-in-situ and invasive carcinoma) of the epithelial lining of the urinary tract (renal pelvis, ureter, bladder and urethra).

Any occupation involving:

(a) Work in a building in which any of the following substances is produced for commercial purposes:—
  (i)   alpha-naphthylamine, betanaphthylamine or methylenebis-orthochloroaniline;
  (ii) diphenyl substituted by at least one nitro or primary amino group or by at least one nitro and primary amino group (including benzidine);
  (iii) any of the substances mentioned in sub-paragraph (ii) above if further ring substituted by halogeno, methyl or methoxy groups, but not by other groups;
  (iv) the salts of any of the substances mentioned in sub-paragraphs (i) to (iii) above;
  (v)   auramine or magenta; or

(b) the use or handling of any of the substances mentioned in sub-paragraph (a)(i) to (iv), or work in a process in which any such substance is used, handled or liberated; or

(c) the maintenance or cleaning of any plant or machinery used in any such process as is mentioned in sub-paragraph (b), or the cleaning of clothing used in any such building as is mentioned in sub-paragraph (a) if such clothing is cleaned within the works of which the building forms a part or in a laundry maintained and used solely in connection with such works.

[(d) exposure to coal tar pitch volatiles produced in aluminium smelting involving the Soderberg process (that is to say the method of producing aluminium by electrolysis in which the anode consists of a paste of petroleum coke and mineral oil which is baked in situ).]

C24
(a) Angiosarcoma of the liver;

(a) Work in or about machinery or apparatus used for the polymerization of vinyl chloride monomer, a process which, for the purposes of this provision, comprises all operations up to and including the drying of the slurry produced by the polymerization and the packaging of the dried product; or

(b) osteolysis of the terminal phalanges of the fingers;

(b) ork in a building or structure in which any part of that process takes place.

(c) non-cirrhotic portal fibrosis.

C25 Occupational vitiligo.

The use or handling of, or exposure to, para-tertiary-butylphenol, para-tertiary-butylcatechol, para-amyl-phenol, hydroquinone or the monobenzyl or monobutyl ether or hydroquinone.

[C26 Damage to the liver or kidneys due to exposure to Carbon Tetrachloride.

Any occupation involving: The use of or handling of, or exposure to the fumes of, or vapour containing, Carbon Tetrachloride.

C27 Damage to the liver or kidneys due to exposure to Trichloromethane (Chloroform).

The use of or handling of, or exposure to the fumes of, or vapour containing, Trichloromethane (Chloroform).

C28 Central nervous system dysfunction and associated gastro-intestinal disorders due to exposure to Chloromethane (Methyl Chloride).

The use of or handling of, or exposure to the fumes of, or vapour containing, Chloromethane (Methyl Chloride).

C29 Peripheral neuropathy due to exposure to n-hexane or methyl n-butyl ketone.

The use of or handling of, or exposure to the fumes of, or vapour containing, n-hexane or methyl n-butyl ketone.]

[C30 Chrome dermatitis, or ulceration of the mucous membranes or the epidermis, resulting from exposure to chromic acid, chromates or bi-chromates.

The use or handling of, or exposure to, chromic acid, chromates or bi-chromates.]

D. *Miscellaneous Conditions*

D1 Pneumoconiosis.

Any occupation—

(a) set out in Part II of this Schedule;

(b) specified in regulation 2(b)(ii).

D2 Byssinosis.

Any occupation involving:

Work in any room where any process up to and including the weaving process is performed in a factory in which the spinning or manipulation of raw or waste cotton or of flax, or the weaving of cotton or flax, is carried on.

D3 Diffuse mesothelioma (primary neoplasm of the mesothelium of the pleura or of the pericardium or of the peritoneum).

[Exposure to asbestos, asbestos dust or any admixture of asbestos at a level above that commonly found in the environment at large.]

[D4 Allergic rhinitis which is due to exposure to any of the following agents—

Exposure to any of the agents set out in column 1 of this paragraph.]

(a) isocyanates;

(b) platinum salts;

(c) fumes or dusts arising from the manufacture, transport or use of hardening agents (including epoxy resin curing agents) based on phthalic anhydride, tetrachlorophthalic anhydride, trimellitic anhydride or triethylenetetramine;

(d) fumes arising from the use of rosin as a soldering flux;

(e) proteolytic enzymes;

(f) animals including insects and other arthropods used for the purposes of research or education or in laboratories;

(g) dusts arising from the sowing, cultivation, harvesting, drying, handling, milling, transport or storage of barley, oats, rye, wheat or maize, or the handling, milling, transport or storage of meal or flour made therefrom;

(h) antibiotics;

(i) cimetidine;

(j) wood dust;

(k) ispaghula;

(l) castor bean dust;

(m) ipecacuanha;

(n) azodicarbonamide;

(o) animals including insects and other arthropods or their larval forms, used for the purposes of pest control or fruit cultivation, or the larval forms of animals used for the purposes of research or education or in laboratories;

(p) glutaraldehyde;

(q) persulphate salts or henna;

(r) crustaceans or fish or products arising from these in the food processing industry;

(s) reactive dyes;

(t) soya bean;

(u) tea dust;

(v) green coffee bean dust;

(w) fumes from stainless steel welding.]

D5 Non-infective dermatitis of external origin (. . . excluding dermatitis due to ionising particles or electro-magnetic radiations other than radiant heat).

Exposure to dust, liquid or vapour or any other external agent [except chromic acid, chromates or bi-chromates,] capable of irritating the skin (including friction or heat but excluding ionising particles or electro-magnetic radiations other than radiant heat).

D6 Carcinoma of the nasal cavity or associated air sinuses (nasal carcinoma).

(a) Attendance for work in or about a building where wooden goods are manufactured or repaired; or

(b) attendance for work in a building used for the manufacture of footwear or components of footwear made wholly or partly of leather or fibre board; or

(c) attendance for work at a place used wholly or mainly for the repair of footwear made wholly or partly of leather or fibre board.

D7 Asthma which is due to exposure to any of the following agents:—

Any occupation involving:

Exposure to any of the agents set out in column 1 of this paragraph.

(a) isocyanates;

(b) platinum salts;

(c) fumes or dusts arising from the manufacture, transport or use of hardening agents (including epoxy resin curing agents) based on phthalic anhydride, tetrachlorophthalic anhydride, trimellitic anhydride or triethylenetetramine;

(d) fumes arising from the use of rosin as a soldering flux;

(e) proteolytic enzymes;

[(f) animals including insects and other arthropods used for the purposes of research or education or in laboratories]

(g) dusts arising from the sowing, cultivation, harvesting, drying, handling, milling, transport or storage of barley, oats, rye, wheat or maize, or the handling, milling, transport or storage of meal or flour made therefrom (occupational asthma

[(h) antibiotics;

(i) cimetidine;

(j) wood dust;

(k) ispaghula;

(l) castor bean dust;

(m) ipecacuanha;

(n) azodicarbonamide]

[(o) animals including insects and other arthropods or their larval forms, used for the purposes of pest control or fruit cultivation, or the larval forms of animals used for the purposes of research, education or in laboratories;

(p) glutaraldehyde;

(q) persulphate salts or henna;

(r) crustaceans or fish or products arising from these in the food processing industry;

(s) reactive dyes;

(t) soya bean;

(u) tea dust;

(v) green coffee bean dust;

(w) fumes from stainless steel welding;

(x) any other sensitising agent.]

D8 Primary carcinoma of the lung where there is accompanying evidence of one or both of the following—

(a) asbestosis;

[(b) unilateral or bilateral diffuse pleural thickening extending to a thickness of 5mm or more at any point within the area affected as measured by a plain chest radiograph (not being a computerised tomography scan or other form of imaging) which—

(i) in the case of unilateral diffuse pleural thickening, covers 50% or more of the area of the chest wall of the lung affected; or

(ii) in the case of bilateral diffuse pleural thickening, covers 25% or more of the combined area of the chest wall of both lungs.]

(a) The working or handling of asbestos or any admixture of asbestos; or

(b) the manufacture or repair of asbestos textiles or other articles containing or composed of asbestos; or

(c) the cleaning of any machinery or plant used in any of the foregoing operations and of any chambers, fixtures and appliances for the collection of asbestos dust; or

(d) substantial exposure to the dust arising from any of the foregoing operations.

[D9 Unilateral or bilateral diffuse pleural thickening extending to a thickness of 5mm or more at any point within the area affected as measured by a plain chest radiograph (not being a computerised tomography scan or other form of imaging) which—

(a) The working or handling of asbestos or any admixture of asbestos; or

(i) in the case of unilateral diffuse pleural thickening, covers 50% or more of the area of the chest wall of the lung affected; or

(b) the manufacture or repair of asbestos textiles or other articles containing or composed of asbestos; or

(ii) in the case of bilateral diffuse pleural thickening, covers 25% or more of the combined area of the chest wall of both lungs.]

(c) the cleaning of any machinery or plant used in any of the foregoing operations and of any chambers, fixtures and appliances for the collection of asbestos dust; or Any occupation involving:

(d) substantial exposure to the dust arising from any of the foregoing operations.

[D10 [Primary carcinoma of the lung]

(a) Work underground in a tin mine; or

(b) exposure to bis(chloromethyl)ether produced during the manufacture of chloromethyl methyl ether; or

(c) exposure to zinc chromate calcium chromate or strontium chromate in their pure forms.]

[D11 Primary carcinoma of the lung where there is accompanying evidence of silicosis.

Exposure to silica dust in the course of—

(a) the manufacture of glass or pottery;

(b) tunnelling in or quarrying sandstone or granite;

(c) mining metal ores;

(d) slate quarrying or the manufacture of artefacts from slate;

(e) mining clay;

(f) using siliceous materials as abrasives;

(g) cutting stone;

(h) stonemasonry; or

(i) work in a foundry.]

[D12 Except in the circumstances specified in regulation 2(d)—

Exposure to coal dust by reason of working underground in a coal mine for a period or periods amounting in aggregate to at least 20 years (whether before or after 5th July 1948) and any such period or periods shall include a period or periods of incapacity while engaged in such an occupation.]

(a) chronic bronchitis; or

(b) emphysema; or

(c) both,

where there is accompanying evidence of a forced expiratory volume in one second (measured from the position of maximum inspiration with the claimant making maximum effort) which is—

[(i) at least one litre below the appropriate mean value predicted, obtained from the following prediction formulae which give the mean values predicted in litres—

For a man, where the measurement is made without back-extrapolation,$(3.62 \times$ Height in metres$)-(0.031 \times$ Age in years$)-1.41$; or, where the measurement is made with back-extrapolation,$(3.71 \times$ Height in metres$)-(0.032 \times$ Age in years$)- 1.44$;

For a woman, where the measurement is made without back-extrapolation,$(3.29 \times$ Height in metres$)-(0.029 \times$ Age in years$)-1.42$; or, where the measurement is made with back-extrapolation,$(3.37 \times$ Height in metres$)-(0.030 \times$ Age in years$)- 1.46$; or]

(ii) less than one litre.

Social Security (Industrial Injuries) (Prescribed Diseases) Regulations 1985, SI 1985/967, Sch 1, Pt I, as amended up to and including SI 2000/1588.

1   There have been many additions to the list of agreed sensitising agents.

Occupations for which pneumoconiosis is prescribed

1. Any occupation involving:
(a) the mining, quarrying or working of silica rock or the working of dried quartzose sand or any dry deposit or dry residue of silica or any dry admixture containing such materials (including any occupation in which any of the aforesaid operations are carried out incidentally to the mining or quarrying of other minerals or to the manufacture of articles containing crushed or ground silica rock);
(b) the handling of any of the materials specified in the foregoing subparagraph in or incidental to any of the operations mentioned therein, or substantial exposure to the dust arising from such operations.
2. Any occupation involving the breaking, crushing or grinding of flint or the working or handling of broken, crushed or ground flint or materials containing such flint, or substantial exposure to the dust arising from such operations.
3. Any occupation involving sand blasting by means of compressed air with the use of quartzose sand or crushed silica rock or flint, or substantial exposure to the dust arising from sand and blasting.
4. Any occupation involving work in a foundry or the performance of, or substantial exposure to the dust arising from, any of the following operations:
(a) the freeing of steel castings from adherent siliceous substance;
(b) the freeing of metal casting from adherent siliceous substance;
    (i) by blasting with an abrasive propelled by compressed air, by steam or by a wheel; or
    (ii) by the use of power-driven tools.
5. Any occupation in or incidental to the manufacture of china or earthenware (including sanitary earthenware, electrical earthenware and earthenware tiles) and any occupation involving substantial exposure to the dust arising therefrom.
6. Any occupation involving the grinding of mineral graphite, or substantial exposure to the dust arising from such grinding.
7. Any occupation involving the dressing of granite or any igneous rock by masons or the crushing of such materials, or substantial exposure to the dust arising from such operations.

8. Any occupation involving the use, or preparation for use, of a grindstone, or substantial exposure to the dust arising therefrom.

9. Any occupation involving:

(a) the working or handling of asbestos or any admixture of asbestos;

(b) the manufacture or repair of asbestos textiles or other articles containing or composed of asbestos;

(c) the cleaning of any machinery or plant used in any of the foregoing operations and of any chambers, fixtures and appliances for the collection of asbestos dust;

(d) substantial exposure to the dust arising from any of the foregoing operations.

10. Any occupation involving:

(a) work underground in any mine in which one of the objects of the mining operations is the getting of any mineral;

(b) the working or handling above ground at any coal or tin mine of any minerals extracted therefrom, or any operation incidental thereto;

(c) the trimming of coal in any ship, barge, or lighter, or in any dock or harbour or at any wharf or quay;

(d) the sawing, splitting or dressing of slate, or any operation incidental thereto.

11. Any occupation in or incidental to the manufacture of carbon electrodes by an industrial undertaking for use in the electrolytic extraction of aluminium from aluminium oxide, and any occupation involving substantial exposure to the dust arising therefrom.

12. Any occupation involving boiler scaling or substantial exposure to the dust arising therefrom.

Social Security (Industrial Benefit) (Prescribed Diseases) Regulations 1985, SI 1985/967, Sch 1, Pt II.

Diseases reportable to the Health and Safety Executive

The following industrial poisonings are reportable to the Health and Safety Executive irrespective of the type of work involved:

28. Poisoning by:
(a) Acrylamide monomer;
(b) Arsenic or one of its compounds;
(c) Benzene or a homologue of benzene;
(d) Beryllium or one of its compounds;
(e) Cadmium or one of its compounds;
(f) Carbon disulphide;
(g) Diethylene dioxide (dioxan);
(h) Ethylene dioxide;
(i) Lead or one of its compounds;
(j) Manganese or one of its compounds;
(k) Mercury or one of its compounds;
(l) Methyl bromide;
(m) Nitrochlorobenzene, or a nitro- or amino- or chloro-derivative of benzene or a homologue of benzene;
(n) Oxides of nitrogen;
(o) Phosphorus or one of its compounds.

The following skin diseases are reportable in the occupations indicated:

1. Inflammation, ulceration or malignant disease of the skin	Work with ionising radiation
35. Chrome ulceration of: (a) the nose or throat; or (b) the skin of the hands or forearm	Work involving exposure to chromic acid or to any other chromium compound
36. Folliculitis 37. Acne 38. Skin cancer	Work involving exposure to mineral oil, tar, pitch or arsenic

45. Occupational dermatitis   Work involving exposure to [certain
                                   specified agents]

There follows a further list of reportable diseases which parallels those
conditions regarded as prescribed for industrial benefit (see Appendix L).

Reporting of Injuries, Diseases and Dangerous Occurrences Regulations 1995,
SI 1995/3163, reg 5(1), Sch 3.

Noxious or offensive substances

The emission of the following from prescribed premises[1] must be prevented by the best practical means (Health and Safety at Work etc. Act 1974, s.5(1)).

Acetic acid or its anhydride
Acetylene
Acrylates
Aldehydes
Amines
Ammonia or its compounds
Arsenic or its compounds
Asbestos
Bromine or its compounds
Carbon disulphide
Carbon dioxide
Carbon monoxide
Chlorine or its compounds
Cyanogen or its compounds
Di-isocyanates
Ethylene and higher olefines
Fluorine or its compounds
Fumaric acid
Fumes or dust containing aluminium, antimony, arsenic, beryllium, cadmium, calcium, chlorine, chromium, copper, iron, lead, magnesium, manganese, mercury, molybdenum, phosphorus, potassium, selenium, silicon, sodium, titanium, tungsten, uranium, vanadium, zinc or their compounds
Fumes or vapours from benzene works, paraffin oil works, petrochemical works, petroleum works, or tar works and bitumen works
Hydrocarbons
Hydrogen chloride
Hydrogen sulphide
Iodine or its compounds
Lead or its compounds

1 Prescribed premises are those in which work detailed in SI 1983/943, Sch 1 is carried out.

Maleic acid or its anhydride
Mercury or its compounds
Metal carbonyls
Nitric acid or oxides of nitrogen
Nitriles
Phthalic acid or its anhydride
Products containing hydrogen from the partial oxidation of hydrocarbons
Pyridine or its homologues
Smoke, grit and dust
Sulphuric acid or sulphur trioxide
Sulphurous acid or sulphur dioxide
Vinyl chloride
Volatile organic sulphur compounds

Some useful equivalents of weight, capacity, length and temperature

Standard measurements in the form of SI units are described in Appendix S. Many reports will, however, refer to more colloquial terms and the following may be found useful as an aid to conversion of these.

Weight
1 gram (g)	= 15.4 grains
1 kilogram (kg)	= 35.2 ounces = 2.2 lb (avoirdupois)
1 grain	= 64.8 milligrams (mg)
1 ounce (avoirdupois)	= 28.3 grams (g)
1 pound (avoirdupois)	= 453.6 grams (g)

Capacity
1 fluid ounce	= 28.4 millilitres (ml)[1]
1 gill	= 5 fluid ounces
1 pint	= 568 millilitres (ml)
1 gallon (Imp.)	= 4.55 litres (l)
1 litre (l)	= 1.76 pints
1 litre (l)	= 35.2 fluid ounces

Length
1 micron (μm)	= 10^{-6} metre (m)[2]
1 inch	= 2.54 centimetres (cm)
1 foot	= 30.5 centimetres (cm)
1 Ångstrom unit	= 10^{-10} metre (m)

Temperature
An interval of 1 degree Centigrade (°C) corresponds to 1.8 degrees Fahrenheit (°F). To convert °F to °C:

$$\frac{F-32}{9} = \frac{C}{5}$$

1 For all practical purposes 1 millilitre is equivalent to 1 cubic centimetre (cc or cm^3).
2 The symbol μ is also used to express the micron.

Some parts of the Electromagnetic Spectrum (wavelength)
Ultraviolet = 100–400 nanometres (nm)
Visible   = 400–800 nm
Infrared   = 800–100 000 nm

Some medical and dental qualifications in the United Kingdom

Primary medical qualifications

LMSSA	Licentiate in Medicine and Surgery of the Society of Apothecaries.
LRCS, LRCP	Licentiate of the Royal College of Surgeons of England and of the Royal College of Physicians of London.
LRCP, LRCS (Edin. or Irel.)	Licentiate of the Royal Colleges of Physicians and Surgeons of Edinburgh or in Ireland.
LRCPS	Licentiate of the Royal College of Physicians and Surgeons of Glasgow.
MB (or BM), BCh (or BS or ChB)	Bachelor of Medicine and Surgery. Graduating degree awarded by the UK Universities with Medical Schools.

Note. All qualifying degrees refer both to medicine and to surgery but not every doctor practises major surgery. Many doctors are also qualified BA (or subsequently MA) or BSc; these are intermediate university degrees taken before clinical training.

Some postgraduate medical degrees

MD	Doctor of Medicine. Obtained by thesis.
MS (or MCh or ChM)	Master of Surgery. Sometimes taken by thesis, sometimes by general examination.
PhD	Doctor of Philosophy. Obtained by thesis after a period of approved scientific research.
MSc	Master of Science. Obtainable in many scientific subjects related to medicine.

Such degrees indicate research in depth of a particular subject. They imply that there is some specific field in which the holder is an authority. Other special masterships are offered—eg in radiology.

Membership of the Royal Colleges and Faculties

Possession of these higher qualifications is certain evidence of specialisation. They are obtained by means of a searching examination; only rarely is 'membership' conferred by virtue of published work or reputation. The Colleges of Physicians in London, Edinburgh and Glasgow (Physicians and Surgeons) at one time conferred individual memberships; examinations are now on a United Kingdom basis. In general, members are elected to be fellows of individual colleges after a delineated period; some colleges, however, confer fellowship by examination.

FRCA	Fellow of the Royal College of Anaesthetists
FRCOphth	Fellow of the Royal College of Ophthalmologists
FRCR	Fellow of the Royal College of Radiologists
FRCS	Fellow of the Royal College of Surgeons
MRCGP	Member of the Royal College of General Practitioners
MRCOG	Member of the Royal College of Obstetricians and Gynaecologists
MRCPath	Member of the Royal College of Pathologists
MRCPsych	Member of the Royal College of Psychiatrists
MRCP	Member of the Royal College of Physicians
MFOM	Member of the Faculty of Occupational Medicine (RCP, Lond.)
MFPHM	Member of the Faculty of Public Health Medicine (RCP, UK)

The colleges will also issue Certificates of Training which indicate that the person has undergone the training needed before he or she can engage in independent medical practice in the specialty. In addition to the specialities indicated by the names of the colleges and faculties, certificates of training can be acquired in paediatrics and clinical oncology.

Postgraduate medical diplomas

The universities and the Royal Colleges issue diplomas on the basis of examination. The role of the diploma in indicating the narrower field of interest and expertise of the holder has been very much reduced by the growth of increasingly specialised Royal Colleges; in many cases, however, they are the sole indication of a particular proficiency while others may be looked upon as 'stepping-stones' to membership. The following list is certainly not exhaustive. Some will have been taken over as Diplomas of the Royal Colleges and are not mentioned below.

DAvMed	Diploma in Aviation Medicine
DipBact	Diploma in Bacteriology
DCH	Diploma in Child Health
DForM	Diploma in Forensic Medicine
DIH	Diploma in Industrial Health

DLO   Diploma in Laryngology and Otology
DMJ   Diploma in Medical Jurisprudence
BAO   Bachelor of the Art of Obstetrics (given in Ireland)
DPhysMed   Diploma in Physical Medicine
DipSocMed   Diploma in Social Medicine
DTM & H   Diploma in Tropical Medicine and Hygiene
DTPH   Diploma in Tropical Public Health

Primary dental qualifications

LDS   Licentiate in Dental Surgery of the Royal Colleges.
BDS   Bachelor of Dental Surgery. Graduating degree awarded by
               most Universities with Dental Schools.

Some postgraduate dental degrees

MDS or MChD   Master of Dental Surgery. Generally only available in
               Universities that do not offer a DDS.
MDentSc   Master in Dental Science.
MCDH   Master of Community Dental Health.
DDS   Doctor of Dental Surgery.
DDSc   Doctor of Dental Science.

Membership of the Royal Colleges and Faculties

MGDS RCS   Membership in General Dental Surgery
MCCD   Membership in Clinical Community Dentistry
MOrth   Membership in Orthodontics
FDS   Fellowship in Dental Surgery
Dental pathologists may also qualify as Members or Fellows of the Royal College
of Pathologists. Many dentists are also medically qualified and may proceed to
higher medical qualifications; these may be specialised—eg FRCS in
faciomaxillary surgery.

Some postgraduate dental diplomas

DCDH   Diploma in Child Dental Health
DDH   Diploma in Dental Health
DDO or DDOrth   Diploma in Dental Orthopaedics
DDPH   Diploma in Dental Public Health
DOrth   Diploma in Orthodontics
DRD   Diploma in Restorative Dentistry

Report to procurator fiscal of death under medical care

To the Procurator Fiscal

....

1. Report on the Death of:
   Full name   .... Date of Birth ....
   Home Address ....
                        (block capitals)

2. Date and Time of Death ....
   Place of Death (specifying exact location) ....
   Date of admission to hospital (if applicable) ....

3. Nature of Disease, Injury or Condition for which medical care was advised.

4. Brief description of clinical findings prior to the procedure, including details of any concurrent pathology.

5. Brief description of medical treatment and preparation of the patient for the procedure. (Please include all medications, doses and times, excluding pre-medication and anaesthetic agents, see para. 9).

6. Was consent obtained for the procedure?

7. PROCEDURE
   (a) Was the procedure elective or emergency? ....
   (b) Nature of procedure (indicate whether proposed, performed, or in progress) ....
   (c) Date and Time: Started: .... Finished ....
   (d) Operator (or doctor involved) ....
                        (block capitals)
   (e) Comments:

8. Was anaesthesia employed (local, regional or general)?
....

9. If so, please give details:
   (a) Pre-medication ....
   (b) Type of anaesthesia ....
   (c) Date and time administration started ....
       stopped ....
   (d) Details of agents and techniques used, including quantities
       ....
       ....
       ....

   (e) Anaesthetist ....
                          (block capitals)
   (f) Comments:

10. Details in chronological order of events immediately preceding death and of resuscitative measures undertaken.

11. Opinion as to cause of death, and any other general observations on the case.

Date   ....   Signature (doctor concerned) ....
                                    (designation) ....
                            Signature (doctor concerned) ....
                                    (designation) ....

NOTES: 1. Deaths to be reported:—
              (a) Cases to be reported would include deaths associated with medication and deaths occurring during or immediately after diagnostic or therapeutic procedures including surgical operations whether anaesthesia was employed or not.
              (b) Deaths which occur in the immediate post-operative period ordinarily not exceeding 12 hours following a general anaesthetic from which consciousness has not been regained.
          2. Wherever practicable this form should be completed in consultation with any other Medical Practitioner specially concerned or specifically mentioned and forwarded to the Procurator Fiscal as soon as possible.
          3. The Death Certificate must not be issued until instructions have been received from the Procurator Fiscal or his representative.
          4. The completion of Question 11 is a matter of discretion. It is to assist the Procurator Fiscal and his Medial Adviser to arrive at a certifiable cause of death.

Notes on the International System of Units (SI Units)

There is a general move to report laboratory results, etc., in terms of SI units (*Système Internationale d'Unités*), many of which will be unfamiliar. The following notes are not exhaustive but may be found useful.

The independent base units of SI are (physical quantity, name of unit, and symbol):

length	metre	m
mass	kilogram	kg
time	second	s
electric current	ampere	A
thermodynamic temperature	kelvin	K
luminous intensity	candela	cd
amount of substance	mole	mol

Decimal multiples and fractions of the units are formed by prefixes, with appropriate symbols:

10^{12}	tera	T	10^{-1}	deci	d
10^{9}	giga	G	10^{-2}	centi	c
10^{6}	mega	M	10^{-3}	milli	m
10^{3}	kilo	k	10^{-6}	micro	μ
10^{2}	hecto	h	10^{-9}	nano	n
10	deca	da	10^{-12}	pico	p
			10^{-15}	femto	f
			10^{-18}	atto	a

Other units can be derived from these—eg the SI unit of area is the square metre (m^2) and of volume the cubic metre (m^3). When there is a combination, the divider ('per') is shown by the use of negative powers. Thus:

Speed = metres per second = $m\ s^{-1}$

acceleration = metres per second per second = $m\ s^{-2}$.

Several derived SI units have been given new and special names. Few of these are of great medical interest save, perhaps:

unit of force = newton = N = $kg\ m\ s^{-2}$ (ie mass $\times$ acceleration)

unit of pressure = pascal = Pa = $N\ m^{-2}$ (ie force per square metre).

Despite this, the common unit of weight (gram = g) and of volume (litre = l) will continue in use.

Slowly, therefore, reports will include less well-known terms—eg:
Blood pressure = 150/75 mmHg = 20/10 kPa
Amount of phenobarbitone = 10 mg/100ml = 430 μmol·l^{-1}.

It is even conceivable that a blood alcohol of 80 mg/100 ml will be reported as 17.4 mmol·l^{-1}.

Temperature on the clinical scale is now preferably referred to in terms of degrees Celsius (°C). The units are identical with degrees centigrade.

Appendix T

Weights of the organs

Organ weights at various ages in grams[1]

Age	Lungs Men	Lungs Women	Brain Men	Brain Women	Heart Men	Heart Women	Kidneys Men	Kidneys Women	Liver Men	Liver Women	Spleen Men	Spleen Women
Newborn	51.7	50.9	353	347	19	20	24	24	124	125	8	6
0–3 mth	68.8	63.6	435	411	—	—	—	—	—	—	—	—
3–6 mth	94.1	93.4	600	534	—	—	—	—	—	—	—	—
6–9 mth	128.5	114.7	877	726	41	36	60	52	300	240	26	25
9–12 mth	142.4	142.1										
1–2 yr	170.3	175.3	971	894	54	48	72	65	400	390	35	34
2–3 yr	245.9	244.3	1076	1012	63	62	85	75	460	450	42	41
3–4 yr	304.7	265.5	1179	1076	73	71	93	84	510	500	48	47
4–5 yr	314.2	311.7	1290	1156	83	80	100	93	555	550	53	52
5–6 yr	360.6	319.9	1275	1206	95	90	106	102	595	595	58	57
6–7 yr	399.5	357.5	1313	1225	103	100	112	112	630	635	62	62
7–8 yr	365.4	404.4	1338	1265	110	113	120	123	665	685	64	67
8–9 yr	405.0	382.1	1294	1208	122	126	128	135	715	745	68	71
9–10 yr	376.4	358.4	1360	1226	132	140	138	148	770	810	73	77
10–11 yr	474.5	571.2	1378	1247	144	154	150	163	850	880	82	85
11–12 yr	465.6	535.0	1348	1259	157	168	154	180	950	950	91	93
12–13 yr	458.8	681.7	1383	1256	180	188	178	195	1050	1080	101	103
13–14 yr	504.5	602.3	1382	1243	202	207	196	210	1150	1180	111	112
14–15 yr	692.8	517.0	1356	1318	238	226	212	222	1240	1270	121	120
15–16 yr	691.7	708.8	1407	1271	258	238	229	230	1315	1330	135	127
16–17 yr	743.3	626.5	1419	1300	282	243	244	236	1380	1360	145	134
17–18 yr	776.9	649.5	1409	1254	300	247	260	240	1450	1380	152	140
18–19 yr	874.7	654.9	1426	1312	310	250	270	244	1510	1395	157	146
19–20 yr	1035.6	785.2	1430	1294	318	251	282	247	1580	1405	160	151
20–21 yr	953.0	792.8	—	—	322	252	290	248	1630	1415	162	155

1 From E Boyd (1962), in Altman and Dittmer *Growth, Including Reproduction and Morphological Development* pp 346–348. Biological Handbooks, Federation of American Societies for Experimental Biology, Washington. Reproduced by permission of the publishers.

Therapeutic and toxic concentrations of some commonly used drugs

Drug	Maximum therapeutic or normal plasma concentration (mg.l^{-1})	Plasma concentration associated with serious toxicity (mg.l^{-1})
Amitriptyline	0.2	1
Amphetamine	0.2	1
Amylobarbitone	5	40
Aspirin	250	750
Butobarbitone	10	80
Caffeine	15	60
Chlordiazepoxide	2	10
Chlormethiazole	2	20
Cocaine	0.3	1
Codeine	0.1	1
Diazepam	2	5
Dihydrocodeine	0.1	1
Dothiepin	0.3	1
Doxepin	0.3	1
Fluoxetine	0.5	1
Fluvoxamine	0.3	5
Imipramine	0.3	1
Iron	1.8	8
Lithium	8	10
Methadone	0.4	1
Methylamphetamine	0.2	1
Methylenedioxymethamphetamine	—	1
Morphine	0.05	0.5
Nortriptyline	0.15	1
Pentobarbitone	5	40
Quinalbarbitone	5	40

Drug	Maximum therapeutic or normal plasma concentration (mg.l⁻¹)	Plasma concentration associated with serious toxicity (mg.l⁻¹)
Temazepam	1	5
Theophylline	20	40
Triazolam	0.02	0.2

These concentrations are approximate only and the figures should be read in the light of the warning note sounded at p 375.

Index